Volume II

UPPER EXTREMITIES

Grabb's Encyclopedia of Flaps

THIRD EDITION

UPPER EXTREMITIES

Grabb's Encyclopedia of Flaps

THIRD EDITION

Editors

Berish Strauch, MD
Professor of Plastic Surgery
Albert Einstein College of Medicine
Bronx, New York

Luis O. Vasconez, MD
Professor of Surgery and Director
Division of Plastic Surgery
University of Alabama Medical Center, Birmingham
Chief Plastic Surgeon
University of Alabama Hospital
Birmingham, Alabama

Elizabeth J. Hall-Findlay, MD
Plastic Surgeon
Banff Mineral Springs Hospital
Banff, Alberta, Canada

Bernard T. Lee, MD
Instructor in Surgery
Harvard Medical School
Division of Plastic and Reconstructive Surgery
Beth Israel Deaconess Medical Center
Boston, Massachusetts

Wolters Kluwer | Lippincott Williams & Wilkins
Health
Philadelphia · Baltimore · New York · London
Buenos Aires · Hong Kong · Sydney · Tokyo

Acquisitions Editor: Brian Brown
Managing Editor: Michelle La Plante
Marketing Manager: Lisa Parry
Project Manager: Bridgett Dougherty
Senior Manufacturing Manager: Benjamin Rivera
Creative Director: Doug Smock
Production Service: Nesbitt Graphics, Inc.

© 2009 by LIPPINCOTT WILLIAMS & WILKINS, a WOLTERS KLUWER business
530 Walnut Street
Philadelphia, PA 19106 USA
LWW.com

Library of Congress Cataloging-in-Publication Data

Grabb's encyclopedia of flaps / editors, Berish Strauch ... [et al.]. -- 3rd ed.
    p. ; cm.
Includes bibliographical references and index.
ISBN 978-0-7817-6432-2
ISBN 978-0-7817-6705-7
1. Flaps (Surgery) I. Grabb, William C. II. Strauch, Berish, 1933- III.
Title: Encylopedia of flaps.
[DNLM: 1. Surgical Flaps. 2. Reconstructive Surgical Procedures. WO 610G727 2009]
RD120.8.G78 2009
617.9'5--dc22

                                                        2008024234

Care has been taken to confirm the accuracy of the information presented and to
describe generally accepted practices. However, the authors, editors, and publisher are not
responsible for errors or omissions or for any consequences from application of the
information in this book and make no warranty, expressed or implied, with respect to the
currency, completeness, or accuracy of the contents of the publication. Application of the
information in a particular situation remains the professional responsibility of the
practitioner.

The authors, editors, and publisher have exerted every effort to ensure that drug
selection and dosage set forth in this text are in accordance with current recommendations
and practice at the time of publication. However, in view of ongoing research, changes in
government regulations, and the constant flow of information relating to drug therapy and
drug reactions, the reader is urged to check the package insert for each drug for any change
in indications and dosage and for added warnings and precautions. This is particularly
important when the recommended agent is a new or infrequently employed drug.

Some drugs and medical devices presented in the publication have Food and Drug
Administration (FDA) clearance for limited use in restricted research settings. It is the
responsibility of the health care provider to ascertain the FDA status of each drug or device
planned for use in their clinical practice.

To purchase additional copies of this book, call our customer service department at (800)
638-3030 or fax orders to (301) 223-2320. International customers should call (301) 223-
2300.

Visit Lippincott Williams & Wilkins on the Internet: at LWW.com. Lippincott Williams &
Wilkins customer service representatives are available from 8:30 am to 6 pm, EST.

10 9 8 7 6 5 4 3 2 1

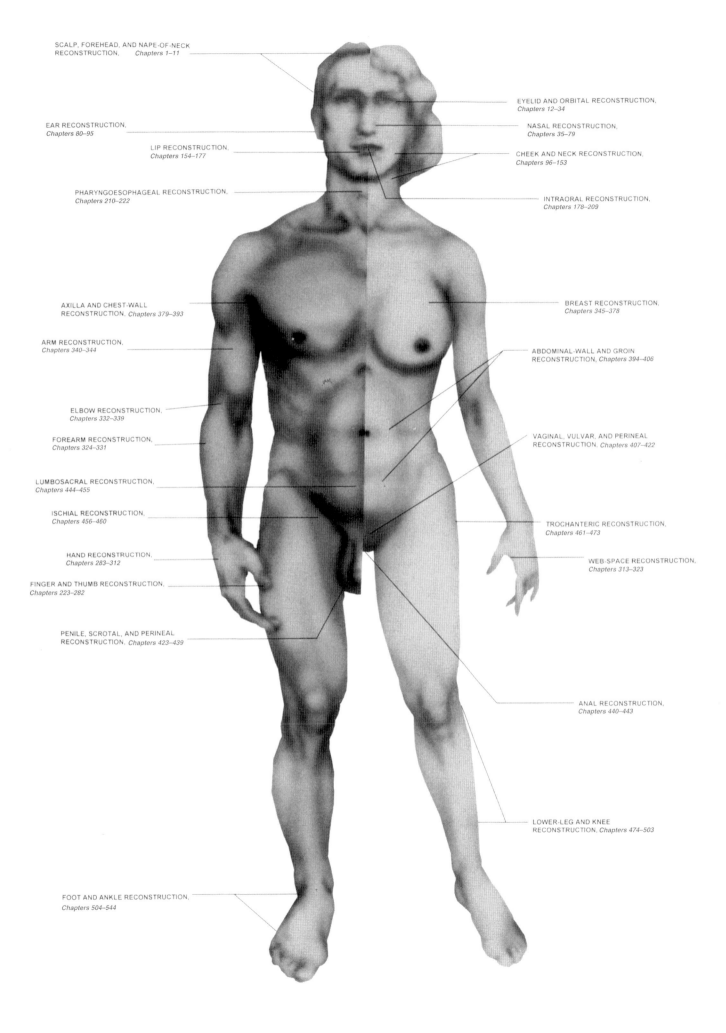

SCALP, FOREHEAD, AND NAPE-OF-NECK RECONSTRUCTION, *Chapters 1–11*

EYELID AND ORBITAL RECONSTRUCTION, *Chapters 12–34*

EAR RECONSTRUCTION, *Chapters 80–95*

NASAL RECONSTRUCTION, *Chapters 35–79*

LIP RECONSTRUCTION, *Chapters 154–177*

CHEEK AND NECK RECONSTRUCTION, *Chapters 96–153*

PHARYNGOESOPHAGEAL RECONSTRUCTION, *Chapters 210–222*

INTRAORAL RECONSTRUCTION, *Chapters 178–209*

AXILLA AND CHEST-WALL RECONSTRUCTION. *Chapters 379–393*

BREAST RECONSTRUCTION, *Chapters 345–378*

ARM RECONSTRUCTION, *Chapters 340–344*

ABDOMINAL-WALL AND GROIN RECONSTRUCTION, *Chapters 394–406*

ELBOW RECONSTRUCTION, *Chapters 332–339*

FOREARM RECONSTRUCTION, *Chapters 324–331*

VAGINAL, VULVAR, AND PERINEAL RECONSTRUCTION. *Chapters 407–422*

LUMBOSACRAL RECONSTRUCTION, *Chapters 444–455*

ISCHIAL RECONSTRUCTION, *Chapters 456–460*

TROCHANTERIC RECONSTRUCTION, *Chapters 461–473*

HAND RECONSTRUCTION, *Chapters 283–312*

WEB-SPACE RECONSTRUCTION, *Chapters 313–323*

FINGER AND THUMB RECONSTRUCTION, *Chapters 223–282*

PENILE, SCROTAL, AND PERINEAL RECONSTRUCTION. *Chapters 423–439*

ANAL RECONSTRUCTION, *Chapters 440–443*

LOWER-LEG AND KNEE RECONSTRUCTION. *Chapters 474–503*

FOOT AND ANKLE RECONSTRUCTION, *Chapters 504–544*

To my wife, and children, and especially to my grandchildren, David Michael, Kimberly Ann, Carolyn Beth, Alexandra Rae, and Matthew Jost.

BERISH STRAUCH, MD

To my wife, Diane, my daughters, Cristina, Nessa and Rachel, and to my grandchildren, Francesca and Elisa, for their continued support and joy they have given me throughout the years.

LUIS VASCONEZ, MD

To my mother, Betty Hall, who has been an inspiration to all her children; and to my own three children, Jamie, David and Elise, who have become very enjoyable young adults.

ELIZABETH J. HALL-FINDLAY, MD

To my wife, Britt, for her unwavering love, support, and sacrifice. I am truly fortunate to be married to such an amazing woman. To my sons, Brodie and Teddy, for the never-ending joy they bring. Finally, to my parents, who share a contagious thirst for knowledge.

BERNARD T. LEE, MD

D. L. Abramson, MD
42A East 74th Street,
New York, New York 10021

W. P. Adams, Jr., MD
Children's Medical Center
Parkland Memorial Hospital
Veteran's Administration Medical Center
Zale Lipshy University Hospital
Baylor Medical Center
5323 Harry Hines Boulevard
Dallas, Texas 75235-9132

J. E. Adamson, MD, FACS (Retired)
P. O. Box 695
Linville, North Carolina 28646

J. Aftimos, MD
Centre Hospitalier D'Agen
Rue des Héros de la Résistance
F-47000 Agen, France

Galip Agaoglu, MD
Department of Plastic Surgery
The Cleveland Clinic Foundation
Cleveland, Ohio

F. C. Akpuaka, MBBS (Ibadan), FRCS (Ed), FRCS (Glasgow), FWACS, FICS
Professor of Plastic Surgery, College of Medicine, Abia State University, Uturu, Nigeria
Director of Plastic Surgery
Plastic Surgery Unit
St. Francis Hospital
2 Richard Street
Asata-Enugu, Nigeria

R. S. Ali, MD
Department of Plastic and Reconstructive Surgery
Castle Hill Hospital
Castle Road
Cottingham, United Kingdom

R. J. Allen, MD
Division of Plastic Surgery
Medical University of South Carolina
Charleston, South Carolina

E. C. Almaguer, MD
Chief of Plastic Surgery, Santa Rosa Medical Center, San Antonio
Baptist Hospital System
343 West Houston, #211
San Antonio, Texas 78205

C. Angrigiani
Posadas 1528 PB
Buenos Aires
Argentina

P. Andrades, MD
Assistant Professor
Division of Plastic Surgery and
Division of Maxillofacial Surgery
University of Chile Clinical Hospital
Hospital del Trabajador
Santiago, Chile

N. H. Antia, FRCSEng, FACSHon (Deceased)

S. Arena, MD (Retired)
125 Greenwood Road
Fox Chapel
Pittsburgh, Pennsylvania 15238

R. V. Argamaso, MD, FACS (Deceased)

L. C. Argenta, MD
North Carolina Baptist Hospital
Bowman-Gray Plastic Surgery
Medical Center Boulevard
Winston-Salem, North Carolina 27157

S. Ariyan, FACS
Yale-New Haven Hospital
Connecticut Center for Plastic Surgery
60 Temple Street, Suite 7C
New Haven, Connecticut 06510

D. P. Armstrong, MD, FACS
Community Memorial Hospital of San Buenaventura
Clinical Faculty, UCLA, Division of Plastic Surgery
168 North Brent Street, Suite 403
Ventura, California 93003

C. Arrunátegui, MD
Department of Plastic Surgery
Hospital da Santa Casa de Misericordia
Belo Horizonte, Brazil

H. Asato, MD
Assistant Professor
Department of Plastic and Reconstructive Surgery
University of Tokyo Hospital
7–3-1 Hongo Bunkyo-ku
Tokyo 113, Japan

E. Atasoy, MD
University of Louisville
Christine M. Kleinert Institute for Hand and Microsurgery
225 Abraham Flexner Way, Suite 700
Louisville, Kentucky 40202–1817

C. Augustin, MD
Centre Hospitalier D'Agen
29, Bd. de la République
F-47000 Agen, France

J. M. Avelar, MD
Albert Einstein Hospital, São Paulo
Al Gabriel Monteiro
Da Silva 620
01442–000 São Paulo-SP, Brazil

K. Azari, MD
Assistant Professor
Division of Plastic Surgery
University of Pittsburgh Medical Center
Pittsburgh, Pennsylvania

H. A. Badran, MB, BCh, FRCS, FRCSEd
Head, Department of Plastic Surgery
Ain Shams University
98 Mohamed Farid Street
Cairo 11111, Egypt

G. J. Baibak, FACS
3634 West Bancroft Street
Toledo, Ohio 43606

B. N. Bailey, MD, FRCS
Oxford Regional Health Authority
Stoke Mandeville Hospital
Mandeville Road
Aylesbury, Buckinghamshire, HP21 8AL
United Kingdom

V. Y. Bakamjian, MD (Retired)
Roswell Park Cancer Institute
Department of Head and Neck Surgery
Elm and Carlton Streets
Buffalo, New York 14263

C. R. Balch, MD
Naples Community Hospital
201 Eight Street, South, Suite 102
Naples, Florida 34102

T. Barfred, MD, PhD
Assistant Professor of Surgery, Odense University
Head of Hand Surgery, Department of Orthopaedic Surgery,
Odense University Hospital, Odense, Sweden
Head of Hand Surgery
Section of Orthopaedic Surgery
Odense University Hospital
500 Odense, Denmark

Marguerite P. Barnett, FACS
530 South Nokomis Avenue, Suite 6
Venice, Florida 34285

R. L. Baroudi, MD
Rua Bahia 969
São Paulo, SP 01244–001
Brazil

J. N. Barron, MS, FRCSEd, FRCSEng (Deceased)

F. E. Barton, Jr., MD
Baylor University Medical Center
Parkland Hospital
Presbyterian Hospital
Mary Shiels Hospital
411 North Washington Avenue, #6000 LB 13
Dallas, Texas 75246–1774

R. M. Barton, FACS
Vanderbilt University Hospital
Nashville Virginia Hospital
Baptist Hospital
Vanderbilt University Hospital
Medical Center South, Room 230
Nashville, Tennessee 37232

J. Baudet, MD
Professor of Plastic and Reconstructive Surgery
University of Bordeaux
Chief of Department of Plastic and Reconstructive Surgery
C.H.U.-Hôpital du Tondu
Groupe Pellegrin-Tondu
Place Amélie Raba-Léon
F-33076 Bordeaux, France

C. Beard, MD (Retired)
University of California, San Francisco
400 Parnassus Avenue, Suite 750-A
San Francisco, California 94143

R. W. Beasly, MD
Professor at NYU Medical Center
Director of Hand Surgery at Bellevue Hospital Center
Hand Surgery Associates
310 East 30th Street
New York, New York 10016–8303

Col. D. W. Becker, Jr., MD
Wilford Hall USAF Medical Center, San Antonio, Texas
2200 Bergquist Drive, Suite 1
Lackland AFB, Texas 78236–5300

H. Becker, MD, FACS
Boca Raton Community Hospital
5458 Town Center Road
Boca Raton, Florida 33486–1009

Professeur T. Bégué, MD
Chirurgie Orthopédique-Traumatologique et Réparatrice de
l'Appareil Locomoteur
Hôpital Avicenne
125, route de Stalingrad
F-93009 Bobigny Cedex, France

F. C. Behan, FRACS, FRCS
91 Royal Parade
Parkville 3052
Melbourne, Victoria
Australia

M. S. G. Bell, MD
Suite 306
340 McLeod Street, South
Ottawa, Ontario, Canada, K2P 1A4

T. Benacquista, MD
Einstein Weiler Hospital
Department of Plastic and Reconstructive Surgery
Albert Einstein College of Medicine and
Montefiore Medical Center
3331 Bainbridge Avenue
Bronx, New York 10467

M. Ben-Bassat, MD
Deputy-Chief
Department of Plastic Surgery
Beilinson Hospital
Tel Aviv, Israel

S. P. Bhagia, MD
Baugh Farzana Plastic Surgery Centre, Agra, India
4/14 Baugh Farzana
Agra 282 002, India

S. K. Bhatnagar, MD
Professor in Plastic Surgery
Department of Plastic Surgery
King George's Medical College
Lucknow 226 003, India

S. Bhattacharya, MS, MCh, FICS
Awadh Hospital, Lucknow
Neera Hospital, Lucknow
Star Hospital, Gorahpur
Consultant Plastic Surgeon and Oncologist
C-907 Mahanagar
Lucknow 226 006, India

S. L. Biddulph, MD
Chief Hand Surgeon, Johannesburg Hospital
Houghton 2050, South Africa

E. Biemer, MD
Department of Plastic Surgery
Technical University of München
Ismaningerstrasse 22
D-81675 München, Germany

J. H. Binns, MD
Wayne State University
540 East Canfield
Detroit, Michigan 48201

R. J. Bloch, MD
R. Sampaio Viana 628
Paraiso-São Paulo 04004–002
Brazil

J. G. Boorman, MD
Queen Victoria Hospital
East Grinstead
West Sussex, RH19 3DZ United Kingdom

L.J. Borud, MD
Instructor in Surgery
Department of Surgery
Harvard Medical School
110 Francis Street, Suite 5A
Boston, Massachusetts 02215

J.-L. Bovet, MD
Unité de Chirurgie de la Main
Clinique Jean-Villar
F-33520 Burges, France

J. B. Boyd, MD, FRCS, FRCS(C), FACS
Cleveland Clinic Hospital, Ft. Lauderdale
Broward General Hospital, Ft. Lauderdale
Holy Cross Hospital, Ft. Lauderdale
Imperial Point Hospital, Ft. Lauderdale
North Ridge Hospital, Ft. Lauderdale
Department of Plastic and Reconstructive Surgery
Cleveland Clinic Florida
3000 West Cypress Creek Road
Ft. Lauderdale, Florida 33309

R. J. Brauer, MD
Greenwich Hospital, Connecticut
49 Lake Avenue
Greenwich, Connecticut 06830–4519

N. K. Breach, MB, FRCS, FDSRCS
Department of Surgery
Royal Marsden Hospital
Downs Road
Sutton SM2 5PT, United Kingdom

T. D. R. Briant, MD, FRCS(C), FACS
Honorary Consultant, St. Michael's Hospital
32 Dale Avenue
Toronto, Ontario, Canada, M4W 1K5

T. R. Broadbent, MD (Retired)
2635 St. Mary's Way
Salt Lake City, Utah 84108

M. Brones, MD, FACS
Grossman Burn Center at Sherman Oaks Hospital,
California
Suite 102
4849 Van Nuys Boulevard
Sherman Oaks, California 91403

M. D. Brough, MD
University College London Hospitals
Royal Free Hospital
The Consulting Suite
82 Portland Place
London W1N 3DH, United Kingdom

E. Z. Browne, Jr., MD, FACS
Cleveland Clinic
Department of Plastic and Reconstructive Surgery
Cleveland Clinic Foundation
9500 Euclid Avenue
Cleveland, Ohio 44195

C. D. Bucko, MD, FACS
Scripps Memorial Hospital, La Jolla, California
Panerodo Hospital
University of San Diego Medical Center
Sheerp Memorial Hospital
Mission Bay, Columbia
Suite B
9900 Genesee Avenue
La Jolla, California 92037

J. Bunkis, MD, FACS
4165 Blackhawk Plaza Circle, Suite 150
Danville, California 94506–4691

G. C. Burget, MD, FACS
Clinical Assistant Professor, Section of Plastic Surgery,
The University of Chicago Hospitals
2913 North Commonwealth Avenue, Suite 400
Chicago, Illinois 60657

J. A. Butler, MD, FACS
Wausau Hospital
Saint Michael's Hospital, Stevens Point, WI
North Central Wisconsin Plastic Surgery, SC
425 Pine Ridge Boulevard, Suite 202
Wausau, Wisconsin 54401

H. S. Byrd, MD, FACS
Baylor University Medical Center
Children's Medical Center
Zale Lipshy University Medical Center
Suite 6000 LB 13
411 North Washington Avenue
Dallas, Texas 75246

D. Calderón, MD
Hospital del Trabajador
Ramon Carnicer, 185-5 Piso
Providencia
Santiago, Chile

W. Calderón, MD
Professor of Surgery
University of Chile
Chief of Plastic Surgery
Service Hospital del Trabajador
Santiago, Chile

M. A. Callahan, MD, FACS
Eye Foundation Hospital
St. Vincent's Hospital
Medical Center East Outpatient Surgery
700 South 18th Street, Suite 511
Birmingham, Alabama 35233

R. R. Cameron, MD (Retired)
38330 Sweetwater Drive
Palm Desert, California 92211–7048

G. W. Carlson, MD
Wadley R. Glenn Professor of Surgery
Department of Surgery
Associate Program Director
Division of Plastic Surgery
Emory University School of Medicine
Atlanta, Georgia

C. E. Carriquiry, MD
Associate Professor, Plastic Surgery, School of Medicine,
Universidad de la República Montevideo-Uruguay
21 de Setiembre 2353 Ap. 201
Montevideo 11200, Uruguay

N. Carver, MS, FRCS, FRCS(Plast)
Department of Plastic and Reconstructive Surgery
Royal London Hospital
St. Bartholomew's Hospital
London, E1 1BB United Kingdom

V. M. Casoli, MD
Department of Plastic and Reconstructive Surgery
C.H.U.-Hôpital Du Tondu
Groupe Pellegrin-Tondu
Place Amélie Raba-Léon
F-33076 Bordeaux, France

P. C. Cavadas, MD, PhD
Head of the Reconstructive Surgery and Microsurgery Unit
Hospital Vírgen del Consuelo
Hand Transplant Surgery Unit
"La Fe" University Hospital
Valencia, Spain

A. Cerejo, MD
Consultant Neurosurgeon
Hospital S. Joao Medical School
Oporto, Portugal
Avenida Vasco Da Gama
Ed. Silva porto, BL.C, 9B
4490 Povoa de Varzim, Portugal

L. A. Chait, MD
Johannesburg Group of Teaching Hospitals
211 Parkland Clinic
Junction Avenue Park
Johannesburg, South Africa

R. Chandra, MS, MCh
Professor, Plastic Surgery
King George's Medical College
Lucknow 226 003, India

R. A. Chase, MD
Professor, Stanford University School of Medicine
Department of Surgery
Stanford, CA 94305

P. Chhajlani, MD
"Ganga Jamuna Apartments"
South Tukoganj, Near Nath Mandir
Indore 452 001, India

D. R. H. Christie, MBChB, FRACR
John Flynn Hopital, Tugun, Australia
Eastcoast Cancer Centre
Inland Drive
Tugun, QLD 4224, Australia

Y. K. Chung, MD
Yonsei University Wonju College of Medicine
Wonju Christian Hospital
Ilsandong
Wonju, Korea

M. E. Ciaravino, MD
Attending Plastic Surgeon
St. Joseph's Hospital
Houston, Texas
3805 West Alabama, #3105
Houston, Texas 77027

B. E. Cohen, MD, FACS
Academic Chief and Director, Plastic Surgery Residency
Program, Cohen and Cronin Clinic
Director, Microsurgical Research and Training Laboratory,
St. Joseph Hospital, Houston
Plastic and Reconstructive Surgery
Cohen and Cronin Clinic
1315 Calhoun, Suite 920
Houston, Texas 77002

C. C. Coleman, Jr., MD, FACS (Retired)
Consultant Plastic Surgeon, Clinical Professor of Surgery,
University of Virginia, Charlottesville, Virginia
Visiting Professor, University of Virginia
P. O. Box 558
Irvington, Virginia 22480–0558

J. J. Coleman III, MD, FACS
University Hospital
Riley Hospital
Wishad Hospital
VA Medical Center
Professor of Surgery
Director, Division of Plastic Surgery
Indiana University
Emerson Hall 235, 545 Barnhill Drive
Indianapolis, Indiana 46202

P. Colson, MD
Head Surgeon
Burn Unit
Saint Luke's Hospital
34, Place Bellecour
F-69002 Lyons, France

M. B. Constantian, MD, FACS
Adjunct Assistant Professor of Surgery, Dartmouth
Medical School
Active Staff, Department of Surgery (Plastic Surgery),
St. Joseph Hospital and Southern New Hampshire
Regional Medical Center
Nashua, New Hampshire
19 Tyler Street, Suite 302
Nashua, New Hampshire 03060

L. M. Cordero, MD (Deceased)

R. J. Corlett, MD
Royal Melbourne Hospital
Preston and North Gate Community Hospital
766 Elizabeth Street
Melbourne 3000, Australia

H. Monteiro Da Costa, MD
Professor and Consultant Plastic Surgeon,
Plastic and Reconstructive Unit, S. Joao Hospital,
Medical School, Oporto
Consultant Plastic Surgeon, Matosinhos and Vila Nova Eaia
Hospitals, Oporto
Professor in Plastic Surgery
Rua do Corvo, 323
Pr. da Granja
4405 Arcozelo VNG, Portugal

E. D. Cronin, MD, FACS
Chief of Plastic Surgery Section, St. Joseph Hospital
Plastic and Reconstructive Surgery
Cohen and Cronin Clinic
1315 Calhoun, Suite 920
Houston, Texas 77002

T. D. Cronin, MD (Deceased)

J. W. Curtin, MD
Rush-Presbyterian-St. Luke's Medical Center,
Chicago, Illinois
1180 Hill Road
Winnetka, Illinois 60093

R. K. Daniel, MD, FACS
Hoag Memorial Hospital/Presbyterian Hospital, California
1441 Avocado Avenue, Suite 308
Newport Beach, California 92660–7704

S. K. Das, MD, FACS, FRCS
St. Dominic's Hospital
River Oaks Hospital
River Oaks East Hospital
University of Mississippi Medical Center
Mississippi Methodist Medical Center
Parkview Hospital, Vicksburg
Division of Plastic Surgery
University of Mississippi Medical Center
2500 North State Street
Jackson, Mississippi 39211

J. E. Davis, MD
Matricula No. 7101
Vincente Lopez 2653, Argentina

R. De la Plaza, MD
Director, Plastic Surgery Department, La Luz Clinic,
Madrid
Clínica de Cirugía Plástica y Estética
Salou, 28
E-28034 Madrid, Spain

A. L. Dellon, MD, FACS
Professor, Plastic and Neurosurgery,
The Johns Hopkins University School of Medicine
2328 West Joppa Road, Suite 325
Lutherville, Maryland 21093

G. H. Derman, MD
Attending Staff, Rush-Presbyterian-St. Luke's
Medical Center
Attending Staff, Evanston Hospital
Assistant Professor, Rush Medical College, Chicago, Illinois
4709 Golf Road, Suite 806
Skokie, Illinois 60076–1258

B. Devauchelle, MD, PhD
Department of Maxillofacial Surgery
Centre Hospitalier Universitaire
Amiens, France

C. J. Devine, Jr., MD
400 West Brambleton Avenue, Suite 100
Norfolk, Virginia 23510–1115

I. K. Dhawan, MD
Department of Surgery
Al Mafraq Hospital
Abu Dhabi, India

Dr. A. D. Dias, MS
Professor Emeritus, L.T.M.G. Hospital, Sion, Mumbai
St. Thereza Hospital, Agashi, Virar
"Shanti Sadan"
157-B Perry Road
Bandra, Mumbai 400 050, India

R. O. Dingman, MD (Deceased)

T. A. Dinh, MD
Division of Plastic Surgery
Baylor College of Medicine
6560 Fannin, Suite 1034
Houston, Texas 77030

M. I. Dinner, MD, FACS
Meridia Hillcrest Hospital
Assistant Clinical Professor
Case Western Reserve Medical School
3755 Orange Plaza
Cleveland, Ohio 44122–4455

B. H. Dolich, MD
Albert Einstein College Hospital and Montefiore
Medical Center
New York Eye & Ear Hospital
1578 Williamsbridge Road
Bronx, New York 10461

R. V. Dowden, MD, FACS
Meridia Hillcrest, Mt. Sinai, University Hospital
6770 Mayfield Road, Suite 410
Mayfield Heights, Ohio 44124

G. A. Drabyn, MD, FACS
Riverside Methodist Hospital
3545 Olentangy River Road, Suite 130
Columbus, Ohio 43214

J. M. Drever, MD, FRCS
Etobicoke General Hospital
Cosmetic Surgery Hospital
135 Queens Plate Drive, Fifth Floor
Toronto, Ontario, Canada, M9W 6V1

J.-L. Ducours, MD
Centre Hospitalier D'Agen
Service de Chirurgie Maxillo-faciale
Centre Hospitalier
86 boulevard Sylvain Dumon
F-47000 Agen, France

G. M. Duncan, MChB, FRACS
Plastic Surgical Unit
Hutt Hospital
Private Bag
Lower Hutt, New Zealand

E. C. Duus, MD
Comanche County Memorial Hospital
Southwest Medical Center
5604 Southwest Lee Boulevard, Suite 310
Lawton, Oklahoma 73505–9663

W. Dzwierzynski, MD
Professor of Plastic Surgery
Medical College of Wisconsin
Milwaukee, Wisconsin

A. S. Earle, MD, FACS
Professor (Emeritus) of Plastic Surgery
Case Western University School of Medicine
1656 Emerald Green Court
Deltona, Florida 32725

D. S. Eastwood, MD (Retired)
St. Kames's University Hospital, Leeds, United Kingdom
Leeds University Hospital
11, North Park Road
Roundhay
Leeds LS8 1JD, United Kingdom

B. W. Edgerton, MD
Kaiser Permanente, West Los Angeles
Plastic Surgery Department
6041 Cadillac Avenue
Los Angeles, California 90034

M. T. Edgerton, MD
University of Virginia Health Sciences Center
Department of Plastic Surgery
Charlottesville, Virginia 22908

P. Egyedi, MD, DMD, PhD
Department of Oral and Maxillofacial Surgery
Utrecht University Hospital
P.O. Box 85500
NL-3508 GA Utrecht, The Netherlands

L. Eisenbaum, MD, PC
Colorado Medical Center of Aurora
Longmont United Hospital
Plastic and Reconstructive Surgery
Esthetic and Hand Surgery
Presbyterian Aurora Medical Center
750 Potomac Street, Suite 201
Aurora, Colorado 80011

M. M. El-Saadi, MD
Assistant Professor of Plastic Surgery
Zagazig University Hospital
Zagazig, Egypt

D. Elliot, MA
Woodlands
Woodham Walter
Essex
United Kingdom

R. A. Elliott, Jr., MD, FACS
P.O. Box 39
Slingerlands, New York 12159

L. F. Elliott, MD
Northside Hospital
St. Joseph's Hospital
Piedmont Hospital
Scottish-Rite Children's Hospital
975 Jonson Ferry, Suite 500
Atlanta, Georgia 30342

N. I. Elsahy, MD, PC, FRCS(C), FACS, FICS
Southern Regional Medical Center, Riverdale, Georgia
6524 Professional Place, Suite A
P.O. Box 1318
Riverdale, Georgia 30274

A. J. J. Emmett, MB, BS, FRCS, FRACS
Honorary Consultant, Princess Alexandra Hospital,
Brisbane, Australia
Woodgreen
128 Osborne Road
Bowral NSW 2576, Australia

D. N. F. Fairbanks, MD
Clinical Professor of Otolaryngology, George Washington
University School of Medicine, Washington, DC
Sibley Memorial Hospital, Washington, DC
3 Washington Circle, Northwest, Suite 305
Washington, DC 20037–2356

G. R. Fairbanks, MD
St. Mark's Hospital
Cottonwood Hospital, Primary Children's Medical Center
Bonneville Surgical Center
1151 East 3900 South, B110
Salt Lake City, Utah 84124

R. S. Feingold, MD
Assistant Clinical Professor in Plastic and Reconstructive
Surgery, Albert Einstein College of Medicine
Long Island Jewish Medical Center
Montefiore Medical Center
New York Hospital Medical Center of Queens
North Shore University Hospital
Winthrop-University Hospital
900 Northern Boulevard
Great Neck, New York 11021

M. Feldman, MD, FACS
Shore Memorial, Somers Point, New Jersey
Feldman Plastic Surgery, P. A.
222 New Road, Suite 6
Linwood, New Jersey 08221

A.-M. Feller, Prof. Dr. med.
Chairman, Department of Plastic Surgery
Behandlungszentrum Vogtareuth
Krankenhausstrasse 20
D-83569 Vogtareuth, Germany

R. J. Fix, MD, FACS
University of Alabama at Birmingham
The Children's Hospital of Alabama
Veterans Administration Medical Center
University of Alabama, Plastic Surgery MEB 524
1813 Sixth Avenue, South
Birmingham, Alabama 35294

A. E. Flatt, MD, FRCS
Baylor University Medical Center, Dallas, Texas
Clinical Professor, SW Medical School, Dallas, Texas
Consultant Emeritus in Hand Surgery,
U.S. Air Force
Director of Education
George Truett James Orthopaedic Institute
Baylor University Medical Center
3500 Gaston Avenue
Dallas, Texas 75246-9990

L. Fonseca Dos Santos, MD
Service d'Orthopedie
Hôpital Trousseau
26 Avenue de Dr. A Netter
F-75012 Paris, France

G. Foucher, MD
Head of SOS Main, Strasbourg
4 Bd. du President
F-67000 Strasbourg, France

M. Fox, MD, FACS
4001 Kresge Way, Suite 320
Louisville, Kentucky 40207–4640

J. D. Franklin, MD, FACS
Erlanger Health System, Memorial Hospital
Hutcheson Medical Center
Plaza Ambulatory Care Center
979 East Third Street, Suite 4002
Chattanooga, Tennessee 37403

A. Freiberg, MD, FRCS(C), FACS
Division of Plastic Surgery
Toronto Western Hospital
399 Bathurst Street
Edith Cavell Wing, 4-304
Toronto, Ontario MST 2S8, Canada

R. Fujimori, MD
Department of Plastic Surgery
Kyoto University
465 Kajii-cho Kawar
Kyoto 602, Japan

T. Fujino, MD, FACS, DrMedSci
Professor and Chairman
Department of Plastic Surgery
Keio University School of Medicine
35 Shinanomachi Shinjukuku
Tokyo 160, Japan

L. T. Furlow, Jr., MD, FACS
Clinical Professor, University of Florida College of Medicine,
Gainesville, Florida
3001 Northwest 28th Terrace
Gainesville, Florida 32605

D. W. Furnas, MD, FACS
University of California, Irvine Medical Center
St. Joseph Hospital, Orange
Childrens Hospital of Orange County
VA Hospital, Long Beach
University of California Irvine Medical Center
Division of Plastic Surgery
101 City Drive
Orange, California 92868–2901

F. N. Gahhos, MD
Venice Hospital
135 San Marco Drive
Venice, Florida 34285

A. Gardetto, MD
Professor of Plastic and Reconstructive Surgery
General Hospital of Brixen
Brixen, Italy

P. M. Gardner, MD
Assistant Professor, Department of Surgery,
Division of Plastic Surgery
University of Alabama at Birmingham
1600 7th Avenue South, ACC 322
Birmingham, Alabama 35233

N. W. Garrigues, MD
Scripps Memorial Hospital
Assistant Professor, University of California, San Diego
3405 Kenyon Street, Ste. 401
San Diego, California 92110–5007

J. S. Gaul, MD (Retired)
Charlotte, North Carolina

K. E. Georgeson, MD
University of Alabama Hospitals
The Children's Hospital of Alabama
1600 7th Avenue, South, ACC 300
Birmingham, Alabama 35233

G. S. Georgiade, MD
Duke University Medical Center—Surgery
P.O. Box 3960
Durham, North Carolina 27710

R. Ger, MD, FRCS
Albert Einstein College of Medicine
1300 Morris Park Avenue
Bronx, New York 10461

V. C. Giampapa, MD, FACS
89 Valley Road
Montclair, New Jersey 07042–2212

A. Gilbert, MD
15 rue Franklin
F-75016 Paris, France

D. A. Gilbert, MD, FRCS(C), FACS
Norfolk General Hospital
Children's Hospital of the King's Daughters
De Paul Hospital
Maryview Hospital
Plastic Surgery Associates, Inc.
400 West Brambleton Avenue, Suite 300
Norfolk, Virginia 23510

R. P. Gingrass, MD, SC
Elmbrook Hospital, Brokfield, Wisconsin
St. Joseph's Hospital, Milwaukee, Wisconsin
Plastic and Reconstructive Surgery
9800 West Bluemound
Milwaukee, Wisconsin 53226

F. Giraldo, MD, PhD
Plastic and Reconstructive Unit, University of Málaga
Regional Hospital "Harlos Haya," Málaga, Spain
Plastic and Reconstructive Unit
Regional Hospital "Carlos Haya"
E-29010 Málaga, Spain

D. W. Glasson, MD, FRACS
Wellington Hospital, Wellington, NZ
Hutt Hospital, Lower Hutt, NZ
Bowen Hospital, Wellington, NZ
Plastic Surgery Specialists
140 Ghuznee Street
Wellington 1, New Zealand

A. M. Godfrey, MB, BCh
Consultant Plastic Surgeon
Nuffield Acland Hospital and Nuffield Orthopaedic Centre, Oxford
The Paddocks Hospital, Bucks, and
The Ridgeway Hospital, Wilts
Felstead House
23 Banbury Road
Oxford OX2 6NX, United Kingdom

R. D. Goldstein, MD, FACS
Assistant Clinical Professor
Albert Einstein College of Medicine
Montefiore Medical Center
Bronx, New York 10461

R. M. Goldwyn, MD, FACS
Clinical Professor of Surgery, Harvard Medical School
Division of Plastic Surgery, Beth Israel Deaconess
Medical Center, Boston, MA
1101 Beacon Street
Brookline, Massachusetts 02146

D. J. Goodkind, MD
Yale-New Haven Hospital
Clinical Instructor of Surgery, Yale University
136 Sherman Avenue, South, Suite 205
New Haven, Connecticut 06511–5236

B. Gorowitz, MD
Department of Plastic and Reconstructive Surgery
C.H.U.-Hôpital Du Tondu
Groupe Pellegrin-Tondu
Place Amélie Raba-Léon
F-33076 Bordeaux, France

L. J. Gottlieb, MD, FACS
Professor of Clinical Surgery, Plastic and
Reconstructive Surgery
Department of Surgery
University of Chicago, Illinois
5841 South Maryland Avenue, MC 6035
Chicago, Illinois 60637

D. P. Green, MD
9150 Huebner Road, Suite 290
San Antonio, Texas 78229

B. M. Greenberg, MD, FACS
833 Northern Boulevard, Suite 115
Great Neck, New York 11021

J. M. Griffin, MD, FACS
Piedmont Hospital
Associate Clinical Professor, Department of Surgery
Emory University School of Medicine
Northside Hospital
Scottish Rite Children's Medical Center
Center for Plastic Surgery
365 East Paces Ferry Road
Atlanta, Georgia 30305–2351

B. H. Griffith, MD, FACS
Northwestern Memorial Hospital
Children's Memorial Hospital
Rehabilitation Institute of Chicago
Chief of Plastic Surgery, Shriners Hospital for Crippled
Children
Northwestern University Medical Center
251 East Chicago Avenue, Suite 1026
Chicago, Illinois 6061–2641

A. R. Grossman, MD, FACS
The Grossman Burn Center
Sherman Oaks Hospital, California
4910 Van Nuys Boulevard, Suite 306
Sherman Oaks, California 91403–1728

P. H. Grossman, MD
Grossman Burn Center
Sherman Oaks Hospital, California
4910 Van Nuys Boulevard, Suite 306
Sherman Oaks, California 91403

J. C. Grotting, MD, FACS
Children's Hospital of Alabama
Baptist Medical Center-Montclair
The Eye Foundation
Baptist Medical Center-Princeton
Health South Medical Center
Brookwood Medical Center
Outpatient CareCenter
McCollough, Grotting & Associates Plastic Surgery
Clinic P. C.
1600 20th Street, South
Birmingham, Alabama 35205

B. K. Grunert, PhD
Medical College of Wisconsin
Froedtert Memorial Lutheran Hospital
Children's Hospital of Wisconsin
9200 W. Wisconsin Avenue
Milwaukee, Wisconsin 53226

C. R. Gschwind, MD
The Centre for Bone and Joint Diseases
Royal North Shore Hospital, St. Leonards
Department of Hand Surgery
Hand and Microsurgery Unit
Royal North Shore Hospital
St. Leonards, NSW 2065, Australia

J. Guerrerosantos, MD
Chairman and Plastic Surgeon-In-Charge
Jalisco Institute for Reconstructive Surgery
Chairman and Professor, Division of Plastic and
Reconstructive Surgery, University of Guadalajara, Mexico
Garibaldi 1793
Col. L de Guevara
Guadalajara, Jalisco, 44680, Mexico

P. J. Gullane, MD
Otolaryngologist-in-Chief, Toronto Hospital, Toronto
Site Leader, Head and Neck Surgery, Princess Margaret
Hospital and Toronto Hospital
Staff Otolaryngologist, Mount Sinai Hospital, Toronto
Consultant Otolaryngologist
North York General Hospital, Toronto
200 Elizabeth Street, East
Toronto, Ontario, Canada, M5G 2C4

J. P. Gunter, MD, FACS
Presbyterian Hospital of Dallas
Parkland Memorial Hospital
Baylor University Medical Center
8315 Walnut Hill Lane, Suite 125
Dallas, Texas 75231–4211

B. Guyuron, MD, FACS
Medical Director of Zeeba Clinic
Clinical Professor of Plastic Surgery
Case Western Reserve University
29017 Cedar Road
Lyndhurst, Ohio 44124

K. F. Hagan, MD, FACS
Vanderbilt University Hospital, Baptist Hospital,
Columbia Centennial, The Atrium
Nashville Surgery Center
Vanderbilt University Medical Center
2100 Pierce Avenue
230, MCS
Nashville, Tennessee 37232–3631

E. J. Hall-Findlay, MD, FRCS
Plastic Surgeon
Banff Mineral Springs Hospital
Suite 340, Cascade Plaza
317 Banff Avenue
Banff, AT TOL 0C0, Canada

G. G. Hallock, MD, FACS
Consultant in Plastic Surgery, The Lehigh Valley and Sacred
Heart Hospitals, Allentown, Pennsylvania
St. Luke's Hospital, Bethlehem, Pennsylvania
1230 South Cedar Crest Boulevard, Suite 306
Allentown, Pennsylvania 18103

S. K. Han, MD, PhD
Professor of Plastic Surgery
Korea University College of Medicine
Seoul, Korea

R. Happle, MD
Department of Dermatology
University of Münster
Schlossplatz 2
D-4400 Münster, Germany

K. Harii, MD
Graduate School of Medicine, The University of Tokyo
Department of Plastic and Reconstructive Surgery
University of Tokyo Hospital
7–3-1 Hongo Bunkyo-ku
Tokyo 113, Japan

D. H. Harrison, MD
Regional Plastic Surgery Centre, Mount Vernon,
Northwood, UK
Flat 33, Harmont House
20 Harley Street
London WIN 1AA, United Kingdom

S. H. Harrison, MD, FCRS (Retired)
The Plastic Surgery
Mount Vernon Hospital
Rickmansworth Road
Northwood HA6 2RN, United Kingdom

C. R. Hartrampf, Jr., MD, FACS
St. Joseph's Hospital
Atlanta Plastic Surgery
Suite 500, 975 Johnson Ferry
Atlanta, Georgia 30342–1619

S. W. Hartwell, Jr., MD
Emeritus Staff, The Cleveland Clinic Foundation
9500 Euclid Avenue, E48
Cleveland, Ohio 44195–5257

A. Hayashi, MD
Assistant Professor, Department of Plastic and
Reconstructive Surgery, Toho University Hospital
Department of Plastic and Reconstructive Surgery
Toho University School of Medicine
6–11–1 Ohmorinishi, Ohta-ku
Tokyo 143, Japan

F. R. Heckler, MD, FACS
Director, Division of Plastic Surgery
Allegheny General Hospital, Pittsburgh, Pennsylvania
Clinical Associate Professor of Plastic Surgery, University of
Pittsburgh, School of Medicine, Allegheny General Hospital
320 East North Avenue
Pittsburgh, Pennsylvania 15212

T. R. Heinz, MD
University of Alabama Hospitals
The Children's Hospital of Alabama
Veteran's Administration Medical Center
University of Alabama at Birmingham
Plastic Surgery
1813 6th Avenue, South (MEB-524)
Birmingham, Alabama 35294–3295

C. Heitmann, MD, PhD
Department of Plastic, Reconstructive and Hand Surgery
Markuskrankenhaus
Frankfurt am Main
Germany

V. R. Hentz, MD
Stanford University Hospital
900 Welch Road, Suite 15
Palo Alto, California 94304

C. K. Herman, MD
Medical Director of Plastic Surgery
Pocono Health Systems
100 Plaza Court, Suite C
East Stroudsburg, PA 18301
Assistant Clinical Professor of Surgery (Plastic Surgery)
Albert Einstein College of Medicine, New York, NY 10467
Private practice, 988 Fifth Avenue, New York, NY 10021

H. L. Hill, Jr., MD
Tallahassee Memorial Medical Center, Florida
Tallahassee Single Day Surgical Hospital
Tallahassee Plastic Surgery
1704 Riggins Road
Tallahassee, Florida 32308

B. Hirshowitz, FRCS
Emeritus Professor of Plastic and Reconstructive Surgery
Faculty of Medicine
Technion-Israel Institute of Technology, Haifa
55 Margalit Street
Mount Carmel
Haifa 34464, Israel

J. G. Hoehn, MD, FACS
St. Peter's Hospital
Samuel Straton Veterans Administration
Albany Medical Center
The Child's Hospital
Albany Memorial Hospital
Albany Plastic and Reconstructive Surgery Center
Four Executive Park Drive
Albany, New York 12203

W. Y. Hoffman, MD, FACS
University of California, San Francisco Medical Center
Associate Professor of Plastic Surgery
University of California, San Francisco
350 Parnassus, Suite 509
San Francisco, California 94117–3608

J. Holle, MD
Institute of Anatomy
Medical University of Vienna
Department of Plastic and Reconstructive Surgery
Wilhelminen Hospital
Vienna, Austria
Krapfenwald G 9
Vienna, A1190, Austria

T. Honda, MD
Department of Plastic and Reconstructive Surgery
Tokyo Women's Medical University
8-1 Kawada-cho, Shinjuku-ku, 162-0054
Tokyo, Japan

C. E. Horton, MD
Sentara Norfolk General Hospital
Bon Secours DePaul Hospital
Children's Hospital of The King's Daughters
229 West Bute Street, Suite 900
Norfolk, Virginia 23510

A. S. Hoschander, MD
Resident
Department of Surgery
Long Island Jewish Medical Center/North Shore University Hospital
Manhasset, New York

W. Hu, MD
Centre Hopitalier Universitaire de Brest
Hôpital de la Cavale Blanche
F-29200 Brest, France

T. Huang, MD
Clinical Professor of Surgery
University of Texas Medical Branch
326 Market Street
Galveston, Texas 77550-5664

D. J. Hurwitz, MD
University of Pittsburgh Medical Center
Children's Hospital of Pittsburgh
Plastic and Reconstructive Surgery
Aesthetic and Craniofacial Surgery
University of Pittsburgh Medical Center
3471 Fifth Avenue
Pittsburgh, Pennsylvania 15213

J. J. Hurwitz, MD, FRCS(C)
Ophthalmological Executive Committee,
University of Toronto
Opthalmologist-in-Chief, Mount Sinai Hospital
Professor of Ophthalmology, University of Toronto
Director of Oculoplastics Programme
University of Toronto
600 University Avenue, Suite 408
Toronto, Ontario, Canada, M5G 1X5

Y. Ikuta, MD
Department of Orthopedic Surgery
Hiroshima School of Medicine
Kasumi 1–2–3
Hiroshima 734, Japan

O. Iribarren, MD
Department of Surgery
Surgery Service and Office of Nosocomial Infections Control
Saint Paul Hospital, School of Medicine
Universidad Catolica del Norte
Larrondo 1080
Videla s/n
Coquimbo. IV Region, Chile

F. Iselin, MD
Director of Hand Service
Department of Surgery, Centre de Chirugie de la
Main-Urgences Mains
Hôpital Nanterre
Paris, France

T. I. A. Ismail, MD
29 Nawal Street
Aguiza-Giza
Cairo, Egypt

Y. Itoh, MD, PhD
National Defense Medical College
Division of Plastic and Reconstructive Surgery
Department of Dermatology
3–2 Namiki
Tokorozawa, Saitama 359, Japan

Y. Iwahira, MD
Department of Plastic Surgery
Toho University Hospital
6–11–1 Ohmorinishi, Ohta-ku
Tokyo 143, Japan

H. Izawa, MD
Associate Professor
Department of Plastic and Reconstructive Surgery
St. Marianna University School of Medicine
2–16–1 Sugao
Myamae-ku, Kawasaki 216, Japan

Z. H. Jabourian, MD
Clinch Valley Medical Center, #2300
Richlands, Virginia 24641

I. T. Jackson, MD, DSc(Hon), FACS, FRCS, FRACS(Hon)
Institute for Craniofacial and Reconstructive Surgery
Diplomate of the American Board of Plastic Surgery
Institute for Craniofacial and Reconstructive Surgery
3rd Floor, Fisher Center
16001 West 9 Mile Road
Southfield, Michigan 48075

R. V. Janevicius, MD, PC
Elmhurst Memorial Hospital, Elmhurst, Illinois
Plastic and Reconstructive Surgery
360 West Butterfield Road, Suite 230
Elmhurst, Illinois 60126

H. Janvier, MD
St. Luke's Hospital
34, Place Bellecour
69002 Lyons, France

V.T. Joseph, MBBS, FRCSEd, FRACS, MMED(Surgery), FAMS
Chairman, Division of Pediatric Surgery
KK Woman's & Children's Hospital
100 Bukit Timah Road
Singapore 229899

B. B. Joshi, MS
Mahatma Gandhi Hospital
Parel
Mumbai 400 012, India

J. Juri, MD
National University
Calle Viamonte 430
Buenos Aires, Argentina 1053

M. J. Jurkiewicz, MD, FACS, FRCS
Emory Affiliated Hospitals
25 Prescott Street, Northeast
Atlanta, Georgia 30308

J. B. Kahl, MD, FACS
Director of Plastic Surgery Residency & Department Head,
Christ Hospital
Head of Department of Plastic Surgery, Mercy Hospital
Active Staff, Bethesda Hospitals
Children's Hospital of Cincinnati
Jewish Hospital and
Deaconess Hospital
President, Montgomery North Plastic Surgery Center
Staffs of Providence, St. Luke, Good Samaritan
Clinical Instructor, University of Cincinnati
10545 Montgomery Rd., #100
Cincinnati, Ohio 45242

W. J. Kane, MD
Mayo Clinic
905 14th Avenue, Southwest
200 1st Street, Southwest
Rochester, Minnesota 55905

E. N. Kaplan, MD
1515 El Camino Real, Suite D
Palo Alto, California 94306

I. Kaplan, MB, ChB
Professor of Surgery and Incumbent of Chilewich Chair of
Plastic Surgery
University of Tel Aviv
Head, Department of Plastic Surgery
Belinson Medical Center
Petah-Tiqva 76 100, Israel

I. B. Kaplan, MD
Plastic Surgery Associates, Inc.
400 West Brambleton Avenue, Suite 300
Norfolk, Virginia 23510–1115

M. R. Karapandžić, MD
Belgrade University
Studenski Trg 1
1101 Belgrade 6, Yugoslavia

A. Karev, MD
Head, Department of Hand Surgery, Kaplan Hospital
Rehovot POBA 76100 Israel

R. B. Karp, MD
Courtesy Staff, Suburban Hospital, Bethesda, MD
11510 Old Georgetown Road
Rockville, Maryland 20852

R. G. Katz, MD
3500 Fifth Avenue
Pittsburgh, Pennsylvania 15213

J. C. Kelleher, MD, FACS
Microsurgery Fellow
Division of Plastic Surgery
Department of Surgery
University of Mississippi Medical Center
Jackson, Missouri

A. F. Kells, MD, PhD
Microsurgery Fellow
Division of Plastic Surgery
Department of Surgery
University of Mississippi Medical Center
Jackson, Mississippi

J. M. Kenkel, MD
University of Texas, Southwestern, Dallas, Texas
5323 Harry Hines Boulevard
Dallas, Texas 75235–9132

C. L. Kerrigan, MD, FRCS
Mary Hitchcock Memorial Medical Center
Lebanon, New Hampshire
Veteran Affairs Medical Center, White River Junction, VT
Dartmouth-Hitchcock Medical Center
One Medical Center Drive
Lebanon, New Hampshire 03756

M. Keyes-Ford, PAC (Deceased)

A. A. Khashaba, MD
Assistant Professor of Plastic Surgery
Zagazig University
4 Dr Ahmed Nada Street
Heliopolis, Cairo, Egypt

R. K. Khouri, MD, FACS
Baptist Hospital, Miami, FL
Doctors Hospital, Miami, FL
Cedars Hospital, Miami, FL
Dermatology and Plastic Surgery Center
328 Crandon Blvd., Suite 227
Key Biscayne, Florida 33149

Y. Kikuchi, MD
Department of Plastic and Reconstructive Surgery
Tokyo Women's Medical University
8-1 Kawada-cho, Shimjuku-ku, 162-0054
Tokyo, Japan

S. K. Kim, MD, PhD
Professor
Department of Plastic and Reconstructive Surgery
Dong-A University School of Medicine
Dong-A University Hospital
Seo-Gu
Busan, Korea

K. S. Kim, MD, PhD
Department of Plastic and Reconstructive Surgery
Chonnam National University Medical School
Dong-gu, Gwangju, Korea

Y. Kimata, MD
Professor
Department of Plastic and Reconstructive Surgery
Okayama University
Graduate School of Medicine, Dentistry and
Pharmaceutical Sciences
Shikata-cho, Okayama, Japan

B. Kirkby, MD
Associate Professor
The Royal Dental College
Copenhagen, Denmark

H. W. Klein, MD, FACS
Mercy Hospitals, Sacramento
Sutter Affiliated Hospitals
University of California, Davis
Suite 202
8120 Timberlake Way
Sacramento, California 95823–5412

S. Kobayashi, MD
Head and Professor of Department of Plastic and
Reconstructive Surgery, Iwate Medical University
19–1 Uchimaru Morioka-shi, Iwate 020
Japan

R. Kolachalam, MD
6848 Tiffany Circle
Canton, Michigan 48187

H. Koncilia, MD
Department of Plastic and Reconstructive Surgery
Wilhelminen Hospital, Vienna, Austria

I. Koshima, MD
Associate Professor of Plastic and Reconstructive Surgery
Plastic and Reconstructive Surgery
Kawasaki Medical School
577 Matsushima, Kurashiki City
Okayama 701–01, Japan

S. S. Kroll, MD, FACS (Deceased)

G. Kronen, MD
1115 Mallard Creek Road
Saint Matthews, Kentucky 40207-2489

J. E. Kutz, MD
Clinical Professor of Surgery (Hand)
University of Louisville School of Medicine
Christine M. Kleinert Institute for Hand and
Micro Surgery
225 Abraham Flexner Way, Suite 850
Louisville, Kentucky 40202

R. Kuzbari, MD
Associate Professor of Plastic Surgery
Wilhelminenspital
Montleartstrasse 37, A-1160
Vienna, Austria

S. Kwei, MD
North Shore Plastic Surgery
4 Centennial Drive, Suite 102
Peabody, Massachusetts 01960

H. P. Labandter, MD, FRCS
Herzlia Medical Center
7 Ramot Yam
Herzlia Pituach, Israel

L. Landín, MD
Assistant Surgeon
Reconstructive Surgery and Microsurgery Unit
Hand Transplant Surgery Unit
"La Fe" University Hospital
Valencia, Spain

V. C. Lanier, Jr., MD
300 Crutchfield Street
Durham, North Carolina 27704

N. Laud, MD
Lokmaya Tilak Municipal General Hospital
and Medical College
Saraswati Nilayam
Hindu Colony, Dadar
Mubai (Mumbai) 14, 400 014 India

S. A. Lauer, MD
Department of Ophthalmology
Albert Einstein College of Medicine and
Montefiore Medical Center
111 East 210th Steet
Bronx, New York 10467

D. Le Nen, MD
Centre Hopitalier Universitaire de Brest, France
Hôpital de la Cavale Blanche
F-29200 Brest, France

B. T. Lee, MD
Instructor in Surgery
Department of Surgery
Harvard Medical School;
Division of Plastic and Reconstructive Surgery
Beth Israel Deaconess Medical Center
Boston, Massachusetts

C. Lefevre, MD
Service d'Orthopedie, C.H.U.
Hôpital de la Cavale Blanche
F-29200 Brest, France

P. Leniz, MD
Burn and Plastic Surgery Unit
Hospital del Trabajador de Santiago
Santiago, Chile

A. G. Leonard, FRCS
Northern Ireland Plastic & Maxillofacial Service
The Upper Ulster Hospital
Dundonald, Belfast BT16 ORH
Northern Ireland, United Kingdom

M. A. Lesavoy, MD, FACS
UCLA Medical Center
Harbor-UCLA Medical Center
Santa Lionica-UCLA Medical Center
VA Medical Center-West Los Angeles
Division of Plastic and Reconstructive Surgery
UCLA School of Medicine
64–128 CHS, Box 951665
Los Angeles, California 90095–1665

M. Lester, MD
Assistant Professor
Department of Plastic and Reconstructive Surgery
University of Florida
Gainesville, Florida;
2 Council Street
Charleston, South Carolina 29401

L. A. Levine, MD
Lake Forest Hospital
Department of Urology
Rush-Presbyterian-St. Luke's Medical Center
1725 W. Harrison Street, Suite 917
Chicago, Illinois 60612

M. L. Lewin, MD (Deceased)

J. R. Lewis, Jr., MD, FACS (Deceased)

V. L. Lewis, Jr., MD
Professor of Clinical Surgery
Northwestern University Medical School
707 North Fairbanks Court
Suite 1210, Chicago, Illinois 60611

R. W. Liebling, MD
Associate Professor
Albert Einstein College of Medicine and
Montefiore Medical Center
Department of Plastic and Reconstructive Surgery
Jacobi Medical Center
1825 Eastchester Road
Bronx, New York 10461

B.-L. Lim, MD
Department of Hand Surgery
Singapore General Hospital
Outram Road
Singapore 0316

Chi-hung Lin, MD
Chang Gung Memorial Hospital
Kweishan
Taoyuan, Taiwan

W. C. Lineaweaver, MD
Professor and Chief, Division of Plastic Surgery
University of Mississippi Medical Center
Jackson, Mississippi

P. C. Linton, MD, FACS
Emeritus Professor of Plastic Surgery
University of Vermont College of Medicine
30 Main Street
Burlington, Vermont 05401

G. D. Lister, MD
Division of Plastic Surgery
University of Utah Medical Center
50 Medical Drive
Salt Lake City, Utah 84132

J. W. Little, III, MD, FACS
1145 19th Street, Northwest, Suite 802
Washington, DC 20036

J. W. Littler, MD (Deceased)

S. Llanos, MD
Burn and Plastic Surgery Unit
Hospital del Trabajador de Santiago
Centre for Health Research and Development
Universidad de los Andes
Chile

P. Lorea, MD
SOS MAIN Strasbourg
Strasbourg, France

M. M. LoTempio, MD
Fellow
Division of Plastic Surgery
Medical University of South Carolina

E. A. Luce, MD, FACS
Chief, Division of Plastic Surgery and Kiehn-DesPrez
Professor at University Hospitals of Cleveland/Case Western
Reserve University
Division of Plastic Surgery
11100 Euclid Avenue
Cleveland, Ohio 44106–5044

H. W. Lueders (Retired)
Community Hospital, Monterey, California
4007 Costado Road
Pebble Beach, California 93953

J. R. Lyons, MD
Yale-New Haven Hospital
Hospital St. Raphael
New Haven, Connecticut
330 Orchard Street
New Haven, Connecticut 06511–4417

S. E. MacKinnon, MD, FACS
Shoenberg Professor and Chief, Division of Plastic and
Reconstructive Surgery, Department of Surgery
Washington University School of Medicine
Division of Plastic Surgery and Reconstructive Surgery
One Barnes-Jewish Hospital Plaza, Suite #17424
St. Louis, Missouri 63110

W. B. Macomber, MD
Albany Medical College
1465 Western Avenue
Albany, New York 12203

N. C. Madan, MD
Associate Professor of Surgery
All India Institute of Medical Sciences
New Delhi, India

K. T. Mahan, DPM
Presbyterian Medical Center of University of Pennsylvania
St. Cigner Medical Center
Bethesda National Naval Medical Center
Pennsylvania College of Podiatric Medicine
The Foot and Ankle Institute
810 Race Street
Philadelphia, Pennsylvania 19107–2496

A. M. Majidian, MD
Grossman Burn Center at Sherman Oaks Hospital, California
2080 Century Park East, Ste 501
Los Angeles, California 90067

S. Malekzadeh, MD
Resident, University of Maryland Medical System,
Baltimore, MD
University of Maryland Medical System
22 S. Greene Street
Baltimore, Maryland 21201

R. T. Manktelow, MD
The Toronto Hospital
Mount Sinai Hospital
Hospital for Sick Children
Etobreske General Hospital
St. Michael's Hospital
The Toronto Hospital
Western Division
399 Bathurst Street 5WW835
Toronto, Ontario, Canada M5T 2S8

C. H. Manstein, MD
Chief, Division of Plastic Surgery, Jeans Hospital,
Philadelphia
Assistant Professor of Surgery, Temple University
School of Medicine, Philadelphia
Manstein Plastic Surgery Associates
7500 Central Avenue, Suite 210
Philadelphia, Pennsylvania 19111–2434

B. Maraud, MD
Centre Hospitalier D'Agen
17, Rue de Strasbourg
F-47000 Agen, France

D. Marchac, MD
Hôpital Necker Enfants Malades, Paris, France
130 rue de la Pompe
F-75116 Paris, France

J. M. Markley, MD, FACS
St. Joseph Mercy Hospital, Ann Arbor
University of Michigan Medical Center, Ann Arbor
Suite 5001–5008
5333 McAulery Drive
Ann Arbor, Michigan 48106

D. R. Marshall, FRACS
Monash University
Wellington Road
Melbourne
Victoria 3618, Australia

D. Martin, MD
Department of Plastic and Reconstructive Surgery
C.H.U.-Hôpital Du Tondu
Groupe Pellegrin-Tondu
Place Amélie Raba-Léon
F-33076 Bordeaux, France

Y. Maruyama, MD
Department of Plastic and Reconstructive Surgery
Toho University School of Medicine
6–11–1 Ohmorinishi, Ohta-ku
Tokyo 143, Japan

Professeur A. C. Masquelet
Chirurgie Orthopédique-Tramatologique et
Réparatrice de l'Appareil Locomoteur
Hôpital Avicenne
125, route de Stalingrad
F- 93009 Bobigny Cedex, France

J. K. Masson, MD
Mayo Clinic
102 Southwest Second Avenue
Rochester, Minnesota 55905–0008

A. Matarasso, MD, FACS, PC
Manhattan Eye, Ear, & Throat Hospital
Albert Einstein College of Medicine and Montefiore Medical
Center
Plastic and Reconstructive Surgery
1009 Park Avenue
New York, New York 10028

S. J. Mathes, MD
University of California, San Francisco Hospitals
and Clinics
Department of Surgery
San Francisco, California 94143–0932

H. S. Matloub, MD, FACS
Professor of Plastic Surgery and Director of Hand Fellowship
Program, Froedtert Hospital
Children's Hospital of Wisconsin
Veteran's Administration Hospital
Department of Plastic and Reconstructive Surgery
Medical College of Wisconsin
9200 West Wisconsin Avenue
Milwaukee, Wisconsin 53226

K. Matsuo, MD
Department of Plastic and Reconstructive Surgery
Shinshu University School of Medicine
3-1-1 Asahi, Matsumoto 390, Japan

J. W. May, Jr., MD, FACS
Chief of Division of Plastic Surgery
Massachusetts General Hospital
Massachusetts General Hospital, Rm. 353
Ambulatory Care Center, Ste. 453
15 Parkman Street
Boston, Massachusetts 02214–3139

J. G. McCarthy, MD, FACS
New York University Medical Center
Bellevue Hospital Center
Manhattan Eye, Ear & Throat Hospital
NYU Medical Center
550 First Avenue
New York, New York 10016

J. B. McCraw, MD, FACS
Professor of Plastic Surgery
University of Mississippi
2500 North State Street
Jackson, Mississippi 39216-3600

I. A. McGregor, MD
7 Ledcameroch Road
Bearsden,
Glasgow G61 4AB, Scotland
United Kingdom

S. Medgyesi, MD
Consultant Plastic Surgeon
Rigshospitalet
Copenhagen, Denmark

J. Medina, MD
Hand surgeon
Department of Orthopedics
Las Palmas
Gran Canaria
Spain

B. C. Mendelson, FRCSE, FRACS, FACS
The Avenue Hospital, Melbourne, Australia
109 Mathoura Road
Toorak, Victoria 3142
Australia

N. Menon, MD
Microsurgery Fellow
Stanford University Medical Center
Division of Plastic Surgery
Palo Alto, California

R. Meyer, MD
Postgraduate Professor ISAPS (IPRAS)
Centre de Chirurgie Plastique
4-Avenue Marc-Dufour
CH-1007 Lausanne, Switzerland

D. R. Millard, Jr., MD, FACS
Jackson Memorial Hospital
Miami Children's Hospital
1444 Northwest Fourteenth Avenue
Miami, Florida 33125

R. L. Mills, MD
751 South Bascom Avenue
San Jose, California 95128–2604

T. Miura, MD
Chukyo University
101 Tokodate, Kaizu-cho
Toyota, Aichi, 470–03, Japan

J. R. Moore, MD
Associate Professor of Orthopedic Surgery
The Johns Hopkins University School of Medicine
1400 Front Avenue, Suite 100
Lutherville, MD 21093–5355

S. C. Morgan, MD
Huntington Memorial Hospital
Arcadia Methodist Hospital
USC-LA County Medical Center
10 Congress Street, Suite 407
Pasadena, California 91105–3023

K. Morioka, MD
Department of Plastic and Reconstructive Surgery
Tokyo Women's Medical University
Tokyo, Japan

A. M. Morris, MD
Dundee University
Dundee, DD1 9SV, Scotland
United Kingdom

W. A. Morrison, MD
Plastic Surgeon and Deputy Director
Microsurgery Research Centre
St. Vincent's Hospital
Melbourne, Australia

H. Müller, MD, DMD (Deceased)

W. R. Mullin, MD, FACS
Jackson Memorial
Cedar Medical Center
Children's Medical Center
Plastic Surgery Centre
1444 Northwest 14th Avenue
Miami, Florida 33125

J. C. Mustardé, MD
90 Longhill Avenue
Ayr, Scotland, KA7 4DF, United Kingdom

F. Nahai, MD
Professor of Plastic Surgery, Emory University
Emory University Clinic
1365 Clifton Road, Northeast
Atlanta, Georgia 30322

J. E. Nappi, MD
Riverside Methodist Hospital
3400 Olentauey River Road
Columbus, Ohio 43214

M. Narayanan, MD
Medical Advisor
Ramalingam Medical Relief Centre
Madras, India

T. M. Nassif, MD
Hospital dos Servidores do Estado
Chief, Department of Reconstructive Microsurgery
Hospital dos Sevidores do Estado
22281 Rio de Janeiro RJ, Brazil

Vu Nguyen, MD
Assistant Professor
Division of Plastic Surgery
University of Pittsburgh Medical Center
Pittsburgh, Pennsylvania

J. M. Noe, MD
Harvard Medical School
25 Shattuck Street
Boston, Massachusetts 02115

K. Nohira, MD
Hokkaido University, Department of Plastic and
Reconstructive Surgery
Keiyukai Sapporo Hospital, Division of Plastic Surgery
Chief of Soshundo Plastic Surgery
Otemachi Building 2F
Minami-1, Nishi-4, Chuo-ku
Sapporo 060, Japan

J. D. Noonan, MD, FACS
Albany Medical Center
St. Peter's Hospital, Children's Hospital
1465 Western Avenue
Albany, New York 12203–3512

M. Nozaki, MD
Department of Plastic and Reconstructive Surgery
Tokyo Women's Medical University
8-1 Kawada-cho, Shimjuku-ku, 162-0054
Tokyo, Japan

K. Ohmori, MD
Department of Plastic and Restorative Surgery
Tokyo Metropolitan Police Hospital
2-10-41 Fujima Chiyoda-ku
Tokyo 102, Japan

S. Ohmori, MD (Deceased)

H. Ohtsuka, MD
Associate Professor
Ehime University Hospital
Surgical Division
Section of Plastic and Reconstructive Surgery
Shitsukawa, Shigenobu-cho,
Onsen-gun, Ehime 791–0295, Japan

C. Orreteguy, MD
Centre Hospitalier-Villeneuve Sur Lot
19, Bd. de la Marine
F-47300 Villeneuve Sur Lot, France

M. Orticochea, MD
Montevideo University School of Medicine
Montevideo, Uruguay

A. I. Pakiam, MD, FACS
Hospital of Saint John and St. Elizabeth
London, United Kingdom

C. E. Paletta, MD, FACS
Associate Professor, Division of Plastic and
Reconstructive Surgery, St. Louis University Hospital
Cardinal Glennon Children's Hospital
Veterans Administration–St. Louis
St. Mary's Health Center
St. Louis University
Associate Professor, Division of Plastic Surgery
3635 Vista at Grand
St. Louis, Missouri 63110–0250

F. X. Paletta, MD, FACS (Retired)
3635 Vista at Grand
St. Louis, Missouri 63110–0250

B. Panconi, MD
Department of Plastic and Reconstructive Surgery
of the Hand
Hôpital Pellegrin-Tondu
Place Amélie Raba-Léon
F-33076 Bordeaux, France

S. D. Pandey, MS, MCh
Professor, Hand Surgery
King George's Medical College
Lucknow 226 003, India

W. R. Panje, MD
Rush-Presbyterian-St. Luke's Medical Center, Chicago, Illinois
1725 Harrison Street, Suite 340
Chicago, Illinois 60612

G. S. Pap, MD, DDS, FACS (Retired)
Plastic and Reconstructive Maxillo-Facial Surgery
2403 Spring Creek Road
Rockford, Illinois 61107

C. Papp, MD
Head, Department of Plastic and Reconstructive Surgery
Hospital of Barmherzige Brüder
Salzburg, Austria

A. M. Pardue, MD, FACS
Los Robles Regional Medical Center
Thousand Oaks, California
1993 West Potrero Road
Thousand Oaks, California 91361

K.J. Park, MD, PhD
Assistant Professor
Department of Surgery
Dong-A University Medical Center
3 go 1, Dongdaesin-dong, Seo-Gu, Busan 602-716
South Korea

S. W. Parry, MD
Tulane Medical Center
Professor of Surgery, Tulane University
Tulane Medical Center Hospital and Clinic
1415 Tulane Avenue
New Orleans, Louisiana 70112–2605

A. Patel, MD
Resident
Department of Otolaryngology
The New York Eye & Ear Infirmary
New York, New York

R. M. Pearl, MD, FACS
Stanford University Hospital
Kaiser Hospital, Santa Clara
Physician-in-Chief
The Permanente Medical Group
900 Kiely Boulevard
Santa Clara, California 95051–5386

James M. Pearson, MD
Chief Resident
Department of Otolaryngology
The New York Eye & Ear Infirmary
New York, New York

I. J. Peled, MD
Chairman, Department of Plastic Surgery
Rambam Medical Center
Technion Institute of Technology, Medical School
Department of Plastic Surgery
Rambam Medical Center
Haifa, Israel

P. Pelissier, MD
Chef de Clinique
Service de Chirurgie Plastique et Reconstructrice
Hôpital du Tondu-Pellegrin
F-33076 Bordeaux, France

A. D. Pelly, MD
Plastic Surgery Unit
The Prince of Wales Hospital
195 Macquarie Street
Sydney 2000, Australia

Y. P. Peng, RWH Pho, FRCS
Consultant
Department of Hand and Reconstructive
Microsurgery
National University Hospital, Singapore;
Emeritus Professor of Orthopaedic Surgery
National University of Singapore

J. O. Penix, MD
Sentard Norfolk General Hospital
Surgical Director of Neurological Surgery
Children's Hospital of the King's Daughters
Neurosurgical Associates
607 Medical Tower
Norfolk, Virginia 23507

J. M. Peres, MD
Department of Plastic and Reconstructive Surgery
C.H.U.-Hôpital Du Tondu
Groupe Pellegrin-Tondu
Place Amélie Raba-Léon
F-33076 Bordeaux, France

M. Pers, DrMed
Head, Department of Plastic Surgery
University of Copenhagen
Rigshospitalet
Copenhagen, Denmark

J. Perssonelli, MD
St. Paul Hay Hospital
Av. Moema 170/111
04082-002 São Paulo SP, Brazil

V. Petrovici, MD
Department of Surgery, University of Cologne
Merheim Hospital
Bachemerstrasse 267
D-50935 Köln, Germany

R. W. H. Pho, MBBS, FRCS
Professor in Orthopaedic Surgery
National University of Singapore
Chief, Department of Hand and Reconstructive Microsurgery
National University Hospital
5 Lower Kent Ridge Road
Singapore 119074

K. L. Pickrell, MD (Deceased)

M. J. Pidala, MD
Western Reserve Medical Center
1930 State Route 59
Kent, Ohio 44240

J. L. Piñeros, MD
President of the Chilean Society of Burns
Burn and Plastic Surgery Unit
Hospital del Trabajador de Santiago
Santiago, Chile

P. Poizac, MD
Centre Hospitalier D'Agen
17, rue de Strasbourg
F-47000 Agen, France

B. Pontén, MD
Department of Plastic Surgery
University of Uppsala
750 14 Uppsala, Sweden

L. Pontes, MC
Plastic Surgery Unit
Department of Surgical Oncology
Portuguese Institute of Oncology
Porto, Portugal

J. A. Porter, MD
Clinical Professor of Surgery
Northeastern Ohio Universities College of Medicine
Summa Health Systems
55 Arch Street, Suite 3D
Akron, Ohio 44304

M. A. Posner, MD
Clinical Professor of Orthopaedics
New York University School of Medicine
Chief of Hand Services, Hospital for Joint Diseases
Chief of Hand Services, Lenox Hill Hospital
2 East 88th Street
New York, New York 10128

Z. Potparic, MD
University of Miami School of Medicine
Division of Plastic Surgery
Miami, Florida 33136

N. G. Poy, MD (Retired)
Scarborough General Hospital, Scarborough, Ont, Canada
4151 Sheppard Avenue, East
Scarborough, Ontario, Canada M1S 1T4

J. N. Pozner, MD
Assistant Clinical Professor of Plastic Surgery
The Johns Hopkins Hospital, Baltimore, MD
Plastic and Aesthetic Surgery
1212 York Road, Suite B101
Lutherville, Maryland 21093

G. Pradet, MD
Centre de Chirugie de la Main-Urgences Mains
Hôpital Nanterre
Paris, France

F. E. Pratt, MD (Retired)
P.O. Box 417880
Sacramento, California 95841

J. J. Pribaz, MD
Brigham & Women's Hospital, Boston
Children's Hospital, Boston
Associate Professor/Chief, Hand and Microsurgery
Department of Surgery/Division of Plastic Surgery
Brigham and Women's Hospital
75 Francis Street
Boston, Massachusetts 02115

J. M. Psillakis, MD
Professor of Plastic and Reconstructive Surgery
University of Sao Paulo, Brazil
Av. Cauaxi 222
Ed. San Martin 703
Barueri 06454-020, Brazil

C. L. Puckett, MD, FACS
University of Missouri Hospital and Clinics
Professor and Head
Division of Plastic and Reconstructive Surgery
University of Missouri
One Hospital Drive
Columbia, Michigan 65212

C. Radovan, MD (Deceased)

S. S. Ramasastry, MD
University of Illinois at Chicago Medical Center
Cook County Hospital, Chicago, Illinois
Mount Sinai Hospital, Chicago, Illinois
820 South Wood Street, (M/C 958) 515 CSN
Chicago, Illinois 60612

O. M. Ramirez, MD, FACS
Greater Baltimore Medical Center
Professor, The Johns Hopkins University
School of Medicine
Franklin Square Hospital, Baltimore
Plastic and Aesthetic Surgery
1212 York Road Suite, B-101
Lutherville-Timonium, Maryland 21093–6240

Y. Ramon, MD
Department of Plastic Surgery
Rambam Medical Center, Haifa
4A Mapu Avenue
Haifa, 34361 Israel

V. K. Rao, MD, MBA
University of Wisconsin Hospital and Clinic
University of Wisconsin Medical School
600 Highland Avenue
Madison, Wisconsin 53792

D. A. Campbell Reid, MD, FRCS
Consultant Plastic Surgeon
Plastic and Jaw Department
Fulwood Hospital
Fulwood
Sheffield, S10 3TD, United Kingdom

R. S. Reiffel, MD, PC, FACS
White Plains Hospital
St. Agnes Hospital
Westchester Medical Center
12 Greenridge Avenue, Suite 203
White Plains, New York 10605

J. F. Reinisch, MD, FACS
Head, Division of Plastic Surgery
Childrens Hospital Los Angeles
University Hospital
Associate Professor of Clinical Surgery, University of
Southern California School of Medicine
Division of Plastic Surgery
Childrens Hospital Los Angeles
4650 Sunset Boulevard, MS #96
Los Angeles, California 90027

A. J. Renard, MD, FACS
3845 Bee Ridge Road
Sarasota, Florida 34233–1160

J. E. Restrepo, MD
Clínica Soma
Medellin, Columbia

C. A. Rhee, MD
2879 Hempstead Turnpike, Suite 204
Levittown, New York 11756

M. Ribeiro, MD
Plastic Surgery Unit
Department of Surgical Oncology I
Portuguese Institute of Oncology
Porto, Portugal

D. Richard, MD
Centre Hospitalier D'Agen
Rue Lamennais
F-47000 Agen, France

R. A. Rieger, MBBS, FRCS, FRACS
327 S. Terrace
Adelaide 5001, Australia

R. Roa, MD
President of the Chilean Burn Association;
Assistant Professor
Medical School, Universidad de los Andes
Santiago, Chile

G. A. Robertson, MD
Victoria Hospital, Winnipeg, Manitoba
Manitoba Clinic
790 Sherbrook Street
Winnipeg R3A 1M3, Canada

J. F. R. Rocha, MD
Laboratoire d'Anatomie de l'UER
Biomedicale de Saint Peres
Hôpital Trousseau
Paris, France

C. Rodgers, MD, FACS
Rose Medical Center
Swedish Hospital
Porter Hospital
Littleton Hospital
4600 Hale Parkway, Suite 430
Denver, Colorado 80220

E. Roggendorf, Dr.sc.med. (Deceased)

M. C. Romaña, MD
Hôpital d'Enfants Armand-Trousseau, Paris
Consultant Surgeon
Department of Orthopaedic and Reconstructive Surgery
for Children
Hôpital Trousseau
26 Avenue A. Netter
F-75012 Paris, France

T. Romo III, MD
Director of Facial Plastic and Reconstructive Surgery
Department of Otolaryngology Head and Neck Surgery
Lenox Hill Hospital
The Manhattan Eye, Ear and Throat Hospital
New York, New York

E. H. Rose, MD
Assistant Clinical Professor (Plastic Surgery)
The Mount Sinai Medical School, New York, NY
Attending Staff, The Mount Sinai Medical Center and
Lenox Hill Hospital, New York, NY
Founder and Director, The Aesthetic Surgery Center,
New York, NY
The Aesthetic Surgery Center
895 Park Avenue
New York, New York 10021

M. Rousso, MD
Senior Lecturer of Surgery
Hadassah Hebrew University, Jerusalem
Head of Hand Surgery and Day Care Surgery
Misgav Ladach General Hospital
POB 90
Jerusalem 91000, Israel

R. T. Routledge, MD, FRCS (Retired)
Chief of Plastic Surgery Department
Frenchay Hospital
Bristol, United Kingdom

R. C. Russell, MD, FACS, FRCS
Memorial Hospital, Springfield, IL
St. John's Hospital, Springfield, IL
Illini Hospital, Pittsfield, IL
Southern Illinois University School of Medicine
Plastic Surgery 1511, P.O. Box 19230
Springfield, Illinois 62794

R. F. Ryan, MD, FACS (Retired)
Emeritus Professor of Surgery (Plastic Reconstructive),
Tulane Medical School, New Orleans, LA
Perido Bay Country Club
5068 Shoshone Drive
Pensacola, Florida 32507

F. J. Rybka, MD, FACS
Mercy Hospital
Sutter Hospital
Professor of Plastic Surgery, University of California, Davis
San Juan Medical Plaza, Suite 350
6660 Coyle Avenue
Carmichael, California 95608–6312

M. N. Saad, MD
Honorary Consultant Plastic Surgeon
Wexham Park Hospital, Slough
Consultant Plastic Surgeon
The Thames Valley Nuffield Hospital, Slough and
The Princess Margaret Hospital
Osborne Road, Windsor
Berks SL4 3SJ, United Kingdom

H. Saito, MD, PhD
Fukui Medical University
Matsuoka-cho, Yoshida-gun
Fukui, Japan

S. Sakai, MD
Associate Professor
Department of Plastic and Reconstructive Surgery
St. Marianna University School of Medicine
2-16-1 Sugao
Myamae-ku, Kawasaki 216, Japan

R. H. Samson, MD
Sarasota Memorial Hospital
Columbia Doctors Hospital
Vascular Associates of Sarasota
4044 Sawer Road
Sarasota, Florida 34233

J. R. Sanger, MD, FACS
Medical College of Wisconsin
9200 West Wisconsin Avenue
Milwaukee, Wisconsin 53226

J.R. Ramón Sanz, MD
Head of Department of Plastic and Reconstructive Surgery
"Marqués de Valdecilla" University Hospital
Santander, Spain

G. H. Sasaki, MD, FACS
St. Luke Medical Center
Huntington Memorial Hospital
Arcadia Methodist Hospital
Plastic and Reconstructive Surgery
800 South Fairmount Avenue, Suite 319
Pasadena, California 91105

K. Sasaki, MD
Chief Professor of Nihon University School of Medicine
Department of Plastic and Reconstructive Surgery
Nihon University School of Medicine, Oyaguchi
Itabashi-ku, Tokyo Japan

R. C. Savage, MD, FACS
Assistant Clinical Professor, Division of Plastic Surgery,
Harvard Medical School
Needham Medical Building
111 Lincoln Street, Suite 3
Needham, Massachusetts 02192

H. Schaupp, MD (Retired)
University ENT Hospital
Frankfurt-am-Main, Germany

L. R. Scheker, MD
Christine M. Kleinert Institute for Hand and Microsurgery
Assistant Clinical Professor of Plastic and
Reconstructive Surgery
University of Louisville
225 Abraham Flexner Way, Suite 700
Louisville, Kentucky 40202–3806

R. R. Schenck, MD, FACS
Associate Professor and Director
Section of Hand Surgery
Senior Attending, Departments of Plastic and
Orthopaedic Surgery
Rush-Presbyterian-St. Luke's Medical Center
1725 Harrison Street, Rm 263
Chicago, Illinois 60612–3828

J. D. Schlenker, MD
Christ
Little Co. of Mary
Palos Community
Holy Cross
Illinois Valley Community Hospital
6311 West 95th Street
Chicago, Illinois 60453

J. Schrudde, MD
University of Köln
Osterriethwed 17
D-50996 Köln, Germany

M. A. Schusterman, MD, FACS
Clinical Associate Professor of Plastic and
Reconstructive Surgery
Baylor College of Medicine, Houston, TX
7505 South Main Street, Suite 200
Houston, Texas 77030

S. P. Seidel, MD
Cullman Regional Medical Center
Woodland Community Hospital
Walker Baptist Medical Center
Seidel Plastic Surgery
2035 Alabama Highway #157
Cullman, Alabama 35055

D. Serafin, MD, FACS
Professor, Chief of Plastic Reconstructive
Maxillary Oral Surgery
Duke University Medical Center
P.O. Box 3372
Durham, North Carolina 27710–0001

R. E. Shanahan, MD, FACS
Emeritus Staff, The Toledo Hospital
Emeritus Clinical Associate Professor of Surgery
Medical College of Ohio at JOCTPC
5945 Barkwood Lane
Toledo, Ohio 43560

L. A. Sharzer, MD, FACS
Albert Einstein College of Medicine and
Montefiore Medical Center
Westchester Square Hospital, NY
Beth Israel Hospital, NY
212 East 69th Street
New York, New York 10021

W. W. Shaw, MD, FACS
Professor, Chief, Division of Plastic Surgery
UCLA School of Medicine
Room 64-140 CHS
10833 LeConte Avenue
Los Angeles, California 90095

R. W. Sheffield, MD, FACS
Cottage Hospital, Santa Barbara, CA
1110 Coast Village Circle
Santa Barbara, California 93108

A. Shektman, MD
332 Washington Street
Suite 355
Wellesley, Massachusetts 02181

S. M. Shenaq, MD, FACS
The Methodist Hospital, Texas Medical Center
St. Luke's Episcopal Hospital, Texas Medical Center
Texas Children's Hospital, Texas Medical Center
Ben Taub General Hospital, Texas Medical Center
Veteran's Administration Hospital, Texas Medical Center
Institute for Rehabilitation and Research, Texas
Medical Center
Diagnostic Center Hospital, Texas Medical Center
Poly Ryan Memorial, Richmond, Texas
Northeast Medical Center Hospital, Humble, Texas
Professor of Surgery, Division of Plastic Surgery
Baylor College of Medicine
6560 Fannin Street, Suite 800
Houston, Texas 77030

G. H. Shepard, MD
Riverside Regional Hospital Medical Center
Newport News, Virginia
Mary Immaculate Hospital
Newport News, Virginia
895 Middle Ground Boulevard, Suite 300
Newport News, Virginia 23606

M. M. Sherif, MD
Associate Professor
Department of Plastic and Reconstructive Surgery
Aim Shams University, Cairo, Egypt
2(A) Al Sayed Abou Shady Street, Flat 606
Heliopolis, Cairo 11361, Egypt

K. C. Shestak, MD
Division of Plastic Surgery
University of Pittsburgh
Pittsburgh, Pennsylvania

Y. J. Shin, MD
Department of Plastic Surgery
College of Medicine
Chungnam National University
640 Taesa-Dong, Jung-ku, Taejeon
301-040 Korea

Y. Shintomi, MD
Soshundo Plastic Surgery Hospital
Director of Soshundo Plastic Surgery
Otemachi Building
Minami-1, Nishi-4, Chuo-ku
Sapporo 060, Japan

G. F. Shubailat, MD, FRCS, FACS
Member of the Senate, Jordan Parliament
CEO and Chairman of the Board, Chief of Plastic Surgery,
Amman Surgical Hospital
P. O. Box 5180
Amman 11183, Jordan

M. Siemionow, MD, PhD, DSc
Professor of Surgery
Director of Plastic Surgery Research
Department of Plastic Surgery
Cleveland Clinic
Cleveland, Ohio

C. E. Silver, MD
Professor of Surgery
Albert Einstein College of Medicne
Chief of Head and Neck Surgery
Montefiore Medical Center
111 East 210th Street
Bronx, New York 10467–2401

R. P. Silverman, MD
Chief, Division of Plastic Surgery
University of Maryland Medical Center
Baltimore, Maryland

F. A. Slezak, MD
Professor of Surgery, Northeastern Ohio Universities
College of Medicine, Department of Surgery
Summa Health Systems, Akron, Ohio
55 Arch Street, Suite 3D
Akron, Ohio 44304

C. J. Smith, MD
Swedish Hospital
Providence Hospital
Northwest Hospital
1221 Madison Street, Suite 1102
Seattle, Washington 98104–1360

E. Durham Smith, MD, FRACS
Senior Associate, University of Melbourne
Melbourne, 3052
Victoria, Australia

R. J. Smith, MD (Deceased)

J. W. Snow, MD
St. Vincent's Hospital
1820 Barrs Street, Suite 701
Jacksonville, Florida 32204

B. C. Sommerland, FRCS
Great Ormond St. Hospital for Children, London
St. Andrew's Hospital, Billeriay, Essex
Consultant Plastic Surgery
The Old Vicarage
17 Lodge Road
Writtle
Chelmsford, CMI 3H4, United Kingdom

J. T. Soper, MD
Professor, Department of Gynecological Oncology
Duke University
Division of Gynecologic Oncology
Duke University Medical Center
Durham, North Carolina 27715–3079

M. Soussaline, MD
Institut Gustave Roussy Villefrief
Clinique Ste. Genevieve
Plastic and Cosmetic Surgery Department
American Hospital
46, Boulevard Saint-Jacques
F-75014 Paris, France

D. Soutar, MD
Clinical Director, Consultant Plastic Surgeon
Honorary Senior Lecturer, University of Glasgow
Plastic Surgery Unit
Canniesburn Hospital
Bearsden
Glasgow, G61 1QL, Scotland, United Kingdom

M. Spinner, MD
557 Central Avenue
Cedarhurst, New York 11516–2136

M. Spira, MD, FACS
Chief of Plastic Surgery, St. Luke's Episcopal Hospital,
Houston, Texas
Baylor College of Medicine
6560 Fannin, Suite 800
Houston, Texas 77030

R. K. Srivastava, MD
Athens Regional Medical Center, Athens, Georgia
180 St. George Place
Athens, Georgia 30606

D. A. Staffenberg, MD, DSc (Honoris Causa)
Chief, Plastic Surgery
Surgical Director, Center for Craniofacial Disorders
Montefiore Medical Center
The Children's Hospital at Montefiore
Associate Professor
Clinical Plastic Surgery, Neurological
Surgery, Pediatrics
Albert Einstein College of Medicine
Bronx, New York

W. R. Staggers, MD
Thomas Hospital, Fairhope, AZ
South Bladwin Hospital, Foley, AZ
188 Hospital Drive, Suite 203
Thomas Hospital Medical Office Center
Fairhope, Arizona 36532

R. S. Stahl, MD, MBA
Associate Chief, Department of Surgery, Yale-New Haven
Hospital
Clinical Professor of Surgery, Yale University School of
Medicine
Yale New Haven Hospital, CB228
20 York Street
New Haven, Connecticut 06504

R. B. Stark, MD, FACS (Retired)
35 East 75th Street, 12C
New York, New York 10021

D. N. Steffanoff, MD (Retired)
114 Via Valverde
Cathedral City, California 92234

H.-U. Steinau, MD
BG-Universitätsklinik Bergmannsheil
Department of Plastic Surgery, Burn Center
Bürkle de la Camp Platz 1
D-44789 Bochum, Germany

M. Steiner, MD
Burn and Plastic Surgery Unit
Hospital del Trabajador de Santiago
Santiago, Chile

H. R. Sterman, MD
Albert Einstein College of Medicine and
Montefiore Medical Center
Holy Name Hospital
870 Palisade Avenue, Suite 203
Teaneck, New Jersey 07666

T. R. Stevenson, MD
Professor and Chief
Division of Plastic Surgery
University of California Davis Medical Center
2315 Stockton Boulevard
Sacramento, California 95817

W. Stock, MD
Ltd. Arzt f. Plast. Chirugie
Chirurgische Klinik
Nussbaumstrasse 2
D-80336 München 2, Germany

M. F. Stranc, MD
Head of Plastic Surgery Section, Health Sciences Center,
Winnipeg, Manitoba
Victoria Hospital, Winnipeg, Manitoba
Manitoba Clinic
790 Sherbrook Street
Winnipeg, Canada, R3A 1M3

W. E. Stranc, MD
Victoria Hospital
Winnipeg, Manitoba, R3A 1M3, Canada

B. Strauch, MD, FACS
Professor
Albert Einstein College of Medicine
5 Flagler Drive Bainbridge Avenue
Rye, New York 10580

V. V. Strelzow, MD, FACS, FRCS(C)
16300 Sand Canyon Avenue, Suite 704
Irvine, California 92618–3707

J. H. Sullivan, MD
Clinical Professor, University of California
San Francisco, California
220 Meridian Avenue
San Jose, California 95126–2903

I. Suzuki, MD
Associate Professor
Department of Plastic and Reconstructive Surgery
St. Marianna University School of Medicine
2-16-1 Sugao
Myamae-ku, Kawasaki 216, Japan

W. M. Swartz, MD, FACS
University of Pittsburgh Medical Center
5750 Centre Avenue, Suite 180
Pittsburgh, Pennsylvania 15206

E.-P. Tan, FRCS(Ed), FRACS
2 St. John's Avenue
Gordon, New South Wales 2072, Australia

M. J. Tavis, MD, FACS (Deceased)

G. Allan Taylor, MD, FRCS(C)
Assistant Professor of Surgery
University of Ottawa Medical School
Chief, Division of Plastic Surgery
Ottawa Civic Hospital
737 Parkdale Avenue
Ottawa, Ontario, Canada K1Y 4E9

G. I. Taylor, MD
Royal Melbourne Hospital
766 Elizabeth Street
Melbourne 3000, Australia

H.O.B. Taylor, MD
Plastic Surgery Resident
Harvard Plastic Surgery Program
Boston, Massachusetts

B. Teimourian, MD, FACS
Attending Surgeon, Suburban Hospital, Bethesda, MD
5402 McKinley Street
Bethesda, Maryland 20817

S. Terkonda, MD
University of Alabama at Birmingham, University Hospital
Instructor, Division of Plastic Surgery
University of Alabama at Birmingham, MEB-524
1813 Sixth Avenue, South
Birmingham, Alabama 35294

J. K. Terzis, MD
Sentara Hospitals
International Institute of Microsurgical Research
Eastern Virginia Medical School
330 West Brambleton Avenue
Norfolk, Virginia 23510

M. R. Thatte, MS, MCh (Plastic)
Mumbai Hospital Institute of Medical Sciences
Shushrusha Citizen's Co-Operative Hospital
Consultant Plastic Surgeon
167-F, Dr. Ambedkar Road
Dadar, Mumbai 400 014, India

R. L. Thatte, MD
Consultant Plastic Surgeon, Bhatia Hospital, Mumbai, India
Apartment 46
Shirish Co-op Housing Society
187 Veer Savarkar Marg
Mumbai 400 016, India

H. G. Thomson, MD, FACS
555 University Avenue, Suite 180
Toronto, Ontario, Canada M5G 1X8

G. R. Tobin, MD, FACS
Professor and Director, Division of Plastic Surgery
University of Louisville Hospitals
Department of Surgery
University of Louisville
Louisville, Kentucky 40292

M. A. Tonkin, MD
Clinical Associate Professor and Head, Hand and Peripheral
Nerve Surgery, Royal North Shore Hospital of Sydney
Department of Hand Surgery
The Royal North Shore Hospital of Sydney
Block 4, Level 4
St. Leonards, New South Wales, 2065, Australia

B. A. Toth, MD
Pacific-Presbyterian Medical Center
Assistant Clinical Professor, University of California, San
Francisco
2100 Webster Street, Suite 424
San Francisco, California 94115–2380

H. Tramier, MD
Service d'Orthopedie - Traumatologie - Chirurgie Pediaturgie
Centre Hospitalier, Aubogne Cedex
41, rue Saint-Jacques
F-13006 Marseille, France

G. Trengove-Jones, MD
Sentara Norfolk General Hospital
Sentara Leigh Hospital
De Paul Hospital
Childrens Hospital of the King's Daughters
Department of Plastic Surgery
Eastern Virginia Medical School
Norfolk, Virginia 23501–2401

W. C. Trier, MD, FACS (Retired)
6321 Seaview Avenue, NW, #20
Seattle, Washington 98107–2671

T.-M. Tsai, MD
Jewish Hospital
Suburban Hospital
Alliant Hospitals
University Hospital
Clark County Hospital, Indiana
Shriners Hospital, Lexington, Kentucky
Audubon Hospital
Caritas Hospital
Christine M. Kleinert Institute for Hand and Micro Surgery
225 Abraham Flexner Way, Suite 850
Louisville, Kentucky 40202

M. Tschabitscher, MD
Department of Microsurgical and
Endoscopic Anatomy
Medical University of Vienna
Vienna, Austria

Y. Ullmann, MD
Deputy Head, Department of Plastic and
Reconstructive Surgery, Rambam Medical Center
Faculty of Medicine (Bruce), Hatechnion, Haifa
Department of Plastic Surgery
Rambam Medical Center
Haifa 31096, Israel

S. Unal, MD
Department of Plastic Surgery
The Cleveland Clinic Foundation
Cleveland, Ohio

J. Unanue, MD
Centre Hospitalier Ter de Villeneuve Sur Lot
19 Bd. de la Marine
F-47300 Villeneuve Sur Lot, France

J. Upton, MD, FACS
Beth Israel Deaconess Medical Center, Boston, MA
Children's Hospital, Boston, MA
830 Boylston Street, Suite 212
Chestnut Hill, Massachusetts 02167

M. L. Urken, MD, FACS
Professor and Chairman, Department of Otolaryngology
Mt. Sinai Medical Center
Box 1189, One Gustave L. Levy Place
New York, New York 10029–6574

E. J. Van Dorpe, MD
Plastic Surgery Department
Onze Lieve Vrouw
Kortrijk, Belgium

F. Van Genechten, MD
Saint Augustinus-Saint Camillus Hospital, Antwerp, Belgium
Virga Jesse Hospital, Masself, Belgium
Oude Maasstraat. 1
B-3500 Hasselt, Belgium

L. O. Vasconez, MD, FACS
Chief Plastic Surgeon
University of Alabama at Birmingham Medical Center
Professor of Surgery and Chief
Division of Plastic Surgery
University of Alabama, Birmingham
1813 6th Avenue, South (MEB-524)
Birmingham, Alabama 35294-3295

T. R. Vecchione, MD
Associate Clinical Professor of Surgery, Division of Plastic
Surgery USSD, San Diego, CA
Senior and Past Chief of Staff, Children's Hospital of San Diego
Senior and Past Chief of Plastic Surgery, Morcy Hospital,
San Diego, CA
Senior and Past Chief of Plastic Surgery, Sharp Memorial
Hospital, San Diego, CA
306 Walnut Avenue, Suite 212
San Diego, California 92103

Professor R. Venkataswami, MS, MCh, FAMS, FRCS (EDIN), DSC (Hon)
Emeritus Professor, Dr M.G.R. Medical University
Chennai, Tamilnadv India
99 Dr. Algappa Chettiar Road
Chennai 600 084, India

R. J. J. Versluis, MD
Department of Otorhinolaryngology and
Head and Neck Surgery
Kennemer Gasthuis Deo
Velserstraat 19
NL-2023 EA Haarlem, The Netherlands

L. Vidal, MD
Department of Plastic and Reconstructive Surgery
C.H.U.-Hôpital Du Tondu
Groupe Pellegrin-Tondu
Place Amélie Raba-Léon
F-33076 Bordeaux, France

C. Vlastou, MD
Director, Department of Plastic and Reconstructive Surgery,
Diagnostic and Therapeutic Center of Athens "HYGEIA"
105-7 Vas Sovias Avenue
Athens 11521, Greece

V. E. Voci, MD, FACS
Presbyterian Hospital, Charlotte, NC
McRoy Hospital, Charlotte, NC
Gaston Memorial Hospital, Gastonia, NC
Voci Center Cosmetic Plastic Surgery, P.A.
2027 Randolph Road
Charlotte, North Carolina 28207–1215

H. D. Vuyk, MD
Gooi-Nord Hospital, Department of Otolaryngology,
Head and Neck Surgery
Rijksstraatweg 1
NL-1261 AN Blaricum, The Netherlands

S. C. Vyas, MD
Oakwood Hospital, Dearborn, MI
22260 Garrison
Dearborn, Michigan 48124

M. Wada, MD
Higasishinagawa Clinic
Higasishinagawa 3-18-8
Shinagawaku, Tokyo, Japan

M. S. Wagh, MS, MCh
Lecturer in Plastic Surgery, LTMG Hospital
Sion, Mumbai 400 022, India
601-602, B-Wing
Shantiwar
Shantivan Housing Complex
Borivali Suite 212(E), Mumbai 400 066, India

R. L. Walton, MD, FACS
University of Chicago Hospitals
University of Chicago - MC 6035
Plastic Surgery
5841 South Maryland Avenue
Chicago, Illinois 60637

A. Wangermez, MD
Centre Hospitalier D'Agen
Rue Lamennais
F-47000 Agen, France

P. H. Warnke, MD
Department of Oral and Maxillofacial Surgery
University of Kiel
Kiel, Germany

H. Washio, MD, FACS
Attending Staff, Plastic Surgery, St. Luke's–Roosevelt
Hospital Center, New York, New York
580 Park Avenue
New York, New York 10021

J. T. K. Wee, MD (Deceased)

F-C. Wei, MD
Professor and Chairman
Department of Plastic and Reconstructive Surgery
Chang Gung Memorial Hospital
199 Tung Hwa North Road
Taipei 10591, Taiwan

A. J. Weiland, MD
The Hospital for Special Surgery, New York, New York
The Hospital for Special Surgery
535 East 70th Street
New York, New York 10021–4872

N. Weinzweig, MD, FACS
Associate Professor of Plastic Surgery and Orthopaedic
Surgery, University of Illinois
Cook County Hospital
Associate Professor of Plastic Surgery and Orthopaedic
Surgery
University of Illinois
Division of Plastic Surgery M/C 958
820 South Wood Street, 515 CSN
Chicago, Illinois 60612–7316

A. W. Weiss, Jr., MD
St. Luke's Hospital
Associate Professor of Surgery, Michigan State University
College of Human Medicine
800 Cooper Street, Suite 1
Saginow, Michigan 48602–5371

M. R. Wexler, MD
Head, Department of Plastic and Aesthetic Surgery, Hand
Surgery and the Burn Unit, and Professor of Plastic Surgery,
Hebron
University, Hadassah Medical Center
Department of Plastic and Aesthetic Surgery
Hadassah University Hospital
Jerusalem 91120, Israel

W. White, MD (Deceased)

J. S. P. Wilson, FRCS
The Cromwell Hospital
London, United Kingdom

C. Windhofer, MD
Department of Plastic and Reconstructive Surgery
Hospital of Barmherzige Brüder
Salzburg, Austria

M. S. Wong, MD
Assistant Professor
Division of Plastic Surgery
University of California, Davis
Sacramento, California

J. E. Woods, MD, PhD, FACS
Mayo Medical Center, Rochester, MN
Emeritus Staff
Division of Plastic and Reconstructive Surgery
Mayo Clinic
200 First Street, Southwest
Rochester, Minnesota 55905

A. P. Worseg, MD
Department of Plastic and Reconstructive Surgery
Wilhelminenhospital
Vienna, Austria

E. F. Worthen, MD (Retired)
3504 Forsythe Avenue
Monroe, Louisiana 71201

Y. Yamamoto, MD, PhD
Assistant Professor, Department of Plastic and
Reconstructive Surgery
Hokkaido University School of Medicine
Kita 15, Nishi 7, Kitaku
Sapporo 060, Japan

N.W. Yii, MD
Division of Plastic Surgery
Wexham Park Hospital
Slough, Berkshire SL2 4HL,
United Kingdom

M. Young, MD
Grossman Burn Center at Sherman Oaks Hospital,
California
4929 Van Nuys Boulevard
Sherman Oaks, California 91403

N. J. Yousif, MD
Froedtert and Memorial Lutheran Hospital
9200 West Wisconsin Avenue
Milwaukee, Wisconsin 53226

P. Yugueros, MD
Mayo Medical Center, Rochester, MN
Division of Plastic and Reconstructive Surgery
Mayo Clinic
200 First Street, Southwest
Rochester, Minnesota 55905

L. S. Zachary, MD, FACS
University of Chicago, Division of Plastic Surgery
5841 South Maryland Ave. P.O. Box MC 6035
Chicago, Illinois 60637–1463

S. Zenteno Alanis, MD
Chief of Service
Department of Plastic and Reconstructive Surgery
Hospital General de Mexico
Providence 400 Penthouse
Mexico 12, D.F.

F. Zhang, MD, PhD
Professor
Division of Plastic Surgery
University of Mississippi Medical Center
Jackson, Mississippi

E. G. Zook, MD, FACS
Memorial Medical Center and St. John's Hospital
Southern Illinois University School of Medicine
Institute for Plastic Surgery
PO Box 19230
747 North Rutlidge Street
Springfield, Illinois 62794–1511

R. M. Zuker, MD, FRCS(C), FACS
Head, Division of Plastic Surgery
The Hospital for Sick Children
Professor of Surgery, Department of Surgery
University of Toronto
Head, Division of Plastic Surgery
The Hospital for Sick Children
555 University Avenue, Suite 1524B
Toronto, Ontario, Canada M5G 1X8

Since our last edition of *Grabb's Encyclopedia of Flaps*, major evolutionary changes have occurred in the field of reconstructive plastic surgery. The explosion of perforator flap sites and the techniques of harvesting the pedicle without extensive sacrifice of the underlying muscles are well represented in this new edition.

In the last ten years, the field of transplantation has also been further advanced by plastic surgeons. Face and hand allotransplantation represents some of the most exciting advances in all of medicine, and we have tried to provide a glimpse of this emerging field with the inclusion of two articles on facial transplantation. What was once science fiction has now become reality and may one day even become commonplace.

The changes in the reconstructive ladder are evident in all arenas. With the widespread success of microsurgery, many defects are currently reconstructed with the most complex free tissue transfers as the primary option, jumping straight to the top of the ladder. On the other hand, negative pressure devices have revolutionized wound care management and, in many cases, has supplanted tissue coverage, moving many potential defects rapidly down the ladder.

More than 12,000 citations in the literature on flaps were reviewed, and 43 new chapters were added to this third edition. Many of the older chapters were revised or brought up to date. The new edition includes flaps, both pedicle and microvascular, for reconstruction of the face, orbits, lips, and nose. The latest techniques in nasal reconstruction, including local mucosal flaps as well as providing total reconstruction of the nasal support and lining with microvascular forearm flaps, have been added. Use of innervated muscle for tongue reconstruction is presented. In the hand volume, many new flaps have been added for reconstruction of the palm, the fingers, and the metacarpals. Breast surgery articles, including the use of medial and lateral pedicles, are new to this edition. A major inclusion has been the addition of the multiple perforator flaps used for breast reconstruction. Articles on reconstruction of the chest and abdomen have been chosen, as have the latest techniques for lower extremity reconstruction.

In adding all of these new choices, the editors were faced with a dilemma. How do we keep the concept of an encyclopedic atlas, while still staying within the confines of hard copy pages and costs of printing? The decision was made to keep all of the previous articles but to list some of the lesser used flaps by chapter title and author only in the printed text so that the reader is aware of these choices. In the online edition, all of the articles, new and old, are presented with full text and illustrations. Of course, editorial opinions at the beginning of the chapters have been maintained to help the reader make prudent reconstructive decisions. To access these complete aricles, go to www.encyclopediaofflaps.com.

The third edition of this encyclopedia would not have been possible without the dedication provided by Dr. R.D. (Lee) Landres. In addition, we would like to thank the editorial staff at Lippincott Williams & Wilkins. To all the authors who contributed new chapters or provided revisions of their original chapters in a timely fashion, we extend our thanks, as we are deeply indebted to them.

Berish Strauch, MD
Luis O. Vasconez, MD
Elizabeth J. Hall-Findlay, MD
Bernard T. Lee, MD

In the last ten years, evolutionary changes in the use of flaps in reconstructive plastic surgery have resulted in increased flap reliability, as well as in more definitive reconstruction of particular defects. Currently, there is much less dependence on the use of flap delays and on random skin flaps. The reconstructive surgeon is now provided with a choice not only of skin flaps, but also of composite flaps which may contain skin and muscle, muscle alone or, in cases where bony defects are also involved, associated bone flaps. There is no longer a requirement for empirical questions about whether or not a particular flap will have an adequate blood supply. We presently think in terms of reliable flaps with a known blood supply and a determinate reliability. Where this is not yet possible, the reconstructive surgeon is likely to consider a free microvascular flap.

Another important change is our independence from the so-called reconstructive ladder, according to which surgeons followed the precept of using the simplest method and then advancing to a more complex one. Nowadays, the objective should always be to utilize the best method first, the one that will fulfill the requirements of the reconstruction, even though it may be the most complex, for example, a microvascular composite flap.

It was impossible for the authors to have included every flap that has been described since the first edition. In fact, considerable care has been taken in choosing proven and reliable flaps. Over 10,000 citations in the literature on flaps were reviewed and 120 new and revised chapters were added to the second edition. A considerable number of chapters describing procedures that have not been proven clinically reliable have been deleted. The editors have also added appropriate editorial comments that should be helpful to the reader wherever these seemed indicated.

Undertaking publication of the second edition of the encyclopedia would not have been possible, had it not been for the dedication and immense help provided by the editorial assistance of Dr. R. D. (Lee) Landres. We would also like to thank the editorial staff at Little, Brown and Company, whose work on this second edition has been taken over by Lippincott-Raven Publishers. Additionally, our sincere thanks to all the authors who contributed new chapters or revision of the original chapters in a timely fashion. We are indebted to them.

B. S.
L. O. V.
E. J. H.-F.

PREFACE TO THE FIRST EDITION

An important and very broad area of plastic surgery entails the coverage of defects throughout the body. These defects are usually covered by flaps, of which we now have a great variety. For approximately 50 years, from the introduction of the tubed flap until the middle 1960s, most flaps were tubed. Although we realized that blood supply was important for survival of the tubed flap, it was not until the end of the 1960s that we began to pay attention to the distinct arterial and venous supplies of different flaps. Axial flaps, musculocutaneous flaps, fasciocutaneous flaps, and microvascular free flaps were introduced in the decade of the 1970s. These were rapidly used in great numbers, with clinical applications throughout the body. The concept of "delay" of flaps has just about been abandoned. It is extremely advantageous that we now have a multitude of flaps that can be applied for the coverage of particular defects.

A flap can be designed and made with an adequate dimension with the knowledge of its exact blood supply; one needs only proper execution to be assured of a consistent, satisfactory, and acceptable result. This great number and variety of the flaps that differ not only in their design, but also in their type, as far as the blood supply is concerned, is "wonderful" for the experienced surgeon, but it also may present a quandary for the student plastic surgeon. The young surgeon may not have the clinical experience of having performed many and different flaps for a similar defect. There is usually no problem with execution of the procedure, but the clinical judgment that some learn by previous clinical errors may be supported by consideration and proper description of available options.

This *Encyclopedia* attempts to provide choices for the closure of particular defects throughout the body. Recognized experts described how to execute a particular flap, and each flap is presented in a uniform format, emphasizing the indications and anatomy, including the blood supply, surgical technique, complications, and safeguards. Selected editorial comments are included as a guide to the reader.

The multiauthored format has been chosen to give each author, often the originator of the flap, an opportunity to explain the procedure, and in each chapter the editors have rewritten only to maintain the uniform format, always attempting to keep the authors' information unchanged.

This *Encyclopedia* is intended to serve as a stimulus to experienced surgeons to refresh their memories about a multitude of options for particular defects so that they may choose what, in their judgment, will give a safe, predictable, and acceptable result. This work also will show the student of plastic surgery the numerous options and will teach him or her to choose the most appropriate one and to consider a great many factors that can play a role in what we call "clinical judgment." Once the proper choice is made, this *Encyclopedia* will refresh knowledge of the clinical aspects of flap execution, as well as the blood supply and the safeguards.

This *Encyclopedia* tends to encompass defects throughout the body and is divided into three volumes. For the reader who wants an increased knowledge of a particular flap, selected references are included at the end of each chapter.

We hope that this work will be helpful to all, including the most experienced surgeons, reinforcing with certainty that a good number of options have been considered and that the best were chosen.

Dr. William Grabb dreamed of a sequel to his book on skin flaps. He had organized and outlined the book and had chosen an initial group of contributors. His foresight encompassed the tremendous influence that microvascular and musculocutaneous flaps would have on the availability of usable flaps. He asked Berish Strauch and Luis O. Vasconez to join him as associate editors, to guide the sections on microvascular and musculocutaneous flaps, respectively. The decision to go forward with the *Encyclopedia* was made in 1981 during the annual meeting of the American Society of Plastic and Reconstructive Surgeons in New York.

Dr. Grabb's untimely death in 1982 halted progress on the work for over nine months. The two associate editors finally decided that the concept of the *Encyclopedia* was too important to plastic surgery for the project not to be completed.

Advice was sought from Lauralee Lutz in Ann Arbor. Lauralee had served as Dr. Grabb's administrative secretary and in-house editor. Her advice resulted in bringing aboard Dr. R. D. (Lee) Landres in New York to help with the editing of the *Encyclopedia*. All the contributors were contacted, and the chapters began to be produced.

The enormity of the task soon became apparent, and Dr. Elizabeth Hall-Findlay, who had worked previously with Drs. Strauch and Vasconez, was asked to join the two editors.

Multiauthored textbooks are often disorganized and repetitive. Faced with well over 400 chapters written in several languages and with various styles, we made a decision: Each chapter was to be reorganized into a similar format—with an introduction, a section on anatomy, and a section on flap design and dimensions, followed by operative technique and clinical results. In general, line drawings were to be the main figures, with some case illustrations. Details of history and research results were to be be omitted. Interested readers would be encouraged to refer to original publications, with each chapter followed by a relevant but not overbearing list of references. We knew we were into at least three volumes and did not want the work to be burdened with unnecessary detail. Despite the rewriting and uniform organization, there was a serious attempt to keep the authors' information unchanged.

This work has already traveled extensively. It has originated from all over the world. The chapters were initially rough-edited and placed on computer disks by Dr. Landres. The disks were sent to Dr. Hall-Findlay in Banff, Alberta, in the Canadian Rocky Mountains. There they were edited directly off the disks, and appropriate illustrations and references were chosen. Most of the chapters spent some time deep in the mountains at one of the most beautiful sites in the world—Lake O'Hara Lodge. There, care had to be taken not to lose any of the text or "work in progress" if the electric generator failed. Further work and refinements always seemed to take ten times longer than expected.

Drs. Vasconez and Strauch reviewed the editorial changes as they progressed and, as well, solicited and received new chapters as delays became prolonged. Meetings were held in Banff, where we closeted ourselves away with "the book," reviewing text and illustrations and discussing editorial comments.

The editors at Little, Brown and Company in Boston have been invaluable in seeing the project to completion. Fred Belliveau had organized and supervised the project from its inception. Curtis Vouwie helped during the seemingly never-ending delays, and Susan Pioli has both encouraged and prodded the work to completion.

Although the delays resulted in criticisms of being out of date, we felt that many of these chapters have stood and will stand the test of time. We tried to keep up with the chapters, without adopting the unproven. Of necessity, we stopped inclusions of new chapters in 1987. We hope that the book will not only be comprehensive, but also useful to surgeons in reviewing options when faced with routine or unusual problems or defects.

We can never thank everyone who has been involved in helping, directly or indirectly, with the *Encyclopedia*. Drs. Strauch, Vasconez, and Hall-Findlay wish to express in common their appreciation to Dr. Lee Landres, who has worked tirelessly for the past seven years on this work. Dr. Hall-Findlay wishes to recognize and thank Cheryl Low and Lynn Enderwick, who helped with many endless secretarial chores while, at the same time, handling patients and managing the office. Checking references accurately would not have been possible without the help of Merle Duncan, librarian at the medical library of the University of Calgary. Patricia Velasquez, Elke Berthold, Doris Freytag, Liesbeth Heynen, and Vickilynn Norton have all helped by being loving and devoted nannies to Jamie, David, and Elise. Dr. Hall-Findlay's mother, Betty Hall, and her in-laws, Jim and Edith Findlay, helped immeasurably with child care during their many visits to Banff, so that work on the *Encyclopedia* could go on. Don Findlay cannot be thanked enough for his understanding and patience.

B. S.
L. O. V.
E. J. H.-F.

INTRODUCTION: THE HISTORY OF VASCULARIZED COMPOSITE-TISSUE TRANSFERS

R. A. CHASE

The compelling drive of human beings to reconstruct deficient or missing parts and the desire of victims to undergo such reconstruction are best appreciated by recognizing the early development and use of pedicle-flap transfers long before the advent of anesthesia. Imagine the tolerance a patient must have had to undergo nasal reconstruction using a forehead pedicle flap without anesthesia. The seminal work of Sushruta (1) in the pre-Christian era must have resulted in meager success; however, the basic principle behind the "Indian flap" is so sound that the procedure is still used in contemporary surgery.

From those early developments, at first slowly, and then like a wild fire in the last four decades, the world has witnessed enormous progress in tissue-transfer surgery. The latter-day developments in anesthesia, antibiotics, hematology, instrumentation, and wound-healing research have given surgeons devoted to reconstruction the opportunity to achieve results that would have been considered miraculous only four decades ago. When immunologic barriers to risk-free transplantation are breached, a whole new wave of applications of existing and developing reconstructive strategies will break upon the world.

PEDICLE TRANSFERS

It is interesting to note, at least from what can be gleaned from recorded history (2), that the first successful transfer of human tissues to heterotopic sites was done by what we now call pedicle techniques. Such transfers are never even transiently, deprived of blood supply. Thus, on a trial-and-error basis, it should not be a surprise that the success of the Hindu Sushruta (1) during the pre-Christian era depended on the use of pedicle flaps of tissue in the face and forehead.

The designation of "Indian flap" for nasal reconstruction has survived, and its use in contemporary surgery testifies to its practicality. It appears to have taken centuries for the principle and procedure itself to travel from its origin in India to Europe—first to the Brancas in Italy, who became known in the fifteenth century for use of the technique and the principle to develop new and imaginative reconstructive procedures. Tagliacozzi in the sixteenth century made use of the printing press to disseminate knowledge of the techniques abroad through his celebrated *De Curtorum Chirurgia* (3) published in 1597.

Nonetheless, the procedures lay dormant for about 200 years until a newspaper, the *Madras Gazette,* and the *Gentleman's Magazine* (4) reported the Indian method for nose reconstruction in 1794. Among others, Carpue (5) in England and von Graefe (6) in Germany further developed the technique in Europe. Zeis, in his 1830 description of the procedure (7), displayed illustrations suggesting the dusky appearance of the flap early after surgery. Warren was the first in the United States to publish this technique in 1837 (8). It appeared in the *Boston Medical and Surgical Journal* (now the *New England Journal of Medicine*).

The pedicle flap principle, initiated by trial and error in pre-Christian history, was established and refined in the nineteenth century and formed the fundamental basis for the spectacular developments in the modern decades of surgery.

I shall mention a few landmarks in the development of tissue transfers during the nineteenth and twentieth centuries. In 1829, Fricke of Hamburg published a book describing many alternate facial flaps (9). Shortly thereafter, Tripier, Malgaigne (10), Burrow, Estlander, von Graefe (6), Abby, Denonvilliere, Rosenthal, Dieffenbach, and Zeis (2)—to name the principals—added further innovations in the shift of tissues to adjacent areas within the face for reconstruction.

Hamilton of Buffalo reported the first successful cross-leg flap in 1854 (12). He also was the first to apply the principle of delay to flap transfer. In 1868, Prince published *A New Classification and a Brief Exposition of Plastic Surgery* (12) with examples of applications of pedicle-flap techniques in plastic surgery. At the Practitioner's Society of New York in 1891, Shrady used an open jump flap cut from one arm and carried after vascularization by the contralateral index finger to fill a cheek contour defect (13). Shortly thereafter, in 1896, the renowned William Stewart Halsted (14) first "waltzed," by end-over-end transfer, a flap from the abdomen up to the neck of a burn victim. He was the first to use the term *waltzed.*

In pedicle-transfer surgery, aside from studies of the delay phenomenon (11,15,16), effects of drugs and radiation (17), and thinning of the flap (18), the refinements during this era were confined largely to the carrying pedicle itself. In 1849, Jobert of Paris, in his two-volume textbook *Chirurgie Plastique* (19), described "the temperature changes in skin flaps and the reinnervation of flaps" and noted that "the size of the pedicle should be proportional to the size of the flap."

The renowned Sir Harold Gillies stated, "In general, a flap should not be larger than the width of its carrying pedicle." In 1920, he added a rider: "A longer flap could be raised if the flap contained in its base a larger vascular pedicle such as the superficial temporal artery" (20).

Gillies' book, *Plastic Surgery of the Face* (21), is a classic in the field and, together with that of John Staige Davis, ushered in the modern era of plastic surgery. Both were based on lessons learned from current works and publications early in the twentieth century, such as those of Vilray Blair (22), and experiences during World War I. Gillies himself had been stimulated and influenced by Morestin, whom he had visited in France. The war experience was very influential on many great contributors to plastic surgery—V. H. Kazanjian, Ferris Smith, R. H. Ivy, Eastman Sheehan, and Sterling Bunnell, to name a few.

As noted by Khoo Boo-Chai (23), John Wood in 1863 had described a flap that, in 1869 (24), he called a "groin flap." He commented on the importance of incorporating known vessels—in his patients, the superficial epigastric vessels.

John Staige Davis, reporting World War I experiences, expanded the uses of pedicle flaps (2,25) and later with William German et al. (26) explored the vascular anatomy of the skin and subcutaneous tissues important in designing such flaps.

John Roberts of Philadelphia pointed to lessons learned in the war and applicable to reparative surgery using pedicle flaps on the hand (27). In 1919, Albee described the surgical construction of an osteoplastic finger substitute using a pedicle flap and a bone graft (28). Also in 1919, at the clinic day of the American Orthopaedic Association at Jefferson Hospital in Philadelphia, P. G. Skillern presented a patient from Polyclinic Hospital in whom a double-pedicle "strap" flap was used for coverage of the dorsum of the right hand (29). Steinler's books appeared in 1923 and 1925 (30,31), at the same time Allen Kanavel's book (32) was published, and later Marc Iselin's *Atlas* (33,34) and Cutler's *The Hand* (35).

In 1931, Jacques Joseph, using illustrations of Manchot from 1889, justified and published illustrations of deltopectoral flaps as vascular-pattern flaps (36,37). The deltopectoral flap was later popularized and used imaginatively by V. Y. Bakamjian, as described in his papers starting in 1965 (38,39). McGregor and Jackson showed its use in hand surgery (40).

A debate between S. H. Milton (41) and P. M. Stell (42) raged in the early seventies on the appropriate base for random flaps. By then, the classification of flaps according to the nature of the pedicle had begun to crystallize. McGregor and Morgan had hinted at it in 1960 (43). Ten years later, McGregor and Jackson proposed that one could outline self-contained vascular territories (44). They referred to work by Shaw, who, together with Payne, had described such a flap based on the superficial epigastric arterial and venous system (45). The technique was developed for care of the wounded during World War II. Other developments in tissue transfer in hand surgery were described in the volumes on hand surgery in World War II (see below).

General plastic surgery as a discipline made enormous strides during this war. For example, at the beginning of the war, there were only four fully experienced plastic surgeons in Great Britain: Gillies, McIndoe, Mowlem, and Kilner. This nucleus of surgeons and their trainees established plastic surgical centers throughout Great Britain, and each made major contributions to the field.

In the United States, Fomon's 1939 *The Surgery of Injury and Plastic Repair* (46) and Barsky's *Principles and Practice of Plastic Surgery* (47) appeared at the beginning of World War II. During the war, Ivy and a group of plastic surgical luminaries wrote two manuals on plastic and maxillofacial surgery for use by military surgeons (48). Plastic surgical centers such as the one at Valley Forge General Hospital were spawning grounds for consolidation of reconstructive strategies. James Barrett Brown, Sheehan, McDowell, Tanzer, Littler, and Cannon exemplify what could be an enormous list of contributors. Books by Sheehan (49), Ivy (50), Kazanjian and Converse (51), May (52), New and Erich (53), Padgett and Stephenson (54), Pick (55), and Smith (56), among others, were published after experiences during the war.

McGregor et al. described the anatomic basis for a flap based on the superficial circumflex iliac vessels (57), the classic McGregor or groin flap. The groin flap has been a mainstay in reconstructive hand surgery (58,59). The terms *random* and *axial* were applied to flaps in McGregor and Morgan's paper in 1973 (60,61).

Early in the twentieth century, the carrying pedicle for random or chance axial pedicle flaps was large and flat. It was refined to a closed tube independently by the Russian Filatov in 1917 (62) and by Gillies at about the same time (20,63,64). Pedicle flaps with identifiable blood vessels had become the rule wherever possible.

Sterling Bunnell's second edition of *Surgery of the Hand* (65) drew heavily from experiences in hand centers during World War II. It was filled with a variety of types of pedicle flaps, as well as his additional technical modifications of the tubed-pedicle flap technique.

William L. White put together an organized review of flap grafts (66) for a meeting that he organized and chaired in Pittsburgh in 1959.

With waltzing, jumping, and tubing, the transfer of tissues from place to place in endless combinations (67), including composites of skin, fascia, muscle (68), and bone, was firmly established (69).

ISLAND PEDICLE FLAP

Since the turn of this century, further refinement of the carrying pedicle had reached the point where flaps are transferred regularly on vascular and neurovascular bundles. The principle of transfer without an intact epithelialized skin pedicle was initiated by Robert Gersuny, of Vienna. In 1887, he published a description of the transfer of a composite flap of soft tissue from the neck to the oral lining of the cheeks (70) carried on a very narrow pedicle of dermis and subdermal vessels from the periosteum of the mandible. This was a one-stage transfer of a pedicle flap without an intact skin pedicle and without specifically identifiable blood vessels.

In August of 1882, Theodore Dunham, of New York, excised a large epidermoid cancer of the cheek and eyelid. He raised a flap from the forehead, and in his publication (71) said, "This flap was so cut as to contain traversing its pedicle and ramifying in it, the anterior temporal artery." Three days after the first procedure, Dunham dissected out the vascular pedicle and buried it beneath the skin of the cheek. The skin pedicle was returned to its donor site. This was the first recorded two-stage island pedicle flap preserving the transferred blood supply intact.

However, it was Monks in 1898 who repaired the defect resulting from an excision of a lower eyelid epithelioma and who first reported a one-stage island pedicle flap (72). He illustrated the procedure that same year in the *Boston Medical and Surgical Journal*. Shelton Horsely beautifully illustrated the use of a forehead flap carried on temporal vessels in a paper in the *Journal of the American Medical Association* in 1915 (73).

J. F. S. Esser, publishing in the *New York Journal of Medicine* in 1917 (74), pointed out that during his care of wounded soldiers in Austria, he often used flaps from the neck directly under the jawline near the external maxillary artery. These flaps had no skin pedicle, but a carrying arm consisting of soft tissue that contained the external maxillary artery. Said Esser, "I called them 'island flaps' because after being placed in the facial defect resulting when scars are removed, they give the effect of a free transplantation."

There was renewed interest in the island pedicle flap for a variety of uses in the sixties (75–80). For example, temporal arterial island flaps found a place in eyebrow reconstruction and for coverage of difficult areas requiring a permanently transferred blood supply.

In this contemporary period of hand surgery, the biologic or island pedicle flap described earlier was first applied to the hand. Erik Moberg (81), discussing a paper by Donal Brooks on nerve grafting (82) at the annual meeting of the American Orthopaedic Association at Bretton Woods, New Hampshire, in 1954, suggested that neurovascular flap techniques were useful in restoring stereognosis to the hand. He showed some exemplary cases. Littler discussed uses of the neurovascular island 2 years later, and Tubiana et al. (79,80), Frackelton and Teasley (83), Holevich (84), Hueston (85), O'Brien (86), Lewin (87), Peacock (78), Winsten (88), and many, many others (89) published ingenious applications of the versatile techniques. Littler reviewed the development in detail during his Monk's Lecture delivered in Boston in 1982 (90).

The versatile island flap (91) could be used as part of a carrier for a nerve transfer to innervate an intact but anesthetic digit tip. It could be used to bring cover and blood supply to a badly damaged devascularized finger. It was useful in transferring composite parts of useless digits to restore others, including whole joints. Many hand surgeons have pointed to its efficacy in the restoration of protective and useful sensibility and blood supply in osteoplastic thumb reconstruction (92–100).

MUSCLE AND MUSCULOCUTANEOUS FLAPS

The first published, planned muscle flap was that of Louis Ombredanne of Paris in 1906 (101). He described a pectoralis minor flap for breast reconstruction, turning down the humeral insertion of the pectoralis minor to recreate a breast mound following mastectomy.

Tanzini introduced a latissimus dorsi muscle flap for breast reconstruction in 1906 (102). The first true musculocutaneous flap was that described in detail in 1912 by Professor Stefano d'Este and published in a monumental paper on chest-wall reconstruction after mastectomy (103). He used the latissimus dorsi and showed the anatomy of both a musculocutaneous flap and an axial flap of skin alone from the same area. Illustrated examples were shown.

The roots, then, were well set at the beginning of the century for refinement of the principles of the modern muscular and musculocutaneous flaps that have become so popular and important in the current era. The interest in muscle and musculocutaneous flaps was renewed when Neal Owens in 1955 suggested the use of a compound neck pedicle composed of the sternocleidomastoid muscle overlying platysma, subcutaneous tissue, and skin in the reconstruction of major facial defects (104).

Ralph Ger, of Capetown, showed the virtue of muscle transfer for coverage of difficult areas in the distal lower limb in a seminal paper in 1966 (105). Shortly thereafter, Miguel Orticochea, of Bogota, Columbia, described the musculocutaneous flap method (106). He presented the technique, using a gracilis musculocutaneous flap as a cross-leg flap with success.

Typically, the empirical but logical use of muscle alone (107) and muscle with overlying skin led to possible application of that principle throughout the body (108–113). For example, after sporadic reports of muscle flaps and musculocutaneous flaps, McCraw and Dibbell outlined possible independent myocutaneous flaps (114); then, fasciocutaneous flaps (115,116) were launched (117–119). Muscles with nutrient vessels are usable as pedicles to carry substantial skin and soft tissue. As an example, the rectus abdominis muscle with its superior epigastric vascular leash may be used to carry a large transverse segment of soft tissue (120), that is axial on its ipsilateral and random on its contralateral side, from the lower abdomen to the breast area.

Credit goes to Elliott and Hartrampf for championing this remarkable transfer of tissue (121). Muscle and musculocutaneous flaps have found multiple uses in upper limb surgery, and even intrinsic muscles are useful as muscle or musculocutaneous carriers (122). Hentz et al. (123) showed the use of the abductor digiti minimi as a musculocutaneous flap within the hand.

FREE COMPOSITE-TISSUE TRANSFER WITH IMMEDIATE REVASCULARIZATION

Once the pedicle for transfer was refined to require only blood vessels with or without sensory nerves, the only remaining deterrent to unlimited anatomic transfer of composite tissues was the length of vascular tether. It followed predictably that the next advance would be an assault on that deterrent. The answer would come from refinements of techniques described by Carrell at the turn of the century (124,125), made possible by the advent of the operating microscope.

Stimulated by the possibilities offered by microsurgery reported by Jacobson and Suarez from Burlington, Vermont (126), Buncke and Schultz (127) worked tirelessly with methods to improve sutures and instruments. Their influence on Berish Strauch, Avron Daniller, Donald Murray, and others in our Stanford laboratories resulted in rat renal transplant developments and rat limb replants.

Clinically, Komatsu and Tamai's thumb replantation in 1968 (128) ushered in the new era of digit replantation (129–132). Buncke et al. reported their one-stage Nicoladoni thumb reconstruction, transferring a big toe to the thumb position in monkeys (133), and Cobbett soon thereafter reported a successful clinical case of such a free digital toe-to-hand transfer (134). The procedure is now well established in hand surgery (135–137).

Berish Strauch and Donald Murray (138), stimulated by the work of Harry Buncke, worked out and reported the transfer of groin skin flaps to the neck in rats.

With that background, and with knowledge of Goldwyn, Lamb, and White's experiments (139) and the vascularized island experiments of Krizek et al. (140), Kaplan, Buncke, and Murray attempted and reported a free flap from the groin to an intraoral site in 1971 (141). The flap survived for 2½ weeks, but it failed to heal to the poorly vascularized recipient bed. Rollin Daniel, after hearing the paper reporting the case, was stimulated to persevere. When the opportunity arose, he and Ian Taylor tried again and reported the first successful free-flap transfer in 1971 (142).

There followed a rash of reports of free groin flap transfers in hand surgery (143–149). The clear advantages of such free flaps are that they supply skin and soft-tissue cover with permanent arterial blood supply and sometimes sensibility in a single stage. Subsequent tendon grafts then may restore extension function. The flap may be a composite of skin and soft tissue with tendons to eliminate the need for later tendon grafting, or it may carry bone as well (150). Morrison et al. have introduced us to the wraparound free composite flap in thumb reconstruction (151)—a modification that Lister, Steichen, and others have used to restore a thumb tip and nail. Free microvascular transfers apply to any part or composite of parts whose viability may be maintained by isolated vessels (152–154).

FREE FUNCTIONAL MUSCLE AND MUSCULOCUTANEOUS FLAPS WITH IMMEDIATE REVASCULARIZATION

The first reported attempts to free transfer skeletal muscle were those of Noel Thompson (155), who startled those attending the Fifth International Congress of Plastic and Reconstructive Surgery in Melbourne in 1971 by showing a technique of free transfer of the palmeris longus or intrinsic foot muscles (the extensor digitorum brevis) to the face (156) without surgical revascularization. After transfer, the patients regained function through muscular neurotization. In 1975, Gerhard Freilinger, of Vienna, did similar free muscle grafts (157), innervating them with nerve grafts from the contralateral facial nerve.

Meanwhile, Tamai and colleagues had been experimenting with free muscle transfers with microvascular and microneural anatomoses in dog rectus femoris muscles (158). They showed survival of the transferred muscles with an interval of denervation atrophy followed by recovery of innervation at about 3 months. They suggested the use of such transfers in humans.

Harii et al. reported free gracilis muscle transfers to the face using microvascular and microneural revascularization and innervation techniques with success (159). They suggested that the principle of free revascularized and reinnervated muscle transfers "would find broad use in recontructive surgery."

Ralph Manktelow, of Canada, having seen some examples of free vascularized muscle transfers at the Sixth People's Hospital in Shanghai and having carried out some animal experiments in his laboratory, started to build a series of free, revascularized, and reinnervated muscle transfers in the upper limb of selected patients. In 1978, at the annual meeting of the American Society for Surgery of the Hand, Manktelow and McKee reported their experience with free musculocutaneous transfers, using a gracilis muscle in one patient and a pectoralis muscle in another, transferred to restore finger flexion (160). The feasibility and growing reliability of these free muscle and musculocutaneous transfers (161–163), as prophetically stated by Harii et al. (159), obviously will have a "wide range of applications in reconstructive surgery."

It has taken the perseverance and faith of a Harry Buncke (164), the energetic aggressiveness of a Bernie O'Brien (165), the patience and technical expertise of Tamai and Harii (166), the organization of the Kleinert (167), Kutz (168), and Lister groups, and the ever-growing list of young microsurgeons (169) to take the early work of Jacobson and Suarez and to place it firmly in the armamentarium of reconstructive surgeons. These pioneers found their greatest pleasure in doing what people said could not be done (170).

Work with venous flaps and arteriovenous flaps is moving from the laboratory to clinical application, one more step toward broadening the armamentarium of the reconstructive surgeon.

There appear to be inexhaustible imaginations among surgeons developing new and innovative flaps for use in every part of the body. Progressive liberation from the large carrying pedicle to the refined vascularized and innervated island flaps to vascularized free flaps has opened the way for near-infinite variations in flap design. New additions to these volumes cover the broad spectrum of composite-tissue transfers in reconstructive surgery. The elders in the field look with a mixture of amazement and envy at surgeons active in the development of new strategies to deal with old problems. In facial, neck, intraoral, esophageal, breast, upper and lower limb, abdominal-wall, genital, and anal reconstruction, there have been new reconstructive techniques added to those in the first edition of this encyclopedia.

The advent of anesthesia opened the way for a flood of new operative procedures in the second half of the 19th century. The evolution of microsurgery in this century has been responsible for the current plethora of new techniques. It is my firm belief that the next wave of innovations will emerge as a result of progress in the related field of transplantation. Solutions for the residual immunologic problems in transplantation will prepare the way for a torrent of procedures based on knowledge of techniques developed by surgeons devoted to the field of composite-tissue transfer.

Meanwhile, exhaustive studies of gross and microscopic vascular anatomy, exemplified by Taylor's mapping of neurovascular territories (171), coupled with anatomic studies to clarify the spectacular advances in imaging, feed into the growing armamentarium available to today's reconstructive surgeons.

References

 1. Wallace AF. History of plastic surgery. *J R Soc Med* 1978;71:834.
 2. Zies E. *The Zeiss index and history of plastic surgery, 900 B.C. to 1863 A.D.*, Vol. 1. Baltimore: Williams & Wilkins, 1977.
 3. Tagliacozzi G. *De curtorum chirurgia per institione*, Vol. 2. Venice: 1597.
 4. *Gentleman's Magazine*. London, October 1974;891.
 5. Carpue JC. An account of two successful operations for restoring a lost nose from the integuments of the forehead. London: 1816.
 6. von Graefe CF. *Rhinoplastik*. Berlin: 1818.
 7. Zeis E. *Handbuch der Plastischen Chirurgie*. Berlin: 1818.
 8. Warren JM. *Boston Med Surg J* 1837.
 9. Fricke JCG. *Die Bildung neuer Augenlider (Blepharoplastik) nach Zerstorungen und dadurch hervorge-brachten Auswartswendungen derselben*. Hamburg: 1829.
10. Malgaigne JF. *Manuel de médecine operatoire*. Brusells: 1834.
11. Hamilton FH. Elkoplasty: on ulcers treated by anaplasty. *NY J Med* 1854.
12. Prince D. *Plastics: a new classification and a brief exposition of plastic surgery*. Philadelphia: Lindsay and Blakiston, 1868.
13. Shrady G. The finger as a medium for transplanting skin flaps. *Med Rec* 1891.
14. Halsted W. Plastic operation for extensive burn of neck. *Johns Hopkins Hosp Bull* 1896.
15. Blair VP. The delayed transfer of long pedical flaps in plastic surgery. *Surg Gynecol Obstet* 1921;3:261.
16. Hoffmeister FS. Studies on timing of tissue transfer in reconstructive surgery. *Plast Reconstr Surg* 1957;19:283.
17. Patterson TIS, Berry RJ, Wiernik G. The effect of x-radiation on the survival of skin flaps in the pig. *Br J Plast Surg* 1972;25:17.
18. Colson P, Houot R, Gangolphe M, et al. Utilisation des lambeaux degraisses (lambeaux-greffes) en chirurgie reparatrice de la main. *Ann Chir Plast* 1967;12:298.
19. Jobert AJ. (de Lamballe). *Traité de chirurgie plastique*. Paris: Bailliere, 1849.
20. Gillies HD. Present-day plastic operation of the face. *J Natl Dent Assoc* 1920;1:3.
21. Gillies HD. *Plastic surgery of the face*. London: Frowde, 1920.
22. Blair VP. *Surgery and diseases of the mouth and jaws*. St. Louis: Mosby, 1912.
23. Boo-Chai K. John Wood and his contributions to plastic surgery: the first groin flap. *Br J Plast Surg* 1977;30:9.
24. Wood J. Fission and extroversion of the bladder with epispadias with the results of 8 cases treated by plastic operations. *Med Chir Trans* 1869;2:85.
25. Davis JS. The use of the pedunculated flap in reconstructive surgery. *Ann Surg* 1918;68:221.
26. Germany W, Finesilver EM, Davis JS. Establishment of circulation in tubed skin flaps. *Arch Surg* 1933;26:27.
27. Roberts JB. Salvage of the hand by timely reparative surgery. *Ann Surg* 1919;70:627.
28. Albee FH. Synthetic transplantation of tissues to form a new finger. *Ann Surg* 1919;69:379.
29. Skillern PG Jr. A surgical clinic at Polyclinic Hospital. *Int Clin* 1919;3:75.
30. Steindler A. *Reconstructive surgery of the upper extremity*. New York: Appleton, 1923.
31. Steindler A. *A textbook of operative orthopedics*. New York: Appleton, 1925.
32. Kanavel AB. *Infections of the hand*, 5th ed. Philadelphia: Lea & Febiger, 1925.
33. Iselin M. *Chirurgie de la main: plaies, infections, chirurgie reparatrice*. Paris: Masson, 1933.
34. Iselin M. *Surgery of the hand, wounds, infections and closed tramata*. Philadelphia: Blakiston, 1940.
35. Cutler CW Jr. *The hand: its disabilities and diseases*. Philadelphia: Saunders, 1942.
36. Gibson T, Robinson DW. The mammary artery pectoral flaps of Jacques Joseph. *Br J Plast Surg* 1976;29:370.
37. Joseph J. *Nasenplastik und sonstige Gesichtsplastik nebst einem Anhang ueber Mammaplastik und einige weitere Operationem aus dem Gebiete der ausseren Korper Plastik*. Leipzig: Verlag von Curt Kapitzsch, 1931.
38. Bakamjian VY. A two-stage method for pharyngoesophageal reconstruction with a primary pectoral skin flap. *Plast Reconstr Sutg* 1965;36:173.
39. Bakamjian VY, Long M, Rigg B. Experience with the medially based deltopectoral flap in reconstructive surgery of the head and neck. *Br J Plast Surg* 1971;24:174.
40. McGregor IA, Jackson IT. The extended role of the deltopectoral flap. *Br J Plast Surg* 1970;23:173.
41. Milton SH. Pedicled skin flaps: the fallacy of the length-width ratio. *Br J Surg* 1970;57:502.
42. Stell PM. The viability of skin flaps. *Ann R Coll Surg Engl* 1977;59:236.
43. McGregor I. Flap reconstruction in hand surgery: the evolution of presently used methods. *J Hand Surg* 1979;4B:1.
44. McGregor IA, Jackson IT. The groin flap. *Br J Plast Surg* 1972;25:3.
45. Shaw DT, Payne RL. One-stage tubed abdominal flaps: single-pedicle tubes. *Surg Gynecol Obstet* 1946;83:205.
46. Fomon S. *The surgery of injury and plastic repair*. Baltimore: Williams & Wilkins, 1939.
47. Barsky AI. *Principles and practice of plastic surgery*. Philadelphia: Saunders, 1938.
48. Ivy RH. *Manual of standard practice of plastic and maxillofacial surgery*. Philadelphia: Saunders. 1942.
49. Sheehan JE. *General and plastic surgery with emphasis on war injuries*. New York: Hoeber and Harper, 1945.

50. Ivy RH, Curtis L. *Fractures of the jaws.* Philadelphia: Lea & Febiger, 1945.
51. Kazanjian VH, Converse JM. *The surgical treatment of facial injuries.* Baltimore: Williams & Wilkins, 1949.
52. May H. *Reconstructive and reparative surgery.* Philadelphia: Davis, 1947, 1958.
53. New GB, Erich JB. *The use of pedicle flaps of skin in plastic surgery of the head and neck.* Springfield, Ill.: Charles C. Thomas, 1950.
54. Padgett EC, Stephenson KL. *Plastic and reconstructive surgery.* Springfield, Ill.: Charles C. Thomas, 1948.
55. Pick JF. *Surgery of repair: principles, problems, procedures,* Vols. 1 and 2. Philadelphia: Lippincott, 1949.
56. Smith F. *Plastic and reconstructive surgery.* Philadelphia: Saunders, 1950.
57. Smith PJ, Foley B, McGregor IA, et al. The anatomical basis of the groin flap. *Plast Reconstr Surg* 1972;49:41.
58. Heath PM, Jackson IT, Cooney WP, et al. Simultaneous bilateral staged groin flaps for coverage of mutilating injuries of the hand. *Ann Plast Surg* 1983;11:462.
59. Lister GD, McGregor IA, Jackson IT. The groin flap in hand injuries. *Injury* 1973;4:229.
60. McGregor IA, Morgan G. Axial and random pattern flaps. *Br J Plast Surg* 1973;26:202.
61. Smith PJ. The vascular basis of axial pattern flaps. *Br J Plast Surg* 1973;26:150.
62. Filatov VP. Plastic procedure using a round pedicle. *Surg Clin North Am* 1959;39:277.
63. Gillies HD. The tubed pedicle in plastic surgery. *NY Med J* 1920;11:1.
64. Webster JP. The early history of the tubed pedicle flap. *Surg Clin North Am* 1959;39:261.
65. Bunnell S. *Surgery of the hand,* 2d ed. Philadelphia: Lippincott, 1948.
66. White WL. Flap grafts to the upper extremity. *Surg Clin North Am* 1960;40:389.
67. Holevich J. Our technique of pedicle skin flaps and its use in the surgery of the hand and fingers. *Acta Chir Plast* 1960;24:271.
68. Hokin JAB. Mastectomy reconstruction without a prosthetic implant. *Plast Reconstr Surg* 1983;72:810.
69. Gilles H. Autograft of amputated digit. *Lancet* 1940;1:1002.
70. Gersuny R. Plastischer Ersatz der Wangenschleimhaut. *Zentralbl Chir* 1887;14:706.
71. Dunham T. A method for obtaining a skin flap from the scalp and a permanent buried vascular pedicle for covering defects of the face. *Ann Surg* 1893;17:677.
72. Monks GH. The restoration of a lower eyelid by a new method. *Boston Med Surg J* 1898;139:385.
73. Horsley JS. Transplantation of the anterior temporal artery. *JAMA* 1915;64:408.
74. Esser JFS. Island flaps. *NY Med J* 1917;106:264.
75. Chase RA. Expanded clinical and research uses of composite tissue transfers on isolated vascular pedicles. *Am J Surg* 1967;114:222.
76. Kuei SJ, Chen EC, Li SY. The use of temporal artery pedicle skin flaps in the repair of facial burns and other deformities. *Chin Med J* 1964;83:65.
77. Murray JF, Ord JVR, Gavelin GE. The neurovascular island pedicle flap: an assessment of late results in sixteen cases. *J Bone Joint Surg* 1967;49A:1285.
78. Peacock EE. Reconstruction of the hand by the local transfer of composite-tissue island flaps. *Plast Reconstr Surg* 1960;25:298.
79. Tubiana R, DuParc J. Restoration of sensibility in the hand by neurovascular skin island transfer. *J Bone Joint Surg* 1961;43B:474.
80. Tubiana R, DuParc J, Moreau C. Restauration de la sensibilité au niveau de la main par transfert d'un transplant cutané heterodigital muni de son pedicule vasculo-nerveux. *Rev Chir Orthop* 1960;46:163.
81. Moberg E. Nerve-grafting in orthopedic surgery. *J Bone Joint Surg* 1955;37A:305.
82. Brooks DM, Seddon HJ. Pectoral transplantation for paralysis of the flexors of the elbow. *J Bone Joint Surg* 1959;41B:36.
83. Frackelton WH, Teasley JL. Neurovascular island pedicle: extension in usage. *J Bone Joint Surg* 1962;44A:1069.
84. Holevich J. A new method of restoring sensibility to the thumb. *J Bone Joint Surg* 1973;45B:496.
85. Hueston J. The extended neurovascular island flap. *Br J Plast Surg* 1965;18:304.
86. O'Brien B. Neurovascular pedicle transfers in the hand. *Aust NZ J Surg* 1965;35:1.
87. Lewin ML. Sensory island flap in osteoplastic reconstruction of the thumb. *Am J Surg* 1965;109:226.
88. Winsten J. Island pedicle to restore stereognosis in hand injuries. *N Engl J Med* 1963;268:124.
89. Rose EH. Local arterialized island flap coverage of difficult hand defects preserving donor digit sensibility. *Plast Reconstr Surg* 1983;72:848.
90. Littler JW, George H. Monks lecture: man's thumb, nature's special endowment. Harvard Medical School, October 2, 1982.
91. Chase RA. *Atlas of hand surgery,* Vol. 1. Philadelphia: Saunders, 1973.
92. Chase RA. An alternate to pollicization in subtotal thumb reconstruction. *Plast Reconstr Surg* 1969;44:412.
93. Dykes ER. Reconstruction of the thumb. *Hawaii Med J* 1967;27:33.
94. Floyd WE. Reconstruction of the thumb. *J Med Assoc Ga* 1968;57:425.
95. Greeley PW. Reconstruction of the thumb. *Ann Surg* 1946;124:60.
96. McGregor IA, Simonetta C. Reconstruction of the thumb by composite bone-skin flap. *Br J Plast Surg* 1964;17:37.
97. Reid DAC. The neurovascular island flap in thumb reconstruction. *Br J Plast Surg* 1966;19:234.
98. Suzuki T, Takahashi T, Chang S, et al. Reconstruction of the thumb. *Jpn Med J* 1967;41:1013.
99. Woudstra ST. Reconstruction of the thumb. *Arch Chir Med* 1967;19:29.
100. Murray JF, Ord JVR, Gavelin GE. The neurovascular island pedicle flap: an assessment of late results in sixteen cases. *J Bone Joint Surg* 1967;49A:1285.
101. Teimourian B, Adham MN. Louis Ombredanne and the origin of muscle flap use for immediate breast mound reconstruction. *Plast Reconstr Surg* 1983;72:905.
102. Tanzini. Sporo il nito nuova processo di aupertozione della menuelle. *Riforma Med* 1906;22:757.
103. d'Este S. La technique de l'amputation de la mamelle pour carcinome mammaire. *Rev Chir* 1912;45:164.
104. Owens N. A compound neck pedicle designed for the repair of massive facial defects: formation, development and application. *Plast Reconstr Surg* 1955;15:369.
105. Ger R. The operative treatment of the advanced stasis ulcer. *Am J Surg* 1966;111:659.
106. Orticochea M. The musculocutaneous flap method: an immediate and heroic substitute for the method of delay. *Br J Plast Surg* 1972;25:106.
107. Minami RT, Hentz VR, Vistnes LM. Use of vastus lateralis muscle flap for repair of trochanteric pressure sores. *Plast Reconstr Surg* 1977;60:364.
108. Carroll RE, Kleinman WB. Pectoralis major transplantation to restore elbow flexion to the paralytic limb. *J Hand Surg* 1979;4A:501.
109. Chase RA, Nage DA. Cosmetic incisions and skin, bone, and composite grafts to restore function of the hand. In: *American academy of orthopaedic surgeons instructional course lectures.* Chap. 6. St. Louis: Mosby, 1974.
110. Hovnanian AP. Latissimus dorsi transplantation for loss of flexion or extension of the elbow. *Ann Surg* 1956;143:493.
111. Jackson IT, Pellett C, Smith, JM. The skull as a bone graft donor site. *Ann Plast Surg* 1983;11:527.
112. Stern PJ, Neale HW, Gregory RO, et al. Latissimus dorsi musculocutaneous flap for elbow flexion. *J Hand Surg* 1982;7:25.
113. Zancolli E, Mitre H. Latissimus dorsi transfer to restore elbow flexion. *J Bone Joint Surg* 1973;55A:1265.
114. McCraw JB, Dibbell DG. Experimental definition of independent myocutaneous vascular territories. *Plast Reconstr Surg* 1977;60:212.
115. Barclay TL, Sharpe DT, Chisholm EM. Cross-leg fasciocutaneous flaps. *Plast Reconstr Surg* 1983;72:843.
116. Fonseca JLS. Use of pericranial flap in scalp wounds with exposed bone. *Plast Reconstr Surg* 1983;72:786.
117. Grabb WC, Myers MB, eds. *Skin flaps.* Boston: Little, Brown, 1975.
118. Mathes SJ, Nahai F. *Clinical atlas of muscle and musculocutaneous flaps.* St. Louis: Mosby, 1979.
119. McCraw JB, Dibbell DG, Carraway JH. Clinical definition of independent myocutaneous vascular territories. *Plast Reconstr Surg* 1977;60:341.
120. Bunkis J, Walton RL, Mathes SJ, et al. Experience with the transverse lower rectus abdominis operation for breast reconstruction. *Plast Reconstr Surg* 1983;72:819.
121. Elliott LF, Hartrampf CR. Tailoring of the new breast using the transverse abdominal island flap. *Plast Reconstr Surg* 1983;72:887.
122. Reisman NR, Dellon AL. The abductor digiti minimi muscle flap: a salvage technique for palmar wrist pain. *Plast Reconstr Surg* 1983;72:859.
123. Chase RA, Hentz VR, Apfelberg D. A dynamic myocutaneous flap for hand reconstruction. *J Hand Surg* 1980;5A:594.
124. Carrel A. La technique operatoire des anastomoses vasculaires et la transplantation des viscere. *Lyon Med* 1920;98:859.
125. Carrel A. Results of the transplantation of blood vessels, organs and limbs. *JAMA* 1908;51:1662.
126. Jacobson JH, Suarez EL. Microsurgery in the anastomosis of small vessels. *Surg Forum* 1960;11:243.
127. Buncke HJ, Schulz WP. Total ear reimplantation in the rabbit utilizing microminiature vascular anastomoses. *Br J Plast Surg* 1966;19:15.
128. Komatsu S, Tamai S. Successful replantation of a completely cut-off thumb. *Plast Reconstr Surg* 1968;42:374.
129. Chen ZW, Meyer VE, Kleinert HE, et al. Present indications for replantation as reflected by long-term functional results. *Orthop Clin North Am* 1981;12:849.
130. Gelberman RH, Urbaniak JR, Bright DS, et al. Digital sensibility following replantation. *J Hand Surg* 1978;3A:313.
131. Weiland AJ, Daniel RK, Riley LH. Application of the free vascularized bone graft in the treatment of malignant or aggressive bone tumor. *Johns Hopkins Med J* 1977;140:85.
132. Vilkki S. Replantation studies on clinical replantation surgery with reference to patient selection, operative techniques and postoperative control. *Acta Univ Tamperensis (A)* 1983;156.
133. Buncke HJ, Buncke CM, Schulz WP. Immediate Nicoladoni procedures in the rhesus monkey, or hallux-to-hand transplantation, utilising microminiature vascular anastomoses. *Br J Plast Surg* 1966;19:332.
134. Cobbett JR. Free digital transfer: report of a case of transfer of a great toe to replace an amputated thumb. *J Bone Joint Surg* 1969;51B:677.

135. Buncke HJ, McLean DH, Geroge PT, et al. Thumb replacement: great toe transplantation by microvascular anastomosis. *Br J Plast Surg* 1973;26:194.

136. O'Brien BM, MacLeod AM, Sykes PJ, et al. Microvascular second toe transfer for digital reconstruction. *J Hand Surg* 1978;3A:123.

137. Ohtsuka H, Torigai K, Shioya N. Two toe-to-finger transplants in one hand. *Plast Reconstr Surg* 1977;60:51.

138. Strauch B, Murray DE. Transfer of composite graft with immediate suture anastomosis of its vascular pedicle measuring less than 1 mm in external diameter using microsurgical techniques. *Plast Reconstr Surg* 1967;40:325.

139. Goldwyn RM, Lamb DL, White WL. An experimental study of large island flaps in dogs. *Plast Reconstr Surg* 1963;31:528.

140. Krizek TJ, Tani R, Desprez JD, et al. Experimental transplantation of composite grafts by microsurgical vascular techniques. *Plast Reconstr Surg* 1965;36:538.

141. Kaplan EN, Buncke HJ, Murray DE. Distant transfer of cutaneous island flaps in humans by microvascular anastomoses. *Plast Reconstr Surg* 1973; 52:301.

142. Taylor GI, Daniel RK. The free flap: composite tissue transfer by vascular anastomosis. *Aust NZJ Surg* 1973;43:1.

143. Ohmori K, Harii K, Sekiguchi J, et al. The youngest free groin flap yet? *Br J Plast Surg* 1977;30:273.

144. Daniel RK, Terzis JK. *Reconstructive microsurgery.* Boston: Little, Brown, 1977.

145. Daniel RK, Weiland AJ. Free tissue transfers from upper extremity reconstruction. *J Hand Surg* 1982;7A:66.

146. Taylor GI, Townsend P, Corlett R. Superiority of the deep circumflex iliac vessels as the supply for free groin flaps: experimental work. *Plast Reconstr Surg* 1979;64:595.

147. Taylor GI, Townsend P, Corlett R. Superiority of the deep circumflex iliac vessels as the supply for free groin flaps: clinical work. *Plast Reconstr Surg* 1979;64:45.

148. Baudet J, LeMaire JM, Guimberteau JC. Ten free groin flaps. *Plast Reconstr Surg* 1976;57:577.

149. Brent B, Byrd HS. Secondary ear reconstruction with cartilage grafts covered by axial, random, and free flaps of temporoparietal fascia. *Plast Reconstr Surg* 1983;72:141.

150. Swartz WM. Immediate reconstruction of the wrist and dorsum of the hand with a free osteocutaneous groin flap. *J Hand Surg* 1984;9A:18.

151. Morrison WA, O'Brien BM, MacLeod, AM. Thumb reconstruction with a free neurovascular wrap-around flap from the big toe. *J Hand Surg* 1980;5A:575.

152. Van Genechten F, Townsend PLG. Free composite-tissue transfer in a compound hand injury. *Hand* 1983;15:325.

153. Taylor GI, Corlett R, Boyd JB. The extended deep inferior epigastric flap: a clinical technique. *Plast Reconstr Surg* 1983;72:751.

154. Fisher J, Cooney WP. Designing the latissimus dorsi free flap for knee coverage. *Ann Plast Surg* 1983;11:554.

155. Thompson N. Treatment of facial paralysis by free skeletal muscle grafts. In: *Transactions of the fifth international congress of plastic and reconstructive surgery.* Melbourne: Butterworth, 1971.

156. Smith JW. A new technique of facial animation. In: *Transactions of the fifth international congress of plastic and reconstructive surgery.* Melbourne: Butterworth, 1971.

157. Freilinger G. A new technique to correct facial paralysis. *Plast Reconstr Surg* 1975;56:44.

158. Tamai S, Komatsu S, Sakamoto H, et al. Free muscle transplants in dogs with microsurgical neurovascular anastomoses. *Plast Reconstr Surg* 1970; 46:219.

159. Harii K, Ohmori K, Torii S. Free gracilis muscle transplantation with microvascular anastomoses for the treatment of facial paralysis. *Plast Reconstr Surg* 1976;57:133.

160. Manktelow RT, McKee NH. Free muscle transplantation to provide active finger flexion. *J Hand Surg* 1978;3A:416.

161. Ikuta Y, Kubo T, Tsuge K. Free muscle transplantation by microsurgical technique to treat severe Volkmann's contracture. *Plast Reconstr Surg* 1976; 58:407.

162. Manktelow RT, Zuker RM, McKee NH. Functioning free muscle transplantation. *J Hand Surg* 1984;9A:32.

163. Terzis JK, Dykos RW, Williams HB. Recovery of function in free muscle transplants using microneurovascular anastomoses. *J Hand Surg* 1978; 3A:37.

164. Bunke HJ. Cobbett JR, Smith JW, et al. *Techniques of microsurgery.* Sommerville, NJ: Ethicon, 1969.

165. O'Brien BM, Miller GDH. Digital reattachment and revascularization. *J Bone Joint Surg* 1973;55A:714.

166. Tamai S, Hori Y, Tatsumi Y, et al. Hallux-to-thumb transfer with microsurgical technique: a case report in a 45-year-old woman. *J Hand Surg* 1977; 2A:152.

167. Kleinert HE, Kasdan ML, Romero JL. Small blood vessel anastomosis for salvage of severely injured upper extremity. *J Bone Joint Surg* 1963; 45A:788.

168. Kutz JE, Dimond M. Replantation in the upper extremity. *Surg Rounds* 1982;14:9.

169. Strauch B. Microsurgical approach to thumb reconstruction. *Orthop Clin North Am* 1977;8:319.

170. Ikuta Y. Free flap transfer: historical review, surgical procedures and some clinical cases. *Hiroshima J Med Sci* 1976;25:29.

171. Taylor GI, Gianoutsos MP, Morris SF. The neurovascular territories of the skin and muscles: anatomic study and clinical implications. *Plast Reconstr Surg* 1994;94:1.

CONTENTS

VOLUME I: HEAD AND NECK

SECTION 1: HEAD AND NECK RECONSTRUCTION

PART A ▪ SCALP, FOREHEAD, AND NAPE OF NECK RECONSTRUCTION

PART B ▪ EYELID AND ORBITAL RECONSTRUCTION

Lower Eyelid

Upper Eyelid

Medial Canthus

Total Eyelid and Socket

Online Chapter

PART C ■ NASAL RECONSTRUCTION

Nasal Tip, Dorsum, and Alae

Nasal Columella

PART E ▪ CHEEK AND NECK RECONSTRUCTION

Cheek and Neck

Online
Chapter

PART G ▪ INTRAORAL RECONSTRUCTION

PART H ▪ PHARYNGOESOPHAGEAL

VOLUME II: UPPER EXTREMITIES

SECTION II: UPPER EXTREMITY RECONSTRUCTION

PART A ▪ FINGER AND THUMB RECONSTRUCTION

Fingertip

Finger

Thumb Tip

Thumb

Online Chapter (icon next to chapter 276)

PART B ■ HAND

PART C ▦ WEB SPACE

PART D ▦ FOREARM

PART E ■ ELBOW

PART F ■ ARM

PART B ■ AXILLA AND CHEST WALL RECONSTRUCTION

SECTION IV: ABDOMINAL WALL AND PELVIC-REGION RECONSTRUCTION

PART A   ABDOMINAL WALL AND GROIN RECONSTRUCTION

PART B ■ VAGINAL, VULVAR, AND PERINEAL RECONSTRUCTION

PART C ■ PENILE, SCROTAL, AND PERINEAL RECONSTRUCTION

PART D ▪ ANAL RECONSTRUCTION

PART E ▪ LUMBOSACRAL RECONSTRUCTION

PART F ▪ ISCHIAL RECONSTRUCTION

PART G ▪ TROCHANTERIC RECONSTRUCTION

SECTION V: LOWER EXTREMITY RECONSTRUCTION

PART A ▮ LOWER LEG AND KNEE RECONSTRUCTION

PART B ▪ FOOT AND ANKLE RECONSTRUCTION

UPPER EXTREMITY RECONSTRUCTION

CHAPTER 223 ■ TRIANGULAR VOLAR SKIN FLAP TO THE FINGERTIP

E. ATASOY

Fingertip amputations are one of the most common injuries, and good judgment should be exercised in selecting the best surgical reconstruction to preserve maximum function.

The ideal procedure should maintain length, and should cover the defect with nontender, well-padded skin that has normal or near-normal sensation. Most methods usually provide good coverage and padding, but not good sensation. The triangular volar skin flap, when indicated and carefully performed, provides good contour and padding, with less scarring of the fingertip than most flaps (1–3). The main advantage of this flap, however, is that it provides normal or near-normal sensation.

INDICATIONS

Among the most common fingertip amputations (Fig. 1), the dorsal oblique amputation is the best indication for this method. In transverse amputations, the remaining part of the distal phalanx must be shortened a few millimeters, in order to facilitate the procedure. However, this is the second-best indication for the triangular volar skin flap. Amputations through the middle or the proximal phalanx also can be treated with this technique.

The triangular volar skin flap is contraindicated for palmar oblique amputations with extensive soft-tissue loss. That defect must be covered by another type of local flap.

ANATOMY

Fibrous septa pass through the subcutaneous tissue, connecting the skin to the periosteum distally and to the flexor tendon sheath proximally. Both the skin and the deep septal attachments must be cut, in order to advance the triangular volar skin flap over the defect. The subcutaneous tissue must be left undisturbed, because it contains the neurovascular supply to the flap.

FLAP DESIGN AND DIMENSIONS

The base of the flap is the cut edge of skin where the amputation has occurred. It should be the width of the amputated edge of the nail matrix. If the base is made much wider, a square fingertip results, rather than the normal round one.

Since a longer flap is easier to advance, the apex of the triangle should be placed at the distal flexion crease. The side

arms of the triangle are not straight, but are drawn as two gently curving lines to the apex (Fig. 2).

OPERATIVE TECHNIQUE

The flap is developed by cutting through the skin completely, but leaving the subcutaneous tissue intact. The flap is then mobilized by separating its deep attachments (fibrous septa) from the periosteum distally and the flexor sheath proximally, especially at the level of the distal flexion crease (Fig. 2).

If these vertical septa are not severed, the flap cannot be adequately advanced. This dissection must be meticulously performed, since preservation of the neurovascular supply to the flap is essential. The dissection should be performed with the aid of a lower-power loupe.

Any excess fatty tissue along the base of the flap should be removed to facilitate closure (Fig. 3). The mobilized flap is advanced distally and is sutured to the edge of the nailbed with 6-0 nylon. The rest of the closure is performed in a V-Y fashion, starting with the proximal end of the incision.

The closure should be performed with little or no tension (Fig. 4). Excessive tension may cause not only partial flap necrosis, but also sensory disturbance in the flap.

In the case of the distally denuded nailbed, the volar triangular flap is performed first. Then the nailbed defect is covered with a reversed dermal graft or, preferably, with a toenail bed graft.

CLINICAL RESULTS

If the indications are taken into account, and if the procedure is properly performed, a satisfactory result can be expected. Reflex dystrophy, hyperesthesia, and sometimes hypoesthesia may occur. These minor complications are usually treated conservatively by medication, exercise, and transcutaneous nerve stimulation.

Partial necrosis of the flap is a major complication, usually caused by suturing the flap under excessive tension. In rare cases it can be caused by injury to the blood supply. The flap should stay viable even if the blood supply on only one side remains intact.

One functionally and aesthetically disturbing late complication is the hook-nail deformity, seen several weeks after the procedure. This deformity results from excessive tension on the flap, which causes the nailbed to curve volarly. The deformity can be corrected by the "antenna" procedure (4).

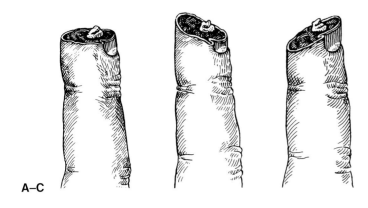

A–C

FIG. 1. **A–C:** The three most common types of fingertip amputations. Only transverse (**A**) and dorsal (**B**) oblique amputations are suitable for the triangular volar skin flap. (From Atasoy et al., ref. 2, with permission.)

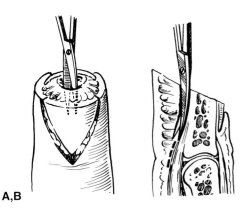

A,B

FIG. 2. **A,B:** The skin is incised, leaving the subcutaneous tissue and vascular supply intact. The fibrous septa are then cut, releasing the flap from the periosteum and the flexor tendon sheath.

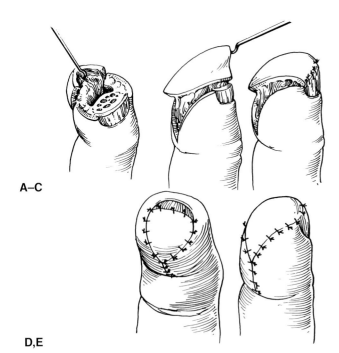

A–C

D,E

FIG. 3. **A–E:** The flap is advanced distally and sutured to the nailbed. Any excess subcutaneous tissue along the base of the flap may be removed to facilitate closure. Starting proximally, the remainder of the incision is closed in a V-Y fashion. It is essential to avoid tension.

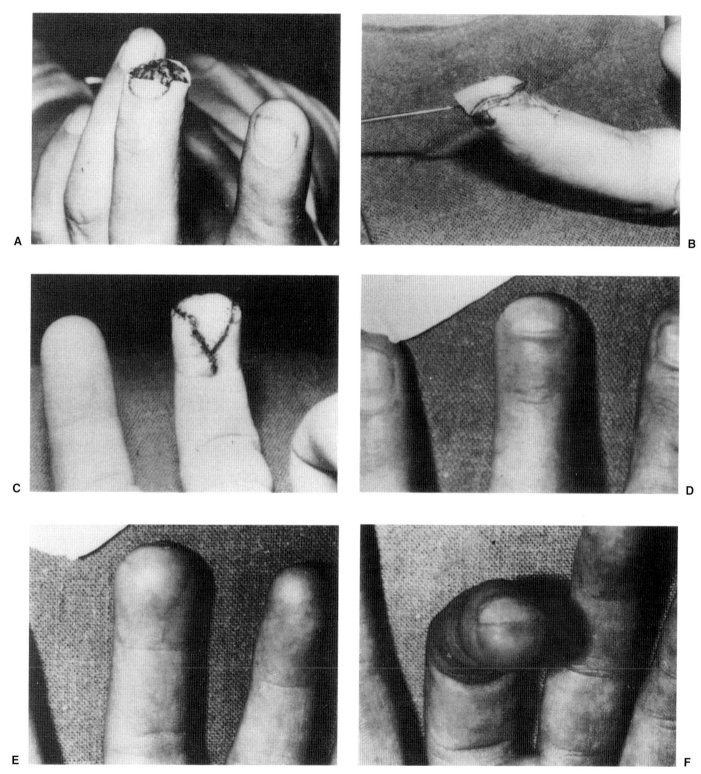

FIG. 4. A–C: Amputation of the dorsal oblique left long fingertip, reconstructed with a triangular volar skin flap. **D–F:** Appearance 4 months postoperatively. (From Atasoy et al., ref. 2, with permission.)

SUMMARY

A triangular volar skin flap can be used to reconstruct transverse or dorsal oblique fingertip amputations.

References

1. Kleinert HE. Fingertip injuries and their management. *Am Surg* 1959;25:41.
2. Atasoy E, Ioakimidis E, Kasdan M, et al. Reconstruction of the amputated finger tip with triangular volar flap. *J Bone Joint Surg* [Am] 1970;52:921.
3. Frandsen PA. V-Y plasty as treatment of finger tip amputations. *Acta Orthop Scand* 1978;49:255.
4. Atasoy E, Godfrey A, Kalisman M. The "antenna" procedure for the "hook nail" deformity. *J Hand Surg* 1983;8:55.

CHAPTER 224 ■ TRIANGULAR LATERAL (KUTLER) SKIN FLAPS TO THE FINGERTIP

A. FREIBERG

EDITORIAL COMMENT

Both this and the previous chapter on the volar sliding skin flap demonstrate excellent methods for covering an amputated fingertip where bone is in excess of soft tissue. These procedures have received bad publicity, primarily because the wounds, incorrectly, are completely closed under tension. The diagrams both in this chapter and in the previous one show all the wounds closed completely. This can be a fundamental error. The two flaps should be readjusted over the distal end and closed loosely, unless they fall together. Secondary contraction will slowly draw the wounds together and provide full-thickness sensible coverage for the tip of the finger.

Partial amputation of the fingertip is one of the most common conditions seen in hand trauma. A paradox of this injury is the magnitude of the potential disability in the context of a relatively small area of the body.

INDICATIONS

Although many methods of repair have been advocated, most fingertip amputations can be treated successfully by allowing the area to heal by secondary intention, or by applying a thin split-thickness skin graft. These are simple methods that allow the surrounding normal fingertip skin to be drawn toward the center of the defect. If a secondary procedure is necessary, the resulting defect may be up to 50% of the original size.

The bilateral V-Y advancement flap method, as originally described by Kutler in 1947 (1), is at present rarely indicated for *primary* repair of the amputated tip. It is, however, a useful method in highly selected situations and a valuable procedure in *secondary* tip revisions (2–6).

Because of the generally excellent aesthetic appearance (Fig. 2) and relatively good sensation, the procedure should be considered for the patient with a true transverse guillotine amputation. Dorsal oblique amputations are, however, better managed by bone shortening and closure, skin grafting, or the triangular volar skin flap. Volar oblique amputations without exposure of bone are best treated by dressings or by thin split-thickness skin grafts.

Bilateral Kutler-type flaps can also be used for more proximal transverse amputations, where further shortening of the digit is not indicated.

Because this procedure uses bilateral, midlateral fingertip tissue, it is ideal for secondary stump revisions with a broad, unsightly tip. The level of revision can be either at the level of the distal phalanx, with or without a nail remnant, or through the distal interphalangeal (DIP) or proximal interphalangeal (PIP) joints, with protruding tissues covering the condyles of the respective phalanges.

ANATOMY

The neurovascular supply courses through the subcutaneous tissue and must be protected during dissection and advancement of the flap. The fibrous septa that connect the skin with the periosteum must be carefully divided. Shepard (7) has pointed out that most of the neurovascular structures are volar, thus allowing the dorsal side to be completely transected.

FLAP DESIGN AND DIMENSIONS

The triangle is based laterally along the edge of the wound. The width of the base will depend on the size of the defect to be covered. The triangle should be about one-half inch long, from the base to the apex.

OPERATIVE TECHNIQUE

After appropriate trimming and debridement, two identical triangular flaps are outlined, and only the skin is incised. By

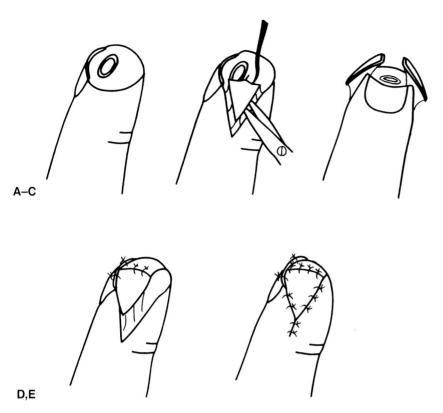

A–C

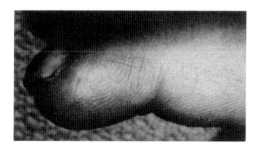

D,E

FIG. 1. Typical transverse amputation with exposed bone. A: The defect. B: The fibrous bands between skin and bone are transected. One must make sure that the neurovascular structures are left intact. C: The flaps are advanced over the defect. D: The flaps are sutured in the midline and to the nail matrix. E: The donor site is closed in a V-Y fashion. (From Freiberg and Manktelow, ref. 3, with permission.)

means of a skin hook and gentle distal traction, the fibrous bands between skin and bone are transected. One must make sure that the neurovascular structures are left intact (magnification at this point is often helpful) (Fig. 1B).

As the fibrous bands are severed, the triangles are gradually advanced over the tip of the finger (Fig. 1C). Further debridement of bone might be required at this stage, to allow for a comfortable tension-free closure. The flaps are sutured in the midline and to the nailbed.

The donor site is closed in a V-Y fashion (Fig. 1E).

Modifications

Occasionally, and especially in the more proximal amputations, the digital neurovascular bundles may be clearly identified at the apex of the triangular flaps. In these cases, the small segmental blood vessels and nerves can be divided completely, and the flaps transferred as true neurovascular islands (see Chap. 228).

Another modification has recently been described that provides greater mobility of the flaps. Shepard (7), using anatomical dissections, has shown that the major nerve and blood

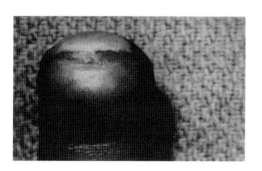

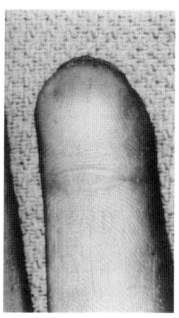

FIG. 2. Postoperative appearance after Kutler repair of a transverse amputation through the level of the middle third of the nailbed. (From Freiberg and Manktelow, ref. 3, with permission.)

supply to these flaps comes from the volar side, therefore rendering the dorsal pedicle redundant. By preserving the pedicle on the volar side only, greater mobility can be achieved (up to 10 mm). Closure is therefore easier, and the need for two flaps can sometimes be eliminated.

CLINICAL RESULTS

These flaps are technically difficult to perform. If the surgeon does not have sufficient expertise, fine instruments, and a good light source, he or she may run the risk of developing flap necrosis.

Occasionally the parrot-beak nail deformity can occur. This is due to suture of the flaps to the sterile matrix and is common to other methods as well.

SUMMARY

Triangular lateral (Kutler) skin flaps are useful mainly for secondary revisions of fingertip amputations. They are indicated only in selected cases for primary repair. A major contribution to this procedure has been the modification proposed by Shepard (see Chap. 225).

References

1. Kutler W. New method for fingertip amputation. *JAMA* 1947;133:29.
2. Fisher RH. The Kutler method of repair of finger tip amputations. *J Bone Joint Surg [Am]* 1967;49(A):317.
3. Freiberg A, Manktelow R. The Kutler repair for fingertip amputations. *Blast Reconstr Surg* 1972;50:371.
4. Weston PAM, Wallace WA. The use of locally based triangular skin flaps for the repair of finger tip injuries. *Hand* 1976;8:54.
5. Gaber M. Kutler repair for the amputated finger tip. *Am Coll Surg Engl* 1979;61:298.
6. Roberts AHM. Kutler repairs for amputated finger tips. *Ann Coll Surg Engl* 1980;62:75.
7. Shepard GH. The use of lateral V-Y advancement flaps for fingertip reconstruction. *J Hand Surg* 1983;8:254.

CHAPTER 225 ■ MODIFIED TRIANGULAR LATERAL SKIN FLAPS TO THE FINGERTIP

G. H. SHEPARD

The Kutler method of lateral V-Y advancement skin flaps to repair fingertip amputations is well known (1). The procedure has not been widely used because of limitations in the distance that the flaps could be advanced. An analysis of the blood supply to this flap has shown that the dorsal pedicle can be incised completely, thus providing much greater mobility to the flap (2–4).

INDICATIONS

This flap is not used as a primary procedure to replace the triangular volar skin flap when the latter is indicated (see Chap. 223). Triangular lateral skin flaps are best used for volar oblique amputations or transverse oblique amputations (5). In the former situation there is not enough skin for a volar advancement flap, and in the latter the volar flap creates an asymmetric finger.

As a secondary procedure, this flap is excellent for remodeling a fingertip that is too broad or that has developed a spoon shape with curvature of the nail.

ANATOMY

Fibrous bands connect the dermis of the distal phalanx to the periosteum. These bands extend outward from the perios-teum, separating the pulp into lobules of adipose cells. The fibrous septa function to prevent gliding of the skin. Cross sections of both monkey and human fingertips show that these bands are considerably thicker laterally and dorsally than the relatively thin bands on the volar pad.

An important observation (Fig. 1) is that the neurovascular bundles are abundant on the volar aspect of the finger and are sparse on the lateral and dorsal areas.

The standard Kutler flaps are greatly restricted dorsally, but the volar side of the flap can be readily elongated. Since the blood supply and cutaneous innervation to the flap are volar structures, preservation of the dorsal pedicle is not only redundant but unnecessarily restricting.

FLAP DESIGN AND DIMENSIONS

The dorsal limb of the flap extends parallel to the bone, from the distal interphalangeal crease to the point at which the lateral margin of the nail emerges from the cover of the lateral nail fold (Fig. 2). The distal width of the flap varies with the level of the amputation, but at the level of the lateral nail fold the flap would be ideally about 7 mm. The length of the dorsal incision should be 2 to 2.5 cm. Therefore in more proximal amputations the apex of the flap may extend into the middle phalanx.

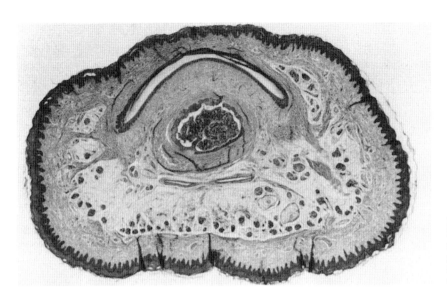

FIG. 1. Cross section of a human finger at the level of the midproximal nail fold. Dense fibrous connective bands are present dorsally and laterally. The neurovascular bundles are abundant in the palmar pulp space. (From Shepard, ref. 4, with permission.)

Kutler originally designed a much smaller flap, with the dorsal limb angulated volarly instead of extending parallel to the bone. This modified flap is larger and a great deal more versatile in reconstruction.

OPERATIVE TECHNIQUE

The dorsal incision is made to the depth of the collateral ligament proximally and to the periosteum distally (Fig. 3). The volar incision is made through skin only. The entire underside of the flap is mobilized from the dorsal incision at the periosteal level. From the underside of the flap, the thickened lateral bands are cut deep to the palmar skin incision. The subcutaneous tissue with its nerves and blood vessels is left intact.

Next the volar aspect of the incision is dissected carefully, by gently cutting the radial bands with the very tips of the scissors. Distal retraction of the flap with a skin hook helps to identify those bands restricting advancement. This dissection is best done with the aid of magnification, in order to preserve the neurovascular structures.

Each flap can easily be mobilized up to 10 mm. When the situation demands, the flap can be elongated to 14 mm by meticulous dissection of the fibrous bands, while preserving the remainder of the pulp. The flaps are advanced to fit the defect. With transverse oblique flaps, the flap on the long side may be advanced a greater distance than the opposite flap, to contour the fingertip into a natural configuration.

The flaps are sutured to each other and the nailbed. The donor site is closed in a V-Y fashion.

CLINICAL RESULTS

Since 1975, 68 of these procedures have been performed. Fifty-two were for traumatic indications and 18 were for elective remodeling of the fingertip. The shaping of the fingertip has been excellent. None of the fingertips has developed the spooning deformity that is occasionally seen with volar V-Y advancement flaps. Irregular pointing with oblique amputations has been eliminated. Sensation has been good in all flaps, and there have been no reoperations for neuroma formation.

There has been one loss of a solitary flap, a unilateral-lateral V-Y advancement flap for an irregular fingertip injury, in which an attempt was made to advance it too far. There have been no other flap losses. In 68 cases, most of them involving bilateral flaps, this represents only one complication in 116 flaps.

SUMMARY

A modification has been made in the triangular lateral skin flap, which allows more flap mobility than the standard Kutler flap. The dorsal pedicle is completely incised, since there is little neurovascular supply dorsally and numerous thick fibrous bands that restrict advancement. This flap is superior to the volar triangular skin flap for volar oblique amputations and for asymmetric transverse oblique amputations.

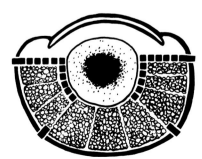

FIG. 2. Cross-sectional diagram. The dotted lines indicate depth of incisions for the bilateral flap. (From Shepard, ref. 4, with permission.)

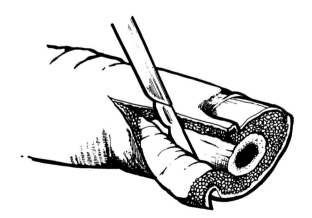

FIG. 3. The dorsal incision mobilizes the flap at the periosteal level. (From Shepard, ref. 4, with permission.)

References

1. Kutler W. A new method for fingertip amputation. *JAMA* 1947;133:29.
2. Wilkerson JL. The anatomy of an oblique proximal septum of the pulp space. *Br J Surg* 1950–1951;38:454.
3. Riordan DC. Functional anatomy of the hand and forearm. *Orthop Clin North Am* 1974;5:199.
4. Shepard GH. The use of lateral V-Y advancement flaps for fingertip reconstruction. *J Hand Surg* 1983;8:254.
5. Atasoy E, Ioakinidis E, Kasdau M, et al. Reconstruction of the amputated fingertip with a triangular volar flap. *J Bone Joint Surg [Am]* 1970; 52(A):921.

CHAPTER 226 ■ TRIANGULAR LATERAL NEUROVASCULAR ISLAND SKIN FLAP TO THE FINGERTIP

S. L. BIDDULPH

Of the industrial accidents reported annually in developed countries, about a third affect the hand, and in the majority of cases only the fingertips are involved. Terminal amputation can leave the digit with a major skin defect and exposed bone (Fig. 1). The triangular lateral neurovascular island flap is a procedure that provides durable skin with normal sensibility in a one-stage operation.

INDICATIONS

Although fingertip lesions are sometimes regarded as minor injuries, they often result in disturbed sensibility and conse-quent loss of function. For this reason it is justifiable to go to great lengths to preserve as much of the sensitive pulp area and overlying skin as possible.

With a more proximal amputation, the bone can usually be shortened another 0.5 cm to obtain more skin, without further sacrificing function of the digital stump. In fact, it can be stated as a general principle that a shorter stump with good skin cover is preferable to a longer stump with disturbed sensibility.

Various techniques have been devised to provide skin cover for the injured fingertip without shortening the digit. The sim-plest of these is the split-thickness skin graft. If, however, the area to be covered is large, this often results in a hypersensitive and fragile area that is adherent to bone.

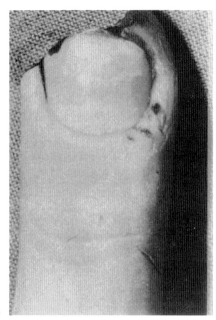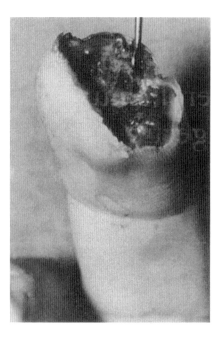

A,B

FIG. 1. A,B: An oblique amputation with bone exposed. (From Biddulph, ref. 5, with permission.)

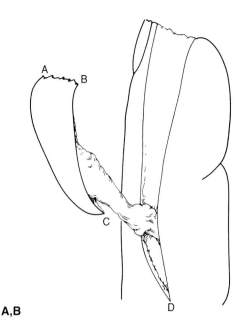 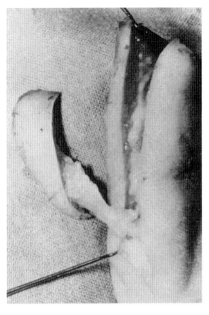

FIG. 2. A: A triangular area *ABC* is mapped out on the ulnar side of the digit or on the side with the longer skin flap. *AB* corresponds to the width of the defect. *C* lies on the midlateral line 3 cm proximally. The neurovascular bundle is identified through an incision *CD* that is 1.5 cm in length. **B:** The triangular island of skin, together with its full complement of subcutaneous tissue and the neurovascular bundle, is completely mobilized. (From Biddulph, ref. 5, with permission.)

Flaps from the palm, neighboring digits, or more distant sites (1–3) require at least two procedures and immobilize the digit in a position that may result in a permanent loss of extension. The flaps may regain some sensation, but this falls well short of what is required in the critical fingertip area (4). The triangular lateral neurovascular island skin flap provides the fingertip with good cover and good sensation, and can be performed in a single stage (5).

ANATOMY

This is an island flap based on one of the digital neurovascular bundles.

FLAP DESIGN AND DIMENSIONS

A triangular area *ABC* (Fig. 2A) is mapped out on the lateral surface of the finger, just volar to the nail fold, preferably on the ulnar side of the digit. In oblique amputations, the side with the longer flap is chosen (Fig. 2B).

The base of the triangle is along the edge of the wound. Its width is dictated by the size of the defect. The length of the flap varies, but usually it extends to the midpoint of the middle phalanx.

OPERATIVE TECHNIQUE

To identify the neurovascular bundle, an incision *CD* (Fig. 2A, B) is made from the apex of the triangle in the midlateral line, extending more proximally for another 1.5 cm. Through this proximal incision the neurovascular bundle is mobilized distally as far as the apex of the triangular skin flap. Great care is taken to preserve the venules that are found in the tissues surrounding the neurovascular bundle. They provide the only means of venous drainage from the flap.

The triangular island is then dissected free down to bone, with its full complement of subcutaneous tissue. The mobility of this flap is sufficient to allow advancement distally for a distance of about 1.5 cm, which usually corresponds to the full width of the tip of the digit. The donor site is closed (Fig. 3) in V-Y fashion (Fig. 4).

Should it still be impossible to achieve full skin cover, the remaining small defect can be covered with a split-thickness skin graft.

The involved digit alone is immobilized until wound healing is complete (usually in about 10 days). Thereafter,

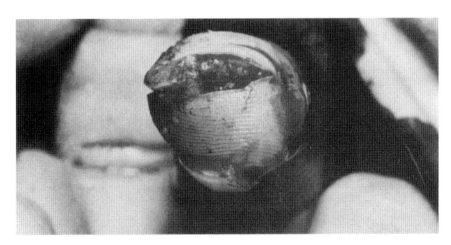

FIG. 3. The flap can be advanced to cover the whole width of the digit. (From Biddulph, ref. 5, with permission.)

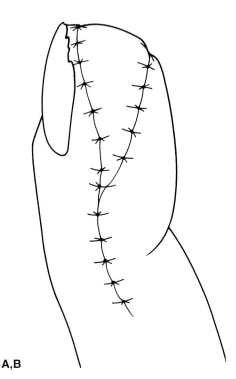 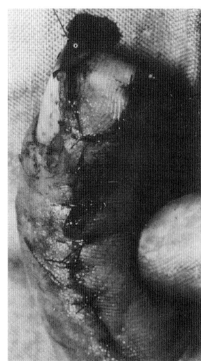

A,B

FIG. 4. A,B: The donor site is closed in a V-Y fashion, requiring no skin graft. (From Biddulph, ref. 5, with permission.)

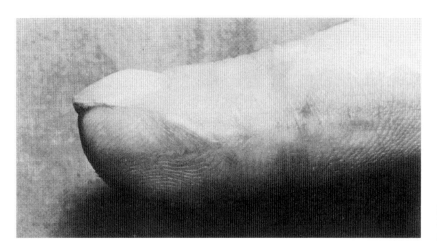

FIG. 5. Healing takes about 10 days and usually leaves a linear scar. (From Biddulph, ref. 5, with permission.)

movement is encouraged to regain full interphalangeal joint function. Normal activities are regained by the third or fourth postoperative week.

CLINICAL RESULTS

This procedure has been carried out on 60 patients, ranging in age from 2 to 60 years. They have been followed for periods of 1 to 5 years.

All adult patients returned to their previous occupations and none complained of tenderness in the operated area. Thirty patients were tested for two-point discrimination. This was found to be normal in every case, when compared with that of the other fingers. None of the patients complained of altered sensation in the flap area, and this did not change with time.

Parrot-beaking of the nail was seen in a few patients and was usually associated with greater bone loss.

In some cases where the flap technique was performed on both sides, necrosis of the intervening volar bridge of skin occurred. This procedure is no longer recommended. With a

unilateral flap any residual shortcoming in skin is best treated with a split-thickness skin graft, which is usually so small that healing occurs by a linear scar (Fig. 5).

SUMMARY

Fingertip amputations can be closed in a single stage with the triangular lateral neurovascular island skin flap. This procedure provides stable cover with normal sensation.

References

1. Flint MH, Harrison SH. A local neurovascular flap to repair loss of the digital pulp. *Br J Plast Surg* 1965;18:156.
2. Hueston J. The extended neurovascular island flap. *Br J Plast Surg* 1965;18:304.
3. Moberg E. Aspects of sensation in reconstructive surgery of the upper extremity. *J Bone Joint Surg [Am]* 1964;46(A):817.
4. Krag C, Rasmussen KB. The neurovascular island flap for defective sensibility of the thumb. *J Bone Joint Surg [Br]* 1975;57(B):495.
5. Biddulph SL. The neurovascular flap in fingertip injuries. *Hand* 1979;11:59.

CHAPTER 227 ■ RECTANGULAR LATERAL NEUROVASCULAR ISLAND SKIN FLAP TO THE FINGERTIP

N. G. POY

The neurovascular island pedicle flap can be used to restore tactile gnosis and durable cutaneous tip coverage to the dominant portions of the affected fingertip (1–5). A neurovascular island flap can be raised from the affected digit itself, using the nondominant portion of the pulp (6).

INDICATIONS

This is a safe, single-stage procedure, requiring minimal immobilization of the affected finger, and it is adaptable to most configurations of tip amputation. The composite nature of the flap actually augments the length of the amputated tip.

The flap can be used for primary coverage of partially amputated digital tips, particularly those involving dominant fingers. As a secondary procedure, the flap is good for coverage of previously scarred, anaesthetic, or painful amputation stumps.

This neurovascular island flap should not be used if there has been a crushing injury to contiguous tissue or a history of previous neurovascular disease or trauma. It is not suitable for use in amputations proximal to the cuticular border of the terminal phalanx.

ANATOMY

The flap is based on one of the neurovascular bundles of the finger.

FLAP DESIGN AND DIMENSIONS

This rectangular-shaped flap is based on the hemipulp of the nondominant portion of the affected digit. The proximal edge of the cutaneous flap should be 2 to 3 mm proximal to the DIP crease (Figs. 1 and 2). A midlateral extension of the flap incision is made to dissect out the neurovascular bundle.

With appropriate dissection and liberation of the neurovascular bundle, advancement of the hemipulp of up to 1.5 mm or slightly beyond is possible. The donor site is subsequently skin-grafted.

OPERATIVE TECHNIQUE

After the skin incisions are made around the flap, an extension is made along the midlateral line of the finger (Fig. 3). Subcutaneous soft-tissue dissection is initially carried out deep to the neurovascular bundle. The hemipulp is then elevated off the periosteum of the terminal phalanx.

Next the subcutaneous dissection along the midlateral line is carried out superficial to the neurovascular bundle. To protect the pedicle, the flap is released while retaining some soft-tissue elements (Fig. 4). Further dissection proximally can be done to advance the flap as necessary (Fig. 5).

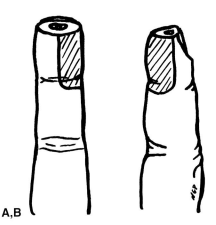

FIG. 1. A,B: Diagram showing the rectangular flap based on one hemipulp (usually on the nondominant side). The proximal edge of the skin flap should be 2 to 3 mm proximal to the DIP joint crease.

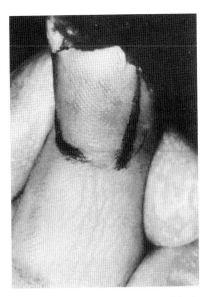

FIG. 2. The flap outlined on the ulnar side of the long finger.

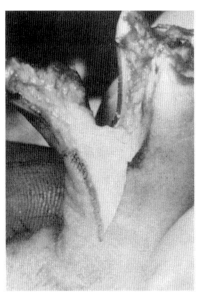

FIG. 3. The incision is extended along the midlateral line, in order to identify and dissect the neurovascular bundle. The hemipulp is elevated off the periosteum of the terminal phalanx.

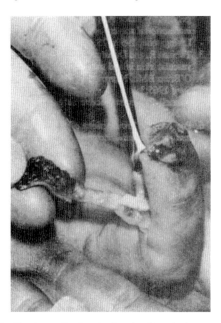

FIG. 4. The flap is totally detached and reflected, showing the abundant retained soft tissue that protects the neurovascular pedicle.

The defect is covered with a split-thickness skin graft. Any soft-tissue or skin revisions to round out the contour are carried out on the flap.

CLINICAL RESULTS

The flap retains good two-point discrimination and actually adds length to the amputated fingertip (Fig. 6). Nailbed support is good, without the tendency toward soft-tissue contracture that can lead to parrot beak nail deformities. Posttraumatic hyperesthesia and stiffness are minimal. The average time away from work is approximately 1 month from the date of surgery.

SUMMARY

The attributes of the neurovascular island, including its ability to retain good sensation and to provide well-padded, robust

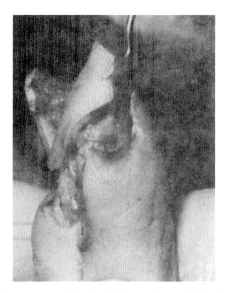

FIG. 5. The neurovascular island flap is advanced distally over the revised terminal phalangeal bone.

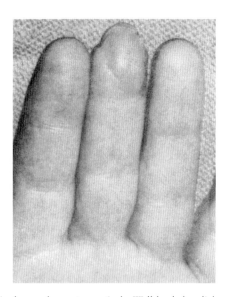

FIG. 6. Twelve weeks postoperatively. Well-healed pedicle, with good nail growth and nailbed support. Note the darker area on the ulnar border of the finger where the donor site was skin-grafted.

cutaneous cover, make it a good flap to cover partially amputated fingertips. It can be used as a single-stage procedure for either primary or secondary closure.

References

1. Moberg E. Transfer of sensation. *J Bone Joint Surg [Am]* 1953;36(A):305.
2. Littler W. Neurovascular skin island transfer in reconstructive hand surgery. In: Wallace AB, ed., *Transactions of the second congress of the international society of plastic surgeons,* London, 1959. London: E&S Livingstone, 1960;175.
3. Tubiana R, Duparc J. Restoration of sensibility in the hand by neurovascular skin island transfer. *J Bone Joint Surg [Br]* 1961;43(B):474.
4. O'Brien BMc. Neurovascular pedicle transfers in the hand. *Aust N ZJ Surg* 1965;3:1.
5. Bunnell S. Reconstructive surgery of the hand. *Surg Gynecol Obstet* 1924;39:259.
6. Poy NG. In: *Transactions of the fifth international congress of plastic and reconstructive surgery.* Melbourne: Butterworths, 1971;542.

CHAPTER 228 ■ OBLIQUE TRIANGULAR SKIN FLAP TO THE FINGERTIP

R. VENKATASWAMI

It is well known that adjacent skin can be the best cover for fingertip amputations. In the method described here, an obliquely placed flap is mobilized on the digital neurovascular pedicle while retaining innervation from both sides (1).

INDICATIONS

This flap is suitable only for oblique amputations of fingertips and thumb tips and for proximal areas in the fingers where further shortening is not advisable.

ANATOMY

The flap consists of the palmar skin and the subcutaneous tissues superficial to the fibrous flexor sheath. The main blood supply to the flap is the neurovascular bundle on the side of the finger, opposite the site of the major portion of the amputation. The flap also receives blood from some branches of the digital vessel on the oblique side. The nerve supply is from *both* digital nerves.

In some cases one may have to divide the fine branches of the blood vessels from the nerve twigs on the oblique side, thereby converting this flap into a true island flap based on one neurovascular bundle.

FLAP DESIGN AND DIMENSIONS

An oblique triangle is marked, with the base equal to the width of the amputated tip and with one side longer than the other (Fig. 1A). The "vertical" side of the triangle is along the midlateral line of the finger. In most cases the flap length, which depends on the amount of advancement necessary, is 1½ to 2 times the base of the triangle. Where the amputation is sloped toward the dorsum, the flap will need to be advanced more than if it is sloped toward the volar surface.

This triangular flap does not move in a V-Y fashion, although its appearance may give that impression. The main advancement occurs because the flap is freed completely from the fibrous flexor sheath and the restricting fibrous bands in the subcutaneous tissue.

OPERATIVE TECHNIQUE

The skin should be incised just enough to expose the globules of subcutaneous fat. With two hooks applied to the base, blunt-pointed straight scissors are used to separate the flap from the fibrous flexor sheath for the whole length of the flap.

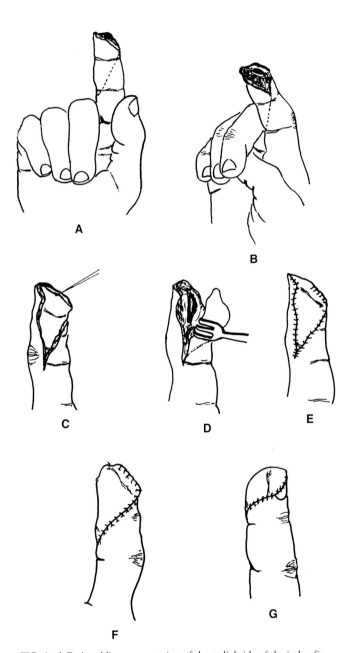

FIG. 1. **A,B:** An oblique amputation of the radial side of the index finger. The oblique triangular flap is marked out over the ulnar side of the finger. Both digital nerves are included in the flap. **C:** The "vertical" side of the triangle extends along the midlateral line of the finger. **D:** The neurovascular bundle on the ulnar side of the finger is included with the flap. As much as possible of the radial neurovascular bundle is also preserved. **E–G.** The flap is advanced and sutured to the nailbed. (From Venkataswami and Subramanian, ref. 1, with permission.)

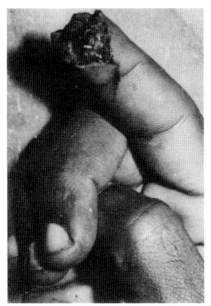
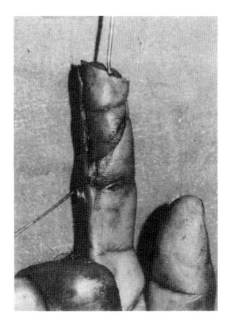

A,B

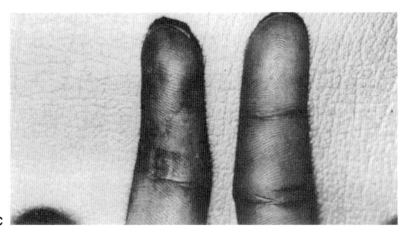

C

FIG. 2. A: An oblique amputation of the tip of the right index finger. B: The oblique triangular flap elevated. The flap is advanced and sutured over the defect. C: Postoperative appearance after 1 year. (From Venkataswami and Subramanian, ref. 1, with permission.)

On the "vertical" side of the triangle, the incision is deepened just dorsal to the neurovascular bundle, which is then included in the flap. When one reaches the apex, the neurovascular bundle is freed by gentle dissection to permit adequate flap mobility.

The minute branches of the neurovascular bundle that enter the flap on the oblique side are carefully dissected, and the fibrous strands are divided. Finally the apex of the flap is lifted, and the fibrous strands holding it are divided. Immediately one can appreciate the free mobility of the flap.

The flap is then advanced and sutured to the nail or the nailbed (Fig. 2).

CLINICAL RESULTS

This procedure has been performed on 78 patients over a 4-year period. The wounds heal in about 10 days, and the majority of patients return to their normal work in approximately 3 weeks. The contour of the fingertip is full and improves with time. There may be some shortening, depending on the extent of the amputation.

Sensation becomes normal within a few weeks, and the initial hyperesthesia that is seen in some instances passes. Marginal flap necrosis occurred in four patients, and some dehiscence at the suture line was seen in three patients. These minor complications were therefore present in 11% to 12% of cases.

SUMMARY

The oblique triangular skin flap is a good method of closing oblique fingertip amputations.

Reference

1. Venkataswami R, Subramanian N. Oblique triangular flap: a new method of repair for oblique amputations of the finger tip and thumb. *Plast Reconstr Surg* 1980;66:296.

CHAPTER 229 ■ VOLAR ADVANCEMENT SKIN FLAP TO THE FINGERTIP

J. W. SNOW

Amputation of the fingertips through a portion of the distal phalanx can be repaired by elevation and advancement of a volar flap.

INDICATIONS

This is a good way to resurface a volar oblique amputation of the fingers, particularly of the index and thumb in adults and of all digits in children (1–6). It also affords a good method for repair of a guillotine amputation.

ANATOMY

Some authors have felt that dorsal necrosis would occur over the middle phalanx, since both neurovascular bundles are carried with the flap. This does not occur, however, if the dorsal branch of the neurovascular bundle is preserved at the proximal interphalangeal joint level. This vessel crosses obliquely to supply the skin over the dorsum of the middle phalanx. It is imperative to preserve this vessel, which is less than 1 mm in diameter, on at least one side of the proximal interphalangeal (PIP) joint.

FLAP DESIGN AND DIMENSIONS

The incision is outlined in the neutral, or midaxial, zone on the radial and ulnar sides of the involved digit. The incision is carried no further than 1 cm proximal to the proximal interphalangeal joint.

OPERATIVE TECHNIQUE

The flap is elevated off the finger, just volar to the flexor tendon sheath. The neurovascular bundles are contained in the flap, and care is taken to preserve intact at least one of the branches at the PIP joint that supply the dorsum of the finger (Figs. 1 and 3).

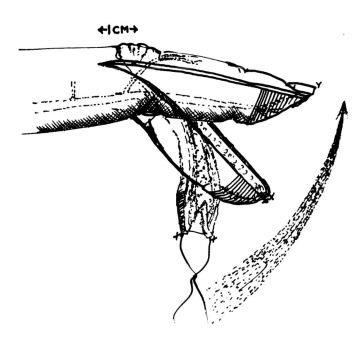

FIG. 1. A volar oblique amputation of an index finger, showing the midaxial incision to 1 cm proximal to the PIP joint. The injury leaves a V-shaped defect with two triangular areas (*shaded*) that are retained and sutured together as shown. Note the dorsal branch of the neurovascular bundle at the level of the PIP joint. This must be preserved on one side at least, in order to avoid dorsal skin necrosis.

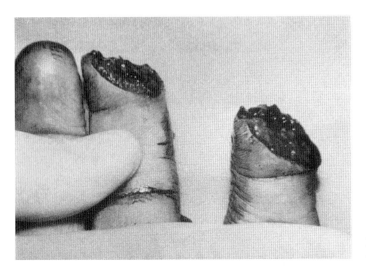

FIG. 2. Slightly angulated volar oblique amputations of the tips of the index and long fingers.

Oblique Amputations

When one is using the volar advancement flap to reconstruct the volar oblique amputation of a finger, the triangles of tissue forming the margins of the avulsion must be preserved for purposes of flap length (Figs. 1 and 2). One cannot advance the most proximal level of a volar oblique amputation all the way to the tip of the finger.

If the lateral triangles of tissue are maintained when the flap is elevated, a V-shaped defect will be created. (I do not make this V-shaped defect, as some have incorrectly stated. It is secondary to the injury.) The V is sutured together in the midline, forming a cup that preserves the length of the flap (Fig. 1) and that creates a suitable contour around the terminal portion of the finger.

Guillotine Amputations

In the case of a guillotine amputation the incision need only go to the proximal interphalangeal joint axis, and it can easily be

advanced to resurface the tip. The initial suture is usually placed through the central portion of the distal aspect of the flap and the midsagittal line of the nail, allowing the interphalangeal joint to flex as the suture is tied down (Fig. 4).

The excess skin and subcutaneous tissue are trimmed while one approaches the sides, so that they fit well into the recipient site. This gives a smooth, well-contoured fingertip without volar scarring. The less lengthy biaxial incisions give better assurance of preserving the dorsal branch of the neurovascular bundle at the proximal interphalangeal joint level.

Modification

A technique has been described that may make it easier for some surgeons to dissect out the flap without damaging the neurovascular bundle and the important dorsal branches. The midaxial incisions are made through the skin alone. The subcutaneous tissue is not incised, but it is carefully dissected up, so that the flap can be advanced and the dorsal branch of the neurovascular bundle at the interphalangeal level can be preserved.

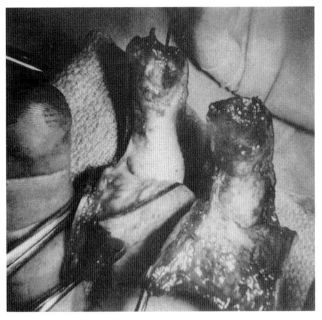

A

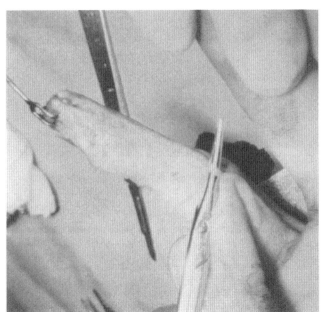

B

FIG. 3. A: Volar flaps elevated and the dorsal branch of the neurovascular bundle demonstrated. Note the V-shaped defect of the index finger. B: Note that the dorsal branch has been dissected and preserved to retain the blood supply to the dorsal skin.

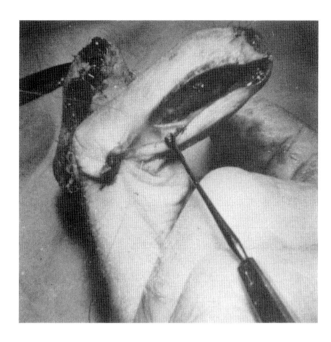

FIG. 4. The flap is advanced, after suturing the V-shaped defect together and allowing the interphalangeal joints to flex. Sutures are inserted in the midaxial incision, so that the flap is advanced from its base.

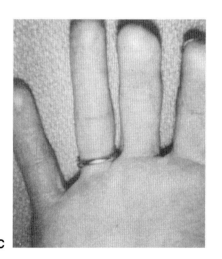 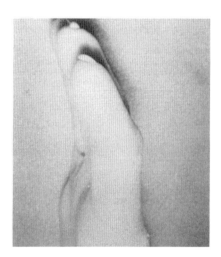 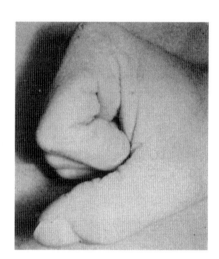

A–C

FIG. 5. A: Postoperative result. B: Note the lack of complete extension of the PIP joint. C: Full flexion of the fingers.

CLINICAL RESULTS

There has not been a single instance of dorsal necrosis in my personal series of 55 cases, because at least one of the branches of the neurovascular bundle that pass dorsally at the level of the PIP joint has been preserved.

In an oblique amputation the two lateral "triangles" created by the injury are sutured together. This creates a midline scar that fortunately has not been particularly troublesome to patients. This repair has been used to resurface a previously grafted fingertip in a blind patient who needed 2- to 3-mm two-point discrimination in order to read Braille (7). After the grafting procedure the patient's ability to read Braille was lost, but it was regained when a volar advancement flap on the index and long fingers was performed.

Physiotherapy is an essential part of this procedure, to avoid flexion contractures at the PIP joint (Fig. 5B).

I do not think it is necessary in most cases to graft the defect and then to do the operation on a healed wound, since infection has not occurred in this series of 55 fingers. It has been my experience that delayed primary repair seems to work best.

SUMMARY

A volar advancement flap can be used to cover thumb tip and other fingertip amputations.

References

1. Moberg E. Aspects of sensation in reconstructive surgery of the upper extremity. *J Bone Joint Surg [Am]* 1964;46(A):817.
2. Snow JW. The use of a volar flap for repair of fingertip amputations: a preliminary report. *Plast Reconstr Surg* 1967;40:163.
3. Posner MA, Smith RJ. The advancement pedicle flap for thumb injuries. *J Bone Joint Surg [Am]* 1971;53(A):1615.
4. Snow JW. Follow-up clinic: the use of a volar flap for repair of fingertip amputations—preliminary report. *Plast Reconstr Surg* 1973;52:299.
5. Kamal MS, et al. Volar advancement flap in fingertip repair. *Egypt J Plast Reconstr Surg* 1979;3:41.
6. Macht SD, Watson HK. The Moberg volar advancement flap for digital reconstruction. *J Hand Surg* 1980;5:372.
7. Joshi BB, Orth MS. Problem of sensory loss in fingertip injuries in the blind. *Br J Plast Surg* 1970;23:283.

CHAPTER 230 ■ VOLAR V-Y "CUP" FLAP

L. T. FURLOW, JR.

The V-Y "cup" flap (1) is a volar V-Y neurovascular flap that provides coverage of fingertip amputations by advancing skin from the volar surface of the distal and middle segments of the digit. The V-Y advancement is done between the distal interphalangeal and proximal interphalangeal flexion creases. The distal end of the flap is cupped to reproduce the contour of the amputated fingertip, a technique first illustrated by Snow (2) (see Chapter 229). The fingertip is reconstructed from volar finger skin that retains its sensation.

INDICATIONS

The volar V-Y "cup" flap is especially useful in cases where the amputation has left the digit shorter volarly than dorsally and the tissue for an Atasoy triangular volar fingertip flap (3) has been amputated. It can also be used for reconstructing the fingertip with insufficient padding, or with beaking of the fingernail.

ANATOMY

The flap is elevated as an island on both digital neurovascular bundles from the underlying distal phalanx and the flexor tendon sheath. The dorsal branches of the digital arteries that arise at the middle phalanx level should be protected, because the distal phalanx and dorsal soft tissues depend on them and may not survive if they are divided.

FLAP DESIGN AND DIMENSIONS

The flap incisions begin distally at the amputation a millimeter or so volar to the lateral nailbed margin, run to the distal interphalangeal (DIP) joint level at or a millimeter volar to the midlateral line, then head directly for the midline of the finger to meet at the PIP flexion crease (Fig. 1A,B; see also Fig. 3A,B).

After elevation on its two neurovascular bundles, the distal end of the flap is cupped by bringing the two distal points of the flap together to form the distal end of the flap into a fingertip shape (Fig. 1C; see also Fig. 3C,D).

OPERATIVE TECHNIQUE

The incisions distal to the DIP joint are made completely through subcutaneous tissue (Figs. 2A and 3A,B). Over the middle phalanx the incisions are initially made just through

dermis to protect the neurovascular bundles. Beginning distally the flap is elevated from the distal phalanx and the flexor tendon sheath (Fig. 3C). The middle phalanx "V" portion of the incisions crosses the neurovascular bundles, which are identified through these incisions and from beneath. Cleland's and Grayson's ligaments, just above and below the neurovascular bundles, are divided at that level, and the attachments of the flap medial and proximal to the neurovascular bundles, in the apex of the "V," are divided to leave the flap attached by only the neurovascular bundles. The flap will now move distally a centimeter or more (Fig. 2B).

The two distal lateral points of the flap are brought together to cup the end of the flap (Fig. 2C and Fig. 3C,D). If the amputation removed more skin volarly, suturing the end of the "cup" will produce a fingertip contour. If the amputation was more transverse, a portion of the volar dog-ear that results from forming the cup may have to be trimmed.

With only slight or no flexion of the PIP and DIP joints the flap is pulled distally and its cupped end brought up and over the transected end of the phalanx and nail. The flap is then sutured in its advanced V-Y position. This part of the closure is nearly always loose, with considerable "gaposis," and the closure of the cup may also be loose (Figs. 2D and 3E). The gaps close very well as the wound heals (Fig. 3F,G).

It is very important that the cup edge of the flap be held dorsal to the nail edge, with the soft tissue of the cup covering bone and nail to prevent beaking of the nail. One or several nylon sutures are passed through the dorsal surface of the nail, then through the distal end of the flap and back to hold the flap up (Fig. 2E,F). As healing progresses the skin margin of the cup of the flap is pulled under the nail end to complete the contouring of the fingertip (Fig. 3F,G).

CLINICAL RESULTS

Since little or no joint flexion is necessary to position the flap, flexion contractures have not been a problem. The cupping method of closure requires the flap to advance no more than 1.0 to 1.5 cm, regardless of the volar skin deficit. The vertical scar from the cupping closure has healed extremely well and has not been sensitive. The dorsal branches of the digital vessels are preserved, maintaining blood supply to the distal phalanx, nailbed, and dorsal tissues.

SUMMARY

The volar V-Y "cup" flap is especially useful for closure of fingertip amputations in cases where the tissue used in the standard Atasoy volar V-Y flap has been amputated. It uses volar skin and preserves sensation—distinct advantages over a cross-finger flap or thenar flap. The donor defect is closed simply, by V-Y advancement.

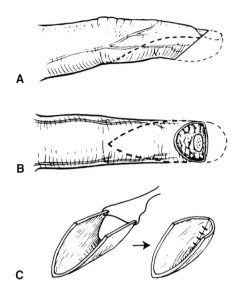

FIG. 1. A,B: Skin incisions. **C:** Cupping the distal end of the flap makes it unnecessary for the volar skin edge to advance to the nail margin. (From Furlow, Jr., ref. 1, with permission.)

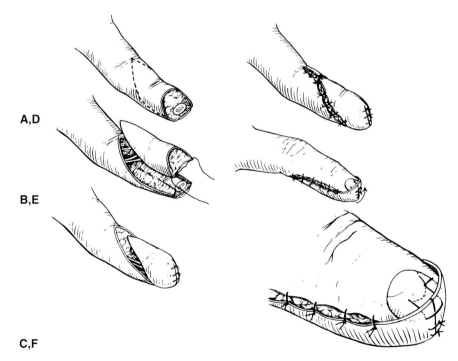

FIG. 2. A,B: Flap elevated from the flexor tendon sheath. **C:** The end of the flap is cupped. **D:** V-Y advancement. **E,F:** It is important that the flap project above the nail edge. Wound contraction will pull the skin to the nailbed margin, contouring the tip. Adequate skin and soft tissue prevent beaking. (From Furlow, Jr., ref. 1, with permission.)

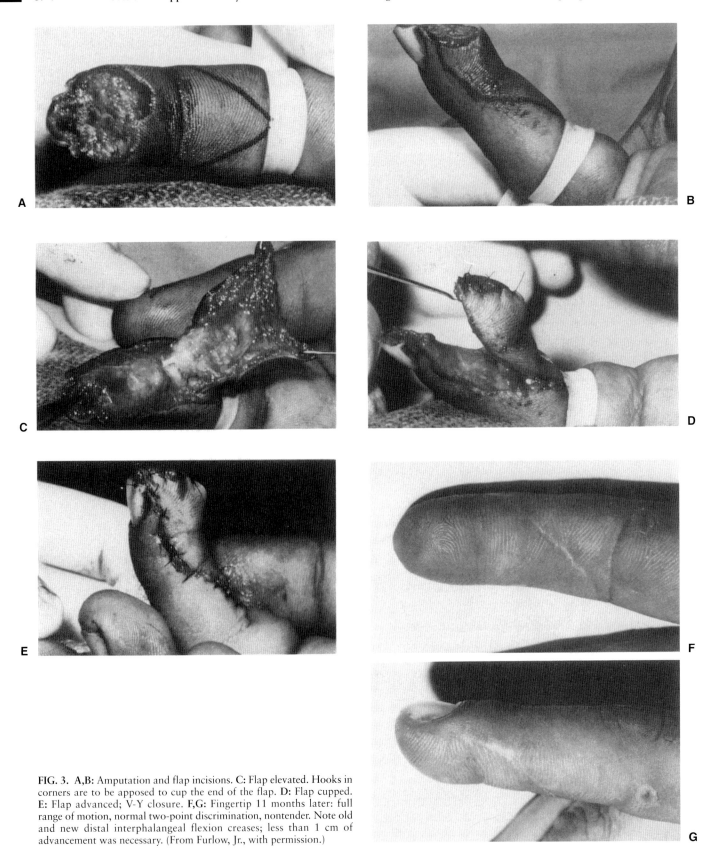

FIG. 3. A,B: Amputation and flap incisions. **C:** Flap elevated. Hooks in corners are to be apposed to cup the end of the flap. **D:** Flap cupped. **E:** Flap advanced; V-Y closure. **F,G:** Fingertip 11 months later: full range of motion, normal two-point discrimination, nontender. Note old and new distal interphalangeal flexion creases; less than 1 cm of advancement was necessary. (From Furlow, Jr., with permission.)

References

1. Furlow LT, Jr. V-Y "cup" flap for volar oblique amputations of fingers. *J Hand Surg* 1984;9(B):253.

2. Snow JW. The use of a volar flap for repair of fingertip amputations—a preliminary report. *Plast Reconstr Surg* 1967;40:163.

3. Atasoy E, Ioakimidis E, Kasdan M, et al. Reconstruction of the amputated finger tip with a triangular volar flap. *J Bone Joint Surg* 1970;52(A):921.

CHAPTER 231 ■ FLAG SKIN FLAP TO THE FINGER

F. ISELIN AND G. PRADET

A flag flap is a square or rectangular flap that originates from the dorsal aspect of a finger. It has a long narrow pedicle that can be twisted, thus proving uniquely versatile for coverage of many nearby defects. It has the appearance of a flag at the top of a flagpole (1–4) (Fig. 1).

INDICATIONS

The length of the pedicle allows the flap to be transferred either to the donor or to an adjacent finger. Because the pedicle can be twisted, the flag flap can be used to cover both dorsal and volar defects.

There are three main indications for this flap (Fig. 2). First, the flap can be used to cover volar defects on the same finger (5–7). Other flaps, such as cross-finger flaps, may be contraindicated, or one may not wish to damage an adjacent digit, especially if ultimate salvage of the injured finger is questionable.

Second, the flap can be used to cover distal digital amputations (5,8,9). It is especially useful, however, for coverage either of thumb amputations (proximal to the nailbed) or of osteoplastic reconstructions. Nerve branches that provide some sensation can be carried with the flap. Since the sensation

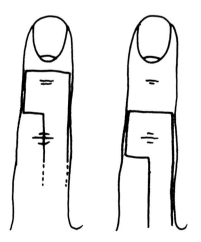

FIG. 1. The flag flap can be designed either distally or more proximally over the dorsum of the donor finger.

is less sophisticated than that of volar skin, it can more easily be retrained to be interpreted as coming from the thumb.

Third, this flap is very useful for dorsal defects, especially over the PIP and metaphalangeal (MP) joints. This is probably its best indication, since both local and volar flaps are inadequate. Whenever the skin quality is not ideal, we routinely use the flap to cover tendon reconstructions in zone 3 (boutonnieres) and resection implant arthroplasties. We have noted that most failures can be attributed to inadequate skin conditions.

The flag flap should not be used unless both volar digital arteries are intact. Otherwise there is some risk of necrosis of the more distal dorsal skin.

ANATOMY

The blood supply of the dorsal aspect of the hand and fingers has been studied (10) by angiography and selective dissection. It has been observed that the dorsal skin of the hand is vascularized by vertical perforating branches originating from the dorsal interosseous arteries. Each vertical ray splits into diverging horizontal branches that have the appearance of vascular stars. The horizontal branches are interconnected through three to four layers of a dermal capillary network.

There are four patterns of blood supply to the fingers. At the level of the web space, some of the horizontal branches from the dorsum of the hand reach the proximal portion of the finger. The area over the rest of the proximal phalanx is vascularized by two commissural arteries originating from the volar digital artery. The middle phalanx is vascularized only by a few small metameric branches originating from the volar digital artery. The distal phalanx is vascularized through the subungual network, which originates from the volar vessels.

There are at least two longitudinal veins with transverse anastomoses that are most prominent over the joints.

It can therefore be seen that any flaps raised from the dorsal aspect of the fingers have a random-pattern blood supply. In standard cross-finger flaps, the longitudinal venous drainage is transected, thus making a wide pedicle necessary. In the flag flap, however, the longitudinal veins are preserved. It is well accepted that good venous drainage is essential to flap survival. Therefore a flap with a long narrow pedicle, even if it is twisted, can survive without ischemia.

A sensory nerve branch can be found beside the longitudinal vein. This should always be preserved with the flap to retain sensation.

FLAP DESIGN AND DIMENSIONS

The dimensions of the flap are more or less determined by the size of the defect to be covered. To place suture lines in neutral

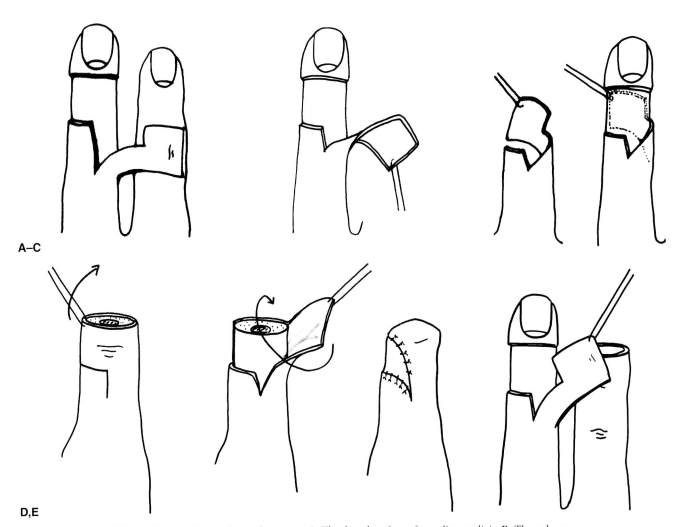

A–C

D,E

FIG. 2. The flag flap can be used to cover: **A:** The dorsal surface of an adjacent digit. **B:** The volar surface of an adjacent digit. **C:** The volar surface of the donor finger. **D:** The tip of the donor finger. **E:** The tip of an adjacent digit.

areas, the flap width will almost always be that of the finger. The length of the flap will vary with the defect (4,6).

A template should always be made first, in order to establish the best position of the flap and of the pedicle. The flap should reach the defect easily, with no more than a 90° twist to the pedicle. The "pole" or pedicle width is half the width of the finger and is located on either side, according to the site the flap must reach.

When both the donor site and the defect are on the same finger (Fig. 2C,D), the flap should be designed with a long enough pedicle to avoid excessive flexion and consequent joint stiffness (7).

If the flap is to be used to cover an amputation tip directly (Fig. 2D,E), care must be taken to avoid including any nail matrix with the flap. If this is not possible, some other form of flap cover should be used. When used for an amputation at the tip of the same finger, this flap does have the advantage of preserving intact the volar skin with its special sensitivity (Fig. 2D). This procedure is used more often in the thumb than in the long fingers.

When the flap is used for dorsal defects, it is outlined on the skin of the adjacent finger, just distal to the joint to be covered. In other words, the flap is taken from the middle phalanx to cover the PIP joint, and from the proximal phalanx to cover the MP joint. The pedicle is situated on the side of the finger next to the recipient digit (Fig. 2A).

OPERATIVE TECHNIQUE

Both the flap and the pedicle are elevated at the level of the extensor tendons, and one must be very careful to leave the paratenon intact, so that it can accept a skin graft. The length of the pole is limited proximally by the longitudinal veins when they merge with the vascular "stars" over the web space. Care is taken to include both the longitudinal vein and the sensory nerve branch in the pedicle (Fig. 3).

When the flag flap is to be transferred to the thumb to cover an amputation, to cover an osteoplastic reconstruction, or to restore sensation after pulp avulsion, both the flag and the pole are shifted radially. A longitudinal incision is made over the dorsum of the thumb, which is widened like a trench to accommodate the pedicle (Fig. 4B). In this case the pedicle is not divided, so that the sensory nerve is retained.

CLINICAL RESULTS

Survival of the transposed flag flap has been achieved in all 50 cases that we have performed. Normal healing is complete within 20 days. In some cases early blistering and marginal crusting have occurred, but there have been no instances of ischemic necrosis.

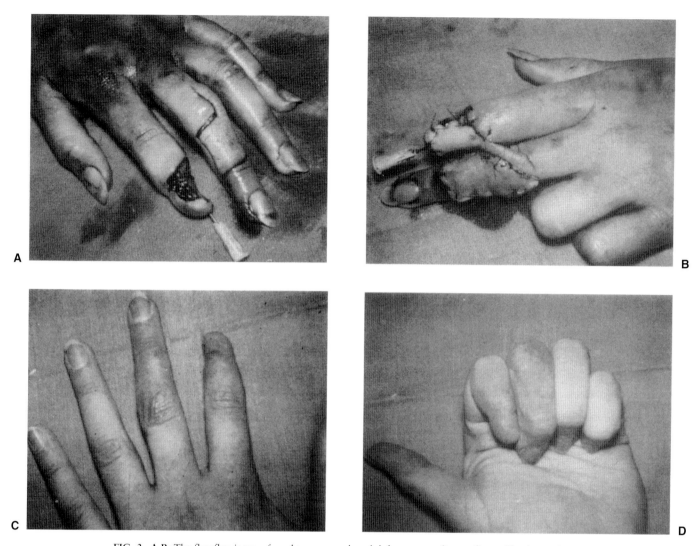

FIG. 3. **A,B:** The flag flap is transferred to cover a dorsal defect on an adjacent finger. The donor site is skin-grafted. **C,D:** Postoperative result.

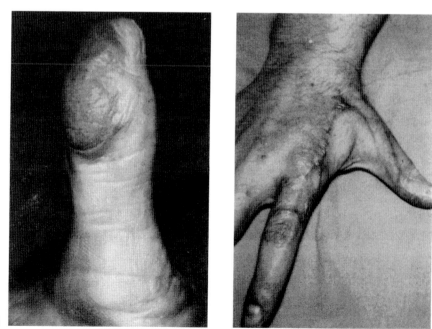

FIG. 4. **A:** The flag flap is used to provide both pulp and sensation to the volar aspect of the thumb. **B:** Note that the pedicle of the flap, which is taken from the index finger, is incorporated into the dorsum of the thumb, so that the sensory nerve can be preserved with the flap. (From Iselin, ref. 4, with permission.)

Provided that the recipient site has been properly prepared, so that the scars lie in neutral zones, the cosmetic result is good. Functional results are more difficult to evaluate, since they depend on the underlying lesion.

The flag flap has been used in 20 cases of fingertip amputation, in two thumb reconstructions, and in eight cases where sensation and coverage were required for the distal thumb. It has been used to cover the volar surface of eight fingers and the dorsal surface of 12 fingers.

SUMMARY

A skin flap that looks like a flag on a flagpole *can* be taken from the dorsum of a finger to cover fingertips, thumbs, and defects on both the dorsal and the volar surfaces of fingers. By including a dorsal sensory nerve in the flap, sensation can be provided to the thumb.

References

1. Vilain R. Technique élémentaire de réparation des pertes de substance cutanées des doigts. *Sem Hop Paris* 1952;29:1.
2. Iselin M, Gosse L. Lelambeau en drapeau, son emploi systématique dans le comblement des pertes de substance limitées des doigts. *Ann Chir Plast* 1962;8:1.
3. Vilain R, Dupuy JF. Use of the flag flap for coverage of a small area on a finger of the palm. *Plast Reconstr Surg* 1973;51:397.
4. Iselin F. The flag flap. *Plast Reconstr Surg* 1973;52:374.
5. Kuhn H. Traitement des amputations en coup de hache des phalanges distales. *Rev Chir Orthop* 1967;53:469.
6. Iselin M, Iselin F. In: *Atlas de technique opératoire de chirurgie de la main*. Paris: Ed. Med. Flammarion, 1971;62–68.
7. Mitz V, Senly G. A propos de l'utilisation du lambeau en drapeau clans la couverture des pertes de substance de is troisième phalange. *Ann Chir Plast* 1975;20:337.
8. Holevich J. A new method of restoring sensibility to the thumb. *J Bone Joint Surg [Br]* 1963;45(B):496.
9. Iselin F, Sedel L, Thevenin R. Resensibilisation du pouce par lambeau de Kuhn et Holevich. *Ann Chir Plast* 1971;16:295.
10. Levame J, Otero C, Berdugo G. Vascularisation arterielle des teguments de la face dorsale de la main et des doigts. *Ann Chir Plast* 1967;12:316.

CHAPTER 232 ■ ON-TOP-PLASTY SKIN FLAP OF THE FINGER

G. J. BAIBAK

EDITORIAL COMMENT

The need for this procedure has been dramatically reduced by the advent of microsurgical toe transfers.

The term *on-top plasty* was coined (1) to describe a technique for transferring a flap from a severely injured digit to a more useful location on the hand as an island vascular flap.

INDICATIONS

The technique of digit migration on neurovascular pedicles is not intended to replace pedicled flaps, bone grafts, or free flap digit reconstruction for hand injuries.

My series has used all fingers of the hand for transfer, the concept being that an injured part is used to increase function of other injured parts (2). If a usable injured finger is available, a normal finger need not be sacrificed for "spare parts."

FLAP DESIGN AND DIMENSIONS

Complete or partial digit migration into the thumb position is quite easily accomplished, even if the distal portion is damaged.

The finger segment is moved along an arc, based at the proximal palmar crease, into the receptor or thumb position. The on-top plasty digit migration concept for gaining length is dependent on MP joint function, i.e., on active and passive flexion and extension (Fig. 1).

Tendons and neurovascular bundles that may have been shortened at the time of migration to a flexed phalanx can gradually be straightened or extended over a period of time. In essence, one gradually stretches the tendons and the neurovascular bundle beyond the initial hook-up length, thus increasing the length and span of grasp of the injured hand (Fig. 2).

OPERATIVE TECHNIQUE

It is assumed that the reader is familiar with the technique of developing and using neurovascular pedicles within the hand (3,4).

The dissection is started in the proximal palm, lest a neurovascular anomaly exist that might preclude transfer. (I have encountered three anomalies in approximately 50 neurovascular islands in the hand). A W-type of incision is used both about the recipient stump and in the donor area, to give good exposure and to prevent linear contractures in the incision and circular contractures around the transposed digit.

The neurovascular pedicles are dissected to include the loose investing areolar tissue. The palmar aponeurosis and the

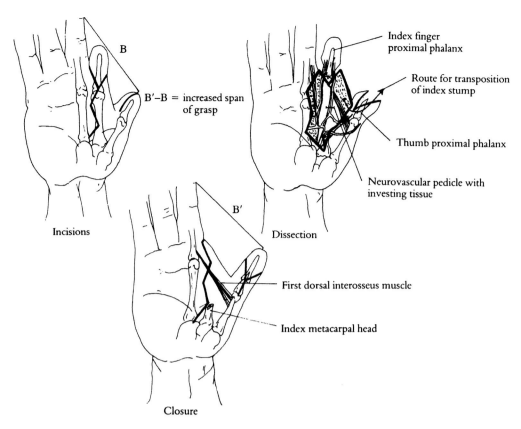

FIG. 1. Migration of index stump to thumb stump. Any other shortened digit may be used in a similar fashion. The long finger stump may be sacrificed to increase the span of grasp in multiple amputations.

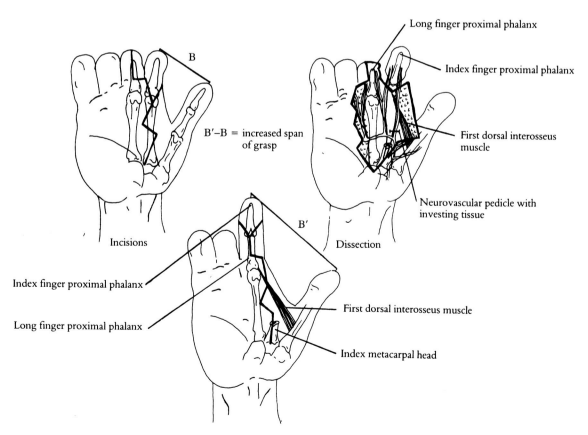

FIG. 2. Migration of the index to long finger stump, illustrating the technique and the increased span of grasp.

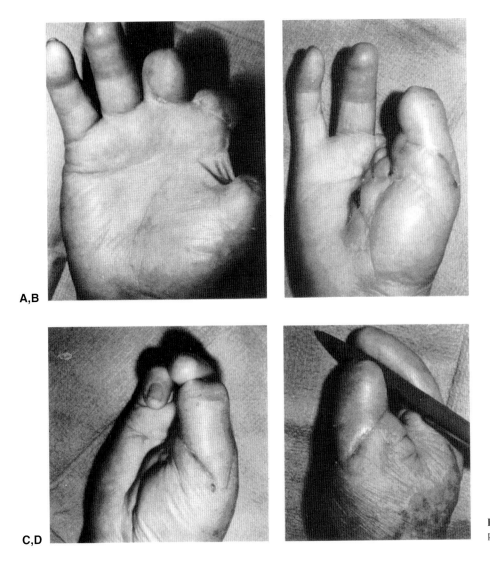

A,B

C,D

FIG. 3. Index to thumb "on-top plasty," showing increased function.

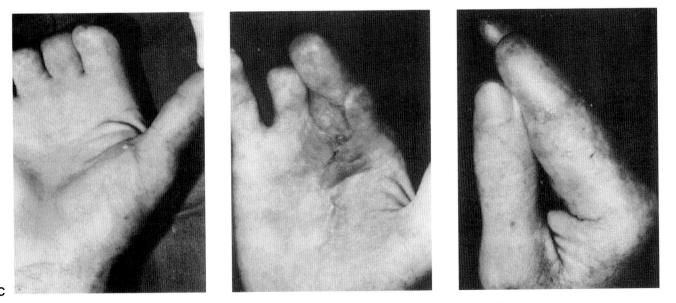

A–C

FIG. 4. Index to long "on-top plasty," illustrating neurovascular pedicles and increased function.

septa extending down to the metacarpals are released from about the neurovascular pedicle of the donor finger and the base of the recipient digit. This release allows for increased freedom of the palmar skin overlying the transplanted neurovascular bundle and reduces the likelihood of vascular constriction to the transposed digit in the subaponeurotic space.

At the time of migration to a finger, the recipient digit is held in 90° flexion while the base of the proximal phalanx of the donor digit is placed "on-top" of the sharpened end of the proximal phalanx of the recipient finger. The thumb, because of its recessed position, need not be flexed for a successful on-top plasty. When one is using the index finger, the first dorsal interosseous muscle is attached to the proximal phalanx of the long finger via a drill hole, in order to reinforce key pinch.

Skin closure is usually accomplished with local skin flaps and/or grafts, as determined by the preexisting defect. At 5 to 6 weeks, when the healing of skin and bone is adequate, the digit is gradually straightened and brought into the fully extended position. Such a period of time allows the nerves and blood vessels to gain length without loss of function (Figs. 3 and 4).

CLINICAL RESULTS

This procedure has been used on ten patients over the past few years. There has been no loss of the migrated digits, nor have there been any significant complications. Sensation of the transposed digits has been maintained at the preoperative level, as measured by two-point tactile discrimination testing. There have been no nonunions requiring secondary procedures at the synostosis.

SUMMARY

Fingers or thumbs that have been shortened by injury and that are useless can be lengthened and made functional by transferring the ends of other injured fingers to the stumps by means of the on-top plasty procedure.

References

1. Soiland H. Lengthening a finger with the "on-the-top" method. *Acta Chir Scand* 1961;122:184.
2. Kelleher JC, Sullivan JG, Baibak GJ, Dean RK. "On top plasty" for amputated fingers. *Plast Reconstr Surg* 1968;42:242.
3. Littler JW. Proceedings of the American Society for Surgery of the Hand. *J Bone Joint Surg* 1956;35(A):917.
4. Frackleton WD, Teasley JL. Neurovascular island pedicle extension in usage. *J Bone Joint Surg* 1962;44(A):1069.

CHAPTER 233 ■ THENAR FLAP

B. W. EDGERTON AND R. W. BEASLEY

EDITORIAL COMMENT

The design of these flaps and the flexion required to the attached finger make one wary of the strong possibility of fixed flexion contractures postoperatively.

Major distal phalangeal amputations are best treated by a local flap from the hand, whenever practicable. The thenar flap has the advantages of near-perfect tissue match, excellent recovery of sensibility, adequate subcutaneous tissue for pulp restoration, and a minimally disfiguring donor site (1–6). Thenar flaps must not be confused with palmar flaps, for which the complication rate is so high as to contraindicate their use (7–18).

INDICATIONS

The major indication for a thenar flap is amputation of the digits distal to the distal interphalangeal joint. No other graft or flap providing adequate subcutaneous tissue for pulp restoration can provide as good a tissue match for texture, appearance, and recovery of sensibility (19). Preservation of finger length provides a functionally and aesthetically superior reconstruction to shortening and closure of the amputation stump, especially if an acceptable fingernail can be salvaged. For those amputations proximal to the distal interphalangeal joint for which reattachment is not possible, a thenar flap may be used for wound closure to preserve length and a functional proximal interphalangeal joint. Positioning becomes more difficult with more proximal amputations, and a volar or dorsal cross-finger flap may then be preferable (see Chap. 246).

ANATOMY

The thenar flap should be raised from a location high on the thenar eminence. Tenderness has not proved to be a problem with scars located in this area. With the flap in this location palmar abduction of the thumb minimizes interphalangeal joint flexion of the injured digit. The distal (or lateral) margin should be placed in the metacarpophalangeal joint crease.

Because the flap has a random blood supply provided by the dermal and subdermal plexuses, it may be raised in any direction. Since subcutaneous tissue is desired in pulp reconstruction, the flap is raised in a plane just superficial to the thenar musculature.

FLAP DESIGN AND DIMENSIONS

The thenar flap may be based in any direction. In most cases of fingertip amputation it is based proximally. The flap may be considered a direct flap, in that the defect is brought to the open surface of the flap. Flaps of approximately 2.25 × 2.25 cm in size are usually necessary to resurface an adult fingertip if contour restoration rather than a flat tip is desired.

Interphalangeal joint contracture of the injured finger is avoided by maximal finger metacarpophalangeal joint flexion and by palmar abduction of the thumb to meet the finger. These procedures usually result in proximal interphalangeal joint flexion of no more than 50° (Fig. 1B). Positioning is more difficult for the index finger and is easier for the more ulnar digits.

A pattern is cut, pressed against the defect, and held against the location of the flap pedicle. A flap to restore fully the round contour of the fingertip must be at least 1½ times larger than the width of the finger (Fig. 1). If the flap is proximally based and extends into the first web, a W-shaped extension is made to avoid a longitudinal scar across lines of tension (Fig. 1A). All flaps should be measured twice and cut once.

OPERATIVE TECHNIQUE

The flap is elevated from the thenar muscles, taking subcutaneous tissue with it. The only vital structure that may be injured underneath this flap is the radial digital sensory nerve to the thumb, which courses along the surface of the flexor pollicis brevis. This nerve should be identified and carefully protected. If the flap is designed distal on the thenar eminence, the motor branch of the median nerve is not vulnerable to injury.

The donor site of the flap may be closed primarily in cases where the flap is less than 2 cm in width, but usually a skin graft is required for closure without thumb restriction. The distal volar wrist crease is a convenient location to obtain a full-thickness, hair-free skin graft of up to 12 mm in width that when divided into two pieces will provide enough skin to cover the defect.

To prevent a bulbous tip and a downward pull on the distal nailbed, only the lateral margins of the flap are sutured to the finger. A carefully shaped gauze packing is placed over the skin graft and the finger is then immobilized with tape to prevent tension on the suture line or flap. A light plaster cast is placed over the hand, with a replaceable window cut in it to allow inspection and wound care.

After 10 to 14 days the pedicle is divided. The flap is never inset at the time of pedicle division, because it will tolerate poorly any handling, tension, or suturing at this time. The wounds are dressed with care not to compress the flap tissues. The wounds are allowed to heal secondarily, but active extension and intrinsic muscle exercises are begun immediately to mobilize the interphalangeal joints. A secondary revision may be performed at a later date for perfection of contour, but it is not required for many cases (Fig. 2).

CLINICAL RESULTS

Flaps taken from the palm have justly earned a bad reputation. One series of 21 palmar flaps reported 24% with tender scars and 38% with stiff joints (12).

A recent careful review of 150 consecutive cases of thenar flaps (18) performed by two surgeons shows that the poor reputation of thenar flaps is not deserved. There were no losses of the flaps and no infections, and excellent contour

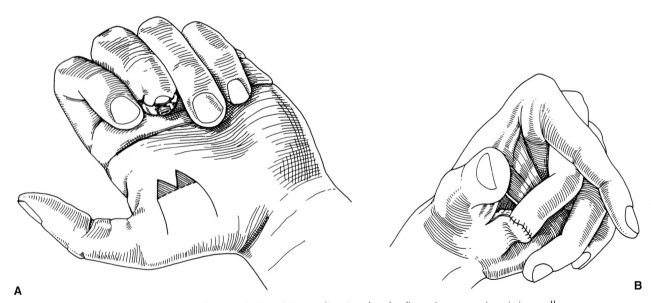

A   **B**

FIG. 1. A: The thenar flap may be based in any direction, but for fingertip amputations it is usually based proximally. To restore the rounded contour of the normal fingertip, the flap should be at least 1½ times the width of the finger. A W-shaped extension can be made to avoid a longitudinal scar across the lines of tension. B: Proximal interphalangeal joint flexion can be a problem with this procedure. Patients should be individually evaluated before choosing this procedure. Positioning is more difficult for the index finger and becomes less of a problem with the small finger.

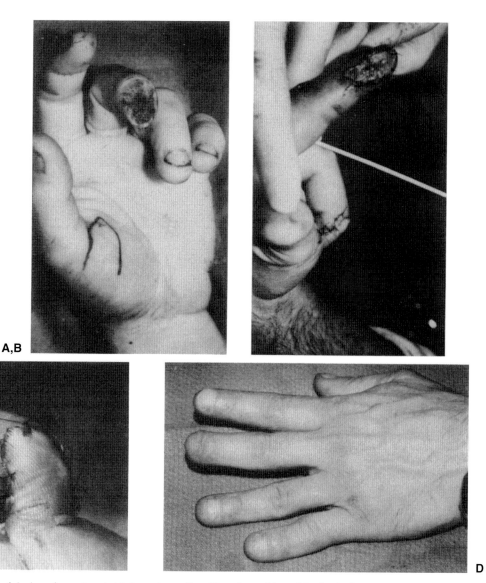

FIG. 2. A: Defect of the long fingertip suitable for a thenar flap. Note the position of the flap high up on the thenar eminence. **B:** Flap in place. Note proximal interphalangeal flexion. **C:** Donor site is covered with a skin graft. **D:** Postoperative result. Note complete proximal interphalangeal extension.

reconstruction was obtained. Only four patients (3%) had any tenderness of the donor site. Only six patients had *any* joint stiffness (there was less than 15° loss of extension in four of the six patients). Recovery of two-point discrimination averaged 7 mm (in agreement with previous authors), and only one patient having repair of the index finger subsequently favored use of the adjacent middle finger. Ninety-four percent of the patients returned to work an average of 11 weeks after injury. (The average was 4.5 weeks in noncompensation cases.) No special difficulties were encountered with children (nine patients) or with older adults (31 patients over the age of 50). Only one of the patients who demonstrated joint stiffening was older than 50 years. The skin grafts to the donor site usually developed some hyperpigmentation, but patients did not find this troublesome.

SUMMARY

The thenar flap is unsurpassed for restoration of major distal phalangeal and selected middle phalangeal digital amputa-

tions. It provides tissue of excellent match, supplies adequate subcutaneous tissue for pulp restoration, and has good recovery of sensibility. When the guidelines are carefully followed the procedure can be performed with minimal morbidity in all age groups.

References

1. Gatewood. A plastic repair of finger defects without hospitalization. *JAMA* 1926;87:1479.
2. Flatt AE. The thenar flap. *J Bone Joint Surg [Br]* 1957;39:80.
3. Gottlieb O, Mathiesen FR. Thenar flaps and cross finger flaps. *Acta Chir Scand* 1961;122:166.
4. Miller AJ. Single fingertip injuries treated by thenar flap. *Hand* 1974;6:311.
5. Barton NJ. A modified thenar flap. *Hand* 1975;7:150.
6. Smith RJ, Albin R. Thenar H-flap for fingertip injuries. *J Trauma* 1976;16:778.
7. Horn JS. The use of full thickness hand skin flaps in the reconstruction of injured fingers. *Plast Reconstr Surg* 1951;7:463.
8. Fusco EM. Fingertip reconstruction with palmar skin flaps. *Am J Surg* 1954;87:608.
9. Barclay TL. The late results of finger tip injuries. *Br J Plast Surg* 1955–1956;8:38.

10. Campbell Reid DA. Experience of a hand surgery service. *Br J Plast Surg* 1956;9:11.
11. Kleinert HE. Fingertip injuries and their management. *Am Surg* 1959;25:41.
12. Sturman MJ, Duran RJ. Late results of fingertip injuries. *J Bone Joint Surg [Am]* 1963;45:289.
13. Smith JR, Bom AF. An evaluation of fingertip reconstruction by cross-finger and palmar pedicle flap. *Plast Reconstr Surg* 1965;3.5:409.
14. Beasley RW. Reconstruction of amputated fingertips. *Plant Reconstr Surg* 1969;44:349.

15. Beasley RW. Local flaps for surgery of the hand. *Orthop Clin North Am* 1970;1:219.
16. Russell RC, Van Beek AL, Wavek P, Zook EG. Alternative hand flaps for amputations and digital defects. *J Hand Surg* 1981;6:399.
17. Beasley RW. *Hand Injuries*. Philadelphia: Saunders, 1981.
18. Melone CP, Beasley RW, Carstens JH. The thenar flap: analysis of its use in 150 cases. *J Hand Surg* 1982;7:291.
19. Porter RW. Functional assessment of transplanted skin in volar defects of the digits. *J Bone Joint Surg [Am]* 1968;50:955.

CHAPTER 234 ■ THENAR H-FLAP

R. J. SMITH*

EDITORIAL COMMENT

The only advantage this procedure provides is a completely closed system when cohering the fingertip. Otherwise a more proximal attachment creates greater flexion constraint than that required in the flap discussed in Chapter 233.

If the distal phalanx protrudes from the wound after a fingertip injury, skin and subcutaneous tissue are needed to provide a functional and aesthetic soft-tissue cover. With a thenar *H-flap* there is a closed system: a graft is not needed to cover the donor site, and scarring and disability at the donor site are negligible (1,2).

INDICATIONS

In infants and small children the wound may heal rapidly by secondary intention. Occasionally a composite graft may survive. For the older child or young adult, however, the thenar flap offers robust and durable skin and subcutaneous tissue that are readily available for direct flap coverage and that require immobilization only of the injured finger.

_____

* Deceased.

The thenar H-flap is indicated for fingertip injuries with protruding bone and with a defect of 1 to 3 cm. It is not usually used in older patients with stiff finger joints or with large soft-tissue defects. It is inappropriate for thumb tip injuries.

FLAP DESIGN AND DIMENSIONS

Regardless of which finger is involved, a palmar flap should always come from the thenar eminence. A hypothenar flap to the little finger forces this finger to assume an awkward position of pronation and flexion, and should not be used.

An H-flap of skin and subcutaneous tissue is elevated from the thenar eminence (Fig. 1A,B). Each of the flaps is about 20% larger than the size of the defect.

OPERATIVE TECHNIQUE

Each flap is sutured to the fingertip and to the other flap (Fig. 1C). Fourteen days later the proximal flap is detached from the palm and sutured to the defect. The distal thenar flap is detached from the finger and advanced to close the donor site (Fig. 1C).

The finger is fully extended on an aluminum splint for 2 or 3 days. Range of motion exercises then are performed for 1 week, during which period the finger is placed in an extension splint at rest.

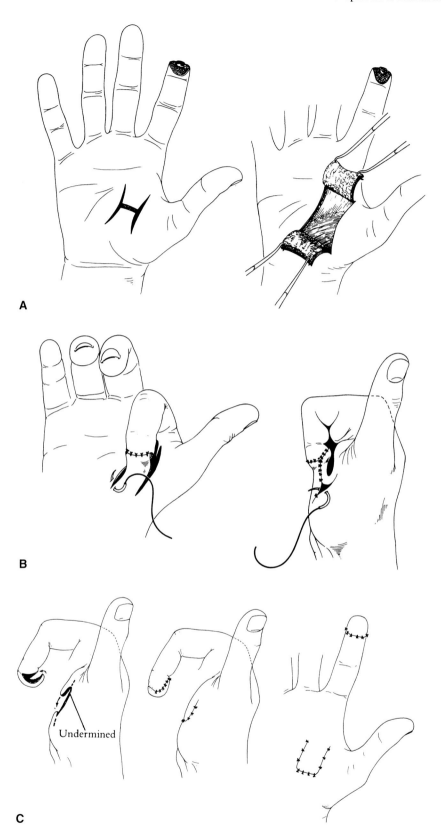

A

B

C

FIG. 1. **A:** An H is incised in the thenar eminence. Each flap is about 20% larger than the defect, with the horizontal limb of the H at the spot where the flexed index finger lies most comfortably. The flaps are elevated down to the thenar fascia. **B:** Both flaps are sutured to the fingertip and to each other. **C:** After 2 weeks, the flaps are detached. One remains with the finger; the other remains on the palm to close the donor site. (From Smith and Albin, ref. 2, with permission.)

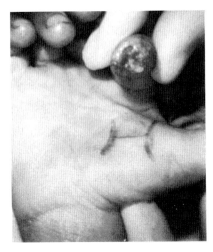 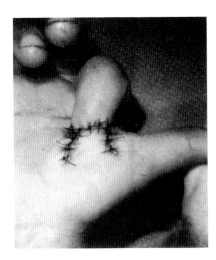 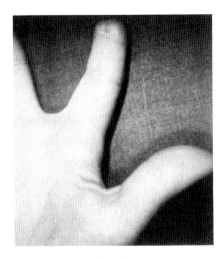

A–C

FIG. 2. A thenar H-flap is used to cover a fingertip defect in an eight-year-old girl. (From Smith and Albin, ref. 2, with permission.)

SUMMARY

The thenar H-flap offers an excellent means of providing aesthetic and functional coverage of deep, medium-sized fingertip defects in younger patients (Fig. 2). One must take care, however, to construct a closed system when applying the flap, and to prevent contracture after the flap has been detached, by appropriate postoperative splinting and exercises.

References

1. Smith JR, Bom AF. An evaluation of fingertip reconstruction by cross-finger and palmar pedicle flap. *Plast Reconstr Surg* 1965;35:409.
2. Smith RJ, Albin R. Thenar H-flap for fingertip injuries. *J Trauma* 1976;16:778.

CHAPTER 235 ■ CROSS THUMB TO INDEX FINGERTIP SKIN FLAP

E. ATASOY

EDITORIAL COMMENT

Early division of the flap must be anticipated. Otherwise there is a danger of joint and first web space contracture. This flap should not be used routinely, but only in the specific situations indicated by the author.

The dorsum of the thumb is not considered an ideal donor site. It can, however, provide excellent coverage in certain cases for fingertip amputations where there is exposed bone.

INDICATIONS

The cross thumb to index skin flap is useful for index fingertip amputations in which there is an associated crushing injury to the dorsum of the long finger (1). With the use of this flap as an elective procedure an unsatisfactory index fingertip stump can be improved in the presence of old multiple finger amputations.

When the index finger is amputated just distal to the proximal interphalangeal joint it is essential to maintain length in order to preserve function. If there are associated amputations of the other fingers at the distal interphalangeal joint level or

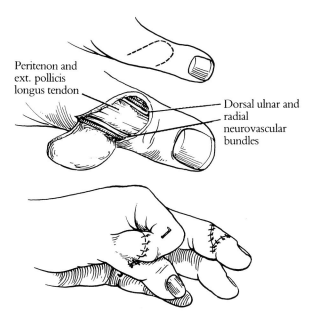

FIG. 1. Schematic representation of the operative technique. (From Atasoy, ref. 1, with permission.)

above, the amputated index fingertip can be covered with a cross-thumb flap, which actually adds a little length (see Fig. 2).

If the long finger is damaged, this flap can be used to cover an index finger in which the complete nailbed and surrounding skin have been avulsed. Otherwise a reversed

cross-finger flap from the long finger would be used to cover the exposed bone and the extensor tendon insertion (see Chapter 247).

ANATOMY

The cross thumb to index flap has a randomly based circulation, but it includes any dorsal veins that are present. Care is taken during the dissection to preserve the peritenon over the extensor pollicis longus tendon, to allow the donor site to be skin grafted. Both dorsal sensory nerves, which should be left intact, run along the edge of the extensor tendon (Fig. 1).

FLAP DESIGN AND DIMENSIONS

A flap that is 3 to 4 mm wider than the defect to be covered is marked on the dorsum of the proximal phalanx of the thumb. The flap can be made twice as long as it is wide. The base of the flap is placed on the radial side of the thumb in a slightly oblique direction (Figs. 1 and 2A).

OPERATIVE TECHNIQUE

A two or three power magnifying loupe is very helpful during this operation. As in ordinary cross-finger pedicles (2–4), full-thickness subcutaneous tissue and dorsal veins should be included in the flap, but the peritenon should be left intact on the extensor tendon.

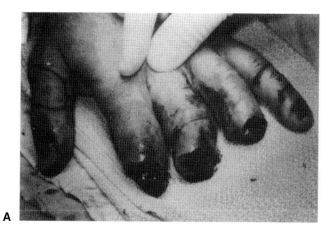

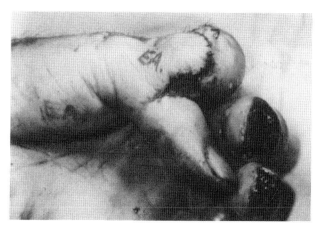

A   B

FIG. 2. A: Severe crushing injury resulting in multiple fingertip amputations. Note the flap outline on the thumb. B: Cross thumb-index flap covering the index finger, which was amputated just distal to the proximal interphalangeal joint. Preservation of length is important in order to retain function. A Kirschner wire is placed across both digits to hold the flap in position, thus avoiding any tension. C,D: Postoperative flexion and extension at 3 months. Note the lack of contracture at the first web space and at the skin-grafted donor site. (From Atasoy, ref. 1, with permission.)

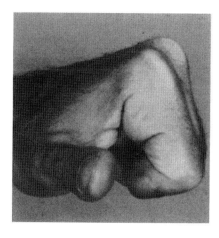

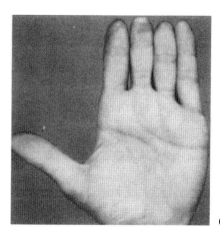

C,D

The defect is covered with a full-thickness skin graft taken from the forearm, upper arm, or groin. The recipient index finger, when positioned on the thumb, will act as a tie-over dressing.

After placing the index finger in the proper position on the thumb, a 0.028 Kirschner wire is inserted through these digits, to maintain the flap in the best position for preventing kinking and stretching. Both ends of the Kirschner wire are bent fairly close to the skin on the thumb and the index finger to prevent migration.

Division of the flap and removal of the Kirschner wire are performed about 2 weeks postoperatively, and gentle manipulation of the first web space and joints is carried out.

CLINICAL RESULTS

Flap necrosis can be avoided by pinning the index finger to the thumb in the optimal position for preventing any vascular embarrassment of the flap.

If both dorsal sensory nerves are preserved intact during the dissection, sensory disturbances at the tip of the thumb should not occur.

First web space contracture and joint stiffness can be prevented by early division of the flap (12 to 14 days postoperatively), and by gentle joint and first web space manipulation, followed by immediate active and passive range of motion exercises.

SUMMARY

The cross thumb to index skin flap is a good method for covering index fingertip defects when there is an associated injury of the long finger that precludes its use as a donor site.

References

1. Atasoy E. The cross thumb to index finger pedicle. *J Hand Surg* 1980;5:572.
2. Cronin TD. The cross finger flap: a new method of repair. *Am Surg* 1951;17:419.
3. Flatt AE. The thenar flap. *J Bone Joint Surg [Br]* 1957;39:80.
4. Kleinert HE. Fingertip injuries and their management. *Am Surg* 1959;25:41.

CHAPTER 236 ■ CROSS-FINGER SKIN-NERVE FLAP

B. E. COHEN

Deep wounds of the fingertip, with excessive loss of skin and subcutaneous tissue, often require flap coverage, particularly if bone or tendon is exposed. Although the cross-finger flap provides durable skin and padding, sensory return is quite variable. To enhance sensibility, an innervated cross-finger flap can be used in which the nerve to the flap tissue is transferred with it and sutured to the end of the digital nerve at the recipient site (1,2).

INDICATIONS

The innervated cross-finger flap should be considered for fingertip reconstruction, since this method has all the merits of the standard cross-finger flap plus the probability of gaining greater acuity of sensation. No further morbidity is incurred, compared with the standard cross-finger flap, because no additional tissues need be denervated at the donor site, and because the nerve used at the recipient site has already been transected by the injury.

This flap should not be used for injuries proximal to the fingertip. Rather, where indicated, a standard cross-finger flap should be chosen and digital nerve continuity to the uninjured fingertip should be either maintained or reestablished.

ANATOMY

In the fingers, the skin over the dorsum of the middle phalanx is innervated by a branch from the proper digital nerve (Fig. 1). This branch originates from the digital nerve just distal to the metacarpophalangeal joint and angles obliquely across the proximal phalanx to the dorsum, where it spreads out to innervate the tissue over the ipsilateral half of the middle phalanx. This nerve is the basis of the innervated cross-finger flap. The proper digital nerve continues to the level of the distal interphalangeal joint, where it ends in dorsal, volar, and tip branches. The volar and tip branches are often transected in severe fingertip injuries requiring flap coverage and serve as recipients for the cross-finger flap nerve.

FLAP DESIGN AND DIMENSIONS

Planning for the flap is done with the use of a pattern made to fit the defect. The flap, situated over the dorsum of the middle phalanx, is generally based on the lateral border of the digit, but may be distally based if that seems to offer a better fit.

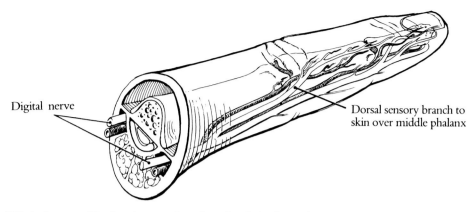

FIG. 1. Anatomy. The dorsal sensory branch used with the flap is shown as it arises from the proper digital nerve and passes to the dorsum of the middle phalanx. A similar branch on the opposite side is not depicted. The proper digital nerve generally begins its terminal branching at the distal interphalangeal joint level. (From Cohen and Cronin, ref. 2, with permission.)

OPERATIVE TECHNIQUE

After cleaning and appropriate debridement of the injured fingertip, an adjacent digit is chosen as the cross-finger flap donor. The middle finger is generally used for resurfacing thumb injuries (Fig. 2).

The sensory nerve to the flap is first sought with the aid of loupe magnification through an oblique incision over its course in the donor finger (Fig. 2A,B). Generally there is a thin layer of subcutaneous fat and fascia overlying the nerve. The nerve is traced to the edge of the planned flap; it is sectioned proximally so that a 2-cm "tail" may be reflected with the flap. The flap is then cut and elevated in the plane of

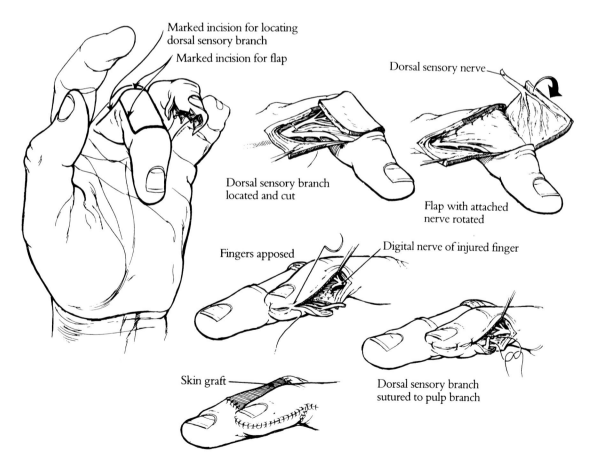

FIG. 2. Operative technique. The steps in the surgical procedure are outlined. See text for details. (From Cohen and Cronin, ref. 2, with permission.)

the extensor tendon paratenon with the nerve in continuity (Fig. 2C).

In the injured finger, on the side opposite the flap donor finger, a short linear incision is made over the digital nerve. The digital nerve is identified proximal to the injury and traced into the traumatic wound (Fig. 2D). Branches to intact tissue are preserved while branches (or, in more proximal injuries, the main nerve trunk) to amputated areas are isolated for nerve junction with the flap sensory nerve.

The flap is transposed to the defect and sutured loosely in place. The operating microscope is then used to perform the neurorrhaphy between the digital nerve (or branch) in the injured finger and the sensory nerve to the flap (Fig. 2E). Careful preparation of the nerve ends prevents occlusion of the axons by overlapping epineurium. A few 9-0 nylon sutures in the epineurium suffice for the nerve junction. The joined nerves are placed in the underlying wound, which is then closed. The remainder of the flap is inset and the flap donor site is grafted (Fig. 2F). The dressing, after-care, and flap division proceed as for a standard cross-finger flap. The nerve junction is opposite the flap base and therefore not in jeopardy at the time of flap division.

CLINICAL RESULTS

In two series almost all fingertips reconstructed with innervated cross-finger flaps gained good sensation and had a better functional result than those reconstructed with standard cross-finger flaps (1,2). In smaller wounds, in which no part of the flap is very distant from well-innervated surrounding tissue, this difference is probably less substantial.

SUMMARY

The innervated cross-finger flap provides cover and good sensation to a fingertip with minimal donor site morbidity.

References

1. Berger A, Meissl, G. Innervated skin grafts and flaps for restoration of sensation to anesthetic areas. *Chir Plast [Berlin]* 1975;3:33.
2. Cohen BE, Cronin ED. An innervated cross-finger flap for fingertip reconstruction. *Plast Reconstr Surg* 1983;72:688.

CHAPTER 237 ■ NEUROVASCULAR ISLAND SKIN FLAP TO THE FINGER AMPUTATION STUMP

R. K. SRIVASTAVA AND J. B. KAHL

EDITORIAL COMMENT

The editors believe that the indications for this procedure are extremely limited. An amputation and closure of the wound would be a simpler procedure and just as efficacious. A ray amputation should also be considered as an alternative.

Once a patient presents with a stiff, nonfunctional, and painful finger, the decision to amputate will often be made. As with all mutilating hand injuries, the philosophy of salvaging any useful tissue from the amputated part of the hand is important.

INDICATIONS

The use of this flap is limited to salvaging the special tactile fingertip skin in case of finger amputation, as long as there are no other digits that need localized sensation. If the amputation is proximal to the PIP joint, the hand may be more functional with

a ray amputation. If the amputation is at, or distal to, the PIP joint, a neurovascular island flap from the distal phalanx can be used to provide good cover and sensation to the stump (1).

If one neurovascular bundle has been damaged during the original injury, the half volar and lateral skin flap based on a single neurovascular bundle is equally good for tactile reception.

ANATOMY

This neurovascular island skin flap is based on one or both neurovascular bundles of the injured finger. The surgically isolated composite bundle should include sufficient areolar tissue to assure independent venous return for the isolated skin flap (2).

FLAP DESIGN AND DIMENSIONS

The area of salvageable volar and lateral skin of the fingertip is outlined (Fig. 1A). The marking is extended proximally for the elevation of standard triangular flaps.

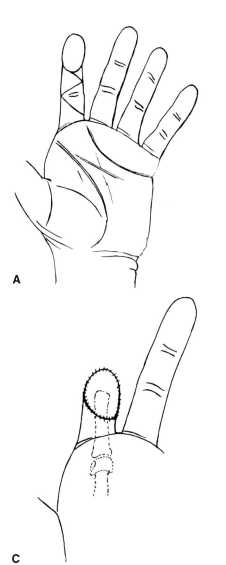

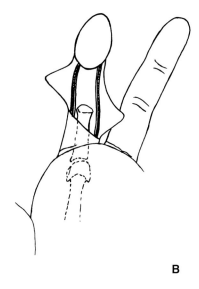

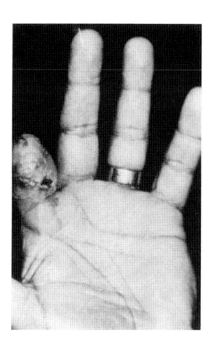

FIG. 1. A: The outline of the volar neurovascular island skin flap and the proximal triangular flaps on the finger that is to be amputated. B: The neurovascular bundles are then isolated and the amputation performed. C: The neurovascular island flap is then sutured loosely into place on the amputation stump. It is essential to avoid any twisting, kinking, or pressure on the pedicle. (From Srivastava and Kahl, ref. 1, with permission.)

FIG. 2. Postoperative result in a 34-year-old man who had an industrial injury to his nondominant left hand. (The injury in the thumb was repaired with a volar V-Y advancement flap.) Despite extensive physiotherapy for 3 months, the index finger was still stiff and painful. After discussion of the alternatives, his finger was amputated at the proximal interphalangeal joint level and the stump was covered by a neurovascular island flap. He did very well after the procedure and returned to work. The sensation over the stump was excellent and central nervous system orientation was achieved in about 6 weeks. (From Srivastava and Kahl, ref. 1, with permission.)

OPERATIVE TECHNIQUE

Beginning proximally at the level of the proposed amputation, the neurovascular bundle or bundles are isolated along with some vein-bearing areolar tissue. The island flap includes the full thickness of skin and padding.

After the amputation is completed, the stump is covered by the island flap without any twisting. It is then sutured in place without any undue pressure on the redundant neurovascular bundle (Fig. 1C).

In the postoperative period, some congestion of the flap may occur, which should clear gradually in 4 to 5 days, as long as the hand is kept constantly elevated.

CLINICAL RESULTS

As long as there is no twisting or kinking of the neurovascular pedicle, and as long as the skin island is large enough to cover the amputated stump loosely, there should be no problem with flap necrosis.

Since the nerve is not sectioned, there is no problem with neuroma formation.

After the flap heals, sensibility in the transferred skin is felt to originate from the tip of the amputated finger, but with time and use (in about 6 to 8 weeks), central nervous system adaptability allows a change in allegiance to the reconstructed unit (Fig. 2).

SUMMARY

The special tactile area of the finger can be preserved as a neurovascular island flap to cover the stump to elective finger amputations.

References

1. Srivastava RK, Kahl JB. Shifting neurovascular island flap for the reconstruction of amputated digital stump. *Plast Reconstr Surg* 1980;66:301.
2. Eaton RG. The digital neurovascular bundle: a microanatomic study of its contents. *Clin Orthop* 1968;61:176.

CHAPTER 238 ■ TRANSPOSITION SKIN FLAP FROM THE SIDE OF A FINGER

D. P. GREEN

A transposition flap consists of a rectangular segment of skin and subcutaneous tissue that is turned on its pivot point to reach the defect to be closed. The side of the proximal phalanx of a finger is an ideal donor site for such a flap because of the redundant skin present there, an observation easily verified by pinching the skin distal to the web. This consistent anatomic feature allows a skin flap 12 to 15 mm wide to be taken from this area and the donor site to be closed primarily without the need for a skin graft (1–10) (Fig. 1).

INDICATIONS

The ideal indication for this flap is an isolated, broad scar crossing the volar aspect of the MP joint (Figs. 1A and 2), but it can also be used, in conjunction with Z-plasties, to deal with more extensive scars involving the entire digit. When the flap is used for more extensive scars, however, careful planning of the extended incisions is necessary, to protect the blood supply of the flaps.

The flap is also useful in patients with Dupuytren's contracture in whom the distance between the volar MP and PIP flexion creases is significantly decreased (Fig. 3) or there is severe skin involvement (dimpling) at the MP level.

FLAP DESIGN AND DIMENSIONS

The flap is drawn on the finger, extending from a point level with the most proximal volar MP crease to the PIP joint (Fig. 1B), a distance of 2.0 to 2.5 cm in the average adult hand. The ulnar side of the finger is preferred as the donor site (10), although if the scar to be released lies more to the radial aspect of the MP flexion crease, the radial side of the finger should be used as the donor site. The proximal half of the flap is 12 to 15 mm in width, gradually tapering to a blunt angle at the distal end. The volar margin of the flap forms a right angle with a relaxing incision in the volar MP crease that is now made across the full width of the finger to allow it to be straightened (Fig. 1B). Of course, care must be taken to protect the neurovascular bundle.

The ideal width-to-length ratio of the flap is 1:1.5 (11), although 1:2 is generally safe. Exceeding this 1:2 ratio is likely to lead to necrosis of the tip of the flap.

OPERATIVE TECHNIQUE

After the scar contracture is released through a transverse volar incision, an elliptical defect remains across the base of the finger (Fig. 1C).

The flap is raised along a plane between the superficial and deep fascia (Fig. 1C), and the base is mobilized sufficiently to allow it to be rotated 90° to cover the elliptical defect. It is not necessary to bring the tip of the flap completely across the base of the finger; in fact, care should be taken to avoid excessive tension on the flap. A longitudinal suture line across the MP crease is avoided by the tapered configuration of the tip of the flap.

The donor site is closed primarily by advancing the volar and dorsolateral skin margins toward each other, leaving the suture line in the desirable midlateral position (Fig. 1D). The use of a skin graft to cover the donor site is not necessary. In some cases it is desirable to leave a triangular defect measuring 2 to 3 mm on each side at the proximal junction where the distal edge of the rotated flap joins the midlateral incision. It is preferable to leave this small area open, rather than to create excessive tension on the flap by attempting perfect closure of the wound. The small defect is usually completely healed by the time the sutures are removed at 10 to 14 days.

No postoperative immobilization is required; active range of motion of the finger is started on the first or second day, after the initial dressing is changed.

CLINICAL RESULTS

In my experience complications have been very infrequent with the proper use of this flap. The donor site heals as a linear scar that does not produce a contracture, since it lies very nearly in the midaxial line of the digit. Necrosis of the tip of the flap may result from excessive tension in closing the donor site and, as noted previously, it is preferable to leave open a small triangular defect at the junction of the flap and the donor site closure, rather than to try to achieve complete skin apposition. Minimal necrosis of the tip of the flap has occurred in a few patients, but these small areas heal by secondary intention. In no patient has a resulting scar contracture across the volar aspect of the MP joint been seen, and in no patient was a subsequent skin graft required.

SUMMARY

A transposition skin flap can be used from the side of the finger to release a volar skin contracture. The donor site can be closed primarily.

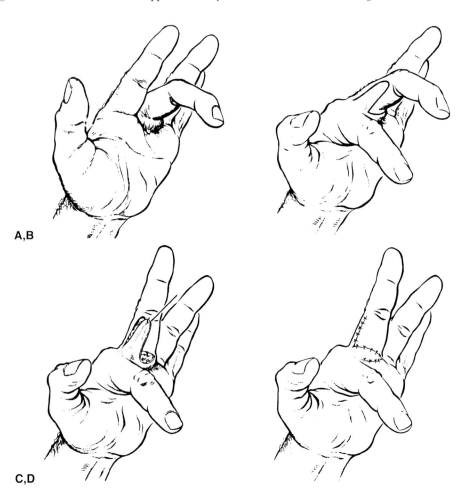

A,B

C,D

FIG. 1. **A:** A scar contracture across the volar aspect of the metacarpophalangeal flexion crease. **B:** The flap is outlined on the side of the digit, its volar limb forming a right angle with a transverse incision across the metacarpophalangeal flexion crease. The flap itself should be approximately 12 to 15 mm in width. **C:** The flap is mobilized on a plane between the deep and superficial fascia. The subcutaneous fat is left attached to the skin flap, and the neurovascular bundle is identified and protected. **D:** The flap is rotated 90° into the elliptical defect created by release of the flexion contracture, and the donor site is closed primarily. No skin graft is required. (From Green and Dominguez, ref. 9, with permission.)

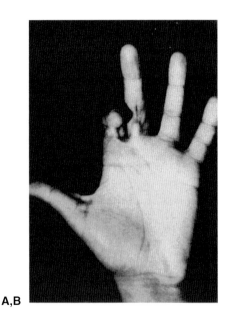
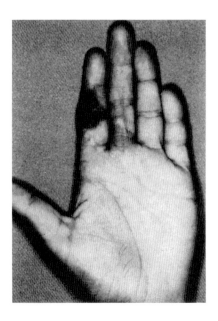

A,B

FIG. 2. **A:** The ideal indication for this flap is a scar across the volar aspect of the metacarpophalangeal flexion crease, as seen in this patient's long finger. The scar in the index finger extends beyond the proximal interphalangeal joint and is too extreme to be corrected with a transposition flap. **B:** The scar in the long finger has been corrected with a transposition flap from the radial side of the finger. A full-thickness skin graft was used to correct the more extensive scar contracture in the index finger.

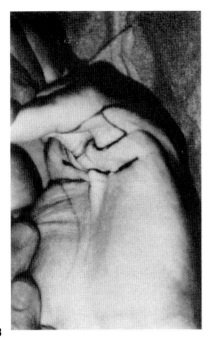 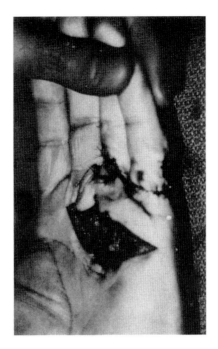

A,B

FIG. 3. **A:** Transposition flaps were used in the ring and small fingers of this patient with Dupuytren's contracture. Note the marked decrease in skin distance between the metacarpophalangeal and proximal interphalangeal creases. **B:** The volar aspects of the metacarpophalangeal creases were covered with transposition flaps from the ulnar side of the small finger and the radial side of the ring finger. The palmar wound was treated with the open technique.

References

1. Tanzer RC. Correction of interdigital burn contractures of the hand. *Plast Reconstr Surg* 1948;3:434.
2. Lewin ML. Digital flaps. *Plast Reconstr Surg* 1951;7:46.
3. Burian, F. *The plastic surgery atlas*. New York: Macmillan, 1968;177.
4. Joshi BB. Dorsolateral flap from the same finger to relieve flexion contracture. *Plast Reconstr Surg* 1972;49:186.
5. Dean RK, Kelleher JC, Sullivan JG, Baibak GJ. Reconstruction of the dorsal and palmar surfaces of the hand with local skin flaps. In: Grabb WC, Myers MB, eds. *Skinflaps*. Boston: Little, Brown, 1975;489–491.
6. MacDougal B, Wray RC, Weeks, PM. Lateral-volar finger flap for the treatment of burn syndactyly. *Plast Reconstr Surg* 1976;57:167.
7. Brinkman JF. Local rotation flap. *American Society for Surgery of the hand correspondence club newsletter*. No. 39, 1978.
8. Howard LD. Rotational flaps. American Academy of Orthopedic Surgeons, Instructional Course Lecture, unpublished.
9. Green DP, Dominguez OJ. A transpositional flap for release of volar contractures of a finger at the MP joint. *Plast Reconstr Surg* 1979;64:516.
10. Russell RC, Van Beek AL, Wavak P, Zook EG. Alternative hand flaps for amputations and digital defects. *J Hand Surg* 1981;6:399.
11. Thompson RVS. Closure of skin defects near the proximal interphalangeal joint, with special reference to the patterns of finger circulation. *Plast Reconstr Surg* 1977;59:77.

CHAPTER 239 ■ LATERAL FINGER ROTATION SKIN FLAP

H. W. LUEDERS

The lateral finger rotation skin flap is used primarily to interrupt a scar on the dorsal surface of the finger, thereby providing the joint surface with good mobile skin (1).

INDICATIONS

The lateral finger rotation flap can be used to reconstruct both the volar and the dorsal surfaces of the finger. Primary uses for the dorsally placed flap are for reconstruction of the fingers after a heavy burn eschar has been excised, for traumatic avulsion of skin over the PIP joint and tendon, and for covering the burned hand early over the PIP joint to prevent the granulomatous rupture of the extensor tendon and hood (2–7).

An advantage of the flap is that it simulates the original skin over the dorsum of the joint and retains some of the inherent qualities of resistance to trauma and of elasticity of motion. It often has sensation. The direction of the rotated flap breaks up the longitudinal scar on the dorsum of the finger.

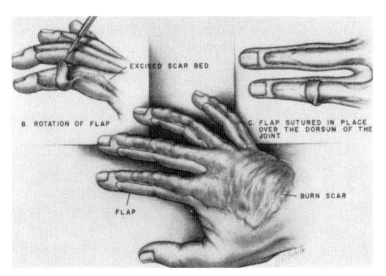

FIG. 1. Flaps are designed over the lateral surfaces of the middle phalanges. Note that the flap includes only undamaged skin. After the dorsal scar is excised, the flap is rotated to cover the proximal interphalangeal adjacent joint. The remaining raw areas are covered with split-thickness skin grafts. (From Lueders and Shapiro, ref. 1, with permission.)

ANATOMY

The circulation of the flap is derived principally from the dorsal digital vessel complex, with minimal contributions from the volar complex.

FLAP DESIGN AND DIMENSIONS

After resection of the burn scar bridle on the dorsum of the hand and finger, the flaps are designed and elevated (Fig. 1). The flaps are proximally based and extend on the lateral side from the proximal interphalangeal joint to or beyond the distal interphalangeal joint. The length of the flap is determined by the width of the finger over the proximal interphalangeal joint, from the midlateral line on the opposite side to the volar line on the flap side. The point of rotation is just proximal to the proximal interphalangeal joint. The width of the flap is from the volar line to the dorsal scar excision.

OPERATIVE TECHNIQUE

With the finger flexed, the flap is rotated over the dorsum of the proximal interphalangeal joint, in such a position as to protect the joint from trauma. The flaps are tested in flexion and extension to see that they do not restrict motion, and then they are sutured.

The donor defect and dorsum are covered with a thick split-thickness skin graft. For the traumatic avulsion injury, a full-thickness graft is preferred. Pressure on the graft is secured by a tie-over bolster dressing, but placing tie-over sutures in the flap should be avoided. The finger is bandaged in the neutral position for 4 to 5 days. The grafts and flaps are examined and, if the grafts are dry, the tie-over dressings are kept in place for another 5 days. If the grafts are stable and the flaps adherent, passive to active motion is allowed.

CLINICAL RESULTS

A disadvantage of this flap is that it requires that the skin on the side of the finger be relatively undamaged. To cover the

joint from one side to another, a flap of great length is necessary. The use of a short radial and ulnar side flap of equal or unequal length could be substituted, but it reintroduces a vertical scar over the dorsal joint surface.

Flap loss has not occurred, and flap morbidity is related to the condition and amount of injury to the lateral skin. Postoperative follow-up shows the flaps to be able to withstand considerable trauma occurring with manual labor, or even with exposure to chemicals. The dog-ear on the proximal side is useful as additional skin, which is necessary for flexion of the finger. After a time the flaps develop transverse wrinkles, just like normal skin, and the hands are left cosmetically acceptable. The most vexing postoperative problem is associated with the skin graft at the junction of the thinner split-thickness graft and the thicker volar palmar skin. The skin graft is intolerant of additional trauma and the junction may crack and become irritated. The callous capability of the skin graft is different and leaves very rough skin that is difficult to clean.

SUMMARY

The lateral finger rotation skin flap is used to cover defects in the dorsum of the finger. It is especially useful for covering the PIP joint in burned hands.

References

1. Lueders HW, Shapiro RL. Reconstruction of burned hands. *Plast Reconstr Surg* 1971;47:176.
2. Flynn JE. Burned and traumatic hands. *Arch Surg* 1947;54:249.
3. Tanzer RC. Reconstruction of the burned hand. *N Engl J Med* 1948; 238:687.
4. Braithwaite F, Watson J. Some observations on the treatment of the dorsal burn of the hand. *Br J Plast Surg* 1949;2:21.
5. Lewin ML. Digital flaps. *Plast Reconstr Surg* 1951;7:46.
6. Peacock EE. Management of the burned hand. *South Med J* 1963;56:1094.
7. Maisels DO. Middle slip or boutonniere deformity in burned hands. *Br J Plast Surg* 1965;18:117.

CHAPTER 240 ■ BIPEDICLE STRAP FLAPS OF THE FINGER

N. W. YII AND D. ELLIOT

EDITORIAL COMMENT

These flaps are particularly useful in longitudinal dorsal defects. Particular attention should be paid to critical aspects of the border digits; flaps should be elevated on the opposite side of the digit first, to avoid potential sensory deficits and painful scars.

Dorsal skin defects in which the loss of integument is longitudinal in shape are not uncommon after injury by rotating machinery and by glass shearing along the length of the digit. This shape of the defect is difficult to reconstruct with commonly used flaps but lends itself to reconstruction by the use of longitudinal bipedicle strap flaps moved across the dorsum of the finger from lateral to medial (1).

INDICATIONS

The procedure is recommended for longitudinal defects on the dorsum of the fingers and thumbs.

ANATOMY

Recent anatomic studies (2–5) have confirmed earlier work by Levame et al. (6), demonstrating that there is an arterial network similar to that of the veins in the dorsal subcutaneous tissue of the digits, with multiple feeding arteries from the palmar digital arteries linking into the dorsal network around the lateral borders of the digit. Although the dorsum does not have such an immediately obvious arterial structure as the palmar aspect of the digits, this network is extensive, explaining the excellent vascularity of longitudinal bipedicle strap flaps.

FLAP DESIGN AND DIMENSIONS

Because the dorsum of the digit is a convex surface, and the injuring object presents a flat surface to this convexity, the deep structures are exposed only along and immediately adjacent to the midline, with the wound becoming progressively shallower laterally (Fig. 1). Adjacent to the central zone of complete loss of the integument is a zone of variable width, in which the subcutaneous fat is preserved with skin loss only. The extreme dorsolateral integument commonly is uninjured. Although portions of the dorsolateral tissues over which the skin is preserved are, by themselves, often too narrow to create bipedicle flaps that can be fabricated successfully in the midline, inclusion of the intermediate zone of the dorsolateral soft tissue, over which only the skin has been lost, makes the longitudinal bipedicle flaps wider, the central defect smaller, and the technique more applicable.

OPERATIVE TECHNIQUE

Dorsal bipedicle strap flaps may be raised on any part of the digit. They may be raised safely to any length, although it is unusual to require reconstructing defects longer than two phalanges in length. A midlateral incision is first made on one side of the digit, and Cleland's ligaments are divided to allow one lateral strap of subcutaneous tissue and skin to move medially (Fig. 2). When possible, we select the "concealed" side of the digit as the donor site of the first flap, although the midlateral incisions heal so well that this is probably an unnecessary precaution. In releasing Cleland's ligaments, care is taken to preserve the dorsal branches of the digital nerve, which provide innervation of the flap. It is not necessary to preserve the dorsal branches of the digital artery if they impede the medial movement of the flap. Through the midline of the dorsal wound, the integument is mobilized in the plane between the extensor paratenon and the undersurface of the subcutaneous fat. If one flap is not sufficient to close the central defect, the other lateral flap is raised in the same manner. The subcutaneous tissue is sutured with an absorbable suture in the midline.

Skin defects, whether on the dorsal or lateral aspects of the digits, are dressed with moist, antiseptic dressings until epithelialization is complete (Fig. 3). This does not impede immediate mobilization of the digits. Another advantage of the open lateral wounds has been the rapid elimination of the edema that always accompanies digital injuries and that is usually retained after reconstruction with flaps in which there is complete skin closure. Complete epithelialization of the dorsal wounds usually takes between 2 and 6 weeks, with the lateral wounds healing within 2 to 4 weeks.

CLINICAL RESULTS

In a series of 28 longitudinal dorsal digital defects, a single flap was used in 9 digits (32%), and both flaps were mobilized in 19 digits (68%) (1). There were no flap failures, complete or partial, and none of the flaps exhibited any feature of circulatory difficulty at any time. The patients were followed up for a mean of 8.4 months (range: 2 to 25 months). All wounds healed uneventfully.

SUMMARY

Dorsal skin defects in which the loss of integument is longitudinal in shape are difficult to reconstruct with commonly used flaps but lend themselves to reconstruction by the use of longitudinal bipedicle strap flaps moved across the dorsum of the finger from lateral to medial. Bipedicle strap flaps are simple and rapid to raise. They add very little time to the procedure,

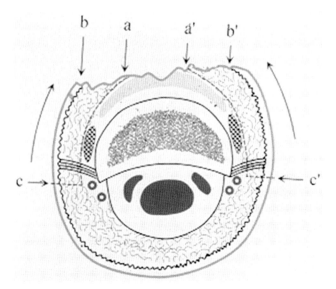

FIG. 1. Transverse section of the finger to illustrate the injury: *a – a'* is the central part of the dorsal wound down to extensor tendon; *b – b'* indicates the width of the skin loss exposing tendon centrally but only subcutaneous fat laterally; *c* and *c'* are the lateral incisions made at surgery, with the dotted lines *c – a* and *c' – a'* indicating the plane of dissection under the bipedicle flaps.

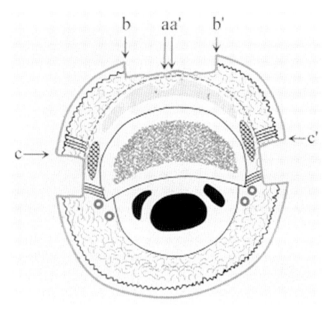

FIG. 2. The same section showing the tissues after movement of the bipedicled flaps medially to allow suture of the subcutaneous fat *(a a')* over the exposed tendon.

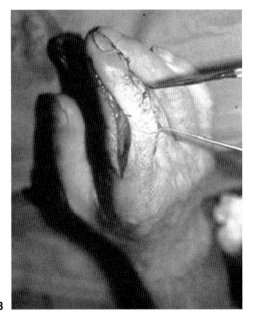

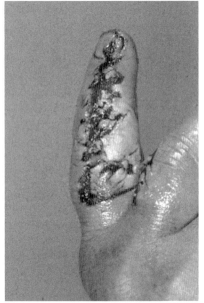

A,B

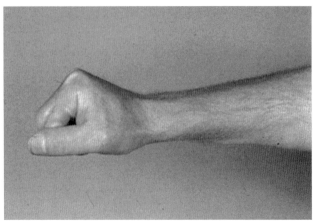

C

FIG. 3. **A:** A single radial bipedicle flap raised and mobilized to cover the exposed extensor tendon dorsally. **B:** The finger several days after reconstruction. The central skin defect dorsally and the lateral wound are dressed three times daily with moist antiseptic dressings, which are removed to allow vigorous mobilization after cleaning. **C:** Late lateral view to show healed wound.

which is useful when reconstruction of the deeper structures has been complex and time-consuming.

Because mobilization is possible from the first postoperative day, the reconstruction contributes little to the functional morbidity of the injury and to surgery. Furthermore, the use of local tissue adjacent to the primary defect, in conjunction with the technique of skin healing by secondary intention on both the dorsal and lateral aspects of the digit, honor the principle of reconstructing "like with like" to a greater degree than with the use of flaps taken from elsewhere, and achieve a good cosmetic result with minimal donor-site scarring. This also obviates the need to disfigure the dorsum of the digits with the bulky and shapeless flaps that have been the hallmark of larger reconstructions of this region in the past.

References

1. Yii NW, Elliot D. Bipedicle strap flaps in reconstruction of longitudinal dorsal skin defects of the digits. *Plast Reconstr Surg* 1999;103:1205.
2. Endo T, Kojima T, Hirase Y. Vascular anatomy of the finger dorsum and new idea for coverage of the finger pulp defect that restores sensation. *J Hand Surg (Am)* 1992;17:927.
3. Del Bene M, Petrolate M, Raimondi P, et al. Reverse dorsal digital island flap. *Plast Reconstr Surg* 1994;93:552.
4. Tremolada C, Abbiate G, Del Bene M, Blandini D. The subcutaneous laterodigital reverse flap. *Plast Reconstr Surg* 1998;101:1070.
5. Strauch B, de Moura W. Arterial system of the fingers. *J Hand Surg (Am)* 1990;15:148.
6. Levame JH, Otero C, Berdugo G. Vascularisation arterielle des teguments de la face dorsale de la main et des doigts. *Ann Chir Plast* 1967;12:316.

CHAPTER 241 ■ AXIAL FLAG SKIN FLAP

G. D. LISTER

EDITORIAL COMMENT

Lengthening the flap pole would maintain the axial vascularity of the flap and, at the same time, would facilitate the transposition and increase the versatility of the flap.

Since the axial flag flap can be rotated like any other island flap through a full circle, it can be brought to cover defects not only over the dorsum of the proximal phalanx or metacarpophalangeal joint of either finger forming the web, but also over the *palmar* surface of the same structures (see Fig. 3A,B). A standard cross-finger flap will cover only one of these eight surfaces, namely the palmar aspect of the proximal phalanx of the adjacent finger (1).

INDICATIONS

The axial flap is of particular value in covering combined lateral and palmar defects (see Fig. 4A).

ANATOMY

The axial flag skin flap, as used thus far, consists of the skin of the dorsal aspect of the proximal phalanx of the finger. The arterial supply comes from the arcade that is formed in the web space by the communication between the proper digital and the dorsal metacarpal arteries (Fig. 1). The dorsal metacarpal arteries arise from the dorsal carpal arch, which is formed by branches of the radial, ulnar, and anterior interosseous arteries (2). They run deep to the extensor tendons on the fascia of the interosseous muscles. At the metacarpophalangeal joint they pass on to the superficial aspect of the extensor hood, where they arborize. One branch passes in a palmar direction through the web space to anastomose with the proper digital artery (3). The other branches of this arcade serve the skin of the dorsal proximal phalanx, communicating thereby with the identical system on the other aspect of the digit. Reliable flow distally goes only as far as the distal extension crease of the proximal interphalangeal joint (2,4). The dorsal metacarpal arteries are not always present in all fingers. In order of decreasing incidence, they appear in the second, first, fourth, and third interspaces. Thus the flap can be raised most confidently on the middle and index fingers.

The venous drainage follows a similar pattern (Fig. 2), the dominant dorsal venous system forming a "bridle" vein, which is an arch over the proximal phalanx some 1 to 2 cm distal to the metacarpophalangeal joint. From this, two dominant veins arise from either end of the arch—that is, on either side of the finger—and pass proximally between the metacarpophalangeal joints, to gain the dorsum of the hand superficial to the extensor tendons. Each of these veins is joined by a web space branch coming from the palmar aspect and, under normal circumstances, carrying flow in that direction (5).

FLAP DESIGN AND DIMENSIONS

With the above anatomic knowledge, an axial flap can be raised, employing the vessels of any web space as the pedicle. (This pedicle on the radial aspect of the index finger supplies the island skin flap to the thumb described in Chap. 273 [4].) Since the pedicle is only as wide as the supplying vessels, the flap can be rotated like any other island flap through a full circle. The selected web space therefore constitutes the pivot point of the axial flag flap (Fig. 3).

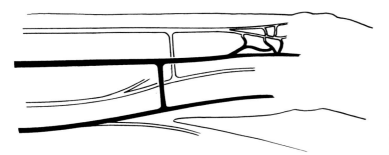

FIG. 1. The dorsal metacarpal artery communicates with the proper digital artery by a web space branch, thereby forming an arcade from which vessels arise to serve the dorsal skin over the proximal phalanx.

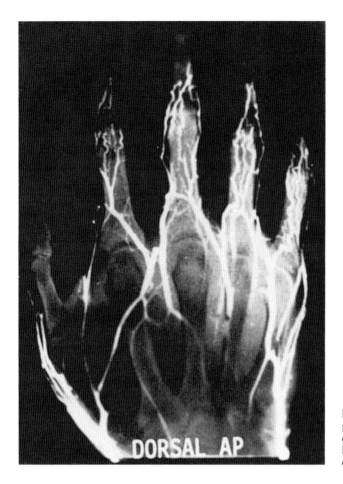

FIG. 2. Here in an injection angiogram the venous drainage of the proximal phalanx can be seen. A number of veins join to form a "bridle" vein over the junction of proximal and middle thirds of the phalanx, from which two major branches proceed proximally on either side of the metacarpophalangeal joint.

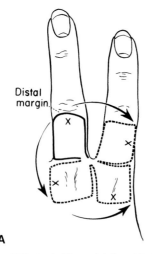

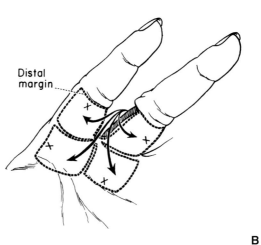

A   B

FIG. 3. A: The axial flag skin flap can be rotated through 360° on the dorsum, thereby covering the proximal phalanx of the adjacent finger and the metacarpophalangeal joints both of that finger and of the donor finger. B: The flap can also be carried down through the web space to cover the palmar aspect of the same four locations. (From Lister, ref. 1, with permission.)

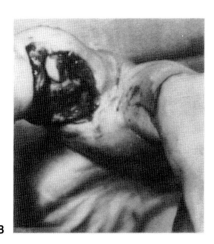
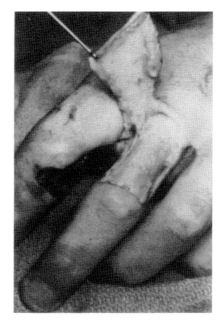

A,B

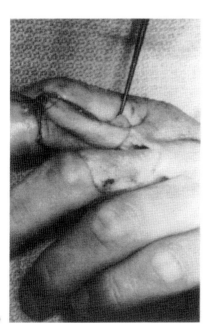
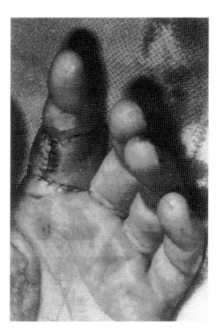

C,D

FIG. 4. **A:** In this case a defect with exposure of the proximal interphalangeal joint on the index finger extends over the lateral and palmar aspects of the index finger. **B:** An axial flag skin flap has been raised on the dorsum of the proximal phalanx of the adjacent middle finger. It is elevated on all four sides, with the exception of a small pedicle at the proximal radial aspect. **C:** The flap is rotated and transposed to cover the defect on the adjacent index finger. **D:** The flap is sutured in position and can here be seen to be well perfused and to cover adequately the palmar as well as the lateral aspect of the defect. A full-thickness skin graft is applied to the secondary defect, and healing occurred uneventfully. (From Lister, ref. 1, with permission.)

The dual palmar and dorsal supply and drainage outlined above offers some security, but before selecting an axial flag flap for coverage of a proximal wound over either aspect of the metacarpophalangeal joint, care should be taken to ensure that the proper digital and dorsal metacarpal arteries have not been injured. The flap is, of course, designed to fit the defect.

The largest flap available extends from midlateral line to midlateral line and from the base of the proximal phalanx to the proximal extension crease of the proximal interphalangeal joint, thereby avoiding the use of a free skin graft over the articulations. This yields a flap of maximum dimensions, 3.5 × 3.5 cm of the middle finger of an 80-kg male. The surgeon should first confirm by reverse planning with a pattern of suitable material that the flap will reach and cover the defect.

OPERATIVE TECHNIQUE

The proximal margin of the flap should be incised first, carrying the incision down to the extensor tendon. The end of the wound that contains the intended pedicle should then be dissected under magnification, if confirmation of the presence of the requisite artery and vein is desired. Once this has been done, the other three margins can be raised exactly in the manner employed for a cross-finger flap, that is, leaving the epitenon on the extensor but taking all veins with the flap. It is safe, from a vascular viewpoint, to incise all four aspects completely, provided that the pedicle is preserved. This gives maximum mobility and makes the use of the flap a one-stage procedure (Fig. 4A–D).

The pedicle does consist, however, of vessels of relatively small caliber, and there is therefore some merit in preserving a 2-mm skin attachment to protect it from stretch and torsion. This attachment can be divided in the office or clinic under local anesthesia and requires no suturing. Once the flap is raised the tourniquet should be released and perfusion confirmed. The flap can then be inset and a full-thickness skin graft applied to the secondary defect (Fig. 5). As with other axial flaps, motion of adjacent joints can be commenced immediately, if appropriate.

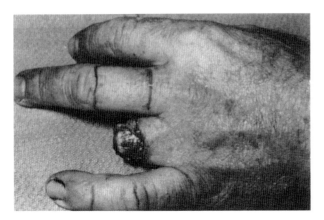 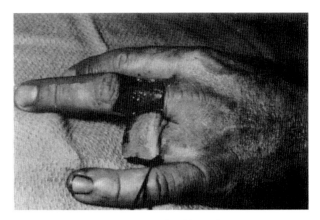

FIG. 5. After grade 3 ring avulsion injury a decision was made that replantation should not be attempted, but maximum length was retained in the amputated digit by employing an axial flag skin flap that covered all aspects of the exposed bone.

CLINICAL RESULTS

All such axial flag flaps have survived in their entirety, barring only one in an 83-year-old patient, which showed superficial necrosis of the distal 20%.

SUMMARY

The axial flag flap consists of the skin on the dorsal aspect of the proximal phalanx of the finger and can be used to cover defects over both the dorsal and volar surfaces of the proxi-mal phalanx or metacarpophalangeal joint of the same or the adjacent finger.

References

1. Lister GD. The theory of the transposition flap and its practical application in the hand. *Clin Plast Surg* 1981;8:115.
2. Johnson MK, Cohen MJ. *The hand atlas.* Springfield: Charles C. Thomas, 1975;55,66.
3. Carlier A, Lister GD. Unpublished data.
4. Foucher G, Braun JB. A new island flap transfer from the dorsum of the index to the thumb. *Plast Reconstr Surg* 1979;63:344.
5. Moss S, Lister GD. Unpublished data.

CHAPTER 242 ■ USE OF THE SEPA FLAP IN THE REPAIR OF DEFECTS IN THE HANDS AND FINGERS

A. D. DIAS

The superficial external pudendal artery (SEPA) flap is an axial-pattern flap based on the superficial external pudendal arteriovenous system. Its usefulness in reconstructive surgery of the hands and fingers has been demonstrated, and it can be raised as a unilateral flap or, when more skin is required, as a bilateral flap.

INDICATIONS

The flap is useful for resurfacing the hand in both dorsal and palmar aspects. When there is a simultaneous loss of both dorsal and palmar skin, the SEPA flap can be used on the dorsum and a flap of the anterior rectus sheath (with split-thickness skin cover) can be used on the palmar side (1,2). The anatomic position of the flap makes it possible to immobilize the hand postoperatively in a more comfortable and natural position than possible with a groin flap. The length and narrowness of the flap allow the patient to move the fingers freely, and also provide considerable freedom during the period of immobilization.

The SEPA flap has also been used in the repair of hypospadias, urinary fistulas, epispadias, degloving injuries of the penis and scrotum, reconstruction of the amputated penis, and following release of groin contractures.

ANATOMY

The superficial external pudendal artery originates from the medial side of the femoral artery at the level of the saphenofemoral junction (3–5). At its origin, the vessel is 2 mm in diameter. It proceeds medially and horizontally, crossing the femoral vein either above the saphenofemoral junction or, with equal frequency, in the angle between the long saphenous and the femoral vein (Fig. 1). Piercing the femoral sheath and the cribriform fascia, it proceeds medially and upward toward the pubic tubercle. Here, it gives off penile, scrotal, or labial branches, and a variable number of small ascending branches toward the superficial inguinal ring. One of the latter branches occasionally enters the inguinal canal. At this point, the vessel is just superficial to Scarpa's fascia.

It then continues upward toward the umbilicus, gradually becoming more superficial (Fig. 2). There are two constant sites of well-developed cross circulation, useful in the bilateral flap: they are at one-quarter and one-half the distance between the symphysis pubis and the umbilicus. Halfway between the symphysis and the umbilicus, the SEPA rapidly branches out into three to four longitudinal vessels, which arborize to form a subdermal plexus in the juxta-umbilical region. On the lateral side, the vessel anastomoses freely with branches of the superficial epigastric artery. The veins follow the arterial pattern, and a pair of venae comitantes accompany the SEPA.

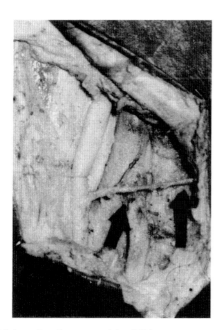

FIG. 1. Origin and early course of the SEPA.

FLAP DESIGN AND DIMENSIONS

The anterior superior iliac spine, the pubic tubercle, and the proximal part of the femoral artery are marked; the full length of the SEPA is marked next (Fig. 3). The midline is marked upward from the pubis to just below the umbilicus. The length of this line can be decreased, according to the requirements of the case. From the upper end of the midline, a horizontal line is drawn laterally for about 3.8 cm. A vertical line is then dropped from the lateral end of the horizontal line; this vertical line reaches down to the level of the pubic tubercle, but stays at least 19 to 25 mm lateral to it. Instead of a horizontal line just described, a sloping line can be outlined for particular digital defects. Using a bilateral flap, similar markings are made on the contralateral side; a bilateral flap can also be designed with halves of unequal length, again meeting the requirements of particular digital defects.

OPERATIVE TECHNIQUE

General anesthesia is commonly used, although local anesthesia has been suitable for unilateral flaps, making it easier to immobilize the hand postoperatively. The flap is cut according to the design and modifications described above. With bilateral flaps, the midline incision is omitted. The length of the flap is adjusted to the requirements of the case; a "cut as you need" approach should be adopted. The thickness of the flap should be in accordance with the anatomy described. As the flap is prepared, perforating vessels of the inferior epigastric artery are encountered on their way to the skin; as many as necessary of these vessels can be cut safely. (No undue postoperative edema has been noted in these flaps, indicating adequate venous and lymphatic drainage.)

The axial vessel is divided on postoperative day 10, and the flap is detached and inset in the third postoperative week. Flap detachment after 15 days is possible, if the initial inset is almost complete. In those cases where the axial vessel cannot be sectioned for technical reasons prior to detachment of the flap, no untoward effect has been noted.

The position of the flap in relation to the hand makes it possible to immobilize the hand postoperatively in a comfortable position. This is especially so when a unilateral flap is used, as it is long and narrow, and can be rotated up to 180° on either side, avoiding the need for rigid postoperative immobilization. A bilateral flap provides a width of about 10 cm. The donor site of a unilateral flap can always be closed by direct suture. With a bilateral flap, the donor site requires a skin graft, after reducing the raw surface by marginal sutures.

The mobility of the flap makes it possible to use it either on the dorsal or palmar surface of the hand. The flap can also be deepithelialized and applied, as required, to the palmar surface of the hand and fingers. Although the presence of hair in the lower part of the flap is a disadvantage, this problem can be decreased, as the upper part of the flap is utilized most of the time. In extreme cases, the hair-bearing skin can be excised, and a split-thickness skin graft applied over the subcutaneous fat.

CLINICAL RESULTS

The SEPA flap has been used to cover exposed tendons, phalanges, metacarpals, and metacarpophalangeal and interphalangeal joints. The unilateral flap is used predominantly on the digits (Fig. 4), while the bilateral flap is used on the hands (Fig. 5). The bilateral flap has also been used as a tubed flap to cover a totally degloved thumb or finger, and for the reconstruction of a new thumb. When used for multiple fingers, these are syndactylized prior to flap application. The flap has

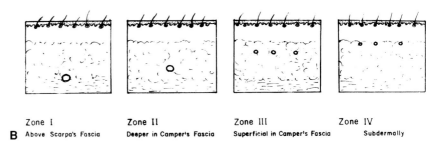

Zone I	Zone II	Zone III	Zone IV
Above Scarpa's Fascia	Deeper in Camper's Fascia	Superficial in Camper's Fascia	Subdermally

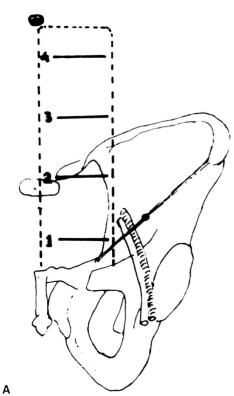

FIG. 2. **A,B:** Progressive depth of the artery. The vessels become more superficial in their course to the umbilicus.

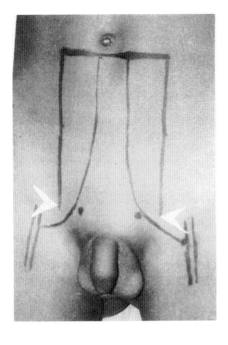

FIG. 3. Design of bilateral SEPA flaps. (From Dias et al., ref. 4, with permission.)

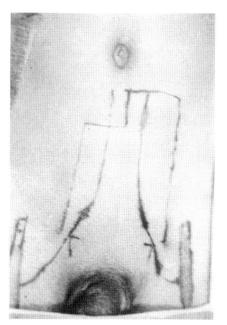
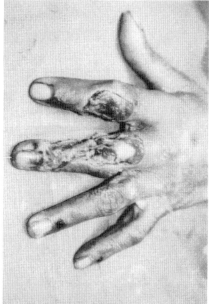
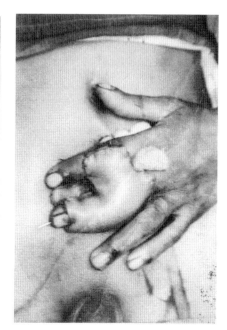

A–C

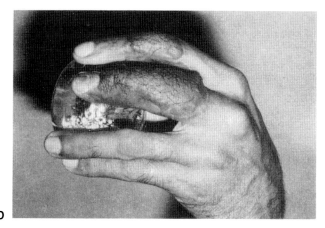

D

FIG. 4. A–D: Use of unequal bilateral flaps for multiple finger sites. (From Dias et al., ref. 4, with permission.)

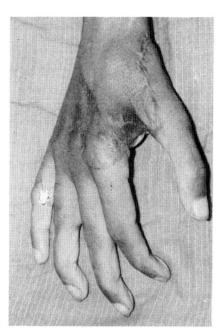
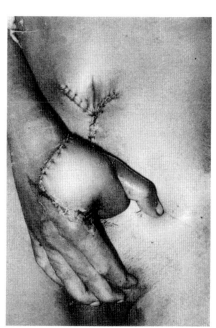
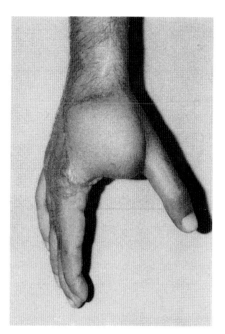

A–C

FIG. 5. A–C: Correction of adduction contracture between thumb and index finger. (From Dias et al., ref. 4, with permission.)

also been utilized in a wraparound fashion for the finger, when both dorsal and palmar surfaces are exposed. The unilateral flap has been used to correct adduction contractures between thumb and index fingers.

The SEPA flap can be used by itself, or combined with a groin flap or a superficial epigastric artery flap, to cover large avulsion injuries of the thumb, fingers, and hand. Its use with the anterior rectus sheath with split-thickness skin coverage has been mentioned previously. For old dorsal injuries of the hand, where extensor tendons are involved in the scar, the skin has been replaced with a SEPA flap, and an anterior rectus sheath flap as a separate layer has been placed under the tendons.

Early mobilization has been vigorously pursued (2). Functional results have been most encouraging, but have varied according to the severity of the injury. The quality of the primary skin coverage contributes greatly to good functional results, and makes any further required reconstructive work on bones or tendons easier. Subsequent defatting of some flaps has been necessary. In the series reported, three flaps were lost due to gross infection from contamination at the time of injury.

SUMMARY

The SEPA flap, which is reliable, safe, and versatile, is a useful addition to the repertoire of the reconstructive surgeon.

References

1. Thatte RL, Patil UA, Dhami LD. The combined use of the superficial external pudendal artery flap with a flap of the anterior rectus sheath for the simultaneous cover of dorsal and volar defects of the hand. *Br J Plast Surg* 1986;39:321.
2. Thatte RL, Patil UA. Flap skin cover in the hand: three new additions. In: Boswick, ed., *Upper extremity surgery and rehabilitation*. Rockville: Aspen, 1986.
3. Patil UA, Dias AD, Thatte RL. The anatomical basis of the SEPA flap. *Br J Plast Surg* 1987;40:342.
4. Dias AD, Thatte RL, Patil UA, et al. The uses of the SEPA flap in the repair of defects of the hands and fingers. *Br J Plast Surg* 1987;40:348.
5. Dias AD. The superficial external pudendal artery (SEPA) axial pattern flap. *Br J Plast Surg* 1984;37:256.

CHAPTER 243 ■ DORSOLATERAL NEUROVASCULAR SKIN FLAP OF THE FINGER

B. B. JOSHI

Local dorsolateral flaps from either side of the finger can be used for volar defects. The flap provides both cover and sensation (1–3). Deficiency of skin from one-half to three-quarters of the proximal or middle segment of the finger can be replaced by local dorsolateral flaps.

INDICATIONS

This flap can be used in multiple finger contractures and in skin loss over the volar aspect of the digits when multiple fingers are involved. It has the advantages of being a one-stage procedure, involving only the injured digit and offering a large and relatively expandable donor area for the reconstruction of the more important volar surface of the fingers.

If a digital vessel is thrombosed, even on one side, the procedure should not be attempted because it may jeopardize the circulation of the finger that is already deficient. Proper selection of cases and establishing the patency of the volar digital vessels are prerequisites for the procedure.

ANATOMY

Adjacent to the base of the proximal phalanx, each collateral volar digital nerve gives off a dorsal branch that joins the dorsal digital branches of the radial or ulnar nerve and supplies the skin on the dorsal surface of the fingers. These are accompanied by branches of the digital vessels. Together these make possible a flap based on a specific neurovascular attachment on either side, over the dorsolateral surface of the finger. This flap can be shaped and swung volarly to provide a fully innervated prehensile surface for the area deficient in skin. The venous drainage of the flap is usually excellent, because most of the veins in the fingers are on the dorsal surface. The vascularity of flaps from the dorsum has already been emphasized by several authors (4,5).

FLAP DESIGN AND DIMENSIONS

Requirements for the size and shape of the flap would depend on the defect that is created after the release of the

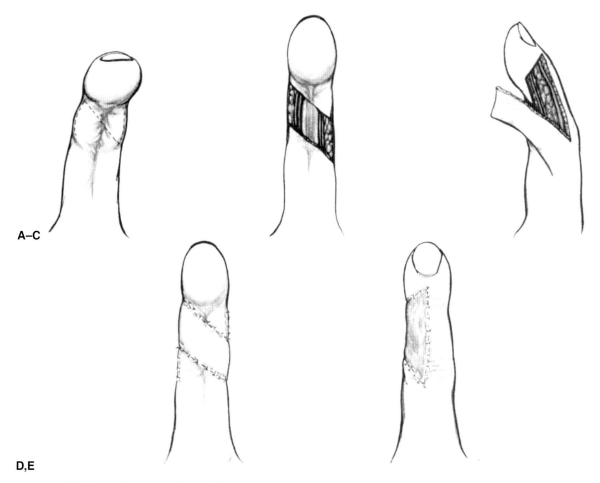

A–C

D,E

FIG. 1. A: Design for release of flexion contracture. B: Resulting defect with exposure of underlying structures. C: Elevation of the dorsolateral flap. D: The flap inset. E: The donor site covered with a split-thickness skin graft. (From Joshi, ref. 1, with permission.)

contracture. It is usually 1.5 to 2 cm in width and 2 to 3 cm in length.

A flap is designed on the dorsolateral aspect of the finger with the midlateral incision as its volar boundary and the dorsal midline as its dorsal boundary. Distally the flap can be extended up to the crease of the distal interphalangeal joint (Fig. 1C).

OPERATIVE TECHNIQUE

Recipient Site

Midlateral incisions are made over either side of the finger, joining the distal interphalangeal and proximal interphalangeal flexion creases. These may be extended proximally and/or distally, if needed, to expose volar digital neurovascular bundles in a healthy area. The neurovascular bundles are freed from scar.

An oblique incision is made over the middle segment of the finger, joining the two midlateral incisions to convert them into an *N* or its reverse, according to the requirements of the dorsoulnar or dorsoradial flap. The scarred skin is not excised. The finger is straightened by dissecting the involved structures and by using gentle force to overcome the contracture (Fig. 2). If a contracture of the flexor sheath needs to be released, the tendon will be exposed.

Donor Site

The flap is raised along with deep fascia, leaving only flimsy areolar tissue over the extensor expansion to envelop and protect the dorsal digital vessels and nerves. Special care should be taken while dissecting near the base of the flap where the vessels and nerves branch off from the volar neurovascular bundle, by limiting dissection on the volar boundary of the flap.

The flap is sutured over the volar aspect and the donor site is covered with a free skin graft held by a tie-over dressing.

The finger is splinted with the interphalangeal joints held in extension and the metacarpophalangeal joint in flexion, to avoid tension on the digital neurovascular bundles.

CLINICAL RESULTS

Necrosis of the transposed flap can occur in a few instances. This may be due to an accidental injury to the dorsal branch of the volar neurovascular bundle at the proximal part of the dissection. Poor selection of cases where dorsal skin has scanty subcutaneous padding can also lead to necrosis of the flap due to insufficient circulation. This is avoidable if a doubtful flap is delayed before transfer and the operation is completed as a two-stage procedure. In about 5% of cases, superficial blister or marginal necrosis of the flap occurs, but these heal subsequently and show some depigmentation of the new skin.

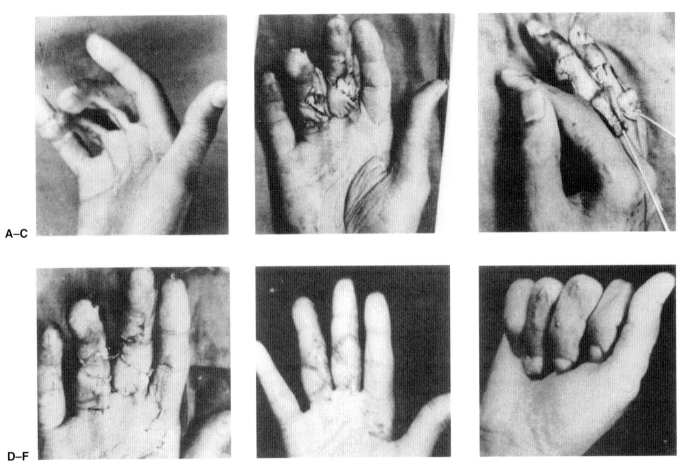

A–C

D–F

FIG. 2. **A:** Flexion contractures of right middle and ring fingers before correction. **B:** Defects on the volar surfaces created after straightening the fingers. **C:** Raised dorsolateral flaps. **D:** The flaps sutured into the volar defects. **E,F:** Postoperative results. (From Joshi, ref. 1, with permission.)

In a series of 156 cases, 95% had satisfactory results following dorsolateral flaps from the same finger, either to release flexion contractures or to cover traumatic wounds on the volar surface of the fingers.

SUMMARY

The dorsolateral skin flap can provide sensory coverage to volar defects or release volar skin contractures over the proximal and middle phalanges of the same finger.

References

1. Joshi BB. Dorsolateral flap from the same finger to relieve flexion contracture. *Plast Reconstr Surg* 1972;49:186.
2. Joshi BB. A local dorsolateral island flap restoration of sensation after avulsion injury of fingertip pulp. *Plast Reconstr Surg* 1974;54:175.
3. Joshi BB. Sensory flaps for the degloved, mutilated hand. *Hand* 1974; 6:247.
4. Flint MH, Harrison, SH. A local neurovascular flap to repair loss of the digital pulp. *Br J Plast Surg* 1965;18:156.
5. Holevich J. A new method of restoring sensibility to the thumb. *Bone Joint Surg* 1963;45(B):496.

CHAPTER 244 ■ ARTERIALIZED SIDE FINGER FLAPS FOR THE PROXIMAL INTERPHALANGEAL JOINT

R. C. RUSSELL AND E. G. ZOOK

Hand burns requiring skin grafts most commonly involve the dorsal surface. Breakdown of a healed split-thickness skin graft over the proximal interphalangeal joint is a difficult problem to manage. The exposed joint is prone to infection that can destroy gliding surfaces and produce chronic osteomyelitis and loss of the finger. Adjacent fingers, when covered with skin grafts, are unavailable as cross-finger flap donor sites. Further skin grafts over the exposed joint are not feasible.

A proximally based arterialized side finger flap, elevated from the lateral/volar surface of the involved digit, can be rotated dorsally to cover the defect, preserving the joint and finger (1).

ANATOMY

Random pattern flaps of a length sufficient to cover the proximal interphalangeal joint would have a marginal blood supply (2,3). Inclusion of the digital artery creates an axial pattern flap with excellent vascularity. The generous flap blood supply aids in the resolution or prevention of infection and helps prevent joint destruction.

FLAP DESIGN AND DIMENSIONS

The flap is centered over the volar digital neurovascular bundle, preferably on the nondominant side of the finger (Fig. 1A). Based proximally and extending 3 to 5 mm past the distal interphalangeal joint flexion crease, the flap incorporates the digital artery but leaves the digital nerve intact (Fig. 1B). Sensation to the fingertip and to the soft tissue over the distal phalanx is therefore preserved.

OPERATIVE TECHNIQUE

A dorsal incision is first made along the midaxial line, with dissection volarly deep to the neurovascular bundle. The volar skin incision begins along the midline of the digit distally. It is angled away from the midline proximally toward the entry point of the digital artery into the finger at the metacarpophalangeal joint flexion crease (Fig. 1A).

The digital artery is carefully separated from the nerve and elevated with the flap (Fig. 1B). Cleland's and Grayson's ligaments are divided along the length of the digit. The venous drainage accompanying the artery and in the base of the flap is carefully preserved by blunt dissection.

The edges of the dorsal defect surrounding the exposed proximal interphalangeal joint are circumferentially excised,

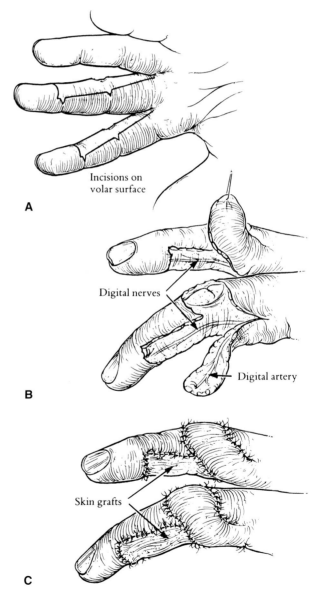

FIG. 1. A: The arterialized side finger flap is centered over the neurovascular bundle on the nondominant side of the finger. The volar incision is darted at the interphalangeal joint flexion creases and angled from the midline distally toward the entry point of the artery into the finger at the metacarpophalangeal joint flexion crease proximally. B: The digital artery is incorporated into the flap, while the digital nerve is left undisturbed. C: Excising the intervening skin bridge, the flap is easily rotated dorsally, to cover the exposed proximal interphalangeal joint.

729

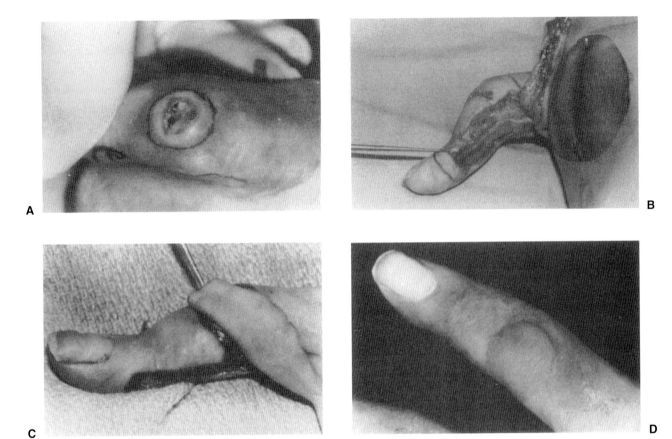

FIG. 2. A: Breakdown of a healed dorsal split-thickness skin graft, with exposure of the proximal interphalangeal joint. **B:** An arterialized side finger flap incorporating the radial digital artery and venae comitantes, but sparing the digital nerve, is elevated from just distal to the distal interphalangeal joint flexion crease. **C:** The flap is rotated dorsally to cover the exposed joint, bringing a generous blood supply to speed healing. **D:** The final result 3 months later, with durable skin and subcutaneous tissue cover. (From Russell et al., ref. 1, with permission.)

including a bridge of skin between the dorsal defect and the flap donor site. The flap is then rotated dorsally and easily covers the proximal interphalangeal joint (Fig. 1C). The donor site is darted at the distal and proximal interphalangeal joint flexion creases, to prevent a straight line volar scar (Fig. 1A).

The donor defect is covered with a full-thickness skin graft from the inguinal flexion crease and secured with a stent dressing. The finger is immobilized for 7 to 10 days to facilitate skin graft survival.

CLINICAL RESULTS

The full-thickness skin graft placed over the retained donor site digital nerve becomes reinnervated and provides stable skin cover. Two-point discrimination to the fingertip on the side of the flap is not affected. In most cases, a full range of digital motion is infrequently achieved, due to prior joint damage, stiffness, or extensor tendon scarring following burn

injury. When indicated, reconstruction of the extensor mechanism can be achieved without difficulty at a later date by reelevation of the flap.

SUMMARY

The arterialized side finger flap provides stable one-step cover for a secondarily exposed proximal interphalangeal joint after breakdown of a healed dorsal split-thickness skin graft (Fig. 2).

References

1. Russell RC, Van Beek AL, Wavak P, Zook EG. Alternative hand flaps for amputations and digital defects. *J. Hand Surg* 1981;6:399.
2. Lewin ML. Digital flaps. *Plast Reconstr Surg* 1951;7:46.
3. MacDougal B, Wray RC, Weeks PM. Lateral-volar finger flap for treatment of burn syndactyly. *Plast Reconstr Surg* 1976;57:167.

CHAPTER 245 ■ TENDOCUTANEOUS DORSAL FINGER FLAP

B. B. JOSHI

The cylindrical shape of the fingers usually confines destruction of tissue on the dorsum, such as that caused by friction injury or contact burn, to a central strip of tissue including the central slip of the extensor mechanism. The lateral bands and the overlying skin are often spared. These unaffected lateral bands, along with the overlying skin with neurovascular connection, are readily available for transfer en masse as a composite flap, not only to cover dorsal defects over the fingers, but also to allow lateral band plasty to achieve active extension of the PIP joint in a single maneuver (1–4).

INDICATIONS

The main clinical use of this flap is salvaging active extension at the PIP joints. It can also be used to provide cover over open PIP joints, since the vascularity of this flap helps in the resolution of infection and joint destruction. In addition, I have used this flap for providing skin cover to heal chronic ulcers over the dorsum of the middle phalanx due to osteomyelitis.

ANATOMY

The dorsal digital branch of the volar digital vessel enters the base of the flap and runs between the skin and the tendon. The skin flap is thus supplied by perforating branches. The transverse and oblique retinacular ligaments arising from the flexor tendon sheath cover these vessels. In this type of pathology, these ligaments are in a contracted state and need to be cut, to allow the dorsal displacement of the lateral bands and exposure of the volar neurovascular bundles. Careful blunt dissection along the flexor digital sheath will make the neurovascular bundle lax enough for lateral displacement along with the flap, and any tension on these delicate branches when the flap is being transferred dorsally will be avoided.

The venous drainage of the flap accompanies the main vessel supplying the flap. It enters at the base of the flap and needs careful dissection. The vascularity of the flap is very good, because the perforating vessels remain undisturbed.

FLAP DESIGN AND DIMENSIONS

The usual measurement of such a flap is about 1 ×3.5 cm. The volar boundary is the anterolateral border of the finger. The dorsal boundary is the junction of healthy skin with scar, and distally it can reach as far as the distal IP joint area.

OPERATIVE TECHNIQUE

An appropriate area of scar tissue to be excised is marked on the dorsum of the finger. A similar area is marked for transfer of the flap from the adjacent skin of the relatively unaffected lateral side of the finger. The volar limit of this flap is the anterolateral joint line; dorsally it starts where scar tissue ends.

The oblique and transverse retinacular ligaments are divided in the long axis of the finger and the lateral band is freed at the distal end of the flap without separating the skin over it. A composite flap of skin and lateral band with the neurovascular connection is thus raised.

The vessels and nerves entering the flap are protected by mobilizing the volar neurovascular bundle and by displacing it laterally, to avoid tension on these delicate structures when the flap is transferred dorsally.

The bed is then prepared by excising the scar tissue and the composite flap is transferred over this defect on the dorsum of the finger. The free distal end of the lateral band in the flap is sutured to the lateral band on the opposite side of the finger, after mobilizing it dorsally from its volarly displaced position (Fig. 1).

The donor site of the composite flap is resurfaced by a split-thickness skin graft with darts on the anterolateral border of the finger, to avoid flexion contracture of the finger from a linear scar.

CLINICAL RESULTS

The tendocutaneous flap has thus far been without vascular problems. A linear scar contracture at the anterolateral border of the finger can be avoided if the donor site is darted at the volar flexion creases and is covered by a thick split-thickness skin graft or a full-thickness skin graft (Fig. 2).

In 28 fingers in which I used the tendocutaneous flap, restoration of healthy skin cover has been achieved in all cases. In cases where the active extensor mechanism could not be restored, the flap improved the condition for future restoration of extension by a tendon transfer or graft. The flap provides a vascularized bed for the grafted tendon.

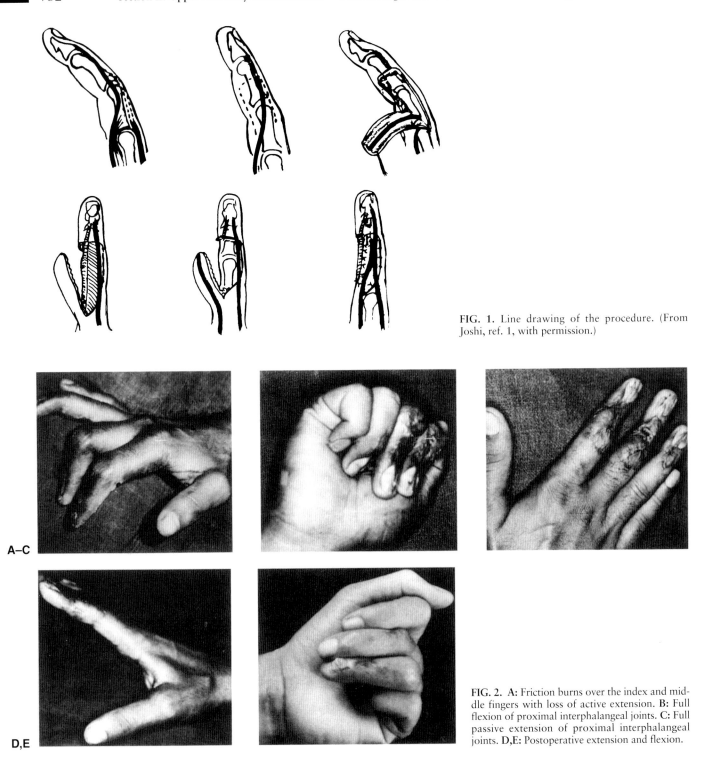

FIG. 1. Line drawing of the procedure. (From Joshi, ref. 1, with permission.)

A–C

D,E

FIG. 2. **A:** Friction burns over the index and middle fingers with loss of active extension. **B:** Full flexion of proximal interphalangeal joints. **C:** Full passive extension of proximal interphalangeal joints. **D,E:** Postoperative extension and flexion.

SUMMARY

The tendocutaneous flap can be used not only to cover the dorsum of the PIP joint, but also to restore active extension.

References

1. Joshi BB. A salvage procedure in the treatment of boutonniere deformity caused by contact burn and friction injury. *Hand* 1982;14:33.
2. Flint MH, Harrison SH. A local neurovascular flap to repair loss of the digital pulp. *Br J Plast Surg* 1965;18:156.
3. Littler JW. Neurovascular pedicle transfer of tissue in reconstructive surgery of the hand. *J Bone Joint Surg* 1956;38(A):917.
4. Joshi BB. A local dorsolateral island flap restoration of sensation after avulsion injury of fingertip pulp. *Plast Reconstr Surg* 1974;54:175.

CHAPTER 246 ■ DORSAL CROSS-FINGER FLAPS

B. W. EDGERTON AND R. W. BEASLEY

The repair of major soft-tissue losses of the digits should be accomplished with local tissues whenever practical. At least 30 authors have made significant contributions to the literature about the clinical applications of cross-finger flaps, comprising experiences with more than 500 cases (1–31).

INDICATIONS

The cross-finger flap is a sturdy, versatile flap that can be used in the following general situations.

Loss of Volar Finger Tissues (see Fig. 2)

Significant loss of volar tissue that requires flap coverage is the prime indication for a laterally based cross-finger flap. In acute traumatic injuries, this will provide necessary coverage of tendons, bones, and joints, to assure primary healing; it will also provide good coverage for secondary reconstruction of the deeper structures. Tumor excisions or the release of post-traumatic, congenital, or Dupuytren's contractures also may expose structures that cannot be covered with local tissues or a skin graft, in which case a laterally based cross-finger flap may offer the best solution.

Loss of Dorsal Finger Tissue (see Fig. 3)

Dorsal tissue loss with exposed tendons or joints has been treated traditionally with distant flaps. When feasible, local flaps are clearly superior. A cross-finger flap, distally based, or in some cases even proximally based, or a "flag flap" with its mobile narrow pedicle (21,22), often can be used for closure of dorsal finger wounds. Occasionally, a deepithelialized cross-finger flap is an alternative to close these wounds (19,23,24).

Major Fingertip Amputations (see Fig. 4)

Many methods have been advocated to treat fingertip amputations, but major amputations with exposed bone (dorsal oblique or guillotine) may be treated with distally based cross-finger flaps. Thenar flaps are generally the best solution for these injuries, but a cross-finger flap may be more practicable in special circumstances. Examples are when the amputation is proximal, when joint stiffness exists, or when there are multiple amputations.

ANATOMY

Dorsal finger skin is basically vascularized by a network of longitudinally oriented vessels that permit a wide latitude of flap design with safety. The proximally based flaps are especially sturdy, because they are based on the axial system of the two dorsal branches of the digital neurovascular bundles. The efficiency of this system is impressively demonstrated by the "flag flap," with which a large block of dorsal tissue is reliably supported by only one of these dorsal branches passing through a very narrow pedicle (see Chap. 231).

This longitudinal orientation of vessels provides excellent retrograde flow, permitting long flaps to be based distally, as is usually required for closure of fingertip amputations. Experience has shown that the vascular network of dorsal skin also permits the flaps to be based laterally (Fig. 1). In laterally based flaps where both axial dorsal branches are divided, circulation is maintained principally through the rich dermal and subdermal plexuses. This blood supply allows the tissue to be de-epithelialized for use as a "reverse dermis" flap (23,24) (see Chap. 247).

FLAP DESIGN AND DIMENSIONS

Dorsal cross-finger flaps are direct flaps, in that the defect is positioned directly under the open surface of the flap (Fig. 2). Distally based flaps up to an approximate size of 3 cm in length by 2 cm in width may be raised from the dorsum of the middle phalanx (Fig. 3). Usually an effort is made not to cross the proximal interphalangeal joint, but it has been demonstrated that this can be done, when necessary, without serious consequences (7). Laterally based flaps can be designed over to the midaxial line opposite the pedicle, giving in the large adult dimensions of up to about 3 cm in length and 6 cm in width. As previously discussed, the axial blood supply of proximally based flaps allows the elevation of almost the entire dorsal surface of a finger as a flap.

Initially the defect to be repaired should be adjusted to a shape that avoids a round scar or longitudinal scars crossing flexion creases, even if the excision of normal tissue is necessary. The finger is always positioned to minimize proximal interphalangeal joint flexion. A pattern of the defect is cut and pressed against the proposed location of the flap pedicle.

The flap must be larger than the defect, and allowance must be made for the length of the pedicle bridge, to avoid tension when it is sutured into place. The base of the flap may be oriented obliquely, to minimize twisting of the pedicle in distally or proximally based flaps. Fingertip injuries require a flap approximately 1½ times the width of the finger, to restore a round contour. All flaps should be measured twice before cutting.

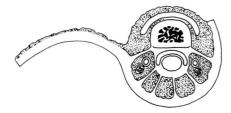

FIG. 1. Level of dissection of a dorsal cross-finger flap. Note that the paratenon is left intact on the donor site. (From Beasley, ref. 20, with permission.)

OPERATIVE TECHNIQUE

Dorsal cross-finger flaps should be elevated just superficial to the paratenon overlying the extensor tendon (Fig. 1), which preserves an adequately vascularized bed for skin grafting and minimizes damage to the network of vessels in the flap. When a long laterally based flap is needed, Cleland's ligaments can be divided and the neurovascular bundle dissected free from the base of the flap (Fig. 4). This not only lengthens the pedicle and adds mobility, but also facilitates safe subsequent flap division. A full-thickness skin graft is used to repair the donor site. When feasible, the graft should also cover the raw surface of the pedicle extending across to the recipient finger.

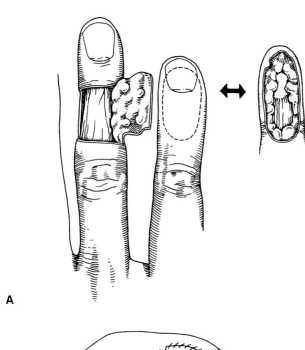

A

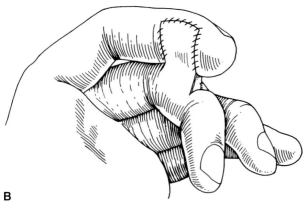

B

FIG. 2. A: Laterally based cross-finger flap used to cover a volar defect. B: Flap in position.

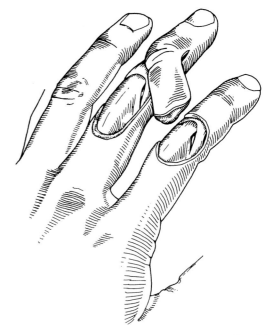

FIG. 3. Distally based cross-finger flap used to cover a dorsal defect.

Immobilization is accomplished with a dressing that provides gentle compression on the skin graft, dry gauze under and around the fingers to prevent maceration, and tape to maintain the carefully selected position. The dressing is covered with a plaster shell in which a window is cut for ongoing inspection. Use of a Kirschner wire to hold the optimal position has been advocated (25) but it has not been necessary in our experience, unless it is required for management of some concomitant problem.

If healing is uncomplicated, the pedicle may usually be divided in 10 to 14 days postoperatively as an office procedure. The donor finger may be compressed with a proximal tourniquet and the vascularity of the flap assessed before division. Flap tissues are intolerant of tension or handling immediately after pedicle division and generally should not be inset at that time. The common exception is in small children who require an anesthetic for pedicle division, and for these patients division is usually deferred until about 21 days. Wounds resulting from division of the pedicle are allowed to epithelialize, as prompt and vigorous efforts are directed to achieve full joint remobilization. When needed, a secondary revision is done several months later.

CLINICAL RESULTS

Of 546 cross-finger flaps reported in the English-language literature, only seven have had any necrosis (usually partial), for a survival rate of 98.7%. Reported complications are infrequent, with authors reporting 47 patients (8.6%) with *any* joint stiffness (most mild); 31 with dysesthesia (5.7%) (most of a minimal degree); 6 (1.1%) with loss of the graft; and 4 (0.7%) with infection. Restoration of well-functioning volar padded skin was almost always achieved. An important parameter of success is the return of sensibility, which generally requires at least 6 months. Seven authors who have carefully evaluated the return of two-point discrimination have found that 80% to 90% of patients have 8 mm or less of static two-point discrimination, which is roughly twice that of a normal finger pulp, but refined enough to be useful to the patient (26–31). These flaps can be used in children with excellent results and in older adults, but every effort to avoid joint stiffness should be made, especially with older patients (27,30).

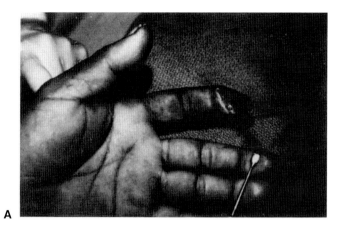
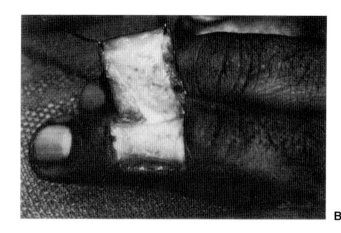
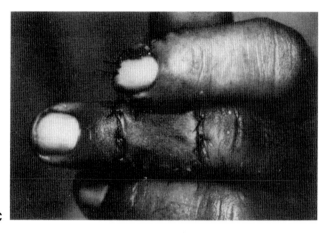
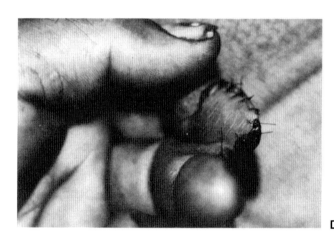

FIG. 4. **A:** Volar fingertip defect. **B:** Elevation of a laterally based dorsal cross-finger flap. Note flap thickness and paratenon left intact on donor site. **C:** Donor site covered with a full-thickness skin graft. **D:** Flap sutured into position.

Limitations of dorsal cross-finger flaps relate to the lack of substantial subcutaneous tissue, the limitations of size, the presence of a dorsal donor site that may be disturbing to some patients, and the occasional presence of hair in the flap, which is unaesthetic when transferred to the volar surface of the hand.

SUMMARY

Cross-finger flaps are valuable procedures and have withstood the tests of time and wide experience. Many variations have been devised by imaginative surgeons to cover volar tissue losses, dorsal tissue losses, and major digital amputations.

References

1. Cronin TD. The cross finger flap in hand surgery. *Ann Surg* 1957;145:650.
2. Gurdin M, Pangman WJ. The repair of surface defects of fingers by transdigital flaps. *Plast Reconstr Surg* 1950;5:368.
3. Horn JS. The use of full thickness hand skin flaps in the reconstruction of injured fingers. *Plast Reconstr Surg* 1951;7:463.
4. Tempest MN. Cross finger flaps in the treatment of injuries to the fingertip. *Plast Reconstr Surg* 1952;9:205.
5. Barclay TL. The late results of fingertip injuries. *Br J Plast Surg* 1955–6;8:38.
6. Campbell Reid DA. Experience of a hand surgery service. *Br J Plast Surg* 1956;9:11.
7. Curtis RM. Cross finger flap in hand surgery. *Ann Surg* 1957;145:650.
8. Kleinert HE. Fingertip injuries and their management. *Am Surg* 1959;25:41.
9. Brody GS, Cloutier AM, Woolhouse FM. The fingertip injury: an assessment of management. *Plast Reconstr Surg* 1960;26:80.
10. Hoskins HD. The versatile cross finger pedicle flap. *J Bone Joint Surg. [Am.]* 1960;42:261.
11. Gottlieb O, Mathiesen FR. Thenar flaps and cross finger flaps. *Acta Chir Scand* 1961;122:166.
12. Sturman MJ, Duran RJ. Late results of fingertip injuries. *J Bone Joint Surg [Am]* 1963;45:289.
13. Woolf RM, Broadbent TR. Injuries to the fingertips: treatment with cross finger flaps. *Rocky Mt Med J* 1967;8:35.
14. Wood RW. Multiple cross finger flaps: "piggy back" technique. *Plast Reconstr Surg* 1968;41:54.
15. Beasley RW. Local flaps for surgery of the hand. *Orthop Clin North Am* 1970;1:219.
16. Artz TD, Posch JL. Use of cross finger flap for treatment of congenital broad constricting bands of the fingers. *Plast Reconstr Surg* 1973;52:645.
17. Wickstrom OW, Bromberg BE. Finger flaps. *Plast Reconstr Surg* 1973;13:481.
18. Kisner WH. Cross finger flaps. *Am Fam Phys* 1979;19:157.
19. Russell RC, Van Beek AL, Wavak P, Zook E. Alternative hand flaps for amputations and digital defects. *J Hand Surg* 1981;6:399.
20. Beasley RW. *Hand injuries.* Philadelphia: Saunders, 1981.
21. Iselin F. The flag flap. *Plast Reconstr Surg* 1973;51:374.
22. Vilain R, Dupuis JF. Use of the flag flap for coverage of a small area on a finger or the palm. *Plast Reconstr Surg* 1973;51:397.
23. Pakiam AI. The reversed dermis flap. *Br J Plast Surg* 1978;31:131.
24. Atasoy E. Reversed cross-finger subcutaneous flap. *J Hand Surg* 1982;7:481.
25. Kislov R, Kelly AP. Cross finger flaps in digital injuries, with notes on Kirschner wire fixation. *Plast Reconstr Surg* 1960;25:312.
26. Smith JR, Bom AF. An evaluation of fingertip reconstruction by cross finger and palmar pedicle flap. *Plast Reconstr Surg* 1965;35:409.
27. Thomson HG, Sorokolit WT. The cross finger flap in children: a follow-up study. *Plast Reconstr Surg* 1967;39:482.
28. Porter RW. Functional assessment of transplanted skin in volar defects of the digits. *J Bone Joint Surg [Am]* 1968;50:955.
29. Johnson RK, Iverson RE. Cross finger pedicle flaps in the hand. *J Bone Joint Surg [Am]* 1971;53:913.
30. Kleinert HE, MacDonald CJ, Kutz JE. A critical evaluation of cross finger flaps. *J Trauma* 1974;14:756.
31. Gelles M, Pool R. Two-point discrimination distances in the normal hand and forearm. *Plast Reconstr Surg* 1977;59:57.

CHAPTER 247 ■ REVERSED CROSS-FINGER SUBCUTANEOUS TISSUE FLAP

E. ATASOY

EDITORIAL COMMENT

This elegant chapter is, in reality, using a fasciocutaneous flap principle. In elevating the flap, care must be taken to maintain the integrity of the subdermal plexus.

The principle of the deepithelialized reversed cross-finger subcutaneous tissue flap from the dorsum of one finger can be widely applied to hand surgery (1–4). It can be used successfully to cover large nailbed defects with exposed distal phalanx, and full-thickness skin defects with exposed tendon and bone.

INDICATIONS

This flap can be used for reconstruction of an avulsed eponychial skin fold and for coverage of exposed tendon near the distal interphalangeal joint (Fig. 1). It can also be used for reconstruction of large full-thickness sterile matrix nailbed defects with exposed bare distal phalanx (Fig. 2), with or without skin loss.

Any contused, repaired, or grafted extensor tendon denuded of peritenon can be covered with this flap, as can a boutonniere deformity with poor quality skin over the proximal interphalangeal joint.

FLAP DESIGN AND DIMENSIONS

The best donor site for this flap is the dorsum of the middle and proximal phalanges. The area over the distal interphalangeal and proximal interphalangeal joints should be avoided because of the thinness of the subcutaneous tissue in these areas.

The skin is marked on the dorsum of the middle phalanx of the adjacent finger approximately 3 to 4 mm larger than the defect (Fig. 1A).

OPERATIVE TECHNIQUE

A thin full-thickness skin flap is elevated under magnification and left attached to the donor finger along the opposite side from the injured finger. Then a full-thickness subcutaneous flap, excluding peritenon, is raised in the opposite direction by placing the base next to the recipient finger (Fig. 1A).

Following meticulous hemostasis, the flap is reversed and sutured to the dermis of the recipient finger. The donor defect is covered with the previously elevated thin full-thickness skin, and a tie-over dressing is applied. A free thin full-thickness skin graft is used to surface the reversed side of the subcutaneous flap, which is covered with a soft dressing, so that there will be no pressure on the flap.

After 2 weeks of immobilization the flap is divided and inset, and gentle mobilization is begun.

For reconstruction of the eponychial skin fold, an area of skin, appropriately sized and shaped to fit the defect, is preserved along the distal portion of the flap (Fig. 1B). This preserved skin forms the inner surface of the reconstructed eponychial skin fold after the reversing and suturing of the flap to the margins of the defect.

When the procedure is used to cover large nailbed defects with exposed distal phalanx and intact germinal matrix, in which there is a good chance for the nail to grow, the reversed flap should not be covered with a skin graft as a permanent procedure. Rather it should be allowed to epithelialize by remaining nailbed. By doing so, the growing nail will have a better chance to adhere to its new bed (Fig. 2).

However, in a case of complete avulsion of the nailbed, germinal matrix, and surrounding skin with exposed bone and extensor tendon, the reversed side of the flap should be covered with a skin graft as a permanent procedure, since there is no chance for the nail to grow.

CLINICAL RESULTS

Complications are very rare if the procedure is done properly and according to the rules of ordinary cross-finger flaps (Fig. 3). Epithelial cyst formation from the reversed dermal elements is rare. These skin elements usually disappear after a few weeks (5). In this series there was no evidence of cyst formation in the several cases that were followed 1 to 3 years postoperatively.

SUMMARY

The reversed cross-finger subcutaneous flap can be widely applied to hand defects, especially to dorsal finger injuries with nailbed defects or with exposed tendon, bone, or joint.

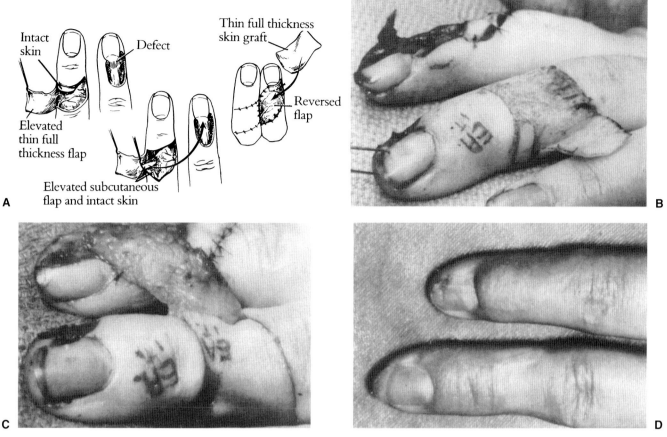

FIG. 1. A: Reconstruction of the eponychium and coverage of the nail root and extensor tendon with deepithelialized reverse cross-finger subcutaneous flap. The small area of preserved skin, after reversing, forms the inner surface of the eponychium. **B:** A flap composed of the full thickness of skin alone is elevated and based along the opposite side of the finger. A subcutaneous flap is elevated and based on the side of the finger next to the defect. Note that the portion of intact skin, once reversed, will form the lining of the eponychial fold. **C:** The subcutaneous flap is reversed onto the defect and then covered with a full-thickness skin graft. The full-thickness skin flap that was elevated off the donor site is then replaced over the intact paratenon and held with a tie-over dressing. **D:** Postoperative result at 1 year. Full nail growth with little deformity. (From Atasoy, ref. 4, with permission.)

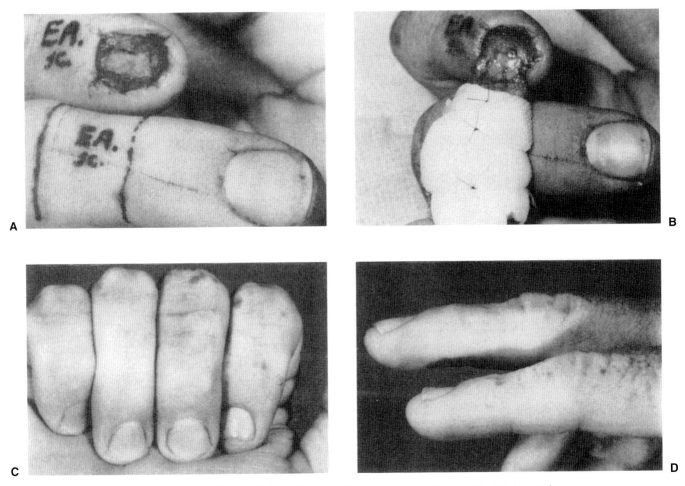

FIG. 2. **A:** Coverage of exposed distal phalanx and reconstruction of large nailbed defect. Defect on small finger and preparation of flap on ring finger. **B:** Reversed subcutaneous flap covering the nailbed defect without skin coverage. Tie-over dressing on the donor site. **C,D:** Six months postoperatively, showing satisfactory nail growth.

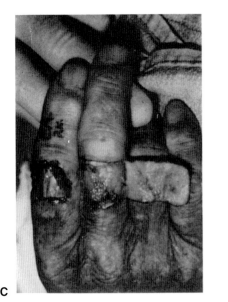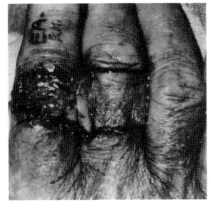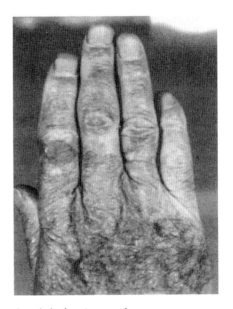

FIG. 3. **A:** Full-thickness skin loss with exposed, lacerated extensor tendon denuded of peritenon of index finger. Elevated full-thickness skin and mobilized flap on the middle finger. **B:** Reversed flap covering the defect and previously elevated full-thickness skin laid down on the donor site. **C:** Six months postoperatively.

References

1. Clodius L, Shamel J. The reversed dermal fat flap: a case report. *Plast Reconstr Surg* 1973;52:85.
2. Pakiam AJ. The reversed dermis flap. *Br J Plast Surg* 1978;31:131.
3. Russell RC, Van Beek AL, Wavak P, Zook EC. Alternative hand flaps for amputations and digital defects. *J Hand Surg* 1981;6:399.
4. Atasoy E. The reversed cross-finger subcutaneous flap. *J Hand Surg* 1982;7:481.
5. Peer LS, Paddock R. Histologic studies on the fate of deeply implanted dermal grafts. *Arch Surg* 1937;37:268.

CHAPTER 248 ■ DORSAL BRANCH OF THE DIGITAL NERVE INNERVATED CROSS-FINGER FLAP

B. B. JOSHI

EDITORIAL COMMENT

Use of the dorsal branch allows transfer of innervated tissue from one finger to the other without sacrificing sensibility to the volar aspects of the tip of the finger.

For full-thickness skin loss over the volar surface of a finger, an ideal repair replaces the tactile surface with skin that has an intact nerve supply and that also produces a satisfactory cosmetic result. The long-term results of cross-finger flaps are generally considered satisfactory. However, after the pedicle is divided from the donor finger, the flap becomes insensitive.

Subsequent restoration of sensation can occur only by reinnervation from the bed and the periphery of the grafted area. The functional quality of these flaps has been questioned. Sensation can be improved by isolating and transposing the dorsal cutaneous branch of the volar digital nerve along with the flap (1).

INDICATIONS

This method is yet another alternative for providing sensibility in repair over the volar aspect of the distal segment of the index finger, which is next in importance to the thumb. The results obtained are comparable to those of the radially innervated cross-finger flaps used for the thumb (see Chap. 272).

I reserve this method for restoring sensibility only in those cases where local neurovascular island flaps are not feasible or where a neurovascular island flap from the other finger is not desired.

ANATOMY

On the radial side of the index and long fingers and on the ulnar side of the small finger, a dorsal branch of the volar digital nerve is well defined (Fig. 1). This dorsal branch on the radial aspect of the long finger arises opposite the base of the proximal phalanx. It accompanies the main volar neurovascular pedicle for about 1 cm, and then it gradually branches off to run obliquely distally and dorsally to supply the dorsal aspect of the middle segment of the long finger. In cases where the nerve does not branch off near the base of the phalanx it can still be seen as a separate fascicle in the volar digital nerve sheath.

OPERATIVE TECHNIQUE

First Stage

To cover a volar defect over the index finger, a radially based cross-finger flap is marked on the middle segment of the long finger. The flap is raised, preserving the dorsal volar nerve branch with its terminal arborizing fibers and with an abundance of areolar tissue protecting the nerve and its fibers (Fig. 1A). The flap is set into the defect of the index finger in the usual fashion (Fig. 1B).

The dorsal digital nerve branch would be seen entering this flap just proximal to the PIP joint. The incision is then carried to sever the oblique fascial bands that attach the skin to the extensor tendon and to the periosteum along the side of the finger. A skin graft is then applied to the donor site.

Second Stage

After 3 weeks or so (depending on the healing at the recipient site) a zigzag incision is made to expose the volar digital neurovascular bundle on the radial aspect of the long finger up to the distal palmar crease. This incision is extended to the index finger in a zigzag fashion, to raise the flap to cover the transposed dorsal branch of the cross-finger flap.

This branch is dissected out, isolated, and transposed onto the index finger along with the detached cross-finger flap (Fig. 2). The length of the dorsal nerve branch is made sufficiently lax

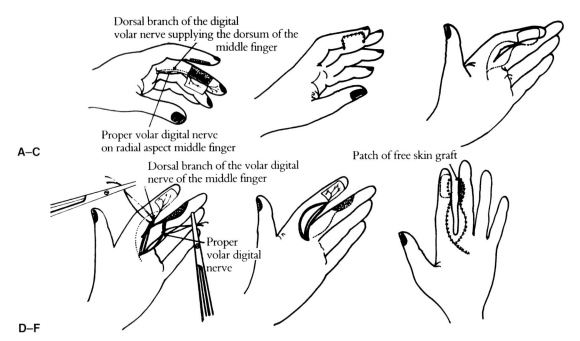

FIG. 1. A: The flap is elevated over the middle phalanx of the long finger. Care is taken to ensure that the dorsal branch of the volar digital nerve is preserved and included in the flap. Loose areolar tissue should be abundant to protect the nerve fibers. **B:** The flap is set into the defect of the index finger. **C:** The incisions are marked for the second stage, which is performed approximately 3 weeks later. **D:** The dorsal branch of the volar digital nerve, which usually arises opposite the base of the proximal phalanx, is dissected proximally. **E:** The nerve branch is then transposed to the index finger. **F:** The donor site may need a skin graft. (From Joshi, ref. 1, with permission.)

by loosening it proximally, to permit this transposition without tension. After closing the skin incision, a small skin graft may be needed on the anterolateral aspect of the long finger.

The nerve may branch away from the main bundle more distally than expected, thus requiring fascicular dissection to isolate and separate it proximally for transposition. This may cause a temporary neurapraxia, which recovers within 3 weeks.

Variations in Technique

The dorsal sensory branch can be transferred along with the flap during the first stage, as shown in Fig. 2. The second stage will then include only division and insetting of the flap.

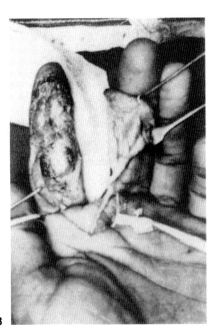
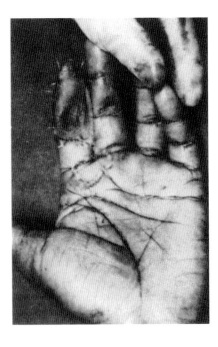

FIG. 2. A: The cross-finger flap has been elevated from the donor site. In this case the dorsal branch of the volar digital nerve has been dissected proximally for transfer to the index finger in the first stage. **B:** The cross-finger flap is inset and will be divided in approximately 3 weeks. The donor site is skin-grafted.

CLINICAL RESULTS

In 17 fingers repaired with this method, the sensation has been considerably better than that expected in standard cross-finger flaps. In 14 fingers the two-point discrimination reached a level of 7.1 to 11 mm. The functional quality of the sensation could not be considered good in the other three fingers, as the two-point discrimination was 13, 15, and 17 mm, respectively.

SUMMARY

The sensory cross-finger flap, based on the dorsal branch of the volar digital nerve, is worth considering for restoring sensibility whenever a cross-finger flap is scheduled for primary coverage of the index finger. It is an alternative to the volar neurovascular island flap from the other fingers (2, 3).

References

1. Joshi BB. A sensory cross-finger flap for use on the index finger. *Plast Reconstr Surg* 1976;58:210.
2. Littler JW. Neurovascular skin island transfer in reconstructive hand surgery. In: *Transactions of the second international congress of plastic surgeons.* Edinburgh: Livingstone, 1960;175.
3. Tubiana R, Du Parc J. Restoration of the sensibility in the hand by neurovascular skin island transfer. *J Bone Joint Surg* 1961;43(B):474.

CHAPTER 249 ■ CROSS-FOREARM SKIN FLAP

D. S. EASTWOOD

EDITORIAL COMMENT

The use of the forearm for fingertip resurfacing not only limits the hand that is attached to the forearm, but also significantly limits the use of the contralateral free hand.

The cross-forearm flap is used to resurface skin defects on the hand, particularly on the fingers (1–4). It has a random blood supply.

FLAP DESIGN AND DIMENSIONS

The flaps are usually more or less rectangular and based on one of the long sides (Fig. 1, flap A), but they may also be based on the narrow end (Fig. 1, flap B). In the latter case a length to width ratio of 1.5:1 should rarely be exceeded. When one is tubing the flap to provide circumferential cover for a digit, the shape is roughly square. When defects on the adjacent surfaces of two fingers are to be covered, as when separating syndactyly with bony fusion, flaps based opposite each other may be required (Fig. 2). Exceptionally, a finger may be inserted into a tunnel under a bipedicled bridge flap.

The use of cloth or paper patterns is advised in planning, especially when more than one flap is to be used. (It is surprising how long a flap may need to be when required to reach up and over a finger.) Further, the flaps should always be made wider (by about 1 to 1.5 cm) than the defect, because they retract when raised.

The best donor site, from a cosmetic viewpoint, is the region of the ulnar border of the forearm; from this site a flap goes well onto either the flexor or the extensor aspect of the fingers (Fig. 3). The flexor aspect of the upper portion of the forearm has the most sensitive skin and is perhaps the easiest site to use. It certainly allows maximum mobility for personal hygiene and other purposes (Fig. 4).

Where several fingers have to be covered, the whole of the forearm is available. One advantage of the forearm is that, being fusiform, the fingers can be spread around it and flaps can be obtained for awkward defects for several fingers at one time (Figs. 5–7). The softer and more adaptable skin of the upper portion of the flexor aspect of the forearm is preferred for this purpose, although the outer aspect is also available. The latter is particularly relevant when skin cover is required for both hands at one time (Fig. 5).

OPERATIVE TECHNIQUE

The portion of the flap intended for the defect on the fingers should be raised at a thickness corresponding to approximately the midpoint of the subcutaneous fat. Cautious thinning with scissors may be required to adapt it to the defect (5,6). As soon as the intermediate, carrying portion of the flap is reached, dissection should be deepened to the fascia, and any further raising of the flap necessary to enable it to reach into the defect should be continued in this plane.

When the flap is to be tubed, it is helpful to close most of the defect directly, because this helps in the tubing. Under other circumstances the temptation to close the defect directly at the time of raising should be avoided, the secondary defect

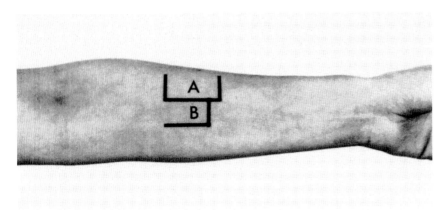

FIG. 1. Basic types of flap.

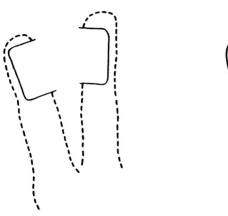
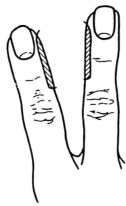

FIG. 2. Flaps with opposed bases used in complex syndactyly with bony fusion.

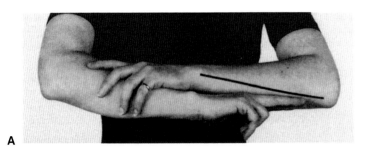

A

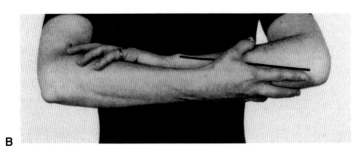

B

FIG. 3. A,B: Positioning for flexor and extensor aspects of finger along ulnar border donor site.

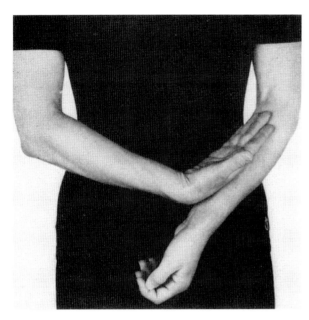

FIG. 4. Use of flexor aspect of forearm. Note position of hand of donor arm.

being grafted with a thin split-thickness skin graft that extends across the pedicle to the margin of the finger defect. If a bridge type of flap is used, the floor of the tunnel must be grafted.

If more than one flap is needed, it is recommended that they should be tentatively planned preoperatively, with the patient conscious. Only one flap is raised at a time and fitted into the defect; the next flap is then raised, because a need for modification may become evident during the procedure.

These flaps are often somewhat inaccessible, and it may be helpful to hold the arms in a raised position by attaching them to the transverse bar of an anesthetic screen that is adjustable for height. This gives good access to what at operation is, in fact, the undersurface of the forearm.

Postoperatively, the arms are immobilized by strapping along the forearms and around the elbows, to hold them in a longitudinal direction, and around the wrists and hand in the other direction (Fig. 5). The tips of individual fingers may be stabilized by sutures through the nails to the skin of the donor arm; superglue may also be used; in children, plaster of Paris slabs may be required. In the recovery room it is helpful to keep the weight of the arms off the abdomen by means of a

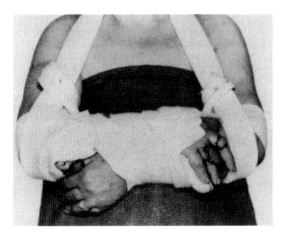

FIG. 5. Flaps for two hands simultaneously. Note spreading of right fingers for multiple flaps.

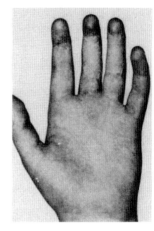

FIG. 6. Serial flaps to ring and middle fingers (burn contracture). (From Eastwood, ref. 4, with permission.)

supporting bridge of Kramer wire; this also helps to maintain the position at this awkward stage. Two or 3 days postoperatively, the amount of strapping may be markedly reduced to free one hand for feeding and toilet procedures.

The flaps are usually separated at 14 days postoperatively. It is often convenient to do this simply under local infiltration anesthesia and to delay formal setting in of the flaps for 48 hours. This acts as a delay tactic and, when practicable, this opportunity may also be used to remove the graft on the secondary defect and to close it directly. Bridge flaps are separated in stages: two-thirds of each pedicle is divided at 10 days, and the rest at 21 days.

In dealing with flexion contractures of the fingers following burn, it is often practical to deal with each finger serially, thus confining the secondary scarring to a linear area along the subcutaneous border of the ulna. When the flaps are placed on the flexor aspect of the fingers, thinning is not usually required, because the movement of the fingers appears to reduce the subcutaneous fat. On the lateral and dorsal aspects of the fingers thinning is often required.

Neurocutaneous Flaps

It is possible to incorporate a cutaneous nerve in a cross-forearm flap, anastomosing its proximal end to the relevant sensory nerve. The superficial branch of the radial nerve becomes subcutaneous some 8 cm proximal to the radial styloid process. It may be incorporated in a proximally based flap

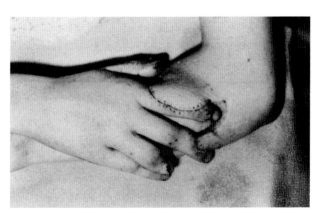

FIG. 7. Flaps for all five digits of one hand (hot press burn).

taken from just above the wrist (7). The medial cutaneous nerve of the forearm runs with the basilic vein and may be identified at the elbow and incorporated in a proximally based flap (8).

There are obvious problems of size and orientation in these flaps. Great care must be taken to ensure that the small branches to the skin itself that arise proximally are not divided. Use of these flaps should be reserved for pulp replacement, where they may be worth the difficulties involved.

CLINICAL RESULTS

Loss of flaps due to deficient circulation is very uncommon. The principal problem is one of separation due to inadequate immobilization and, above all, to faulty planning in multiple flaps when digits are placed in a position that results in tension on the flap bases. Children up to the age of 3 years present a special problem, because of their tendency to curl their fingers into flexion. Under these circumstances a bridge type of flap is indicated.

The main practical problems are those associated with nursing patients with limited or absent use of both hands (incidentally an excellent practical cure for smoking). Children tolerate the procedure well, being used to intimate attention and being capable of playing with their feet. Adults are prone to shoulder stiffness; the joints must be put through as full a range of movement as possible while the arms are joined, preferably under the direction of a physiotherapist who will also supervise recovery of movement after separation.

SUMMARY

The forearm is a good donor site for flap coverage of one or more fingers. It can be modified to become a sensory flap, when indicated.

References

1. Campell Reid DA. Experience of a hand surgery service. *Br J Plast Surg* 1956;9:11.
2. McCash CR. Cross-arm bridge flaps in the repair of flexion contractures of the fingers. *Br J Plast Surg* 1956;9:25.
3. Teich-Alasia S, Barberis ML. The value of the cross-arm flap in reconstructive surgery of the hand. *Chir Plast [Berlin]* 1972;1:134.
4. Eastwood DS. Cross-forearm flaps. *Hand* 1974;6:62.
5. Thomas CV. Thin flaps. *Plast Reconstr Surg* 1980;65:747.
6. Colson P, Janvier H. Primary total defatting of flaps. *Ann Chir Plast* 1966;11:11.
7. Dolich BH, Olshansky J, Babar AH. Use of cross-forearm neurocutaneous flap to provide sensation and coverage in hand reconstruction. *Plast Reconstr Surg* 1978;62:550.
8. Paneva-Holevich E. Sensory cross-forearm neurocutaneous flap. *Acta Chir Plast [Prague]* 1980;22:86.

CHAPTER 250 ■ CROSS-HAND HYPOTHENAR SKIN FLAP TO THE FINGER

C. ARRUNÁTEGUI

The hypothenar flap can be used effectively to cover denuded fingertips on the opposite hand (1). The flap provides skin similar to that which is lost, while resulting in minimal donor site morbidity. One of the main advantages of this flap is that the pedicle can be divided in 3 to 5 days.

INDICATIONS

The advantages of this technique are (1) the procedure is easy to perform; (2) there is a minimal period of immobiliza-tion; (3) the cosmetic and functional results are excellent; and (4) the donor site is hidden and an insignificant scar results. Among the disadvantages are that only about 5 to 6 mm² of donor area can be used, on average, to avoid problems in the donor hand, and that both hands are simultaneously immobilized.

ANATOMY

There is a clear line of demarcation between the palmar and the dorsal skin over the hypothenar eminence (2). The palmar skin is used for the flap. The subcutaneous tissue is divided into compartments that cushion the area. The trabeculae that run between the dermis and the fascia overlying the hypothenar muscles help to resist friction. These are all characteristics that make the flap ideal for fingertip coverage.

On both sides of the ulnar border are branches of the ulnar nerve to the little finger. In the distal and proximal parts of the

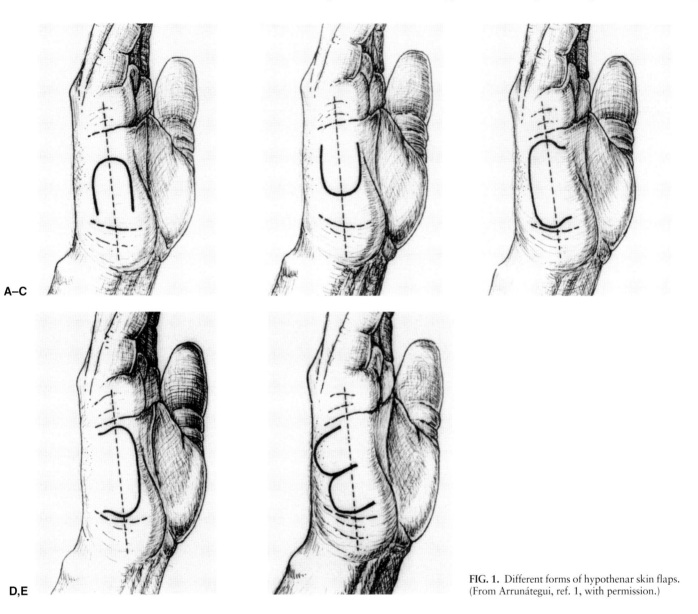

A–C

D,E

FIG. 1. Different forms of hypothenar skin flaps. (From Arrunátegui, ref. 1, with permission.)

hypothenar skin there are two natural creases that limit the surgical field.

The fingertips have an interconnecting dermal-subdermal plexus containing arteriovenous shunts, similar to hypothenar skin. This rich anastomotic network on both sides allows circulation into the flap from the fingertip to be established quickly. It is for this reason that the pedicle can be divided as early as 2 to 3 days.

FLAP DESIGN AND DIMENSIONS

The flap must be designed preoperatively so that the hands lie in a comfortable position. Care must be taken to orient the flap so that the pedicle can lie over the remaining nailbed. In this way, after division of the pedicle, the raw area will be at the level of the nailbed and secondary healing will enhance the fixation of the nail as it grows.

The flap should be designed larger than the recipient area and should be situated as much as possible over the palmar skin. Depending on the requirements, flaps can be designed to cover two fingertips simultaneously (Fig. 1E).

OPERATIVE TECHNIQUE

Once the hands are positioned comfortably and the flap sutured into place, the hands may be held together by dressings or even sutures.

The pedicle was initially divided at only 2 days, with excellent results. Currently I feel it is safer to divide the pedicle at 3 days in most cases. It may be better to wait 4 days in laborers who have a thick keratin layer. In those patients with a poor bed with exposed tendons and bone, the pedicle should not be divided for 5 days.

The pedicle is not inset, but secondary healing is allowed to take place. This produces a better cosmetic result than would follow grafting (Figs. 2 and 3).

CLINICAL RESULTS

After flap integration and complete healing have occurred, all properties and characteristics of the transferred skin are surprisingly recovered. The color match, texture, and all tests of

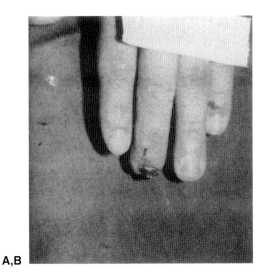
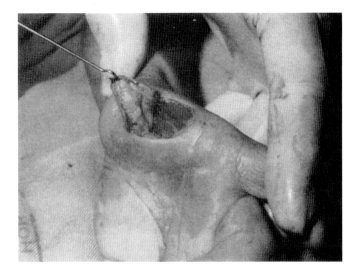

A,B

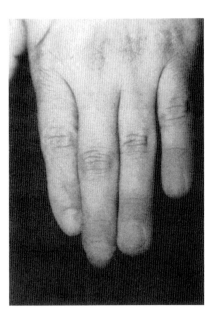
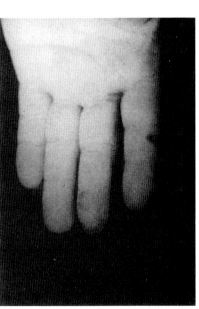

C–E

FIG. 2. A 26-year-old man with large loss of pulp and nail. **A:** Twenty-five days after injury. The finger-tip has already undergone both a skin graft and a local flap. **B:** Elevation of the flap. **C:** Immediately after application of hypothenar skin flap. The pedicle was divided after 2 days. **D:** Forty-five days postoperatively. Dorsal side. **E:** Forty-five days postoperatively. Palmar side. (From Arrunátegui, ref. 1, with permission.)

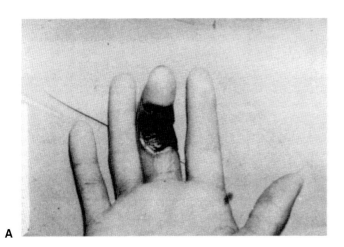

A

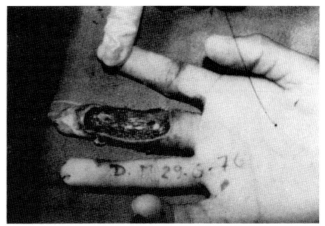

B

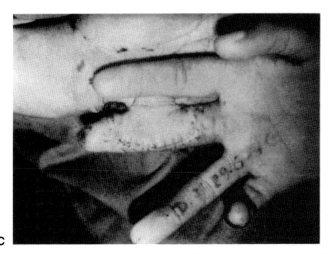

C

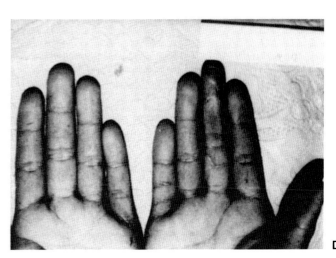

D

FIG. 3. A 14-year-old girl with necrosis produced after a glass injury. **A:** Fifteen days after injury. **B:** The necrotic tissue, including the deep flexor tendon, was removed. **C:** Immediately after application of a large hypothenar skin flap. The pedicle was divided after 4 days. **D:** One year postoperatively. (From Arrunátegui, ref. 1, with permission.)

sensitivity of the new fingertip are positive after 2 to 6 months. In some patients, it can even be difficult to identify the injured finger 1 year later.

SUMMARY

A cross-hand hypothenar skin flap can be used to cover fingertip defects on the opposite hand.

References

1. Arrunátegui C. El colgajo hipotenar. *Revista de cirugía estética* 1976;1:67.
2. Bargmann W. *Histologia y anatomia microscopica humans.* Spanish translation of the 3d German edition. São Paolo, Brazil: Labor S. A., 1961; 675–690.

CHAPTER 251 ■ CROSS-HAND, CROSS-FINGER NEUROVASCULAR SKIN FLAP

M. R. WEXLER AND I. J. PELED

EDITORIAL COMMENT

This complex procedure would have limited applications. Since other microsurgical techniques are available, the same objective perhaps can be accomplished in a more expeditious manner.

Restoration of sensation of the finger pulp in hand trauma is important for hand function. This is especially important in reconstruction of the thumb and index finger.

INDICATIONS

In cases of subtotal loss of the volar aspect of the fingers, for instance following deep burns, coverage is initially undertaken using skin flaps. The best flap for this purpose is the cross-arm flap that supplies good skin coverage with a supple, delicate layer of subcutis. The cross-hand, cross-finger neurovascular island flap can be used when the volar aspect of all the fingers is lost (1).

To restore sensation, continuity of the sensory nerves and organs is needed, the density of which is relatively higher in digits and the tips of digits than elsewhere. For this reason neurovascular flaps from the fingers or toes are superior to most other neurovascular flaps for restoring sensibility.

Restoration of sensation is important along the radial side of the index and middle fingers and along the ulnar side of the thumb, enabling two-finger and three-finger pinch. The whole length of the donor finger should be included in the neurovascular island flap (2); this increases the amount of sensitive skin in the recipient finger along its whole length (Fig. 1).

OPERATIVE TECHNIQUE

The injured fingers have previously been covered with a cross-arm flap. The donor site is usually the ulnar side of the ring finger: the flap is outlined along the midlateral ulnar line (1), using the end of the interphalangeal creases as a landmark (Fig. 2).

The skin is incised along with Cleland's ligament down to the areolar plane over the tendon sheath. The recipient index finger, covered previously with a flap taken from the arm, is incised along its midlateral radial side under the flap to the middle of the finger all along its length. The two hands are then brought together, the donor flap is sutured to the recipient finger along its radial aspect, and the primary covering flap is crossed over to the donor finger along its ulnar side.

The hands are bandaged together with light Elastoplast and left in this position for 12 to 14 days.

In a second operation the neurovascular island is dissected, consisting of half of the finger width. It is advised to take it in a zigzag fashion to prevent flexion contracture. Care should be taken to leave the neurovascular bundle attached to the skin and to leave its surrounding fatty tissue attached to it. At the web space care must also be taken to avoid damage to the arteries where the common digital artery branches into the two proper digital arteries. The branch of the neighboring finger is dissected, ligated, and cut. The artery is then dissected further proximally to the superficial palmar arch, where it is ligated and severed.

The digital nerve is dissected by separating the common digital nerve as proximally as needed. It is then sharply severed and the proximal end of the nerve is buried into muscle or bone. At this stage the neurovascular island flap is connected all along the ulnar side of the recipient finger. The flap that was taken from the injured finger and is now connected all along the ulnar side of the donor finger is severed in a zigzag fashion from the volar aspect of the recipient finger. The two hands are thus separated, each having a longitudinal flap that was originally on the other finger.

The palm of the recipient finger is then opened to the proximal palmar crease, and further if needed. The artery is sutured to any available artery with an end-to-end anastomosis or to the superficial palmar arch in an end-to-side anastomosis, using microvascular technique. The artery could be elongated by interposing a vein graft, if necessary. The digital nerve is sutured to its corresponding proximal severed nerve.

It should be mentioned that this crossed-over island neurovascular flap can survive as a random flap without this microvascular anastomosis, but the enhanced perfusion can decrease any symptoms related to vascular insufficiency.

CLINICAL RESULTS

Circulatory difficulties of neurovascular island flaps are almost always due to venous insufficiency (3). Sensation does spread eventually beyond the island flap. A cross-hand, cross-finger neurovascular skin flap can provide durable integument with maximal sensation, without impairment of sensory pathways (1). Because of the anatomy of the human finger, in which most of the arteries are on the volar aspect and most of the veins are in the dorsum, the usual neurovascular island flap is difficult to use as a free flap, because veins for drainage may be lacking. At least one neurovascular bundle should be left at the donor finger, to avoid damage to this finger.

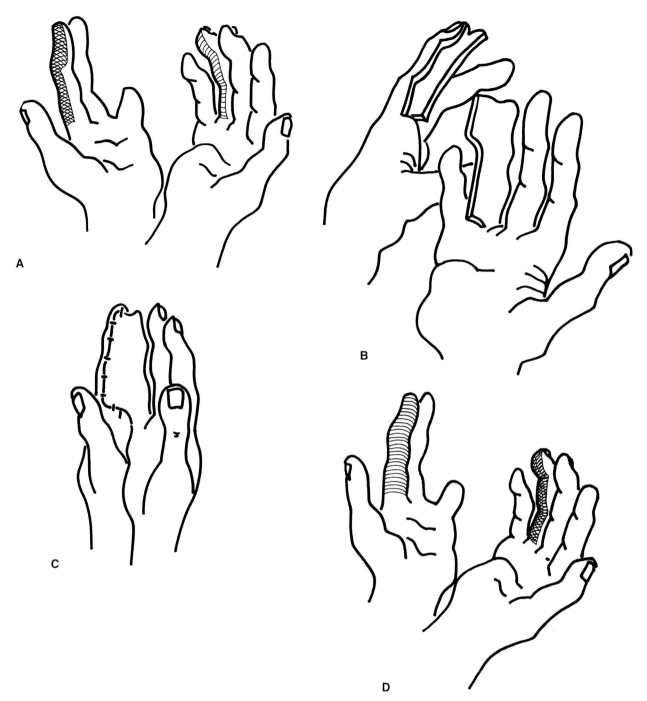

FIG. 1. **A:** Sensory loss of the volar aspect of the index and middle fingers of the left hand after mangle injury. The right hand was covered with a cross-arm flap. The planned cross-hand, cross-finger neurovascular flap to be taken from the ulnar side of the right ring finger is outlined. **B:** A flap based on the ulnar side of the left index finger is raised to cover the ulnar defect of the right ring finger. Note neurovascular island flap still based on its vascular supply and the whole length of the radial side of this finger, before crossing it over to cover the radial side of the left index finger. **C:** The two hands are "glued" together through the two crossed-over flaps. One is a neurovascular flap from the right ring finger, sutured to the radial aspect of the left index finger. This is hidden behind another flap taken from the left index finger to the right ring finger donor site. **D:** The two flaps after separation. At this stage, microsurgery was used for arterial anastomosis and digital neurorrhaphy (see text).

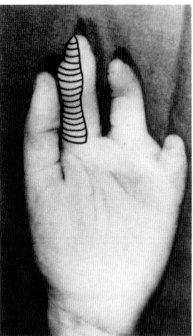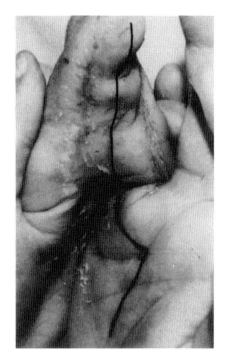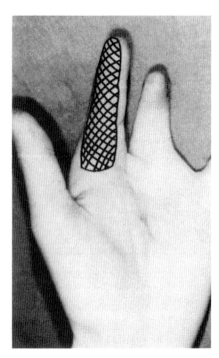

A–C

FIG. 2. **A:** Injured hand with index and long fingers covered with a thin cross-arm flap. There was no sensation in these fingers. The area to be covered with a cross-hand, cross-finger neurovascular island flap is outlined. **B:** A cross-hand, cross-finger neurovascular island flap. The recipient is the left index finger and the donor is the volar aspect of the right ring finger. To avoid injury to the distal phalanx of the donor finger, it is recommended that only half the volar aspect be used, i.e., one neurovascular bundle and its skin as island flap. (From Wexler and Neuman, ref. 1, with permission.) **C:** The neurovascular island flap following its separation, marked with criss-cross lines.

SUMMARY

The cross-hand, cross-finger neurovascular skin flap can be used to provide sensation, with correct cortical orientation to the fingers. It is especially useful when most or all of the volar aspect of the fingers of one hand has been damaged.

References

1. Wexler MR, Neuman Z. Cross hand, cross finger neurovascular flap: a preliminary report. *Br J Plast Surg* 1975;28:216.
2. Milford L. Neurovascular island grafts. In: Grenshaw AH, ed. *Campbell's operative orthopaedics.* St. Louis: Mosby, 1971;81–82.
3. Peacock EE. Island pedical gymnastics. In: Cramer LM, Chase RA, eds. *Symposium on the Hand.* St. Louis: Mosby, 1971;209–221.

CHAPTER 252 ■ LOUVRE SKIN FLAP

A. J. J. EMMETT

This is a multiple broad dermal-thickness flap for the resurfacing of finger defects (1–3). Skin loss from the surface of a number of adjacent fingers will involve a wider area than could be provided by resurfacing with a continuous single flap (Fig. 1A). In order that a greater surface area of cover can be provided for a number of adjacent digits, separately based flaps are simultaneously raised and placed on the defects (Fig. 1B).

INDICATIONS

Full-thickness burns with loss of cover over the extensors are suitable for this type of repair. I have used it similarly on the flexor surface as well. The donor sites have been the abdomen or the opposite arm, or flexor or extensor surface of the upper arm. The cross-arm flap on the lateral surface of the upper arm is suitable when the fingers have some degree of fixed flexion, which then fits that contour.

ANATOMY

The flaps have a random pattern blood supply, depending on the dermal, subdermal, and subcutaneous vascular plexus.

FLAP DESIGN AND DIMENSIONS

After excision of the finger burn or scar, the extent of skin replacement required can be determined. This total area can be measured and the required area projected to the proposed donor site.

The spread of skin required will be wider than the possible span of the fingerbreadth, and it is planned that the donor site will extend beyond each finger progressively (Fig. 2B). The natural elastic recoil of each finger tends to pull it back into each pedicle base, helping with the snug fit of flap to finger. The flaps are initially all raised together, and the donor sites are skin grafted primarily.

The fingers must fit comfortably into the flap or there will be too much tension on the stitch line and poor healing. In planning the flap situation and the hand position to be maintained for 2 to 3 weeks, it is wise to have the patient's agreement to that position.

OPERATIVE TECHNIQUE

The flaps are raised as thinly as possible; this is reasonably safe because they have such a broad base in relation to their length. Atraumatic sharp dissection is used to raise the flap with skin hooks and scalpel blade. I avoid using vasoconstrictors and diathermy on the flaps: they always ooze, to a degree.

Tapering an increasing thickness of subcutaneous tissue into the flap pedicle as the flap is raised makes for a better blood supply and produces an even fit around the side of the finger. Keep in mind that this subcutaneous tissue then must be thinned when the flap is divided and inset, so that it should be thicker mainly at the base. A two-thirds healed inset is needed for safe insetting of the remaining one-third of the base at the time of flap division (Fig. 2). In general, I have left the flap attached for 3 weeks before dividing it, because an extra week has produced better healing and blood supply, allowing me to do more insetting safely at the time of flap division.

The flap is divided at 3 weeks, the subcutaneous tissue is trimmed from the base of the pedicle, and the pedicle inset to the side of the finger to produce an even contour (Fig. 2C). This involves a little undermining of the flap, which is safe only if there is a well-healed primary attachment of two-thirds to three-quarters of the flap. If delayed healing occurs with the flap initially, the pedicle base only is best divided and left to inset itself, with a secondary recontouring later.

Some months later, when the flaps are supple and the joints have been restored to as much movement as can be achieved with active therapy, a secondary repair is carried out, as necessary (Fig. 2D). Some excess of flap always seems to develop, and this needs to be removed.

FIG. 1. A: The curved surface of the fingers in a cross section required more skin than a flat application could provide. B: Lower abdominal wall plan for the flap, planned for an area where the hand can rest comfortably. Fingers are spread apart to a width that will provide the area of skin required for each finger flap. This is then marked on the abdominal wall. These are broadly based thin flaps. C: The dermal-thickness flaps with subcutaneous tissue pedicle are each raised from what is the base of the preceding flap. Since only dermis is raised, the circulation is left to support the pedicle of the next flap. The pedicle thickens toward the base of each flap, and the subcutaneous thickness is drawn up on the side of the finger as the flap is sutured on. It helps if the finger is supple and can rotate a little. (From Emmett, ref. 3, with permission.)

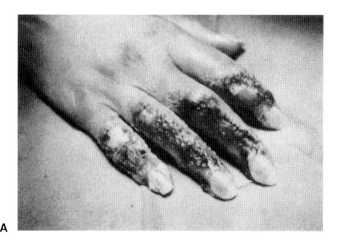

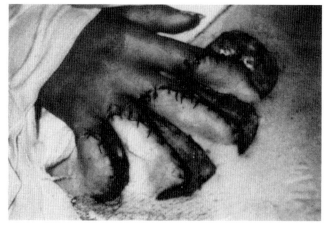

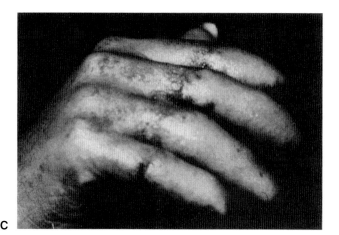

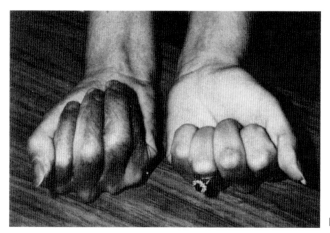

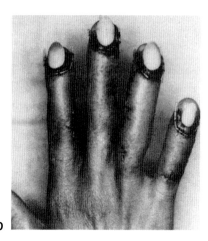

FIG. 2. A: Full-thickness hot press burns of the dorsum of the fingers with loss of the skin, subcutaneous tissue, extensor tendons, and nailbeds, as well as burn of dorsal joint capsules. **B:** The dorsal joint capsules were preserved to be vascularized by the flap. Primary repair was by louvre flap only. At 4 days, the bread-thin louvre flaps were sewed on each finger after excision of deep burn. Donor sites were skin-grafted. Fingers were rotated a little to shorten the flap pedicle. Note that the flap for the index finger was taken wide of the position in which the finger can sit, and the finger then lay back into the flap pedicle. This applied to each other finger to a lesser degree, least with the little finger. **C:** One week after flap division from the abdomen. The thicker subcutaneous tissue in the pedicle base of each flap was thinned out before insetting that base. The broad attachment and close coaption of flap to finger gave a blood supply adequate to allow this thinning at the time of inset. The flap had been attached 3 weeks. **D:** Secondary later reconstruction. A zigzag side incision along each finger side allowed excess skin to be removed, and extensor tendons have been inserted as grafts. Nailbed folds were made with flap underlap, and artificial nails were used to stent these folds. One joint arthrodesis was held with Kirschner wire. **E:** Flexed hands showing quite good proximal interphalangeal joint movement. Distal interphalangeal joint movement is limited, and the distal interphalangeal joint of the middle finger is fused. Nail folds can be seen. Extensor grafts are pulling through well. Fine abdominal hairs are showing. (From Emmett, ref. 3, with permission.)

CLINICAL RESULTS

The scar left at the donor site is rather unsightly initially, but it fades and flattens and is acceptable to patients who have had adequate explanation prior to the operation.

SUMMARY

Skin flaps from the abdomen or the arm can be used to cover either the flexor or the extensor surfaces of the fingers. Louvre skin flaps are elevated to cover each finger separately and simultaneously. This provides more tissue than a single skin flap.

References

1. Barron JN, Emmett AJJ. Subcutaneous pedicle flaps. *Br J Plast Surg* 1965;18:51.
2. Colson P, Houot R, Gangolphe M, et al. Utilisation des lambeaux degraisses (lambeaux greffes) en chirurgie reparatrice de la main. *Ann Chir Plast* 1967;12:298.
3. Emmett AJJ. Finger resurfacing by the multiple subcutaneous pedicle or louvre flaps. *Br J Plast Surg* 1974;27:370.

CHAPTER 253 ■ DERMO-EPIDERMAL FLAP

P. COLSON AND H. JANVIER

The dermo-epidermal flap was developed to solve two basic problems in coverage of hand defects (1–4): Coverage needs to be thick enough to retain normal elasticity, so that fingers can pass through their full range of motion. At the same time, coverage needs to be thin enough to avoid bulkiness (5).

ANATOMY

The flap is completely separated from the subdermal fat. It is therefore nourished only by the most superficial portion of the dermal-subdermal plexus. However, the flap is thick enough to retain nerve endings and most of the sensory organs (6,7).

FLAP DESIGN AND DIMENSIONS

With such a tenuous random vascular supply, one would assume that the flap would be limited to only small defects. However, whole hand defects can be covered by using either a single or a bipedicled flap.

The flap should not be longer than it is wide (base). To cover one or two fingers, the flap does not need to be longer than 8 to 10 cm. A bipedicle flap can be as large as 15 to 18 cm (Figs. 1 and 2).

It is unwise to use the inside of the arm to cover the volar surface of the fingers, since pressure on the chest wall may interfere with circulation to the flap. If several fingers are to be covered, they should be widely spaced, so that there is enough tissue at the time of division to cover the lateral surfaces of the fingers (Fig. 3).

OPERATIVE TECHNIQUE

The flap is elevated just below the dermis and it must be securely fixed to the defect. Although joint mobilization can be preserved, especially with the cross-arm position, shearing forces must be avoided (Fig. 4). Otherwise, in-growth of vessels may be prevented, resulting in loss of the flap.

CLINICAL RESULTS

The dermo-epidermal flap looks bright red initially (Fig. 5), and then takes on a cyanotic hue. These variations are felt to be due to changes in the vasomotor system and to short circuits occurring in the arteriovenous anatomoses in the flap. The cyanosis persists for 4 to 5 days and the skin then takes on a more reassuring appearance.

Text continues on page 757.

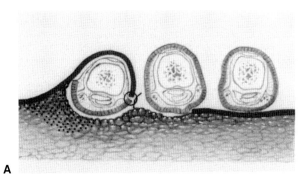

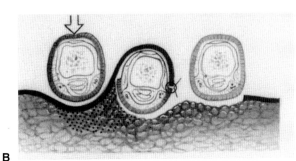

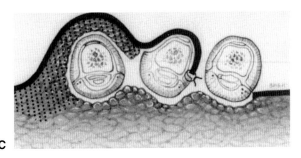

FIG. 1. Various techniques to cover one finger with the dermo-epidermal flap. A: Coverage of a single outside finger. B: Coverage of a single inside finger should *not* be done this way. Compression from the outside finger can lead to necrosis of the flap. C: The outside finger should lie underneath the base of the flap.

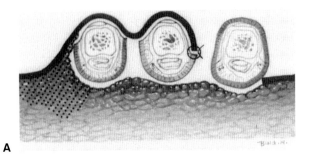

A

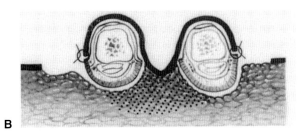

B

FIG. 2. **A,B:** Various techniques to cover two fingers.

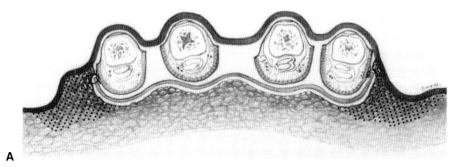

A

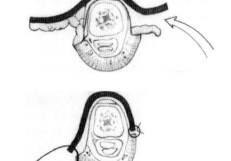

B,C

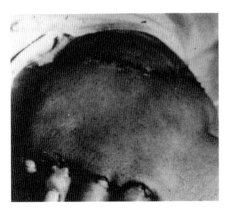

FIG. 3. **A:** Coverage of multiple fingers. The donor site is covered first with a split-thickness skin graft. **B,C:** The fingers should be spaced widely apart, to have enough tissue at division for covering the lateral aspect of the fingers.

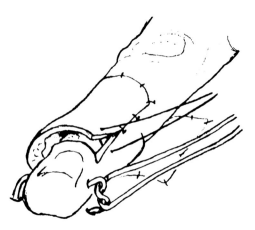

FIG. 4. Shearing forces should be avoided. One way to fix the finger is to suture it, as shown.

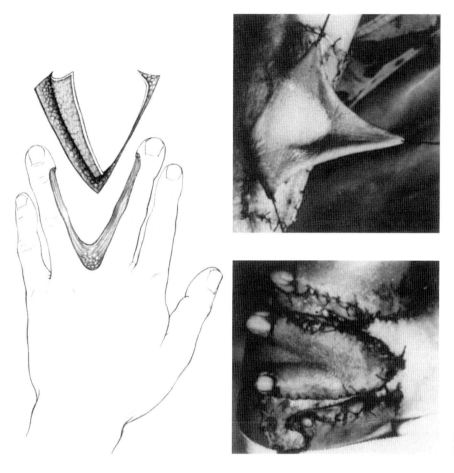

FIG. 5. Coverage of two adjacent digits, including the web space.

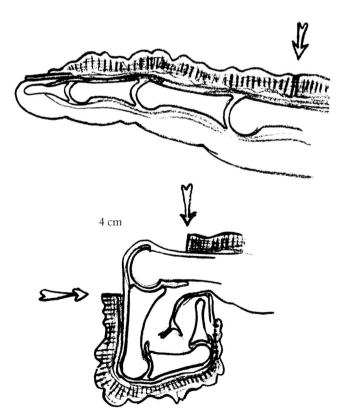

4 cm

FIG. 6. The dermo-epidermal flap can provide skin with normal elastic properties that are not provided with skin grafts.

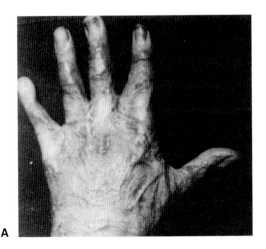

A

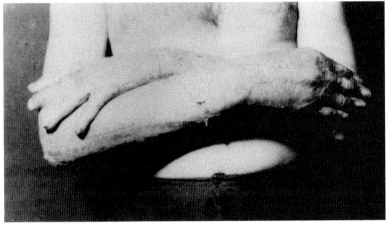

B

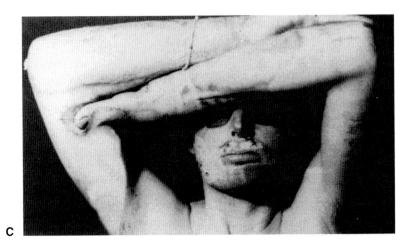

C

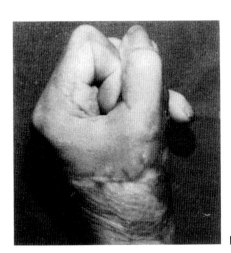

D

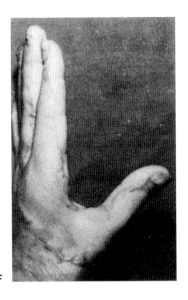

E,F

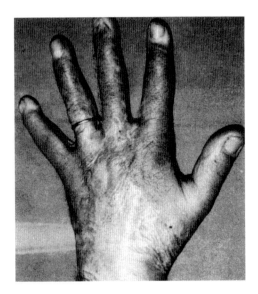

FIG. 7. A: Burned hand. B,C: Positioning.
D,E: Result of dermo-epidermal flap coverage.
F: Result 4 years later.

The skin cover provided by the dermo-epidermal flap is thicker and more elastic than full-thickness skin grafts. This extra mobility is of prime importance in covering hand defects (Figs. 6 and 7).

The donor site must be covered with a split-thickness skin graft. Judicious choice of donor site can minimize the cosmetic deformity.

SUMMARY

The dermo-epidermal flap can be used to provide thin, durable coverage for hand defects.

References

1. Colson P, Janvier H. Le dégraissage primaire et total des lambeaux d'autoplastie à distance. *Ann Chir Plast* 1966;11:11.
2. Colson P, Janvier H, Gangolphe M, Laurent J. Brûlures du dos de la main. Problèmes posés par la réparation secondaire de la région des commissures. *Ann Chir Plast* 1970;15:14.
3. Kelleher JC, Sullivan JG, Dean RK. Use of a tailored abdominal pedicle flap for surgical reconstruction of the hand. *J Bone Joint Surg* 1970; 52(A):1552.
4. Arlon HG. Couverture d'une perte de substance cutanée post traumatique de la jambe par "cross-legs" utilisant un lambeau dégraissé selon la technique de Colson. *Bulletin et memoires de la Société des Chirurgiens de Paris* 1973;63:167.
5. Ionescu OG, Polovici A, Ciomei G. Valeur du lambeau sous claviculaire dégraissé dans les reconstructions digitales. *Acta Orthop Belg* 1975;41:3355.
6. Burton AC. *Physiology and biophysics of the circulation*. Paris: Masson, 1974;51, fig. 24.
7. Martineaud JP, Seroussi S. *Physiologie de la circulation cutanée*. Paris: Masson, 1977;59.

CHAPTER 254 ■ SUPRACLAVICULAR INNERVATED FLAP TO THE FINGER

B. C. SOMMERLAD AND J. G. BOORMAN

EDITORIAL COMMENT

This is an elegant procedure the surgeon might wish to consider for the totally desensitized hand.

When the hand has sustained significant skin loss, a flap is frequently required to provide sturdy cover and to allow maximal function. Many innervated flaps have been described for use in the hand (1–5), but most provide only a limited quantity of skin with one sensory nerve. The supraclavicular innervated flap (6) provides a larger area of skin innervated by three or more nerves, thus giving it advantages over other flaps in cases where larger areas are to be resurfaced. The procedure allows multiple digits to be resurfaced by one flap, but with separate innervation.

INDICATIONS

The flap is indicated in cases of extensive skin loss, for example, after degloving injuries or severe burns, when no suitable local flap is available. For smaller areas of loss it may be advisable to use another flap (1–3,5), such as those from the foot or the contralateral hand (4), that are thinner and may provide better sensation. The flap may be used as a primary procedure (in which case the relative simplicity of the first stage may be advantageous for an emergency operation), or for secondary reconstruction.

ANATOMY

The cervical plexus gives rise to a branch that emerges from behind the sternomastoid muscle and thereafter divides into the supraclavicular nerves. From a point slightly below the midpoint of the muscle close to the external jugular vein, these nerves radiate toward the clavicle. They supply the skin area superior to, overlying, and inferior to the clavicle as far as the second rib, extending from the midline to the point of the shoulder.

We found (6) that although three was the commonest number, up to five distinct and significant branches could be identified at a level just above the clavicle, any or all of which may be sutured separately to recipient nerves in the hand. The nerves are 1 to 2 mm in diameter and typically contain two to five bundles. In nonobese subjects the nerves may be palpated as they cross the clavicle (Fig. 1A).

The blood supply of this skin area is from three main sources: (1) the transverse cervical artery (superficial branch) (7); (2) the internal mammary artery (perforating branches) as is used for the deltopectoral flap (8); and (3) the thoracoacromial artery. The possibility thus exists of raising these innervated flaps on an axial pattern blood supply or as free flaps. An innervated deltopectoral flap has been used for pharyngeal reconstruction (9), but this flap is supraclavicularly innervated only in its upper half.

FLAP DESIGN AND DIMENSIONS

The maximum size of a supraclavicular innervated flap is approximately 20 × 12 cm, depending on the patient's size. Its

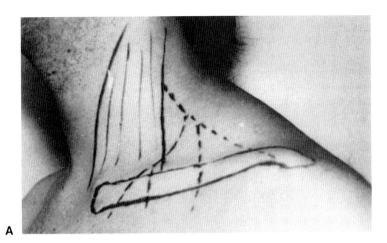
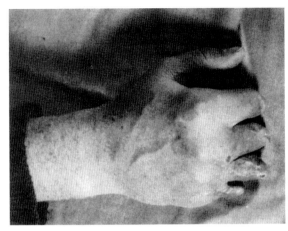
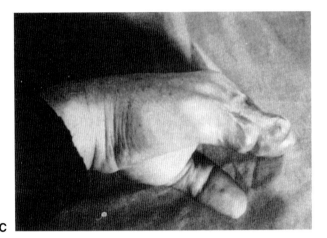
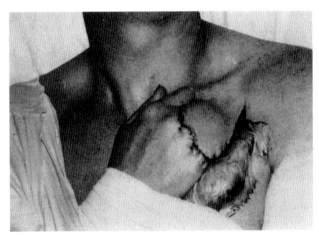

FIG. 1. **A:** Surface anatomy of main supraclavicular nerve branches (*broken lines*) in relation to ster-nomastoid and clavicle. **B,C:** A 28-year-old laborer with insensitive skin cover of his middle, ring, and little fingers. The skin broke down frequently with minor trauma, and movements at the metacarpopha-langeal joints were restricted (0° to 45°). This was the result of an accident 7 months earlier, when his hand had been caught between two heavy rollers, producing a crushing and degloving injury. (**B** is repro-duced from Sommerlad and Boorman, ref. 6, with permission.) **D:** A flap measuring 12 × 12 cm based superiorly was designed and inset onto the dorsal surface of the stumps.

thickness is moderate: greater than foot flaps, but less than groin flaps, both these other types being alternative sensory flaps for hand resurfacing. The flap is not appropriate in obese subjects.

Flap design is dictated by the orientation of nerves for suture in the recipient hand. In its most useful application—resurfacing both dorsal and volar surfaces together—it is con-venient to base the flap superiorly and to inset it onto the dor-sal surface (Fig. 1B–D). At the stage of flap division the nerves are identified and are sutured to digital nerves as the flap is inset on the palmar aspect of the hand.

OPERATIVE TECHNIQUE

To ensure inclusion of the nerves, the flap should be raised to include the deep fascia, especially in its superior portion. The nerves are readily identified on the deep surface of the flap. They pierce the fascia 1 to 2 cm above the clavicle, and then lie between fascia and platysma. To make nerve suture easier, a length of nerve proximal to the flap may be taken with the flap (Fig. 1E,F).

When more than one digit is to be resurfaced, subsequent separation can be safely achieved if the web spaces have been marked by a short length of rubber tubing (Fig. 1F).

CLINICAL RESULTS

The donor site of this flap may be closed directly or, if a larger area of skin is needed, may require grafting. There is no inter-ference with shoulder movements, and no loss of sensation in the remaining skin has been detectable. Scarring in this area is less acceptable to women patients. We have used this flap only in men, who more commonly sustain the type of injury for which the use of this flap is indicated.

SUMMARY

The supraclavicular innervated flap can provide a large area of sensory skin to the hand. The flap can be used to resurface multiple fingers while providing each with separate inner-vation.

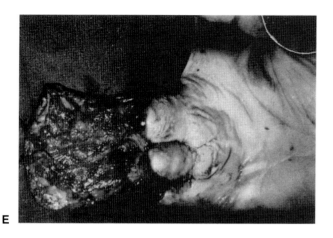

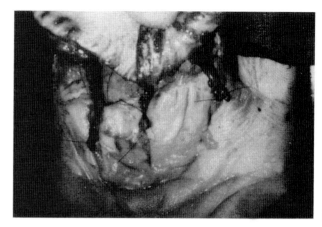

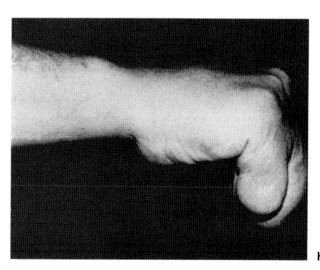

FIG. 1. *Continued* **E:** The flap was divided 4 weeks later (and 1 week after a preliminary delay). **F:** Three nerves were identified and sutured to the digital and common digital nerves (one nerve per finger). The web spaces had been marked with rubber tubing, and the fingers had subsequently been released and thinned. **G,H:** The patient was able to return to his previous employment as a laborer. His metacarpophalangeal joint range improved to a range of 0° to 90°. He has good light touch and pinprick sensation and localization. He is also able to detect hot and cold temperatures, which could not be done previously. He has suffered no further breakdown or ulceration of the skin.

References

1. Daniel RK, Terzis JK, Midgley RD. Restoration of sensation to an anaesthetic hand by a free neurovascular flap from the foot. *Plast Reconstr Surg* 1976;57:275.
2. Ohmori K, Harii K. Free dorsalis pedis sensory flap to the hand with microneurovascular anastomoses. *Plast Reconstr Surg* 1976;58:546.
3. May JW, Chait LA, Cohen BE, O'Brien BM. Free neurovascular flap from the first web of the foot in hand reconstruction. *J Hand Surg* 1977;2:387.
4. Dolich BH, Olshansky KJ, Babar AH. Use of a cross-forearm neurocutaneous flap to provide sensation and coverage in hand reconstruction. *Plast Reconstr Surg* 1978;62:550.
5. Strauch B, Tsur H. Restoration of sensation to the hand by a free neurovascular island flap from the first web space of the foot. *Plast Reconstr Surg* 1978;62:361.
6. Sommerlad BC, Boorman JG. An innervated flap incorporating supraclavicular nerves for reconstruction of major hand injuries. *Hand* 1981;13:5.
7. Lamberty BGH. The supraclavicular axial pattern flap. *Br J Plast Surg* 1979;32:207.
8. Bakamjian VY. A two stage method for pharyngo-esophageal reconstruction with a primary pectoral skin flap. *Plast Reconstr Surg* 1965;36:173.
9. David DJ. Use of an innervated deltopectoral flap for intra-oral reconstruction. *Plast Reconstr Surg* 1977;60:377.

CHAPTER 255 ■ MICROVASCULAR TRANSPLANTATION EN BLOC OF THE SECOND AND THIRD TOE

E. BIEMER

The second and third toes can be transferred en bloc to the hand (1–5). Indications are limited to special cases such as (1) amputation of all fingers, when only a thumb is left, and (2) total hand amputation, where the procedure is used in combination with single toe transfer for thumb reconstruction.

ANATOMY

Transfer of the second and third toes en bloc depends on an intact dorsalis pedis artery, as does the transfer of the big toe or of a single second toe. In the region of the tarsometatarsal joints, the dorsalis pedis artery gives rise to the arcuate artery at the lateral border of the foot. From the arcuate artery arise the dorsal metatarsal arteries, which divide at the level of the metatarsophalangeal joints into the dorsal digital arteries. These latter, in turn, divide to supply each side of the neighboring toe.

When the second and third toes are elevated, the second metatarsal artery as well as the first must be included, in order to have a good blood supply for the third toe. It should be noted, however, that in about 15% of cases the dorsalis pedis artery is not available.

To attain dorsal sensitivity in the toes, the deep peroneal nerve, which runs parallel to the artery, must be included. The plantar digital nerves normally run far more superficial to the flexor tendon than do the digital nerves in the fingers. For venous drainage, the venae comitantes are included and, just to be safe, a superficial vein from the venous arch of the dorsum of the foot.

OPERATIVE TECHNIQUE

Donor Site

The vascular supply to the donor area should be clarified by palpation, Doppler sonography, or angiography. It is important to ascertain whether the posterior tibial artery will supply the forefoot after removal of the dorsalis pedis artery.

In most instances the vascular connection in the recipient hand will be done in the snuffbox area. Therefore, quite a long vascular pedicle is needed. In addition to marking the course of the artery, the appropriate veins draining the toe superficially on the dorsum of the foot should be marked and should be elevated with the transplant, in case there is difficulty preparing the venae comitantes. It should also be decided if

incorporation of the dorsalis pedis flap for soft-tissue coverage of the hand is necessary. The use of a paper model is recommended for this purpose.

After raising the neurovascular trunk and incorporating the extensor tendons of the toe, an osteotomy is done. Then, by lifting the toes, the plantar nerves and the flexor tendon are separated and divided. If this preparation is done from the dorsum of the foot, a scar can be avoided on the plantar side of the foot that extends as far as the weight-bearing surface of the sole of the foot. The tendons taken with the transplanted toes are always somewhat longer than initially required.

The donor defect of the foot is closed with the objective of putting the heads of the first and fourth metatarsal as close together as possible. The ends of the metatarsal bones are carefully covered by local small muscles. Finally the whole defect is covered with a split-thickness skin graft.

Recipient Site

At the recipient site, the bones of the stumps (mostly third and fourth metatarsal bone) are exposed by two dorsal palmar fish-mouth incisions, which are connected by incising through the included web space so that an H-incision results. In cases where all the metacarpal bone is lost, alterations of the incision depend on the individual situation. The functional structures such as tendons and digital nerves are then identified, and the recipient vessels, mostly in the snuffbox area, are prepared.

The transplantation starts with bone fixation. In most of my cases I use Kirschner wires with transosseous wiring. This is an almost always stable and applicable procedure. The metatarsophalangeal joints of the toes are fixed in a slightly flexed position by Kirschner wire, to avoid hyperextension of the new finger. When only the head of the metatarsal bone is needed, this can also be achieved by a palmar flexion of the metatarsal head of up to 60°. One can thereby achieve useful flexor function in the metatarsophalangeal joint, or the use of that joint just for elongation of a new finger.

After tendon repair, the nerves are sutured and finally the arterial and the venous anastomoses are done. The decision to anastomose either a vena comitans or a superficial vein depends on the best venous reflux after opening the arterial anastomosis. Occasionally two venous anastomoses are done primarily.

The hand is not elevated as in replantation cases, but placed even somewhat lower than heart level. The donor foot is put in a light cast that allows both good stabilization of the foot and early mobility after the third or fourth day. In our experience, it normally takes up to 3 months until the donor area is completely healed.

CLINICAL RESULTS

There were no vascular complications in seven cases (Figs. 1–3). All transplanted toes survived very well. As to the mobility of the new "fingers," I found the motivation of these highly handicapped patients was so immense that in all instances extremely good functional results were achieved. The mobility of the second toe was always somewhat greater than that of the third toe. Most of the flexion and extension occurred in the proximal interphalangeal joint of the toes. Sensitivity steadily increased up to a two-point discrimination of 6 to 10 mm over 3 years. This is an interesting result, because two-point discrimination in a normal toe in an adult is 22 to 26 mm. All of the patients were pleased with the result, and

would ask again for the same procedure under the same circumstances. In two cases, a tenolysis was done as a secondary procedure, to improve hand flexion.

Mobility of the donor foot is comparatively limited. In my experience, patients need a specially made inlay to support the destroyed transverse arch of the foot, for up to 2 years. After this period, they could all wear normal shoes without difficulty. There was no breakdown or reulceration in the donor area, but it must be pointed out that the age of the patients ranged between 16 and 31 years.

An alternative to the procedure discussed is transferring only a single toe (6,7) and building up only one long finger. This leads to a lobster hand, and with this grip it is very difficult to stabilize a telephone receiver or to write—results that are easily achieved with the two-toe en bloc transplantation, which also yields superior aesthetic results.

SUMMARY

Although there are very limited indications, two-toe en bloc transplantation has its place in reconstructive hand surgery.

A–C

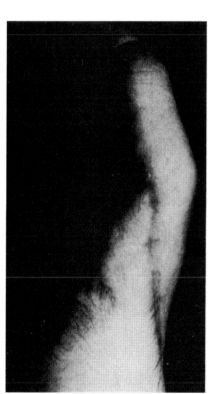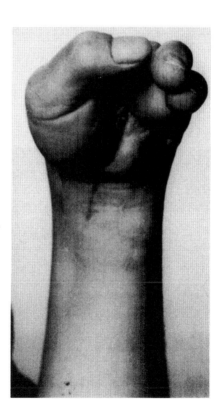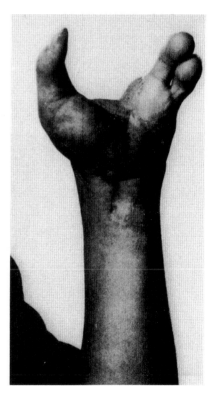

FIG. 1. A: Condition after an explosion injury of the left hand in a 16-year-old boy. Only the thumb was left. **B,C:** Good functional result 2 years after two-toe en bloc transplantation and shortening of the thumb. (From Biemer and Duspiva, ref. 5, with permission.)

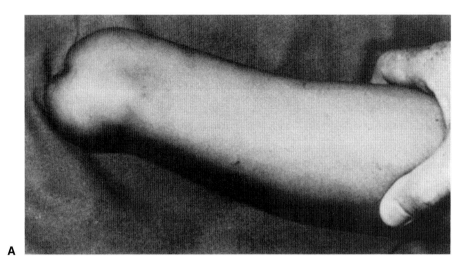

A

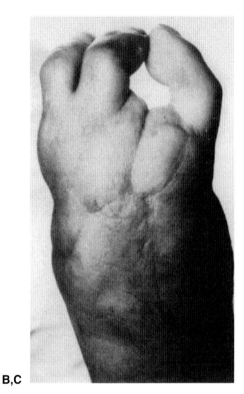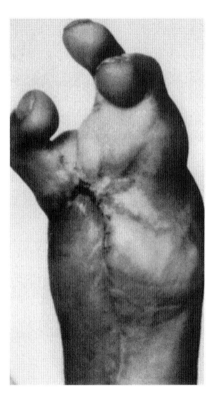

B,C

FIG. 2. **A:** Amputation of all four fingers of both hands. **B,C:** Functional results at 5 months after finger reconstruction of the right hand by two-toe en bloc transplantation. (From Biemer and Duspiva, ref. 5, with permission.)

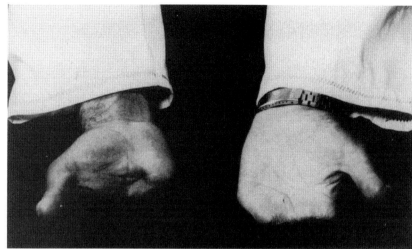

FIG. 3. A: Double hand amputation in a 23-year-old man. B,C: Reconstruction of one hand by three toes. (From Biemer and Duspiva, ref. 5, with permission.)

A

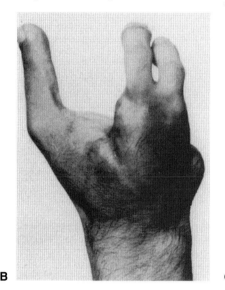

B

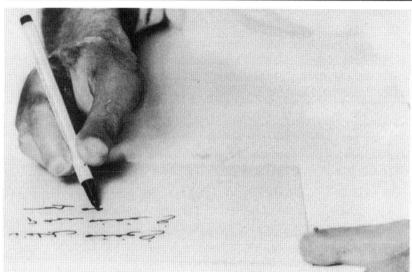

C

References

1. O'Brien BM, McLeod AM, Sykes PJ, Donahoe S. Hallux-to-hand transfer. *Hand* 1975;7:128.
2. Biemer E. In: Lie TS ed. *Toe transfer for thumb and finger replacement microsurgery*, Vol. 17. Amsterdam, Oxford: Excerpta Medica, 1979.
3. Biemer E, Stock W, Herndl E, Duspiva W. Reconstruction of the hand by free tissue transfer. *Int J Microsurg* 1980;2:159.
4. Biemer E. Daumenreconstruction. *Hefte zur Unfallheilkunde* 1982;158:428.
5. Biemer E, Duspiva W. *Reconstructive Microvascular Surgery*. New York: Springer, 1982.
6. Ohmori K, Harii K. Transplantation of a toe to an amputated finger. *Hand* 1975;7:134.
7. Biemer E. Zehentransplantation. Presented at the Third Congress of the European Section of the International Confederation for Plastic and Reconstructive Surgery, The Hague, May 22–27, 1977.

CHAPTER 256 ■ MICROVASCULAR FREE TRANSFER OF TOE JOINTS

J. E. KUTZ, H. W. KLEIN, T.-M. TSAI, AND B.-H. LIM

The problem of finger joints rendered stiff, painful, or unstable by trauma or disease presents the most vexing of dilemmas managed by the hand surgeon. While arthrodeses, fusions, and prosthetic joint replacements all have their indications and successes, these procedures are limited by the very problems for which they are used, i.e., poor motion, instability, and limited function. We have transferred an autologous joint by free microvascular techniques in 10 patients, and both clinical and experimental results indicate that a biological joint best meets the needs of motion, durability, and stability (1–5). In addition, the advantages of longitudinal growth may be added when the joint is transferred with its epiphysis in a growing child. In some situations more than one joint requires reconstruction. In two cases we have successfully used both the proximal interphalangeal (PIP) joint and metatarsophalangeal (MTP) joint of the second toe for a double joint microvascular free transfer on multiple metacarpophalangeal (MCP) joint damage based on a single pedicle (6,7).

INDICATIONS

We believe that the indications for this transfer are (1) traumatic joint loss in young active patients who need joint motion, (2) juvenile cases with epiphyseal damage and growth arrest, and (3) multiple joint injuries. These indications presume the presence of a good distal finger. The transfer should be attempted only in patients with adequate motivation to understand and maintain the postoperative care required.

ANATOMY

The blood supply of the transfer is based on the dorsalis pedis and the plantar digital arterial system. The digital arteries of the toes form transverse arterial branches at the MTP, PIP joint, and the distal interphalangeal (DIP) joint, which in turn branch to the articular surface and metaphyseal areas of the phalanges. At the level of the transverse artery, the vessel continues dorsally to supply the skin over the joints.

OPERATIVE TECHNIQUE

A dorsal incision is made over the donor foot to identify and preserve the dorsalis pedis, the first dorsal metatarsal arch, and the dorsal venous arch. The extensor hallucis brevis sometimes needs to be divided to expose the arterial system adequately. The incision is carried onto the second toe, so that an island of skin can be harvested over the PIP joint as a monitor of the subsequent vascular status of the joint transfer.

The digital artery of the medial (tibial) side is divided at the DIP joint, taking care to preserve the articular and metaphyseal branches. The lateral (fibular) branch is preserved, after carefully ligating the metaphyseal branches. The dissection is done with 3× to 4× loupe magnification. After mobilizing the vessels, the DIP joint is disarticulated, and an osteotomy is performed at the midpoint of the proximal phalanx taking care not to damage the medial metaphyseal branch of the proximal phalanx (Fig. 1B).

The extensor tendon and the skin island are preserved as a unit. At this point, complete mobilization of the transfer is possible (Fig. 1A). The circulation is checked, the pedicle length is measured, and the corresponding lengths of dorsalis pedis artery and dorsal vein are harvested.

Prior to the harvest, the recipient site in the hand is prepared (Fig. 1C). Scar tissue is excised, the bone ends are freshened, tendons are mobilized, and the recipient vessels are identified.

The transfer is performed by first stabilizing the bone with interosseous wiring and a bone peg taken from the anterior tibia (Fig. 1D). A longitudinal Kirschner wire also may be used. A bone peg graft is used to fuse the toe joint in the foot (Fig. 1E). In our experience, end-to-side arterial anastomosis has been the most useful method of reconstruction, especially if a vessel size mismatch occurs (Fig. 1F). Two veins are anastomosed. Both the superficial system and the venae comitantes (deep system) can be used. Postoperative temperature and color are monitored in the skin island and are indicators of a viable transfer.

In the double joint transfer, the second toe, including the MTP joint, is harvested together with a skin paddle from the tibial aspect of the big toe (Fig. 2A). The medial (tibial) digital artery is mobilized by dividing metaphyseal and articular branches to the PIP joint. The articular and metaphyseal branches over the lateral (tibial) side of the MTP joint are divided to free the fibular digital vessel. The distal commissural vessels at the distal phalanx are preserved to maintain vascular continuity (Fig. 2B). The mobilization of the digital vessels in this manner increases the interjoint pedicle length. This allows the reconstruction of two adjacent MCP joints based on a single pedicle (Fig. 2C,D).

CLINICAL RESULTS

Possible complications include (1) arterial or venous failure resulting in loss of the vascularized advantage, with the joint acting merely as an elaborate arthrodesis; (2) delayed union; and (3) malposition and misalignment.

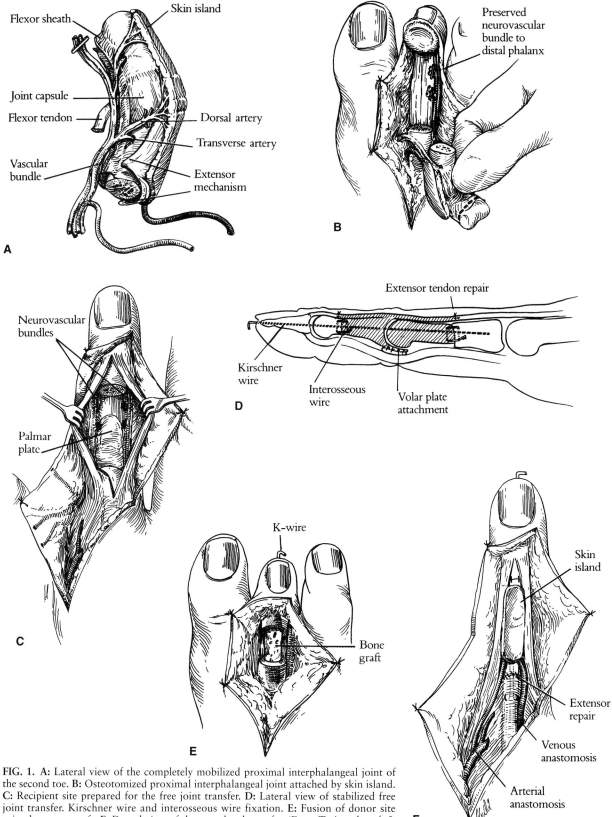

FIG. 1. A: Lateral view of the completely mobilized proximal interphalangeal joint of the second toe. B: Osteotomized proximal interphalangeal joint attached by skin island. C: Recipient site prepared for the free joint transfer. D: Lateral view of stabilized free joint transfer. Kirschner wire and interosseous wire fixation. E: Fusion of donor site using bone peg graft. F: Dorsal view of the completed transfer. (From Tsai et al., ref. 5, with permission.)

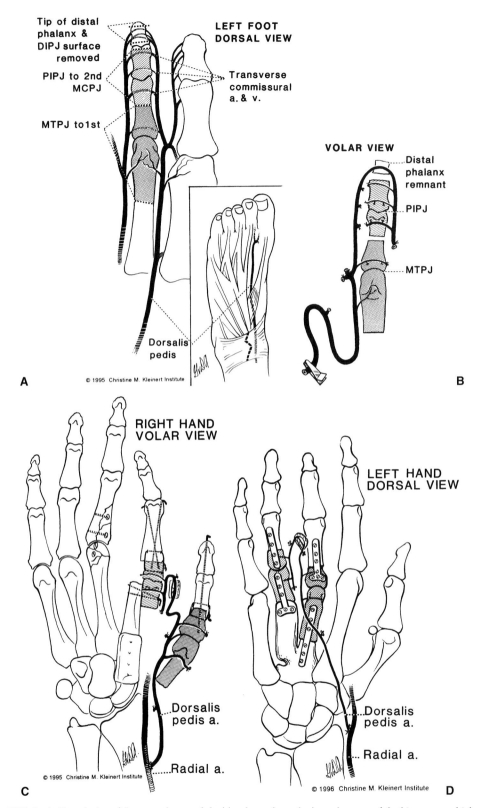

FIG. 2. A: Vascularity of the second toe and the blood supply to the lateral aspect of the big toe on which the skin paddle for monitoring is based. **B:** Mobilization of the medial vascular branches to the PIP joint and lateral vascular branches at the MTP joint, with preservation of the distal commissural branches. **C:** Transfer of the PIP joint of the second toe to reconstruct the second MCP joint and the MTP joint to reconstruct the first MCP joint (case 1). **D:** Transfer of the PIP joint and MTP joint of the second toe to reconstruct the third and fourth MCP joint of the left hand, respectively.

To 1993, all of our 10 transfers have been successful, followed from 1 to 3 years. Our mean operative time was 8 hours, and the mean hospital stay 9 days. The articular space was preserved in all cases. The mean ranges of motion were 22.1° to 54.9° active and 7.3° to 64.1° passive. All joints transferred were free of pain, and all but one have stable union. In two patients with open epiphyses there was radiological evidence of longitudinal growth. Additional required operations included extensor and flexor tenolysis in two cases, reconstruction of a radial collateral ligament in one patient, and a transposition skin flap in one patient.

Recently we had two cases that required a double joint transfer. The PIP joint and the MTP joint of the second toe were used to reconstruct two adjacent MCP joints in the hand based on a single vascular pedicle. In both cases at 6 months and 4 months follow-up the joint architecture and spaces were maintained, and sound union of the joint transferred was achieved. The first case will require further staged reconstruction because of the complexity of the injury. In the second case, at 4 months' follow-up the active range of motion of the transferred PIP joint to the long MCP joint is 3° and the passive range of motion is 30°. The MCP joint to the ring has an active range of motion of 26° and 37° of passive motion. We have seen no evidence of functional deficit in the donor foot in any of the single or double joint transfers.

SUMMARY

Transfer of a microvascular toe phalangeal joint can be used for traumatic finger joint loss or for a juvenile with epiphyseal damage and joint arrest. In multiple joint loss, it is possible to reconstruct two joints with a single toe and a single vascular pedicle.

References

1. Erdelyi R. Experimental auto-transplantation of small joints. *Plast Reconstr Surg* 1963;31:129.
2. Hurwitz PH. Experimental transplantation of small joints by microvascular anastomoses. *Plast Reconstr Surg* 1979;64:221.
3. Snowdy HA, Omer GE, Sherman FC. Longitudinal growth of a free toe phalanx transplant to a finger. *J Hand Surg [Br]* 1980;5:71.
4. Tsai TM, Ogden L, Jaeger SH, Okubo K. Experimental vascularized total joint autografts: a primate study. *J Hand Surg [Br]* 1982;7:140.
5. Tsai TM, Jupiter J, Kutz JE, Kleinert HE. Vascularized autogenous whole joint transfer: a clinical study. *J Hand Surg [Br]* 1982;7:335.
6. Tsai TM, Lim BH. Single toe double joint transfer using a vascular pedicle. Proceedings of the 12th Symposium of International Society of Reconstructive Microsurgery, 1996.
7. Tsai TM, Lim BH. Free vascularized transfer of the metatarsophalangeal and proximal interphalangeal joints of the second toe for reconstruction of the metacarpophalangeal joints of the thumb and index finger using a single vascular pedicle: a case report. *Plast Reconstr Surg* 1996;98(6):1080.

CHAPTER 257 ■ VOLAR THUMB ADVANCEMENT SKIN FLAP

M. A. POSNER

The objectives in the treatment of thumb tip injuries are to preserve length, restore normal sensibility, maintain joint mobility, and provide a tip that is well padded and free from tender scars. Advancement of a volar skin flap will satisfy these objectives in the primary and secondary treatment of many injuries involving the distal segment of the thumb (1–4).

INDICATIONS

The procedure is particularly applicable to avulsion injuries of the volar pulp tissue or to resurfacing a scarred, tender thumb tip where most of the distal phalanx remains intact.

ANATOMY

Both neurovascular bundles remain with the volar flap, thereby retaining its sensibility and blood supply regardless of its length. The dorsal strip of skin remains viable, since it receives its circulation from the first dorsal metacarpal artery arising from the dorsal carpal arch that is formed by dorsal branches of the radial and ulnar artery (5). This pattern of circulation to the dorsal skin is different in fingers where the dorsal skin (particularly at the level of the distal segment) is dependent on the volar digital vessels. The risk of dorsal skin necrosis is therefore far greater following a volar advancement flap in a finger than in a thumb (see Chap. 229).

OPERATIVE TECHNIQUE

Midaxial incisions are made on the radial and ulnar sides of the thumb (Fig. 1A,B). The volar skin with its subcutaneous tissue and both neurovascular bundles are elevated from the underlying tendon sheath of the flexor pollicis longus (Fig. 1C).

Advancement of the flap is obtained primarily by interphalangeal joint flexion. Flexion of the interphalangeal joint will permit the flap to be advanced up to 1.5 to 2 cm, if it is elevated to the flexion crease of the metacarpophalangeal joint (Fig. 1D).

With amputations through the distal phalanx, the bone should be contoured. Similarly, the end of the advancement skin flap itself should be contoured to approximate it closely to the dorsal skin. Postoperatively a dorsal plaster splint is applied, immobilizing the wrist in neutral position and the thumb in slight flexion, to relieve any tension on the skin sutures. Active thumb flexion can be instituted immediately postoperatively and active extension exercises encouraged when the splint is discontinued in 7 to 10 days.

CLINICAL RESULTS

Necrosis of the dorsal skin or flexion contractures of the interphalangeal joint have not been encountered in any case treated with this procedure. The ability to hyperextend the interphalangeal joint is sometimes lost postoperatively, but this has no clinical significance (Fig. 2).

SUMMARY

Restoration of padding with skin of normal sensibility is the predictable outcome for the primary or secondary treatment of thumb tip injuries.

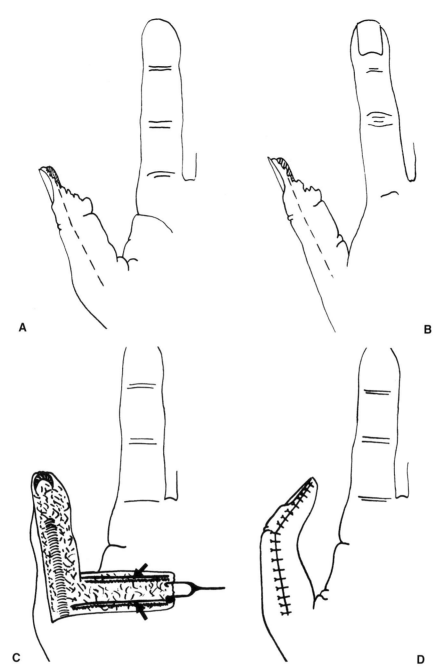

FIG. 1. **A,B:** Midaxial incisions are made on the radial and ulnar aspects of the thumb to the metacarpophalangeal flexion crease. **C:** The entire volar skin flap with both neurovascular bundles (*arrows*) is elevated from the underlying flexor tendon sheath. **D:** Advancement of the flap is primarily obtained by flexion of the interphalangeal joint. (From Posner and Smith, ref. 2, with permission.)

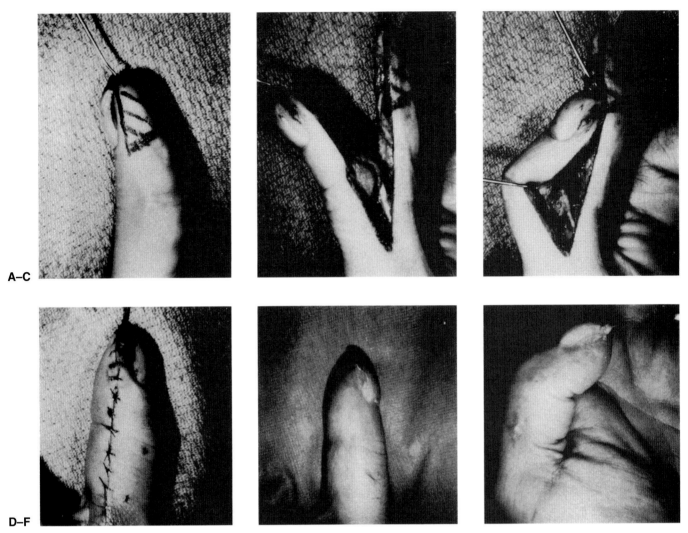

FIG. 2. A: This patient had an area of hypersensitivity over the distal 1.5 cm of the thumb tip after a crushing injury. **B,C:** The volar skin flap was elevated from the underlying tendon sheath and was easily advanced by flexion of the interphalangeal joint. **D:** Immediately postoperatively, after the area of hypersensitive skin was excised and the volar flap advanced. The distal portion of the flap was trimmed to follow the contour of the nail. **E,F:** Several months postoperatively, the patient had a painless thumb tip with normal padding and sensibility. Interphalangeal flexion was not limited and extension was to the neutral position. (From Posner and Smith, ref. 2, with permission.)

References

1. Moberg E. Aspects of sensation in reconstructive surgery of the upper limb. *J Bone Joint Surg* 1964;46(A):817.
2. Posner MA, Smith RJ. The advancement pedicle flap for thumb injuries. *J Bone Joint Surg* 1971;53(A):1618.
3. Keim HA, Grantham SA. Volar-flap advancement for thumb and finger tip injuries. *Clin Orthop* 1969;66:109.
4. Millender LH, Albin RE, Nalebuff EA. Delayed volar advancement flap for thumb tip injuries. *Plast Reconstr Surg* 1973;52:635.
5. Macht SD, Watson HK. The Moberg volar advancement flap for digital reconstructions. *J Hand Surg* 1980;5:372.

CHAPTER 258 ■ ROTATION ADVANCEMENT SKIN FLAP TO THE THUMB TIP

R. V. ARGAMASO

The thumb has a greater range of motion than any other finger and is indispensable to the prehensile function of the hand. Because the thumb is endowed with only two phalanges, the complete loss of the distal phalanx compromises its ability to encompass large objects with the opposing fingers. Conserving length should be the formost objective in selecting methods of wound closure in cases involving amputation injuries distal to the interphalangeal joint.

INDICATIONS

The treatment of choice should be to use the amputated segment if it is replantable. However, this course is not always possible in many injuries. The distal phalanx, even when projecting beyond the level of soft-tissue loss, should not be sacrificed simply to achieve direct skin suture. Rather, as much bone stock as can possibly be covered with a skin flap should be preserved.

An ideal flap is one that closely resembles palmar digital skin in appearance and texture. More important, it should possess good tactile sensation. Direct advancement of a volar skin flap with both neurovascular bundles satisfies these criteria (1). Stretching the volar skin, however, is limited to a few millimeters. Often a successful coverage by this method is accomplished only in conjunction with flexion of the thumb at both metaphalangeal (MP) and interphalangeal (IP) joints (2). There is a risk of causing a flexion contracture in older patients.

Flexion contraction may be overcome by transferring an island skin flap with a neurovascular pedicle from one side of a finger to the thumb tip (3). Obviously a skin graft is needed to resurface the donor defect. In this instance, there is loss of sensation at the donor site, and the sensation at the thumb tip needs to be reoriented at a cortical level.

A method is described for rotating the entire volar skin of the thumb, keeping its innervation intact (4,5). A second flap from the first web on the dorsum of the hand is transposed, to close the secondary defect at the base of the thumb. This method offers several functional and aesthetic advantages: discriminative sensibility and texture quality of the skin remain the same, the scar lines are in a location away from the tactile surface of the thumb, and full-range joint motions are not compromised.

The technique described here is ideal for sharp or guillotine-type amputations of the thumb tip, but is also suitable for crushing injuries in which the soft tissues of the stump are not seriously damaged.

ANATOMY

The flap is elevated on the ulnar side of the thumb and then back-cut along the volar surface at the MP crease. Both neurovascular bundles are dissected to allow rotation and advancement of the flap, but they are preserved. In this way the thumb retains good sensation that is correctly represented on the cerebral cortex.

FLAP DESIGN AND DIMENSIONS

The flap is based on the radial side of the thumb, but the blood supply comes through both neurovascular bundles. The flap is elevated from the defect just dorsal to the midaxial line of the ulnar side of the thumb. At the level of the MP crease, a back-cut is made to allow the flap to rotate and advance into the defect (Fig. 1). The pivot point of the flap is at the radial side of the MP crease.

Once the flap is inset, a triangular-shaped defect is created at the base of the thumb. The open area may be resurfaced by a skin flap transposed from the dorsal skin of the first web. This triangular flap (Fig. 1) is planned slightly larger in dimension than the secondary defect on the volar surface of the thumb. One side of the flap is an extension of the midaxial thumb incision. It runs almost parallel to the fold of the web skin, and its apex is at the lateral side of the index finger, where it turns back parallel to the index metacarpal. The flap can be 2 cm in width.

OPERATIVE TECHNIQUE

If necessary, any small remnants of nail matrix should be removed. Tiny residues of fingernail regenerating in an abnormal fashion can cause discomfort.

Once the incision from the defect to the MP crease has been made, a gradual back-cut is done. The digital neurovascular bundles are identified and kept intact. The proper digital nerves and arteries are found proximally on the palmar side of the flap. They move toward the midaxial planes as they course distally. The neurovascular bundles are raised carefully with the volar skin flap (Fig. 2A). It may be necessary to dissect these bundles in the palm, to allow the skin flaps more mobility to rotate and stretch over the stump.

Once the triangular flap is transposed into the defect left by the rotation advancement flap, the defect on the side of the index finger is closed by direct skin approximation. For more

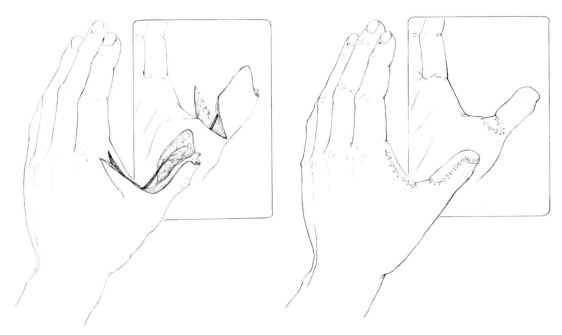

FIG. 1. Volar thumb and dorsal web skin flaps elevated and inset. (From Argamaso, ref. 4, with permission.)

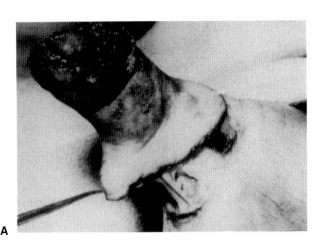

A

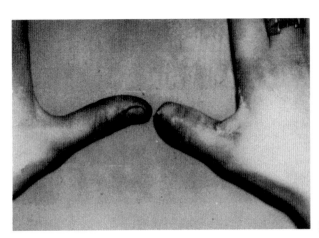

B

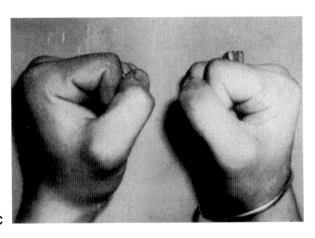

C

FIG. 2. A: Crush-type amputation across the middle of the distal phalanx. The neurovascular bundles are elevated with the flap. **B:** Postoperative radial abduction and extension of interphalangeal and metacarpophalangeal joints. **C:** Postoperative flexion of interphalangeal and metacarpophalangeal joints. (From Argamaso, ref. 4, with permission.)

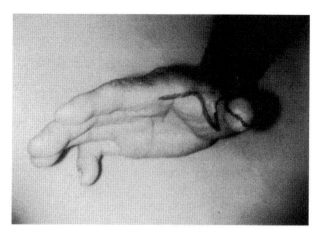

FIG. 3. The postoperative position of the flaps is outlined with ink. Note that the scars are away from areas of contact during pinch or grasp. (From Argamaso, ref. 4, with permission.)

distally located tip injuries, where only a short distance of volar skin advancement is required, the secondary defect at the thumb base is usually amenable to simple direct closure by mobilizing the loose dorsal and palmar skin.

The thumb is kept in palmar abduction for about 10 to 14 days. Thereafter active exercises are started.

Online Chapter

CHAPTER 259. Extended Palmar Advancement Flap

A. L. Dellon

www.encyclopediaofflaps.com

CLINICAL RESULTS

Tender scars have not been observed in the cases presented in this report. In general, scars on contact areas, such as the web skin and opposing sides of the thumb and index finger, should be avoided (Fig. 3). The pigmented dorsal web skin that is transposed to the volar side of the thumb has not caused any aesthetic problems.

SUMMARY

A volar rotation advancement flap can be used to close thumb tip injuries. Good cover and normal sensation are provided and the donor defect can be easily closed with a transposition flap from the index finger.

References

1. Moberg E. Aspects of sensation in reconstructive surgery of the upper limb. *J Bone Joint Surg* 1964;46(A):817.
2. Posner MS, Smith RJ. The advancement pedicle flap for thumb injuries. *J Bone Joint Surg* 1971;53(a):1618.
3. Littler JW. In: Converse JM, ed. *Reconstructive plastic surgery.* Philadelphia: Saunders, 1964;1638–1639.
4. Argamaso RV. Rotation-transposition method for soft tissue replacement on the distal segment of the thumb. *Plast Reconstr Surg* 1974;54:366.
5. Joshi BB. One-stage repair for distal amputation of the thumb. *Plast Reconstr Surg* 1970;45:613.

CHAPTER 260 ■ VOLAR CROSS-FINGER FLAPS

R. W. BEASLEY AND B. W. EDGERTON

Maintenance of maximum length is axiomatic in the treatment of thumb amputations. Whenever possible, wound closure without shortening should be accomplished with local tissues or those from an adjacent digit. The volar cross-finger flap has several advantages for repair of distal thumb amputations (1,2). Positioning is much easier than with a dorsal cross-finger flap from the index finger, and the donor site is hidden on the volar side of the finger. Local tissue of near-perfect match with the ability to recover an excellent degree of sensibility is used,

adequate padding is restored, and there is minimal donor site morbidity.

INDICATIONS

The volar cross-finger flap is an excellent method of reconstruction for dorsal oblique, guillotine, or volar amputations of the distal thumb. The volar advancement flap (3) is a good

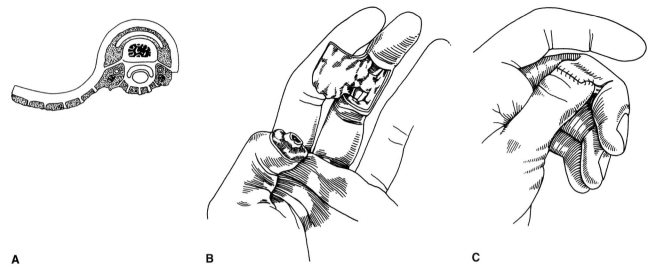

A   **B**   **C**

FIG. 1. **A:** The volar cross-finger skin flap. Note that the neurovascular bundle is left attached to the base of the pedicle. A formal dissection of the neurovascular bundle is required when the flap is divided. The flap is dissected in a plane just superficial to the tendon sheath, thereby preserving an adequate bed for skin grafting. **B:** Volar flap prepared for transfer. **C:** Flap in place on the amputated thumb tip. (From Beasley, ref. 2, with permission.)

alternative to this flap for dorsal oblique amputations; but the volar cross-finger flap is a better alternative for major volar losses, because it provides excellent tissue replacement without any traction on the vessels or nerves of the thumb that may result in dysesthesia. The volar cross-finger flap also provides sufficient skin and subcutaneous tissue under no tension for support of the fingernail and for proper tip contour (Fig. 1).

ANATOMY

The volar skin of the digits has a vertically oriented blood supply with only short horizontal interconnections. This differs from the dorsal skin, which has a longitudinal orientation of vessels. This difference must be respected and there is a limit to the size of volar flaps that can be safely elevated. During the elevation of the flap, the neurovascular bundle must not be dissected free from the pedicle (Fig. 1A), in contrast to dorsal cross-finger flaps, because this will seriously jeopardize the blood supply to the flap. A formal dissection of the neurovascular bundle in a bloodless field is necessary at the time of pedicle division. These flaps are direct flaps, in that the defect is positioned directly under the open surface of the flap.

FLAP DESIGN AND DIMENSIONS

The thumb is placed in opposition to the volar surface of the long finger, and a decision is made whether to use the proximal or middle phalanx and whether to base the flap on the radial or ulnar border of the finger. If the tissue has been lost only on the volar surface of the thumb, the volar cross-finger flap should be based ulnarly. Most cases of guillotine or dorsal oblique thumb amputations are more suitably handled by a flap based on the radial side of the finger (Fig. 1B). Positioning is more favorable with respect to the joints when tissues overlying the middle phalanx are used, but a flap overlying the proximal phalanx will provide a greater bulk of subcutaneous tissue. A maximum-sized flap of 2 × 2 cm may be raised from the volar surface of either the proximal or the middle phalanx of the long finger.

A pattern of the defect is created and placed on the donor surface. The flap is outlined to include extra length of the base, and the margins are carried to lines of neutral skin tension just as with elective incisions, even if part of the flap must be discarded. Care should be taken to minimize flexion of the proximal interphalangeal joint (Fig. 1C). All flaps should be measured twice before cutting.

OPERATIVE TECHNIQUE

The flap is elevated in a plane just superficial to the tendon sheath, which preserves an adequate bed for skin grafting (Fig. 2A,B). The flap must be dissected free from the opposite underlying neurovascular bundle, but the neurovascular bundle at the base of the flap must not be dissected from the pedicle. After obtaining meticulous hemostasis, a full-thickness skin graft is sutured into the volar defect and the flap is then sutured to the thumb (Fig. 2C). A carefully fitted compressive dressing is placed over the skin graft and the thumb and finger are secured together with tape before applying a light plaster shell with a window to allow inspection.

With progressive healing, the pedicle of the flap may be divided in 10 to 14 days as a formal operative procedure. Care must be taken not to injure the neurovascular bundle in the pedicle when the base of the flap is severed. Sutures may be used gently to approximate the donor site after division and for hemostasis, but the flap should not be sutured or inset further at the time of severance. The flap tolerates handling or any tension poorly at this stage. A noncompressive dressing is applied and mobilization of joints is begun at once. The wound is allowed to epithelialize and a secondary revision is required for an occasional patient.

CLINICAL RESULTS

Volar cross-finger flaps have been used on our service in 20 cases (Fig. 2D). No instances of flap loss, infection, or donor site complications have occurred.

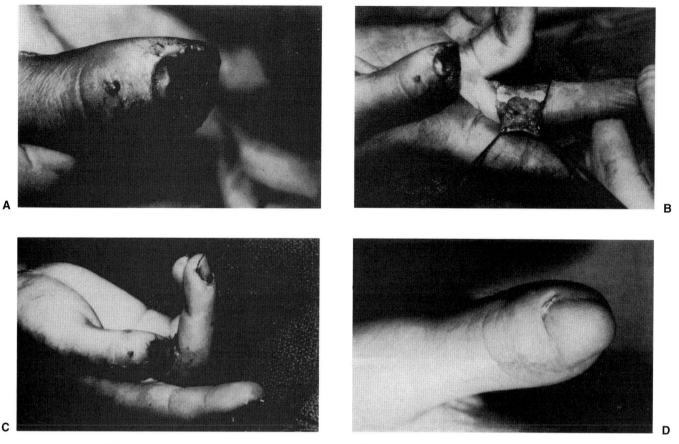

FIG. 2. **A:** Dorsal oblique amputation of the thumb tip. **B:** Dissection of the flap, leaving the neurovascular bundle attached to the base of the flap. **C:** The flap in place. The donor site is covered with a full-thickness skin graft. **D:** Postoperative appearance. Note that thumb length has been preserved.

SUMMARY

The volar cross-finger flap is an excellent reconstructive method for dealing with major distal amputations of the thumb, whether dorsal oblique, guillotine, or volar oblique. The flap furnishes well-padded volar skin of near-perfect tissue match to preserve maximum thumb length and support of the nailbed.

References

1. Beasley RW. Principles of managing acute hand injuries. In: Converse JM, ed. *Reconstructive plastic surgery*. Philadelphia: Saunders, 1977; 3027.
2. Beasley RW. *Hand injuries*. Philadelphia: Saunders, 1981.
3. Moberg E. Aspects of sensation in reconstructive surgery of the upper extremity. *J Bone Joint Surg [Am]* 1964;46:817.

CHAPTER 261 ■ SIDE FINGER SKIN FLAP TO THE THUMB TIP

R. C. RUSSELL AND E. G. ZOOK

EDITORIAL COMMENT

Although this flap is valuable for thumb tip reconstruction, the extreme flexion of the finger while it is attached to the flap may result in significant residual stiffness of the finger.

A cross-finger flap can be elevated from the side of the proximal phalanx to cover thumb tip amputations (1). This flap has certain advantages over previously described techniques for this difficult problem (2–16).

INDICATIONS

A side finger flap elevated from the index or long finger will easily reach thumb tip amputations distal to the interphalangeal joint in all age groups. More proximal amputations may be difficult to reach in less supplely working hands.

FLAP DESIGN AND DIMENSIONS

The flap is proximally based and centered dorsal to the midaxial line over the proximal phalanx of the donor finger. It can extend slightly beyond the proximal interphalangeal joint flexion crease distally, and may be as wide as 2 cm, depending on the circumference of the donor digit. Elevation from the ulnar side of the finger is best, to decrease donor site deformity. The ulnar sides of the digits are hidden from view during most hand use and at rest.

The injured thumb tip is first manipulated next to the proposed donor site to assess ease of positioning. With the fingers flexed, the midaxial line is next marked along the top of the interphalangeal joint flexion creases. The flap is then outlined with the finger extended, so that two-thirds of the flap lies dorsal to the midaxial line (Fig. 1A).

OPERATIVE TECHNIQUE

Elevation is begun dorsally, by incision through the skin and subcutaneous tissue to the underlying extensor tendon mechanism. The flap is dissected in a volar direction preserving the peritenon, until the neurovascular bundle is identified.

The distal and volar skin incisions are then completed to a level superficial to the underlying digital artery and nerve. The flap is then elevated proximally to the volar metacarpophalangeal joint flexion crease.

The dorsal incision may be extended further into the interphalangeal web space, to permit greater flap mobility. Large dorsal veins seen entering the base of the flap should be preserved by gentle scissor dissection, dividing only persistent fibrous tissue.

If the donor defect is to be closed primarily, the dorsal and, to a lesser degree, volar skin edges are undermined and approximated toward the base of the flap (Fig. 1). Care should be taken to avoid excessive tension of the soft tissue at the base of the flap. Larger donor defects are closed with a full-thickness skin graft from the inguinal flexion crease, using a stent dressing. The flap is then rotated 90° volarly or dorsally over the thumb (Fig. 1C).

Postoperatively, the injured and donor digits should be immobilized, to facilitate neovascular ingrowth into the flap and, when necessary, the take of the skin graft. Flaps are divided in 12 to 18 days, followed by immediate active and passive range of motion exercises.

CLINICAL RESULTS

Side finger flap donor sites form fine scars away from the grasping surface of the digit, and these scars have been uniformly nontender. Skin-grafted donor sites may remain depressed or become hyperpigmented with time. However, when placed on the ulnar side of the finger, the deformity is much less visible and is cosmetically superior to that seen following standard dorsal cross-finger flaps.

Residual stiffness of the injured or donor digits has not occurred in our patients, and all flaps have provided stable cover.

SUMMARY

The side finger skin flap is an excellent choice for thumb tip amputations, when a more cosmetically acceptable donor site is desired.

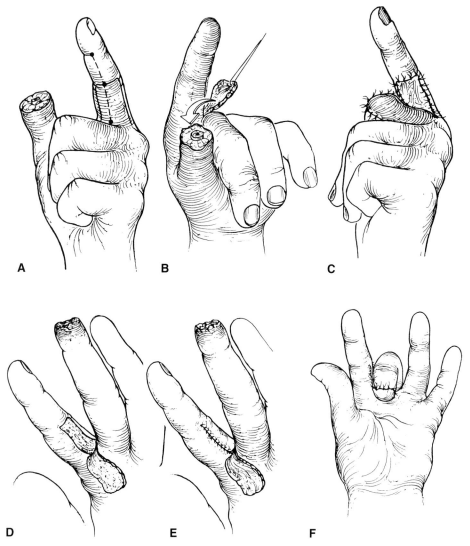

FIG. 1. A side finger flap from the ulnar side of the donor finger is centered above the midaxial line (**A**) and can be rotated 90° volarly to cover an amputated thumb tip (**B,C**). The side finger may be rotated to cover an amputated fingertip (**D–F**). (From Russell et al., ref. 1, with permission.)

References

1. Russell RC, Van Beck AL, Wavak P, Zook EG. Alternative hand flaps for amputations and digital defects. *J Hand Surg [Am]* 1981;6:399.
2. Atasoy E, Ioakimidis E, Kasdan ML, Kutz JE, Kleinert HE. Reconstruction of the amputated finger tip with a triangular volar flap: a new surgical procedure. *J Bone Joint Surg [Am]* 1970;52:921.
3. Barton NJ. A modified thenar flap. *Hand* 1975;7:150.
4. Bennett JE. Fingertip avulsions. *J Trauma* 1966;6:249.
5. Flatt AE. The thenar flap. *J Bone Joint Surg [Br]* 1957;39:80.
6. Gatewood. A plastic repair of finger defects without hospitalization. *JAMA* 1926;87:1479.
7. Hoskins HD. The versatile cross-finger pedicle flap: a report of twenty-six cases. *J Bone Joint Surg [Am]* 1960;42:261.
8. Kutler W. A new method for finger-tip amputation. *JAMA* 1947;133:29.
9. Littler JW. Principles of reconstructive surgery of the hand. In: Converse JM, ed., *Reconstructive plastic surgery.* Philadelphia: Saunders, 1964; 1612–1673.
10. Miller AJ. Single fingertip injuries treated by thenar flap. *Hand* 1974;6:311.
11. O'Brien BM. Neurovascular island pedicle flaps for terminal amputations and digital scars. *Br J Plast Surg* 1968;21:258.
12. O'Brien BM. Neurovascular pedicle transfers in the hand. *Aust N Z J Surg* 1965;35:2.
13. Robins RHE. Fingertip injuries. *Hand* 1970;2:119.
14. Smith RJ, Albin R. Thenar "H-flap" for fingertip injuries. *J Trauma* 1976;16:778.
15. Tempest MN. Cross-finger flaps in the treatment of injuries to the fingertip. *Plast Reconstr Surg* 1952;9:205.
16. Woolf RM, Broadbent TR. Injuries to the fingertips: treatment with cross-finger flaps. *Rocky Mt Med J* 1967;35:1195.

CHAPTER 262 ■ COCKED HAT (GILLIES) THUMB SKIN FLAP

D. A. CAMPBELL REID

The *cocked hat flap* was first suggested by Gillies (1) in 1946 as a possible technique for lengthening the partially amputated thumb.

INDICATIONS

This flap is usually used for lengthening a thumb amputated in the region of the metacarpophalangeal joint (2–4). It may be used only as a reconstructive procedure. By the time this is undertaken, scarring following primary surgery for the amputated thumb will have matured and softened.

The cocked hat flap can be used when all four fingers are intact if it is not considered justifiable to pollicize a finger. It can also be used in the mutilated hand if no suitable digit is available for pollicization.

ANATOMY

This is a distally based flap. The blood supply is from the vessels that are distributed to the thumb, the radial side of the index finger, and the adjoining web. The princeps pollicis artery arises from the deep palmar arch and divides into the two proper digital arteries to supply the volar aspect of the thumb.

The first dorsal metacarpal artery arises from the radial artery just before it passes between the two heads of the first dorsal interosseous muscle, and divides almost immediately into the two branches that supply the back of the thumb and the adjacent side of the index finger. Branches of the radialis indicis artery will also supply the flap. This vessel arises either from the deep palmar arch or from the princeps pollicis artery. There is a considerable anastomotic network between these various component vessels to supply the skin of the thumb/index web.

Veins accompany these arteries, and it is these that are responsible for the venous drainage of the flap, since the superficial veins on the dorsal aspect of the hand must be divided when raising the flap.

FLAP DESIGN AND DIMENSIONS

In the average-sized adult hand, the width of the flap at its base measures 7 to 8 cm. The length of the flap from base to apex measures 5 to 6 cm. The pivot of the flap is the radial side of the index finger, where it joins the first web space (Fig. 1).

A U-shaped flap is marked out, commencing on the dorsal aspect opposite the neck of the second metacarpal and curving around the base of the thumb over the carpometacarpal joint onto the thenar region of the palm. The palmar part of the flap then extends distally, parallel to, and about 1 cm on the

radial side of, the thenar crease, ending at a point corresponding to the beginning of the flap on the dorsum.

OPERATIVE TECHNIQUE

Dissection of the flap starts on the dorsal aspect and at the level of the deep fascia. Superficial veins encountered in the dissection are ligated or coagulated. As the end of the stump is reached, great care must be taken not to damage the skin, which will almost certainly be adherent to the stump. Dissection is made directly on the bone, thus freeing the skin.

Further dissection is then extended onto the palmar aspect, until the flap is completely free and may be displaced over the end of the stump (Fig. 2A,B). Branches of the median nerve to the stump are preserved. Radial nerve branches on the dorsum must be sacrificed, and the proximal ends are coagulated with bipolar diathermy, in an attempt to prevent neuroma formation.

The thumb stump is then cleared of soft tissue and, if the thumb has been amputated through the metacarpophalangeal joint, the cartilage is removed from the metacarpal head. Otherwise, sclerotic bone is cut away to leave a healthy bone surface. Once the tourniquet is released, the flap may initially appear somewhat congested.

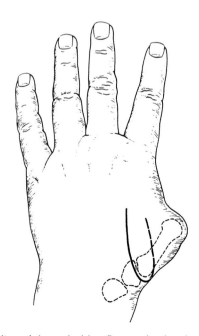

FIG. 1. Outline of the cocked hat flap on the thumb stump. (From Campbell Reid, ref. 4, with permission.)

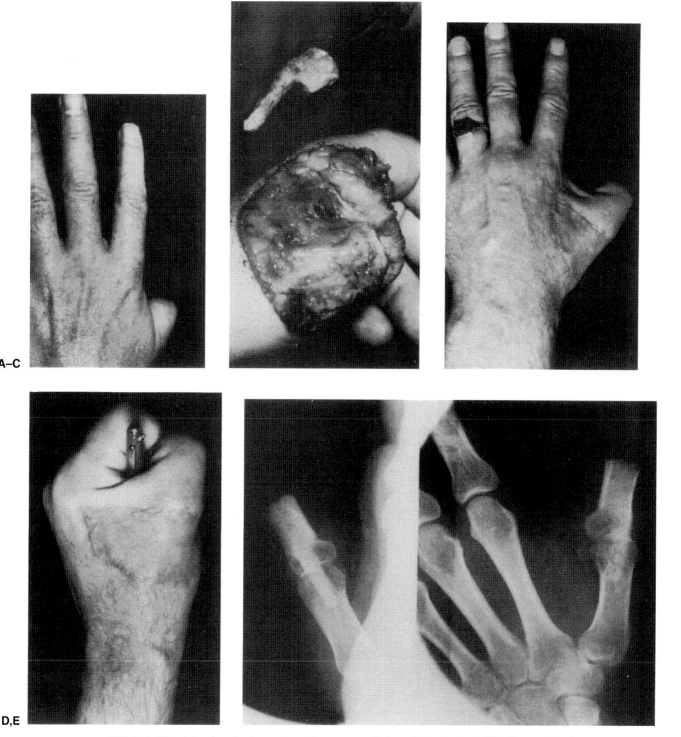

A–C

D,E

FIG. 2. A: Thumb loss just distal to an immobile metacarpophalangeal joint. **B:** Cocked hat flap raised and displaced over the metacarpal head, with iliac bone graft about to be inserted. **C,D:** Postoperative result with donor site skin-grafted. The thumb was lengthened 2.5 to 3 cm, and good sensation was present over the tactile surface. **E:** X-ray demonstrates incorporation of bone graft 6 months later. (From Campbell Reid, ref. 4, with permission.)

The bone graft is taken as a 5-cm segment from the full thickness of the iliac crest. The proximal 2.5 cm of graft is made into a peg using the cortical bone, while the remaining part is shaped to size (Fig. 2B). The bone on the dorsal aspect will be cortical, continuous with the peg, while the rest will be cancellous, providing the necessary bulk. The cortical bone gives the graft its strength. The metacarpal is then reamed out to receive the peg, which is securely inserted for its full length (Fig. 2E). No other fixation is required.

The skin flap is then draped over the bone graft, which must not be of such bulk or length as to imperil the blood supply of the flap. If that part of the flap overlying the end of the graft remains blanched, then the bone graft is either too long or too bulky. The bone graft in that case must be removed, further reduced, and rounded off.

The flap must completely cover the bone graft. The resultant defect is skin-grafted. The first dressing is changed about 10 days later. Early use is encouraged, as this appears to hasten consolidation of the bone graft.

CLINICAL RESULTS

The author has had no failures due to loss of the skin flap. Initially the flap may be a little congested and the surface may blister, but with elevation for 2 to 3 days it soon settles.

Complications occasionally occur, but these are related to the bone graft. Resorption has occurred in one case. In another case a bone graft extruded, but this was in an early case where the graft was taken from the upper end of the ulna.

It is not possible to obtain a graft of adequate bulk from this site, and the bone is almost entirely cortical. The rather narrow bone graft ulcerated through the end of the thumb flap, became infected, and had to be removed. Subsequently, the grafts were all taken from the iliac crest, as has been described, with satisfactory results.

The secondary defect covered with a thick split-thickness skin graft heals well, with no functional deficit. There have been no problems with neuromata where the radial nerve fibers have been severed.

This operation does displace the thumb/index web distally, but, should it be required, the web may subsequently be deepened by a Z-plasty.

SUMMARY

Thumb lengthening can be achieved by covering a bone graft with the Gillies cocked hat flap.

References

1. Gillies H. "Cocked hat thumb flap." Paper presented at the Annual Meeting of the British Association of Plastic Surgeons, 1946.
2. Hughes NC, Moore FT. A preliminary report on the use of a local flap and peg bone graft for lengthening a short thumb. *Br J Plast Surg* 1950;3:34.
3. Campbell Reid DA. In: Pulvertaft RG, ed., *Operative surgery: the hand.* 3d Ed. London: Butterworths, 1977.
4. Campbell Reid DA. The Gillies' thumb lengthening operation. *Hand* 1980;12:123.

CHAPTER 263 ■ THUMB PULP NEUROVASCULAR ISLAND FLAP

R. W. H. PHO

The thumb pulp flap is a local neurovascular island flap based on the volar radial digital neurovascular bundle of the thumb, to resurface extensive pulp loss of the thumb when tendon and bone are exposed. The flap offers excellent skin coverage with adequate soft-tissue padding and near-normal sensibility (1–3) (see Chap. 265).

INDICATIONS

This flap can be used to preserve thumb length in cases of traumatic amputation. It is also excellent for replacing either pulp or skin loss on the volar surface of the thumb (Figs. 1 and 2) or of the first web space.

The thumb pulp flap is a flexible flap that is not technically difficult. The preservation of the dorsal skin bridge to retain its alternative blood supply is a method of salvaging the flap if the vascular pedicle is accidentally damaged, thrombosed, or congenitally absent. The flap can then be replaced in its original bed or converted into a transposition flap with the dorsal skin bridge as its base.

There is an added advantage in that the flap retains relatively normal sensibility. There is none of the sensory disorientation that is seen in the neurovascular island flap that is taken from other digits.

ANATOMY

The skin over the dorsoradial side of the thumb receives sensory innervation from both the radial nerve and the volar digital nerve (Fig. 1A,B) (4–6). The volar digital nerve on the

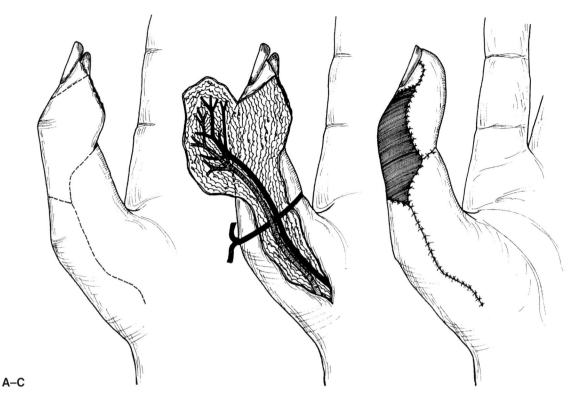

A–C

FIG. 1. **A:** Outline of the flap. Note the proximal extension used to isolate the neurovascular bundle. **B:** The flap has been raised, but with the dorsal skin bridge left intact. A digital tourniquet has been applied, excluding the isolated neurovascular bundle. **C:** The dorsal skin bridge has been divided. The island flap is then advanced distally and the donor defect covered with a full-thickness skin graft. (From Pho, ref. 3, with permission.)

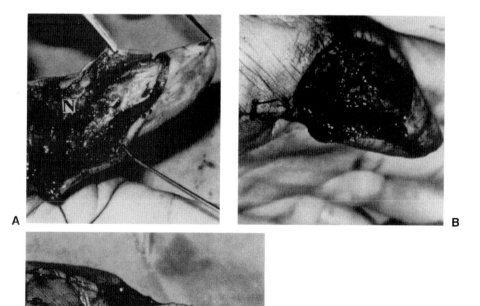

FIG. 2. **A:** The flap is raised with an intact neurovascular bundle (*N*) and with the dorsal skin bridge still intact. **B:** After division of the dorsal skin bridge, the island flap has been raised, showing the donor defect (which is skin-grafted). **C:** The island flap is advanced to cover the pulp defect. (From Pho, ref. 3, with permission.)

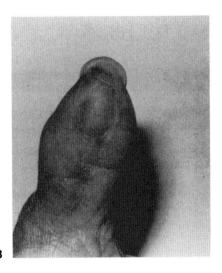
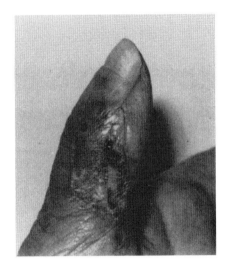

FIG. 3. A,B: Pulp loss with unhealthy tender scar. (From Pho, ref. 3, with permission.)

radial side normally sends its minute dorsal branches distal to the interphalangeal joint.

The main trunk is accompanied by the volar digital artery, which has a relatively constant location just distal to the first metacarpophalangeal joint. The artery is invariably dorsal and deep to the digital nerve and lies just superficial to the fibrous flexor sheath. It normally sends a branch dorsally at the level of the neck of the proximal phalanx and forms a cross-anastomosis with the ulnar digital artery.

FLAP DESIGN AND DIMENSIONS

An island flap based on the volar digital neurovascular bundle can be raised from the metacarpophalangeal joint proximally to within 3 mm of the nail fold distally. Similarly, the flap can be extended across the midline dorsally. However, the sensory innervation provided by the radial volar digital nerve to the skin proximally and across the midline is limited (Fig. 1).

The island flap to be raised is outlined with methylene blue, corresponding to the size of the defect to be resurfaced.

OPERATIVE TECHNIQUE

A preliminary identification of the volar radial neurovascular bundle is made by a midlateral incision at the level of the metacarpophalangeal joint. The bundle should be raised with the surrounding fatty tissue (Fig. 2A). The plane of dissection should be superficial to the fibrous flexor sheath.

The neurovascular bundle together with the skin flap is raised, leaving only a midline skin bridge connecting it to the surrounding dorsal skin as its base, to obtain its alternative blood supply (Fig. 2A). The neurovascular bundle is traced as far proximally in the palm as is necessary to obtain adequate length for advancement.

A digital tourniquet is then placed around the thumb, excluding the isolated neurovascular bundle. The main arm tourniquet is then released.

If the pedicle has been raised successfully, there will be initial bleeding confined to the wound edges of the raised flap. Subsequently, due to cross anastomosis along the intact dorsal skin bridge, the remaining thumb will become pink. Once this is confirmed, one can safely divide the dorsal skin bridge and convert the flap into an island flap (Fig. 2B), advancing it distally to cover the pulp defect (Fig. 2C).

The donor area should always be resurfaced with a full-thickness skin graft, to provide a cosmetically stable scar. The loss of sensation over the donor area is not significant, because it is not the critical area where precise prehension is required.

A dorsal plaster slab is used in the first 2 weeks, with the metacarpophalangeal joint and the interphalangeal joint flexed to avoid undue stretching of the pedicle.

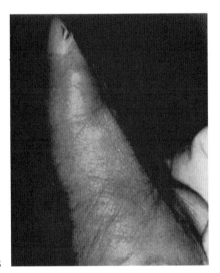
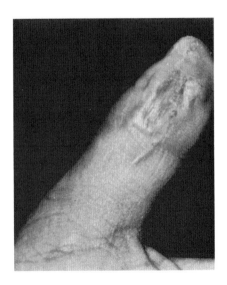

FIG. 4. A,B: Postoperative result showing the donor area and the newly reconstructed pulp. (From Pho, ref. 3, with permission.)

CLINICAL RESULTS

This technique was used in six thumbs with extensive pulp loss. Three cases were done as primary procedures; three cases were done as secondary procedures for residual tender scarring on the pulp that affected pinch strength (Figs. 3 and 4).

In five cases the flap was raised successfully. In one case, done as an elective procedure and as my second attempt at using this technique, the flap showed no evidence of circulation before division of the dorsal skin bridge. It was decided that it would be too risky to convert it into an island flap. Instead it was used as a rotation flap to narrow the gap that had to be closed.

All five patients in whom flaps were converted into island flaps successfully achieved primary wound healing within 2 weeks. Each was able to return to his or her original work within 6 weeks.

The results were assessed 9 to 40 months after operation. None of the patients experienced hyperesthesia, pain, or autonomic disturbance such as cold sensitivity or excessive sweating in the flap or donor area. The flap was supple with no induration along the margins.

Sensibility was evaluated by light touch, two-point discrimination, and ninhydrin printing. All patients responded well to light touch with cotton wool, but they seemed to have delayed responses to pin pricks, as compared with the response in the surrounding digits.

The two-point discrimination test was recorded as varying from 3 to 6 mm. One patient had an initial record of 15 mm at 2 weeks after the operation, but improved to 6 mm by 9 months later. In all of the other patients, there was no alteration of two-point discrimination from the initial recording immediately after operation to that measured several months later.

Two patients, in whom strength of pulp-to-pinch was assessed before and after operation, showed significant improvement in pinch strength.

SUMMARY

The thumb pulp flap is a neurovascular island flap that is useful for covering defects of the thumb tip with well padded sensory skin.

References

1. Joshi BB. Local dorso-lateral island flap for restoration of sensation after avulsion injury of the finger tip. *Plast Reconstr Surg* 1974;54:175.
2. Pho RWH. Restoration of sensation using a local neurovascular island flap as a primary procedure in extensive pulp loss of the finger tip. *Injury* 1976;8:20.
3. Pho RWH. Local composite neurovascular island flap for skin cover in pulp loss of the thumb. *J Hand Surg* 1979;4:11.
4. Coleman SS, Anson BJ. Arterial patterns in the hand based upon a study of 650 specimens. *Surg Gynecol Obstet* 1961;113:409.
5. Wallace WA, Coupland RE. Variation in the nerves of thumb and index finger. *J Bone Joint Surg [Am]* 1975;57:491.
6. Parks BJ, Abelaez J. Medical and surgical importance of the arterial blood supply of the thumb. *J Hand Surg* 1978;3:383.

CHAPTER 264 ■ DORSAL TO VOLAR TRANSPOSITION SKIN FLAP OF THE FINGER

S. H. HARRISON AND D. H. HARRISON

The dorsal skin flap is designed to provide neurovascular cover to the dynamic sensory areas of the hand (1): the ulnar side of the thumb pulp, the radial side of the index and middle pulps, and the ulnar side of the pulp of the little finger.

INDICATIONS

The area to be covered is greater than that treatable by small local flaps and would normally qualify for a cross-finger or neurovascular island flap (2). A disadvantage of the cross-finger flap is the lack of sensation. With the neurovascular island flap the patient can have difficulties with cortical sensory representation. The dorsal to volar transposition flap has been further developed by converting it into an island on the same neurovascular pedicle (3). It can then cover the whole of the terminal pulp in length and three-quarters of the width.

ANATOMY

The blood supply of the terminal segment is shown in Fig. 1 (4), demonstrating how large vessels arise from the digital artery in the middle segment of the finger to supply the dorsal skin. A rich anastomosis occurs around the nailbed. Distally there is free communication between the dorsal vessels and the vessels of the pulp. The blood supply will permit the elevation of a long and fairly narrow flap based on the main dorsal branch of the digital artery that arises in the

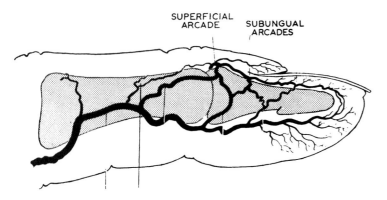

FIG. 1. Vascular supply to the finger. (From Flint and Harrison, ref. 1, with permission.)

middle segment of the finger. This artery arises from the volar digital artery, within the neurovascular tunnel created by Grayson's ligament anteriorly and Cleland's cutaneous ligament posteriorly (Fig. 2). The dorsal branch of the digital nerve accompanies the dorsal branch of the digital artery.

FLAP DESIGN AND DIMENSIONS

The incision along the side of the dorsum curves just proximal to the proximal interphalangeal joint crease, and the length is therefore the distance between the proximal interphalangeal joint crease and the nail fold (see Fig. 3B). The width of the flap is the entire dorsum of the finger. The nailbed is not at risk from ischemia, because of the excellent anastomosis around the nailbed.

OPERATIVE TECHNIQUE

As the dissection proceeds toward the base of the flap, it is essential to divide Grayson's ligament (Fig. 2). This will allow the dorsal branch and the main digital vessel to turn toward the midline of the finger, to avoid kinking and to reduce tension on the main vascular pedicle. It is important to elevate the flap at a critical level between the vascular field and the paratenon and, at the same time, to free the dorsal branch and

the main digital branch from the fascial compartment, in order to prevent kinking of the main artery (Fig. 3B).

To offset the effect of crush and to allow the vascular tree to recover, a delayed primary repair can be performed on the fifth day, after a primary toilet and debridement.

CLINICAL RESULTS

The success of this flap depends on careful anatomic dissection and design, supplemented by magnification. If there has been an element of crush in the primary injury (as distinguished from a slicing injury), it is desirable to defer primary repair for delayed primary or secondary, using a split-thickness skin graft for physiologic cover.

The complications of all such flaps are ischemia and infection. If there is any doubt about the viability of the flap it should be replaced. If it survives it can be used as a delayed flap.

A functional deficit is the loss of sensation in the skin-grafted donor site on the dorsum of the finger.

SUMMARY

The dorsal neurovascular skin flap can provide both cover and sensation to volar pulp losses.

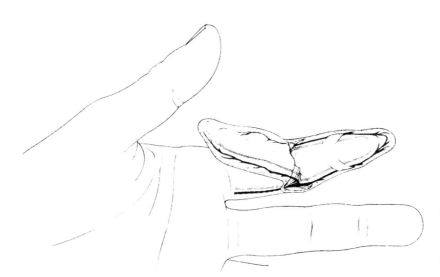

FIG. 2. Drawing showing the anatomy of Cleland's ligament, which lies dorsal to the neurovascular bundle, and Grayson's ligament, which lies volar. Release of these ligaments will avoid kinking and excess tension on the vessels. (From Flint and Harrison, ref. 1, with permission.)

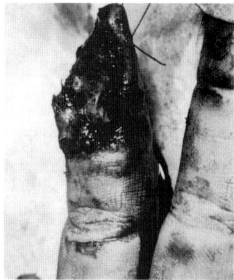
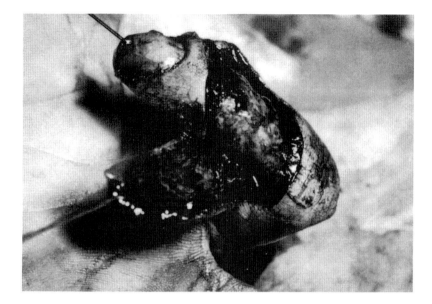

A,B

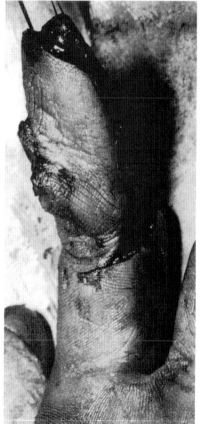
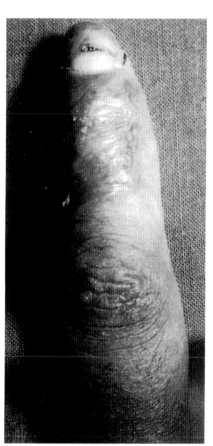
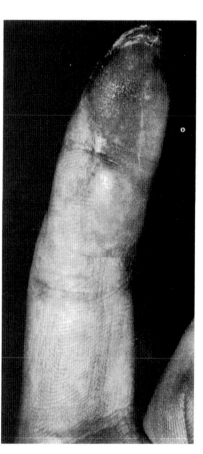

C–E

FIG. 3. **A:** Pulp defect suitable for a dorsal transposition flap. There is almost a total loss of the terminal pulp skin and subcutaneous tissue. **B:** The flap elevated from the dorsum of the finger. The dissection lies in the critical area between the paratenon and the neurovascular plateau. **C:** The flap adequately covers the defect. **D,E:** Postoperative result. A split-thickness skin graft is used to cover the donor site. (From Flint and Harrison, ref. 1, with permission.)

References

1. Flint MH, Harrison SH. A local neurovascular flap to repair loss of the digital pulp. *Br J Plast Surg* 1965;18:156.
2. Littler JW. Neurovascular pedicle transfer of tissue in reconstructive surgery of the hand. *J Bone Joint Surg* 1956;38(A):917.
3. Joshi BB. A local dorsolateral island flap restoration of sensation after avulsion injury of fingertip pulp. *Plast Reconstr Surg* 1974;54:175.
4. Flint MH. Some observations on the vascular supply of the nailbed and terminal segments of the finger. *Br J Plast Surg* 1955;8:186.

CHAPTER 265 ■ DORSOLATERAL ISLAND SKIN FLAP TO THE FINGERTIP AND THUMB TIP

B. B. JOSHI

EDITORIAL COMMENT

Retention of the dorsal vein is most likely unnecessary and probably limits the mobility of the flap. The neurovascular bundle itself will provide sufficient venous drainage for the flap. This operation is still an extremely useful procedure. It is one of the better nonmicrovascular reconstructions of the thumb that provides a very useful and functional digit (see Chap. 263).

The fingertip can be reconstructed by using a flap from the dorsolateral surface of the finger (1). This flap is based on the volar digital vessels and their dorsal branches, thus providing good sensory tissue to cover pulp loss.

INDICATIONS

The dorsolateral island flap is suitable for repair of those defects that are too large to be covered by such procedures as the volar advancement flap or the volar V-Y advancement flap.

The dorsolateral island flap does not have the problem of cortical reorientation, and is therefore preferred over an island flap transfer from another finger (2,3). It has better sensibility than palmar flaps or cross-finger flaps, as the latter are essentially insensitive flaps that depend on subsequent innervation from the bed and periphery of the grafted area.

Since the donor site is dorsolateral, the functional deficit is minimal. Volar skin is left essentially undisturbed, and there is no danger of producing a flexion contracture.

The only contraindication would be thrombosis of the digital artery.

ANATOMY

The skin over the distal two phalanges of the finger is supplied mainly by segmental branches of the volar digital arteries and nerves, with many anastomoses among the dorsal and volar branches.

Small island flaps that contain only distal phalangeal skin do not have good circulation. Subsequently the island flaps are extended to include the skin over two distal segments; one must be careful to include both the most proximal dorsal branch of the volar digital vessels and a vein over the dorsum of the finger. The accompanying nerves are also included in the pedicle.

The flap can be taken from either side of the finger or thumb. The dorsal branches of the radial artery and nerve are usually quite separate from the volar branches in the thumb. Vessels and nerves need to be preserved and dissected proximally, as do the branches of the volar digital neurovascular bundles.

FLAP DESIGN AND DIMENSIONS

The flap is extended proximally in an oblique direction, from the edge of the defect to the midlateral border of the finger at the level of the proximal interphalangeal joint crease. Distally, the flap extends along the margin of the defect to the tip, and then turns dorsally, leaving a border of skin measuring 2 to 5 mm next to the nail. The flap extends proximally along the midline of the dorsum of the finger, and then turns obliquely to join the midlateral line at the proximal interphalangeal joint crease (Fig. 1).

This flap will usually cover the full length of the defect and about three-quarters of the width of the pulp.

OPERATIVE TECHNIQUE

An incision is made along the midlateral line proximal to the flap outline. The volar digital vessels and the nerves in the pedicle area are dissected to their entrance into the flap. Care must be taken to preserve the branches of the neurovascular bundle that arise at the proximal interphalangeal joint level. The pedicle must be dissected sufficiently to allow adequate advancement of the flap. This may involve extending the incision proximally into the palm (Fig. 1A).

The flap as outlined above is raised from the volar aspect initially. The neurovascular bundle and its branches are preserved within the flap (Fig. 1C). Before the dorsal incisions are made, the tourniquet should be released and the circulation checked. A dorsal vein should be included with the flap as the incisions are completed (Fig. 1D). If there is a separate dorsal neurovascular bundle, as in the thumb, it should also be dissected and preserved.

After the flap is advanced into the defect, the donor site is covered with a skin graft (Fig. 1E,F). The finger is immobilized for 2 weeks with partial flexion at the metacarpophalangeal joint (Figs. 2 and 3).

CLINICAL RESULTS

Partial necrosis occurred in two early cases, when small island flaps were raised. Once the flap was enlarged to cover both the middle and distal phalanges and to include the neurovascular

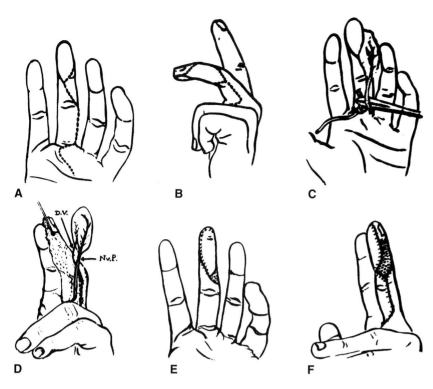

FIG. 1. A: The flap outline extends proximally in an oblique direction from the edge of the defect to the junction of the proximal interphalangeal joint crease and the midlateral line. B: The flap outline extends distally along the edge of the defect. A border of skin of about 2 to 5 mm should be left along the margin of the nail. The incision then runs proximally down the midline of the dorsum of the finger and then turns obliquely to join the midlateral line at the level of the proximal interphalangeal joint crease. C: The neurovascular bundle is dissected proximally to allow advancement of the flap into the defect. D: A dorsal vein and the branches of the neurovascular bundle, as they cross dorsally at the proximal interphalangeal joint, are included with the flap. E: The flap is advanced into the defect. F: The dorsolateral donor site is skin-grafted. (From Joshi, ref. 1, with permission.)

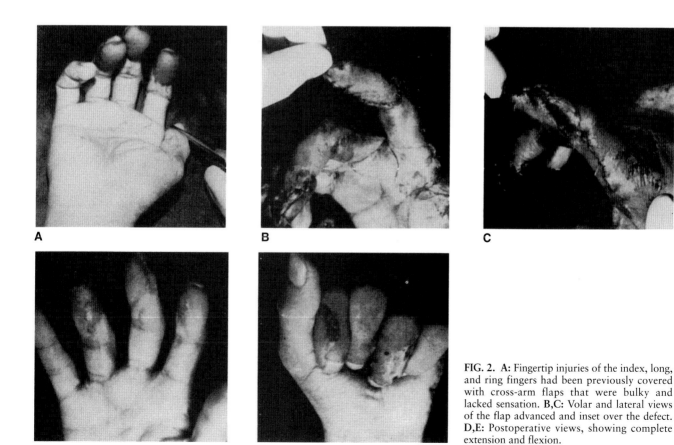

FIG. 2. A: Fingertip injuries of the index, long, and ring fingers had been previously covered with cross-arm flaps that were bulky and lacked sensation. B,C: Volar and lateral views of the flap advanced and inset over the defect. D,E: Postoperative views, showing complete extension and flexion.

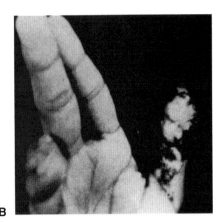
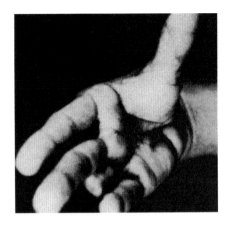

A,B

FIG. 3. A: Dorsolateral island flap after transposition and advancement to the thumb. B: Final result.

branches as they cross dorsally at the proximal interphalangeal joint, flap circulation has not been a problem.

More than 200 dorsolateral island flaps have been done at my center. The sensation obtained in these island flaps has been excellent, with a two-point discrimination of 3 to 4 mm (Fig. 2).

SUMMARY

Fingertip or thumb tip injuries can be repaired with an island flap based on one of the dorsolateral surfaces of the same digit. This leaves a minimal donor site defect and provides good padding and sensation to the volar pulp.

References

1. Joshi BB. A local dorsolateral island flap restoration of sensation after avulsion injury of finger tip pulp. *Plast Reconstr Surg* 1974;54:175.
2. Littler JW. Neurovascular pedicle transfer of tissue in reconstructive surgery of the hand. *J Bone Joint Surg* 1956;38A:917.
3. Flint MH, Harrison SH. A local neurovascular flap to repair loss of the digital pulp. *Br J Plast Surg* 1965;18:156.

CHAPTER 266 ■ DIGITAL NEUROVASCULAR ISLAND SKIN FLAP

J. W. LITTLER AND J. M. MARKLEY

EDITORIAL COMMENT

This is the "classic" procedure described by Littler in the late 1950s. Its use both as an island transfer and, more recently, as a free transfer, provides sensibility to another part of the hand. If it is transferred as a pedicle, it requires reeducation, which may be difficult for some patients.

The anatomic specificities of various regions allow particular reconstructive techniques. The spoke-like digital neurovascular bundles that radiate from the central palm into the fingers allow the lateral transfer of an innervated and well-perfused composite skin island to a critical site deprived of special coverage.

INDICATIONS

The finger neurovascular composite skin island can provide durable corniferous glabrous skin with excellent perfusion and functional sensibility (1–3). It is particularly useful for resurfacing defects in the critical functional contact areas of the thumb or index finger after loss of their terminal surfaces, in various reconstructions of the thumb by osteoplastic methods, or to enhance a reunited amputated part.

Although usually used as a secondary procedure after initial healing with a free skin graft or distant flap, primary reconstruction with a digital neurovascular island flap may be advantageous in carefully selected cases (4). Use of the neurovascular island flap for relief of a chronically painful digit with inadequate skin and soft tissue and poor sensibility should be undertaken with caution, because disabling dysesthesia persists with distressing frequency in such cases despite technically good and well-healed flaps (5).

The neurovascular island transfer of composite tissue is adaptable to reconstructive problems when part or all of a digit is to be discarded. For example, when the index, due to injury or disuse, could serve better as a source of composite tissue, it may be removed with transfer of its tactile corniferous skin as a neurovascular island, to resurface the thumb web or other area in need of durable cover.

Microsurgical techniques make possible potentially useful variations on the neurovascular island transfer of digital skin. In cases of replantation or revascularization of digits in which insufficient length of vessel or nerve is available, the deficiency may be met by transfer, without skin, of artery and nerve from a donor site of lesser advantage (6). Also, the problem of reorientation of localization of sensibility may be partially solved by vascular island transfer with division of the donor nerve and microsurgical fascicular anastomosis with a remaining recipient site sensory nerve. The latter maneuver demands careful management of the proximal stump of the donor digital nerve to reduce the possibility of painful neuroma.

ANATOMY

The radial arrangement of the digital arteries and nerves from the central palm to the digits is the basic anatomic feature permitting transfer of a neurovascular island between any two digits (Fig. 1). The center of the arc of transfer of this flap is thus a small midpalmar zone approximated by the points of intersection of the palmar midline axes of the fully extended and abducted digits. Variations in vessel and nerve anatomy occur, obligating the surgeon to be aware of potential

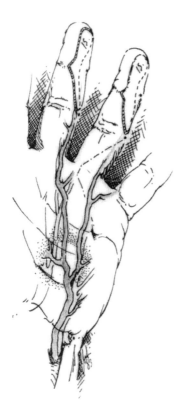

FIG. 1. The radial arrangement of the volar digital arteries and nerves from the central palm to the digits is the basic anatomic feature permitting transfer of a neurovascular composite island.

anatomic pitfalls (7). Preoperative wrist and digital Allen's tests and Doppler tracing of the digital vessels are sufficient to identify cases where a technically troublesome anomaly may be present. In such cases, comprising 2% to 3% of hands, angiography may be indicated (8). The flap depends on multiple small veins in the soft tissues adjacent to the artery and nerve for venous drainage (9).

FLAP DESIGN AND DIMENSIONS

The ulnar aspects of long or ring fingers are the usual donor areas. Selection is based on surface area required, vascular integrity, preexisting digital injury or affliction, and choice between median and ulnar innervated skin. Patterns of innervation may be checked preoperatively by selective local anesthetic nerve blocks. A digital Allen's test is used to confirm perfusion of the finger adjacent to the donor finger by the contralateral digital artery that will not be divided in dissection of the flap.

The flap should include the skin of the distal segment of the donor finger nearly to the hyponychial ridge, in order both to transfer the domain of critical sensibility and to avoid occurrence of a painful neuroma at the distal end of a too proximally based flap. The most volar edge of the flap should be the digital volar midline, with darts at the interphalangeal flexion creases (Fig. 2A). The most dorsal edge of the flap should be determined by flap size requirements and may extend to the dorsal digital midline, without darts. Generally, the maximum width flap is desirable; this requires preservation of the dorsal branch of the digital nerve in the flap. The proximal limit of the flap is determined by the dimensions of the recipient defect.

OPERATIVE TECHNIQUE

It is advisable to defer definitive preparation of the recipient area until after the flap dissection if this involves creation of an open defect not already present. The configuration of the donor composite tissue determines that of the recipient site.

The palmar incisions radiate in zigzag fashion from the central palm to the bases of the flap and recipient sites. The neurovascular leash should be transferred entirely through open incisions without tunneling (Fig. 2B).

Dissection begins in the palm. The common digital artery and nerve to the flap are identified. At the bifurcation to proper digital arteries, the proper artery to the adjacent finger is isolated. Care must be taken to avoid denuding the digital artery and nerve of the small vein-bearing soft tissue loosely attached to them.

After the initial palmar dissection has verified suitability of the neurovascular anatomy for transfer, the margins of the flap are incised. The flap is elevated by sharp dissection from its distal end proximally, leaving the thin areolar layer over the extensor tendons and the flexor sheath. It will be necessary to isolate, divide, and ligate the transverse-oblique vincular and articular branches of the digital artery at each interphalangeal joint. The dorsal branch of the proper volar digital nerve is preserved with the flap.

On reaching the proximal end of the flap, the nerve-vessel pedicle is dissected into the palm, preserving the adherent fatty areolar tissue. The identity of the proper digital artery to the adjacent finger is reconfirmed, and this vessel is then severed and ligated, freeing the common digital artery. Slightly more proximally, the dorsal interosseous branch of the common digital artery must also be divided, as well as several small arterial branches. The proper digital nerve is carefully separated from the common nerve by epineural incision using

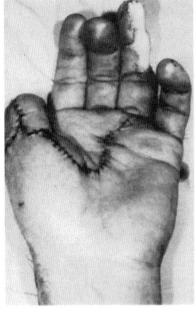
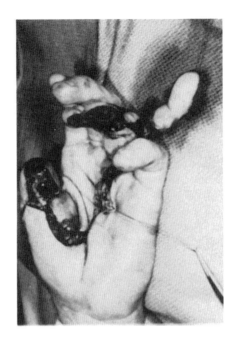

A,B

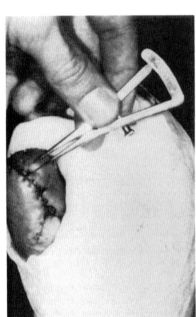
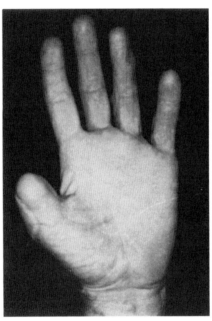

C,D

FIG. 2. **A:** The distal and volar margins of this donor area skin graft outline the correct incisional configuration. An even broader base for the interphalangeal dart may be desirable. **B:** Use of open incisions without tunneling assists transfer of the neurovascular leash without torsion, tension, or kinking. **C:** The completed flap in a case of traumatic loss of distal phalanx and denudation of proximal phalanx of thumb. Early preservation of two-point sensibility. **D:** One year postoperatively.

loupe magnification. The digital nerve and artery with their attendant areolar investment are thus mobilized to the central palmar rotation point from the superficial arterial arch.

The incision from rotation point to recipient bed is opened. Beneath the zigzag flaps, a straight subcutaneous course at least 1 cm in width is prepared for the neurovascular pedicle. The flap is transferred to the recipient site. If any tension, torsion, or kinking of the pedicle occurs, it must be corrected. The recipient defect is then prepared. The flap is sutured in place. The palmar and digital incisions are closed, taking care to ensure that the neurovascular pedicle is not compressed or kinked. The donor defect is resurfaced with a free graft. This may later be replaced with a corniferous graft from the pedal instep, if desired. A nonconstricting longitudinally oriented dressing with plaster shell or splint support is applied.

Attention to specific details of design and transfer of the digital neurovascular composite skin island seems to enhance

the preservation of sensibility (10). The surgical technique and variations in technical details may account for the differing results cited. We feel that the essential surgical features are:

1. The flap should always encompass the specific sensory area of the proper volar digital nerve, including the territory of its dorsal branch. It should extend to the tip of the digital phalanx to avoid the painful neuromata that may occur if the nerve is severed more proximally.
2. As much soft tissue as possible should be left with the neurovascular pedicle, avoiding separation of vessels from nerves.
3. Tension and compression of the neurovascular bundle should be avoided, as these are known to interfere with nerve function, causing neurapraxia, and may be responsible for cases of gradual loss of two-point discrimination (11). This may be prevented by open

exposure of the final path of the neurovascular bundle, rather than transfer by subcutaneous tunneling.

4. Incisions, especially the donor area margins, must be designed to avoid secondary interphalangeal joint contracture deformity.

5. Such procedures should be done only by surgeons experienced in reconstructive surgery of the hand and well versed in the details of hand anatomy. Loupe magnification is recommended.

CLINICAL RESULTS

With proper attention paid to careful dissection and handling, this is a sturdy, highly reliable flap. We are unaware of any occurrences of necrosis of the digital neurovascular island skin flap.

Flexion contracture of the donor digit may result if the volar line of union of skin graft with normal skin is not adequately broken by darts at the interphalangeal joint creases. The donor finger should be mobilized rapidly, as soon as the reparative graft has taken. Dynamic splinting may occasionally be needed if flexion contracture develops.

Nearly all surgeons with experience in digital neurovascular island skin composite transfer state that durable skin, sensibility, and improved circulation can reliably be provided. The question concerning maintenance of discriminatory touch is controversial. Widely varying results are reported, including preservation of normal static two-point discrimination (10,12–14), complete loss of two-point discrimination (5,15), and early preservation with later decrease in two-point sensibility below critical levels (16,17). Present neurophysiologic information suggests that moving touch is of great significance to normal tactile perception. Our experience continues to suggest that attention to the details of design and execution of this flap as discussed above will lead in most cases to preservation of useful functional sensibility in the flap.

Recent studies suggest that sensibility should be evaluated by moving two-point discrimination and vibration (18,19). To date, no series of digital neurovascular island skin transfers have been evaluated by this method. Although the successful transfer of normal sensibility is highly desirable, it is not necessarily tantamount to useful function. The independent thumb resurfaced with durable skin will nearly always be used to advantage, despite decreased sensibility, as long as it is not dysesthetic.

Furthermore, the change in conscious localization of feeling from the donor to the recipient area is variable, often difficult, and sometimes fails to occur (18,20,21). When attained, it may be temporarily lost by immobilization of the hand or in moments of severe stress. Distortion of cortical patterns of sensory events following peripheral nerve repair is known to occur. Conflict between tactile, proprioceptive, and visual perception may result in such distortions in patients

with neurovascular island flaps. An organized program of sensory reeducation (18,21) may result in improved quality and relocalization of sensibility and is recommended postoperatively for patients with digital neurovascular island skin transfers.

SUMMARY

The digital neurovascular island skin flap in its various forms is a useful technique to restore sensibility and therefore function to the thumb and the index finger.

References

1. Moberg E. Transfer of sensation. *J Bone Joint Surg* 1955;37(A):305.
2. Littler JW. Neurovascular island transfer in reconstructive hand surgery. In: *Transactions of the second congress of the international society of plastic surgeons.* London: Livingstone, 1960; 175–178.
3. Littler JW. Principles of reconstructive surgery of the hand. In: Converse JM, ed. *Reconstructive plastic surgery.* Philadelphia: Saunders, 1964; 1612–1673.
4. Chase RA. Early salvage in acute hand injuries with a primary island flap. *Plast Reconstr Surg* 1971;48:521.
5. Murray JF, Ord JVR, Gavelin GF. The neurovascular island pedicle flap. *J Bone Joint Surg* 1967;49(A):1285.
6. Doi K. Replantation of an avulsed thumb, with application of a neurovascular pedicle. *Hand* 1976;8:258.
7. Lignon J, Le Tenneur J, Ratcliffe H, et at. Lambeau en ilot digital muni de son pedicule vasculo-nerveux. *Ann Chir* 1976;30:917.
8. Coleman SS, Anson BJ. Arterial patterns in the hand based upon a study of 650 specimens. *Surg Gynecol Obstet* 1961;113:409.
9. Eaton RG. The digital neurovascular bundle: A microanatomic study of its contents. *Clin Orthop* 1968;61:176.
10. Markley JM Jr. Preservation of two-point sensibility in digital neurovascular island flaps. *Plast Reconstr Surg* 1977;59:812.
11. Lundborg G. Structure and function of the intraneural microvessels as related to trauma, edema formation, and nerve function. *J Bone Joint Surg* 1975;57(A):938.
12. Chase RA, Iverson RE. Commentary. In: *Symposium on the hand,* Vol. 3. St. Louis: Mosby, 1971; 221.
13. Tubiana R, Duparc J. Restoration of sensibility in the hand by neurovascular skin island transfer. *J Bone Joint Surg* 1961;43(B):474.
14. Stice RC, Wood MB. Neurovascular island skin flaps in the hand: function and sensibility evaluations. *Microsurgery* 1987;8:162.
15. Reid CAC. The neurovascular island flap in thumb reconstruction. *Br J Plast Surg* 1966;19:234.
16. Krag C, Rasmussen KB. The neurovascular island flap for defective sensibility of the thumb. *J Bone Joint Surg* 1975;57(B):495.
17. Omer GE, Day DJ, Ratcliffe H, et al. Neurovascular cutaneous island pedicles for deficient median nerve sensibility. *J Bone Joint Surg* 1970;52(A):1181.
18. Dellon AL. *Evaluation of sensibility and re-education of sensation in the hand.* Baltimore & London: Williams & Wilkins, 1981.
19. Wall PD. Two transmission systems for skin sensations in sensory communication. In: Rosenblith WA, ed. *Sensory Communication.* Cambridge, Mass.: MIT Press, 1961; 475–496.
20. Paul RL, Goodman H, Merzenich M. Alterations in mechanoreceptor input to Brodmann's areas 1 and 3 of the post-central hand area of Macaca mulatta after nerve section and regeneration. *Brain Res* 1972;39:1.
21. Parry CW, Salter M. Sensory re-education after median nerve lesions. *Hand* 1976;8:250.

CHAPTER 267 ■ REVERSE DIGITAL ARTERY FLAP TO THE FINGERTIP

S. K. HAN

EDITORIAL COMMENT

It is important that this flap be used only in the reconstruction of defects distal to the distal interphalangeal (DIP) joint. In addition, although this flap can be designed as a sensate flap, long-term follow-up has shown minimal benefit and therefore innervation is no longer recommended.

Fingertip injuries represent the most common type of injuries seen in the upper extremity. Their management is functionally and aesthetically important but, at the same time, controversial. The goals of fingertip reconstruction are preservation of functional length and sensibility, prevention of symptomatic neuromas and of adjacent joint contracture, and minimization of aesthetic deformity. The usefulness and postoperative results of the reverse digital artery flap for fingertip reconstruction are reported. This relatively simple and time-saving procedure is done in one stage, maintains the finger length with sufficient soft-tissue padding, provides thin and hairless skin, avoids uncomfortable immobilization, and shortens the hospital stay. Excellent sensory restoration is possible, the donor-site scar can be hidden, flap size is unlimited, cosmetic results are acceptable, and the flap can be used in multiple fingertip amputation cases.

INDICATIONS

The distally based arterial island flap was first described in 1973 (1). Since then, several authors have introduced modifications, including the reverse digital artery flap, which has many advantages over the more conventional flap (2). The reverse digital artery flap is indicated in any cases with amputations or tissue defects distal to the DIP joint of the fingers. However, this flap is contraindicated in cases with injuries proximal to the DIP joint.

ANATOMY

Regarding the digital arterial system, the existence of sufficient arterial anastomoses between the digital arteries from both sides has long been known (3–6). According to Strauch and de Moura's findings (6), there are three transverse digital palmar arches in the fingers and their locations are constant: that is, at the level of the proximal cruciate ligament, distal cruciate ligament, and just distal to the flexor digitorum profundus insertion. Therefore, this flap is perfused from the contralateral side proper digital artery through the middle transverse palmar arch at the level of the distal cruciate ligament, and then from the ipsilateral proper digital artery. In addition, an abundant number of vascular communications in the pulp of the distal phalanx exist, and these communications enable the reverse digital artery flap, with a more distally skeletonized pedicle, to gain its retrograde blood supply without any trouble (Fig. 1).

Regarding the venous system, the reverse digital artery flap is drained through the tiny venules and capillaries contained in the perivascular soft tissue (7).

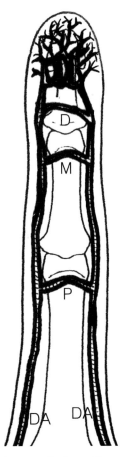

FIG. 1. Digital arterial system of a finger. Three transverse digital palmar arches between digital arteries and abundant vascular communications in the pulp of a distal phalanx exist. DA, digital artery; P, proximal palmar arch; M, middle palmar arch; D, distal palmar arch.

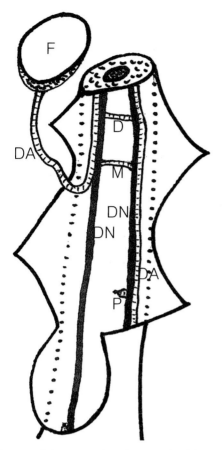

FIG. 2. Diagram of the reverse digital artery island flap. The flap is perfused from a contralateral side proper digital artery through a middle transverse palmar arch and then an ipsilateral proper digital artery. F, reverse digital artery island flap; DA, digital artery; DN, digital nerve; P, divided proximal palmar arch; M, middle palmar arch; D, distal palmar arch.

FLAP DESIGN AND DIMENSIONS

The flap is designed in a stellate shape to avoid scar contracture on the ulnar or radial side of the proximal phalanx of the finger, with a digital artery as the central axis (according to the size and shape of the defect); however, the least-used side of the finger is chosen, if possible.

Reviewing the sizes of the flap I have used, the length and width of flaps ranged from 1.6 to 3.2 cm and 1.0 to 2.5 cm, respectively, with a maximum size of 3.2 × 2.5 cm. In extended flaps, the dorsal skin over the metacarpophalangeal joint, as well as the lateral skin of the proximal phalanx, can be included (8).

OPERATIVE TECHNIQUE

The procedure is carried out under regional block or general anesthesia. After minimal debridement of the wound, the size and shape of the defect are measured.

After pneumatic tourniquet inflation, a skin incision is made, and the flap is elevated carefully with the aid of surgical-loupe magnification. The digital artery is first identified, and then separated from the proper digital nerve to the level of about 5 mm proximal to the DIP joint, to transfer the flap freely but, at the same time, not to injure the middle transverse

digital palmar arch. However, the digital artery may be dissected more distal to the level of the DIP joint in cases where enough finger pulp remains, to include vascular communications between radial and ulnar proper digital arteries.

I usually consider the center of the fingerprint as an indicator. If this remains at the recipient site, the digital artery can be dissected more distally. This maneuver enables the flap to move to the very distal part with ease.

A generous cuff of subcutaneous tissue is maintained around the vascular pedicle, to preserve the tiny perivascular venules. The digital artery at the proximal end of the flap is ligated and divided.

In cases of sensate flaps, the dorsal branch of the digital nerve or the superficial sensory branch of the radial or ulnar nerve attached to the flap is identified and dissected, then microanastomosed to the digital nerve at the defect by an epineurial technique. However, I no longer use sensate flaps, because the long-term results do not show a significant difference between sensate and insensate flaps, and additional operating time is required for innervated flaps. Sensory recovery in the insensate flaps comes from collateral sprouting from adjacent intact nerves and central adapting mechanisms (9).

The flap is transferred and sutured to the defect loosely, so as not to compress the pedicle. A skin graft is applied to the donor defect. Postoperatively, the operated on hand is elevated, and no anticoagulants are used (Fig. 2).

CLINICAL RESULTS

One hundred forty fingers with defects of the distal phalanx were reconstructed using reverse digital artery flaps (2,10). Survival of the flaps was successful in all fingers, except for one. In 20 fingers, postoperative congestion developed but subsided spontaneously within 2 to 3 days in all of them (Fig. 3). Postoperative sensory recovery in all cases was excellent. All the evaluated flaps had the ability to detect light touch, temperature, and sharp stimuli. Regarding scar contracture, no patient required an additional operation for further improvement of the fingertip shape, although a mild irregularity was seen at the flap edge in three of the patients.

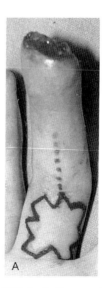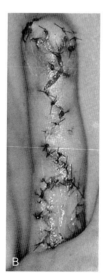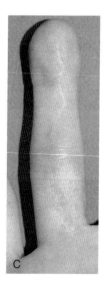

FIG. 3. A: Preoperative design of an insensate reverse digital artery flap. **B:** Immediate postoperative view after flap transfer by extensive dissection of the digital artery to the level of the distal interphalangeal (DIP) joint. **C:** One year following the operation.

SUMMARY

The reverse digital artery flap is an excellent choice for coverage of fingertip defects because it is a safe and reliable procedure with a high survival rate.

References

1. Weeks PM, Wray RC. *Management of acute hand injury.* St. Louis: Mosby, 1973;140.
2. Han SK, Lee BL, Kim WK. The reverse digital artery island flap: clinical experience in 120 fingers. *Plast Reconstr Surg* 1998;101:4.
3. Brockis JG. The blood supply of the flexor and extensor tendons of the fingers in man. *J Bone Joint Surg* 1953;35:131.
4. Edwards EA. Organizations of the small arteries of the hand and digits. *Am J Surg* 1960;99:837.
5. Zbrodowski A, Gajisin S, Grodecki J. The anatomy of the digitopalmar arches. *J. Bone Joint Surg* 1981;63:108.
6. Strauch B, de Moura W. Arterial system of the fingers. *J Hand Surg* 1990;15:148.
7. Lai CS, Lin SD, Yang CC. The reverse digital artery flap for fingertip reconstruction. *Ann Plast Surg* 1989;22:498.
8. Lai CS, Lin SD, Chou CK, Tsai CW. A versatile method for reconstruction of finger defects: reverse digital artery flap. *Br J Plast Surg* 1992;45:443.
9. Jaaskelainen SK, Peltola JK. Electrophysiologic evidence for extremely late sensory collateral reinnervation in humans. *Neurology* 1996;46:1703.
10. Han SK, Lee BL, Kim WK. The reverse digital artery island flap: an update. *Plast Reconstr Surg* 2004;113:1753.

CHAPTER 268 ■ STAGED NEUROVASCULAR ISLAND SKIN FLAP FROM THE MIDDLE FINGER TO THE THUMB TIP

R. VENKATASWAMI

EDITORIAL COMMENT

The concept of reinnervating the island sensory flap with the nerves in the thumb is a good one. The author executes the procedure in a staged manner; however, the editors feel that if the donor site were on the ulnar side of the ring or long finger, the integrity of the radial side of those fingers would be retained. Perhaps an even further advancement would be to take the entire flap from the big toe and do both a nerve repair and a vessel repair without violating any of the structures in the fingers.

For covering acute skin loss over the thumb tip and the adjacent terminal phalanx, an island flap of skin and subcutaneous tissue based on the radial neurovascular bundle is transferred from the middle finger in the first stage. During the second stage of division of the flap from its donor finger, the digital nerve of the flap is anastomosed to the digital nerve of the thumb.

INDICATIONS

The neurovascular island flap can be used to cover thumb tip injuries in two stages. This procedure differs from other neurovascular island flaps (1–3), in that the nerve to the flap is divided and anastomosed to the nerve in the thumb. The patient therefore gains his original cortical sensory orientation.

This flap can also be used to cover the dorsal aspect of the proximal interphalangeal joint when there is compound tissue loss.

ANATOMY

The flap is initially based on the neurovascular bundle of the middle finger, as are the classical neurovascular island flaps. In the second stage, however, the bundle is completely divided. This means that the vascular supply to the flap is dependent on neovascularization from the thumb. The nerve is anastomosed to the stump of the nerve in the thumb, thus providing more accurate cortical representation.

FLAP DESIGN AND DIMENSIONS

A cloth pattern of the defect is laid on the radial side of the middle finger. The radial side of the middle finger is chosen because this brings the donor finger and thumb into the most convenient and comfortable position for the patient.

The flap is usually taken from the middle phalanx. If a larger flap is needed, it is extended onto the proximal phalanx, leaving the distal phalanx untouched (Fig. 1).

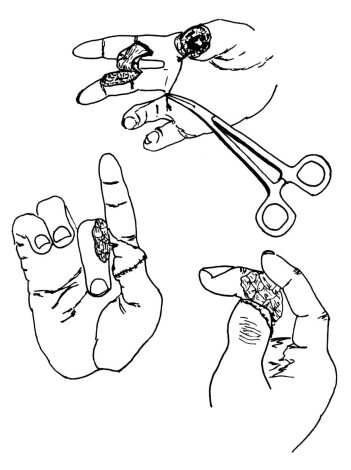

FIG. 1. Schematic outline of the staged neurovascular island skin flap that is used to cover thumb tip amputations.

If a wide flap is needed, the dorsal and volar incisions can extend just beyond the midline.

OPERATIVE TECHNIQUE

First Stage

During debridement of the thumb tip one of the digital nerves is dissected for a centimeter proximally and the end is tagged with 6-0 nylon for later identification.

After the flap has been designed and marked, the volar and dorsal incisions are made. The volar incision is deepened to the flexor sheath and the dorsal incision is deepened to the paratenon covering the extensor tendon. Then the distal incision is made and the neurovascular bundle is divided.

The flap is mobilized proximally, keeping the neurovascular bundle well protected by the retinacular fibers. Once the proximal limit of the flap is reached, the skin alone is divided and the neurovascular bundle is dissected to convert the flap into an island flap (Fig. 2A).

The donor defect is then covered with an intermediate split-thickness skin graft. To prevent scar contracture of the volar and dorsal incisions, one or two oblique cuts are made and these flaps are shifted distally to create a zigzag scar line.

The middle finger is then flexed to bring it near the recipient defect. This entails a flexion of 80° to 90° at the metacarpophalangeal joint and 40° to 50° of flexion at the proximal interphalangeal joint. This is a comfortable position for most patients. The flap is sutured to the defect and the neurovascular bundle is covered either by the skin graft or by the skin flap (Fig. 2B).

Second Stage

After 2 to 3 weeks, the neurovascular bundle is dissected proximally in the middle finger for a few millimeters and then divided. The extra length may be useful for a tension-free anastomosis. The digital artery is divided and ligated. The nerve is then repaired microsurgically (Fig. 2B–D).

SUMMARY

This staged neurovascular island flap provides both cosmetic and functional skin cover to thumb tip amputations. By anastomosing the donor and recipient nerves, a better cortical sensory orientation can be achieved than with the classical neurovascular island flaps.

A,B

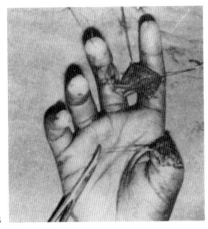
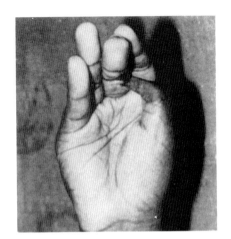

C,D

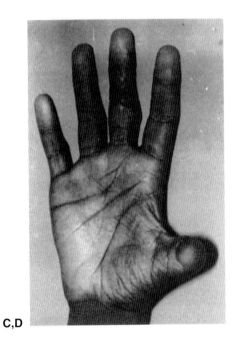
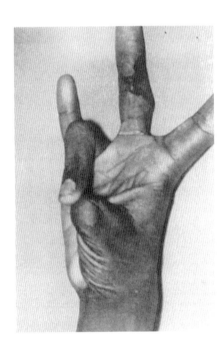

FIG. 2. **A:** The radial digital nerve and artery comprise the pedicle of this island flap. **B:** The island flap covers the thenar amputation stump. **C:** Appearance of the hand 2 months postoperatively. **D:** The thumb length is adequate to permit pinch.

References

1. Moberg E. Transfer of sensation. *J Bone Joint Surg* 1955;37(A):299.
2. Littler JW. Neurovascular skin island transfer in reconstructive hand surgery. In: *Transactions of the second congress of the international society of plastic surgeons.* London: Livingstone, 1960;175–179.
3. O'Brien BM. Neurovascular pedicle transfers in the hand. *Aust N Z J Surg* 1965;35:2.

CHAPTER 269 ■ MODIFIED PALMAR SKIN FLAP TO THE FINGERTIP

K. S. KIM

EDITORIAL COMMENT

It is important to understand the anatomy of the transverse palmar arterial branches for flap design. Identification of the vessel on the opposite side of the digit will help to accurately design the pedicle as well.

The modified palmar skin flap to the fingertip is a homodigital, normograde, neurovascular island flap based on the transverse palmar branch of the digital artery. The stability of palmar skin is critical for finger function; however, the use of a palmar skin flap can be justified for fingertip reconstruction, because the fingertip is a most important tactile area and contributes much to finger power. In addition, palmar digital island flaps can be used to resolve some problems arising with the use of several other flap techniques, despite the sacrifice of important palmar skin.

INDICATIONS

The so-named palmar digital island flap (1) has earned a place in the armamentarium of reconstructing fingertip defects, although the palmar surface of the finger is not usually considered a flap donor site (2). Reattachment of fingertip parts is the best method of preserving both length and the normal nail complex anatomy. If this is not possible, several flap techniques may be used to resurface the defect, but each method has some disadvantages. Local advancement flaps (3,4) provide soft-tissue coverage of similar quality to that of normal glabrous skin but cannot always be used because of distance limitations regarding flap advancement. Regional (4,5) and distant flaps (6) provide enough tissue for reconstruction, but prolonged immobilization can lead to stiffness of the injured digits. Several homodigital island or subcutaneous pedicled flaps (7–14) have been developed to avoid the disadvantages of local, regional, and distant flaps, but even these have some disadvantages of their own.

The palmar digital island flap can be used to reconstruct all defects of the finger, although it is used mainly to reconstruct fingertip and palmar defects, particularly large palmar defects of the fingertip, thus justifying the sacrifice of important palmar skin. This flap offers the advantages of both proximally and distally based homodigital island flaps, including a constant and reliable blood supply without sacrificing a major artery, excellent sensory recovery because of the digital nerve branches contained in this flap, coverage of the palmar defect with skin that has similar qualities in a single operative field, less venous congestion because of a proximally based and normograde flap, a

one-stage procedure for both functional and aesthetic preservation of the fingertip, and the avoidance of long hospitalization and hand immobilization.

This procedure is also versatile, as it can be raised on any transverse palmar branch of the proper digital artery, and it is easy to plan because it can reach the wound by means of rotating the adjacent palmar tissue. An important problem with the flap is palmar scar contracture resulting from the sacrifice of palmar skin. Skin graft loss may aggravate the palmar scar, because a tie-over bolster dressing is not applied to prevent direct compression of the pedicle. When a transverse palmar branch is located on the rim of tissue adjacent to the wound, a flap based on the branch may not be raised because of the possibility of vascular injury.

ANATOMY

According to Strauch and De Moura (15), there are three major transverse palmar branches (or arches) in each digit: the proximal, middle, and distal transverse palmar branches. The locations of these branches are constant, and the proximal and middle transverse branches are always associated with the limbs of the proximal and distal cruciate ligaments. The distal transverse palmar branch lies just distal to the insertion of the profundus tendon (Fig. 1A) and is approximately the same size as the middle branch, which is about 1.5 times larger than the proximal transverse palmar branch. There are, on average, four palmar branches of the proper digital arteries from each side at the level of the proximal and middle phalanges. Many small branches from the proper digital arteries and transverse palmar branches are connected to the palmar arterial network.

Although there may be some exceptions, many hand surgeons have reported not being able to find the venae comitantes running with the proper digital artery (1,16–18). In fact, the perivascular cuff tissue of the proper digital artery contains tiny venules, but not the venae comitantes (7). Therefore, the palmar digital island flap is perfused from the proper digital artery through the transverse palmar branch, and is drained through tiny venules and capillaries in the perivascular soft tissue (Fig. 1).

FLAP DESIGN AND DIMENSIONS

Palmar digital island flaps can be designed at distal, middle, or proximal phalangeal areas of the long fingers according to defect patterns. If possible, a flap should be designed on the lateral or medial palmar skin of the finger, to maximally preserve the palmar skin. Although the flap can be oriented in any direction, the transverse palmar branch is placed carefully

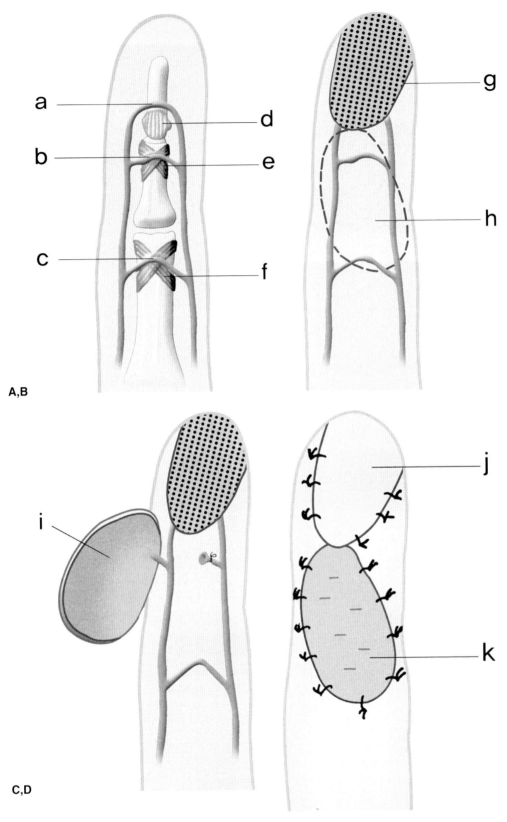

A,B

C,D

FIG. 1. **A:** Surgical anatomy. **B–D:** Operative technique. *a*, distal transverse palmar branch; *b*, middle transverse palmar branch; *c*, proximal transverse palmar branch; *d*, insertion site of the profundus tendon; *e*, distal cruciate ligament; *f*, proximal cruciate ligament; *g*, pulp defect; *h*, flap design; *i*, elevated flap; *j*, transposed flap; *k*, skin graft to the donor defect. (From Kim KS, Yoo SI, Kim DY, et al. Fingertip reconstruction using a palmar flap based on the transverse palmar branch of the digital artery. *Ann Plast Surg* 2001;47:263, with permission.)

in the distal region of the flap, and the flap is based on the proximal side of the wound for fingertip reconstruction (Fig. 1B). Even though the flaps are based distally, actual blood flow always adopts a normograde pattern (Fig. 1C). Therefore, the flap can include nearly the entire palmar surface of the finger and may be 2.5 cm in width and 5 cm in length. However, the usual dimensions are less than 2.0 cm in width and 3.5 cm in length.

OPERATIVE TECHNIQUE

After a tourniquet has been applied at the base of the finger, a skin incision is made from the side opposite the vascular pedicle. The flap is elevated carefully, with the aid of a loupe or the operating microscope, to leave the paratenon in situ to ensure skin-graft take. The transverse palmar branch is first identified, then ligated and divided at the distal midportion of the flap. The neurovascular pedicle can be best found where the transverse palmar branch derives from the proper digital artery of the side opposite the vascular pedicle.

The transverse palmar branch and the branch of the proper digital nerve in the pedicle area are then dissected to enable entrance into the flap. As the dissection proceeds toward the proper digital artery and nerve, it is essential to divide Grayson's ligament, but Cleland's ligament can be preserved. To avoid kinking and to reduce tension on the vascular pedicle, fibrous septae should be freed, by scissors dissection, from underlying bone and tendon sheath. To enable a free range of flap transposition, the pedicle can be dissected safely to the proximal level to the point where the transverse palmar branch derives from the proper digital artery. During dissection, a generous cuff of subcutaneous tissue is maintained around the vascular pedicle to preserve tiny perivascular venules (Fig. 1C).

The raised flap is then transposed and sutured loosely to the defect, and the donor site is covered with a split-thickness skin graft from the hypothenar or plantar area. A tie-over bolster dressing is not applied, to prevent direct compression of the pedicle (Fig. 1D).

The hand is elevated to minimize postoperative venous congestion, but anticoagulants are not used. The finger is splinted for 1 week to ensure graft success, after which both passive and active mobilization can be carefully started. In addition, a light protective dressing is worn for approximately 2 weeks.

CLINICAL RESULTS

Although sometimes temporary venous congestion and desquamation in the skin may develop, flap necrosis due to arterial or venous complication is rare. More than 70 palmar digital island flaps have been performed at the Chonnam National University Medical School during the past 10 years, and all flaps have survived well. This high success rate is attributed to an excellent blood supply and careful selection and preservation of the vascular pedicle. Moreover, long-term follow-up shows good flap durability and elasticity, and although

sensory recovery depends on the severity of digital nerve damage, flap sensibility is usually near-normal to normal, compared to intact contralateral fingers and the donor site.

Occasionally, temporary cold intolerance, hypersensitivity, or paresthesia develops, but long-term follow-up demonstrates complete recovery in most patients. The donor site is usually covered with a split-thickness skin graft from the hypothenar or plantar area, to achieve a better color match with adjacent skin areas. In addition, it should be noted that donor-site care is important for early finger mobilization, and that skin grafts may fail to take, partially as a result of subgraft hematoma, because compressive dressing is difficult at the palmar side. However, scar contracture at most flap donor sites is minimal.

SUMMARY

Although palmar digital island flaps require the sacrifice of important palmar skin, they provide excellent padding and sensation for fingertip reconstruction. Therefore, despite some difficulties, they appear to be suitable for fingertip reconstruction and, in particular, are indicated for patients with large palmar defects of the fingertip.

References

1. Kim KS, Yoo SI, Kim DY, et al. Fingertip reconstruction using a palmar flap based on the transverse palmar branch of the digital artery. *Ann Plast Surg* 2001;47:263.
2. Kutler W. A new method for fingertip amputation. *JAMA* 1947;133:29.
3. Atasoy E, Ioakimidis E, Kasdan ML, et al. Reconstruction of the amputated fingertip with a triangular palmar flap—a new surgical procedure. *J Bone Joint Surg (Am)* 1970;52A:921.
4. Tempest MN. Cross-finger flaps in the treatment of injuries to the finger tip. *Plast Reconstr Surg* 1952;9:205.
5. Miller AJ. Single fingertip injuries treated by thenar flap. *Hand* 1974;6:311.
6. McGregor IA, Jackson IT. The groin flap. *Br J Plast Surg* 1972;25:3.
7. Lai CS, Lin SD, Yang CC. The reverse digital artery flap for fingertip reconstruction. *Ann Plast Surg* 1989;22:495.
8. Kojima T, Tsuchida Y, Hirase Y, Endo T. Reverse vascular pedicle digital island flap. *Br J Plast Surg* 1990;43:290.
9. Niranjan NS, Armstrong JR. A homodigital reverse pedicle island flap in soft tissue reconstruction of the finger and the thumb. *J Hand Surg (Br)* 1994;19B:135.
10. Del Bene M, Petrolati M, Raimondi P, et al. Reverse dorsal digital island flap. *Plast Reconstr Surg* 1994;93:552.
11. Kayikçioğlu A, Akyürek M, Safak T, et al. Arterialized venous dorsal digital island flap for fingertip reconstruction. *Plast Reconstr Surg* 1998;102:2368.
12. Joshi BB. A local dorsolateral island flap for restoration of sensation after avulsion injury of fingertip pulp. *Plast Reconstr Surg* 1974;54:175.
13. Venkataswami R, Subramanian N. Oblique triangular flap: a new method of repair for oblique amputations of the fingertip and thumb. *Plast Reconstr Surg* 1980;66:296.
14. Tsai TM, Yuen YC. A neurovascular island flap for palmar-oblique fingertip amputations. *J Hand Surg (Br)* 1996;21B:94.
15. Strauch B, De Moura W. Arterial system of the fingers. *J Hand Surg (Am)* 1990;15A:148.
16. Eaton RG. The digital neurovascular bundle; a microanatomic study of its contents. *Clin Orthop Rel Res* 1968;61:176.
17. Lucas GL. The pattern of venous drainage of the digits. *J Hand Surg (Am)* 1964;9A:448.
18. Cormack GC, Lamberty BGH. *The arterial anatomy of skin flaps.* London: Churchill Livingstone, 1986:186–193.

CHAPTER 270 ■ REVERSE DORSAL DIGITAL AND METACARPAL FLAPS

P. PELISSIER

Reverse dorsal digital and metacarpal (DMD) flaps use the dorsal skin of the digital or metacarpal areas, and they are based on the arterial branches anastomosing the volar and dorsal arterial networks of the fingers. These flaps are transposed as reverse island flaps. Dissection of the flap is easy and rapid, and preserves the collateral nerve and artery to the fingertip.

INDICATIONS

The DMD flap is actually a proximal extension of previously described flaps (1–3). These flaps combine the advantages of an extended skin paddle and a versatile pivot point on the phalanx, and they allow coverage of wide and distal defects.

ANATOMY

The dorsal vascular network is known to vascularize the dorsal aspect of the hand and fingers (4,5). This network is made of terminal branches of the dorsal metacarpal arteries and dorsal branches of the collateral digital arteries (Fig. 1). Anastomosing branches between the palmar and dorsal vascular systems are present in all three phalanges (4). Four of them, located at the middle and distal third of the proximal phalanx, the middle of the second phalanx, and at the level of the distal interphalangeal joint, are larger and represent a constant communication between the volar and dorsal vascular systems. These branches are potential pivot points for reverse dorsal flaps. Venous drainage depends on a parallel venous system surrounding the arterial pedicle.

FLAP DESIGN AND DIMENSIONS

Flaps may be harvested from the dorsum of the proximal phalanges or the dorsum of the commissure; they are supplied by the anastomosing branches. Blood flow is then orthograde in the collateral digital artery and retrograde in the dorsal vascular network. In addition, the vascular territory of the flap possibly extends up to the metacarpal area (6), thus increasing both the size of the flap and its arc of rotation. The flap is designed on the dorsal aspect of the metacarpal area or the dorsal aspect of the finger. The estimated emerging point and direction of the communicating branch is also marked; it theoretically represents the pivot point of the flap (Fig. 1). Design includes marking the subcutaneous pedicle that will be raised with the flap. Ideally, it should be almost as wide as the skin paddle to make vascularization safer.

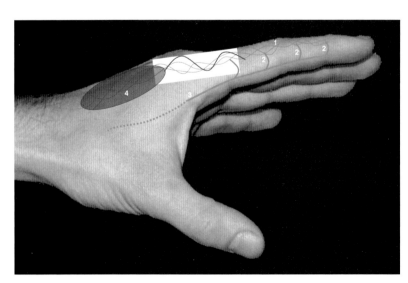

FIG. 1. Arterial blood supply of fingers and flap design. White area indicates the subcutaneous pedicle to be included in the dissection. *1*, dorsal arterial network; *2*, anastomosing branches; *3*, collateral digital artery; *4*, skin paddle.

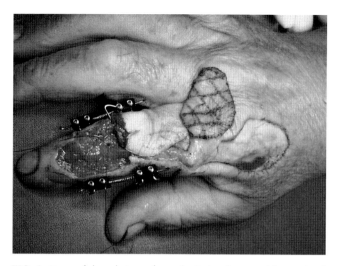

FIG. 2. Loss of dorsal tissue from the index finger, with proximal interphalangeal joint and extensor tendon avulsion and bone exposure. Reverse metacarpal flap harvested with a large subcutaneous pedicle. This patient also had an associated extensor fixation and joint immobilization with an external fixator.

OPERATIVE TECHNIQUE

The technique is safe and easy (7). Dissection begins with a "lazy S" incision above the pedicle area. The skin is undermined, exposing the subcutaneous pedicle. The skin paddle is then incised deep to the paratenon, in continuity with the lateral edges of the subcutaneous pedicle as far as the pivot point (Fig. 2). It is useless and potentially dangerous to try to visualize the pedicle when dissecting the flap. To protect the pedicle, soft tissue is taken in a block from the subcutis to the paratenon. The flap is then harvested from proximal to distal, and dissection stops just before the pivot point. The tourniquet is released with the flap in its original position, to ensure adequate refill of the vascular pedicle. The flap is then rotated and sutured with a few stitches.

CLINICAL RESULTS

Average time for flap dissection is usually less than 20 minutes. Over a series of 48 cases, two partial flap necroses were reported that did not impair the final result. The outcome was satisfactory in all patients. Donor-site morbidity was minimal. The wound was either primarily closed or skin-grafted. No patient complained about the resulting scars. The pedicle is reliable enough to be twisted over 180 degrees, and although venous drainage could be considered tenuous, no venous congestion was observed. These flaps, however, do not seem suitable for restoring sensibility, even when a branch of a dorsal sensitive nerve is included and anastomosed with a collateral digital nerve.

SUMMARY

Reverse dorsal digital and metacarpal flaps are recommended for coverage of dorsal defects, as they use skin from the dorsum of the hand or fingers and do not require the sacrifice of a collateral digital artery. The reported procedure combines an extended skin paddle and a versatile pivot point on the phalanx and allows coverage of wide and distal defects. Dissection is rapid and not complex, as there is no need to look for the vascular pedicle. Moreover, the surgical technique is easy to handle, because residents performed half of the procedures.

References

1. Del Bene MD, Petrolati M, Raimondi P, et al. Reverse dorsal digital island flap. *Plast Reconstr Surg* 1994;93:552.
2. Valenti P, Masquelet AC, Begue T. Anatomic basis of a dorso commissural flap from the 2nd, 3rd and 4th intermetacarpal spaces. *Surg Radiol Anat* 1990;12:235.
3. Masquelet AC, Valenti P. Les lambeaux dorso-commisuraux. *Ann Chir Plast Esthét* 1994;39:287.
4. Strauch B, De Moura W. Arterial system of the fingers. *J Hand Surg (Am)* 1990;15:148.
5. Coleman SS, Anson BJ. Arterial patterns in the hand based upon a study of 650 specimens. *Surg Gynecol Obstet* 1961;113:409.
6. Bakhach J, Martin D, Baudet J. Le lambeau paramétacarpien ulnaire: Un experience de dix cas cliniques. *Ann Chir Plast Esthét* 1996;41:269.
7. Pelissier P, Casoli V, Bakhach J, et al. Reverse dorsal digital and metacarpal flaps: a review of 27 cases. *Plast Reconstr Surg* 1999;103:159.

CHAPTER 271 ■ MICROVASCULAR FREE TRANSFER OF THE NAIL

G. D. LISTER

Toe-to-hand transfer has become a reliable method of thumb reconstruction and its anatomic bases have been well established. The entire toe is not always required, and successful microvascular transfer of neurovascular islands and of composites of pulp and nail—the wraparound flap—has been successfully developed (1). It might appear that the hemipulp must be included to ensure integrity of the arterial supply to the transfer. However, by application of the anatomy detailed below, transfer of the nail with a rim of perionychium can be achieved in those rare cases in which the nail alone has been lost in a patient to whom it has unusual significance.

INDICATIONS

The important properties of the nail are well recognized—protection, prehension, and cosmesis. Loss of the nail alone inflicts a significant disability, and attempts to restore the entire structure by free composite transfer have not been uniformly successful (2,3). Considerable though the disability may be, rarely does it warrant a lengthy and complex reconstructive procedure. Where the demands of special skills do justify it, microvascular free transfer of the nail offers the possibility of complete survival and a perfect functional result.

ANATOMY

The blood supply of the nailbed has been described in detail (4). There are three arterial arcades (Fig. 1): a superficial one at the base of the distal phalanx dorsally, just distal to the extensor tendon insertion, which receives contributions from both the middle and distal phalangeal segments of the proper digital artery; a proximal subungual arcade, which runs across the dorsal surface of the phalanx at the level of its narrow waist; and a distal subungual arcade, which lies at the base of the ungual process. Both of these latter arcades derive from the digital arteries at their cruciate anastomosis on the palmar aspect of the terminal phalanx via branches that pass through the rima ungualum, which is the space between the waist of the phalanx and the lateral interosseous ligament (Fig. 2).

The lateral interosseous ligament, which attaches to the ungual spines distally and the lateral tubercles of the distal phalanx proximally, serves as the strong lateral attachment of the nailbed (5). The means by which the nailbed is adherent to the phalanx are not clarified in available texts. Certainly common experience shows that once disrupted, that attachment is rarely reestablished satisfactorily.

OPERATIVE TECHNIQUE

The procedure is performed as a combined simultaneous dissection, the radial artery being exposed with the cephalic vein just distal to the snuffbox, while the dorsalis pedis artery and the first dorsal metatarsal artery are dissected on the foot. In nail transfers to a finger other than the thumb and in the 20% or more of cases where the dorsal arteries of the foot are unsatisfactory, the microarterial anastomosis can be between digital arteries. In the thumb, however, access is much superior when the anastomosis is made more proximally. Once satisfactory vessels have been isolated, preparation of the transfer and of its bed can proceed. This occurs in three stages.

Skin Incisions

Since the nail of the toe is somewhat larger than that of the thumb, the defect created in excision of the thumbnail remnant must be enlarged somewhat, without discarding uninjured and sensate pulp tissue. This is achieved as follows. The incisions that skirt the distal and lateral aspects of the nail on the toe are made gently convex toward the nail and their length C is measured. Similar but straight skirting incisions are made on the thumb and their length A is measured (Fig. 3A).

Back-cuts of length B are then made from the corners at which the thumb incisions meet, in such a way as to make $A + 2B = C$. The incision proximally from the nail fold of the thumb is of a zigzag nature, exposing distal branches of the radial nerve. No skin is discarded from the thumb, other than that immediately adjacent to the nail. The proximal skin incisions in the toe are designed to excise a V, the apex

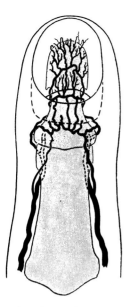

FIG. 1. There are three dorsal arterial arcades that supply the nailbed (see text). (From Flint, ref. 4, with permission.)

of which lies over the web space some 3 to 4 cm proximal to the nail (Fig. 3C). This permits dissection of veins and branches of the superficial and deep peroneal nerves. The flap so created must be elevated in the plane between these nerves and veins and the underlying extensor tendon, out to a point just distal to its insertion. This point must also be exposed in the thumb.

Arterial Mobilization

The appropriate digital artery is mobilized from the skeleton of the toe by coagulating all of its branches to the midline of the toe, leaving the digital nerve intact on the toe. Once the

distal phalanx is reached, it is necessary to free the artery sufficiently to permit safe access to the bone for osteotomy. This is achieved by dissecting the palmar surface of the phalanx until the two attachments of the lateral interosseous ligament can be seen and divided (Fig. 2). This permits the lateral margin of the nail to be lifted sufficiently to allow bone cuts.

Osteotomy (see Fig. 3B)

Identical osteotomies are performed in the distal phalanges of toe and thumb. First, an anteroposterior transverse cut is made one-half way through the phalanx just distal to the insertion of the extensor tendon. Care should be taken that this is of equal depth across its full breadth and that the dorsal vessels are not disturbed in the process. Then a coronal cut is made in such a way as to join the first osteotomy and thereby remove the dorsal half of the phalanx distal to the extensor tendon.

The transfer is then performed (Fig. 3C), rigid fixation of the bone being achieved with Kirschner wires (Fig. 3D,E), and the artery, vein, and dorsal nerves are joined.

CLINICAL RESULTS

The outcome is pleasing in both appearance and function (Fig. 3F,G). The nail is of normal stability, this being assured by the early union of the large area of cancellous bone that is placed in contact by the technique of osteosynthesis described above.

SUMMARY

Loss of the nail can have unusual significance to some patients. By application of the anatomy described above, microvascular free transfer of the nail from the foot to the hand can be achieved.

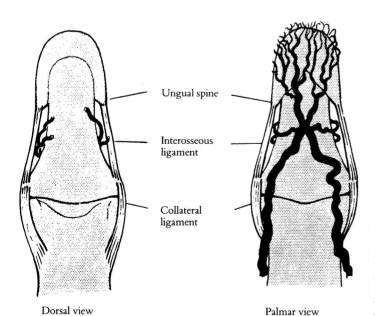

Ungual spine

Interosseous ligament

Collateral ligament

Dorsal view   Palmar view

FIG. 2. The digital arteries form a cruciate anastomosis from which pass the branches to the proximal and distal subungual arcades through the rima ungualum, which lies between the waist of the phalanx and the lateral interosseous ligament. It should be noted that the interosseous ligament passes from the lateral tubercles to which the distal end of the collateral ligament of the distal interphalangeal joint attaches, to the ungual spines distally. (From Flint, ref. 4, with permission.)

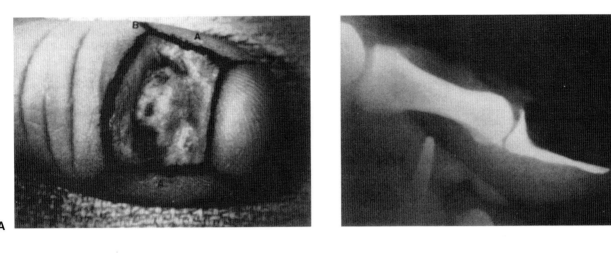

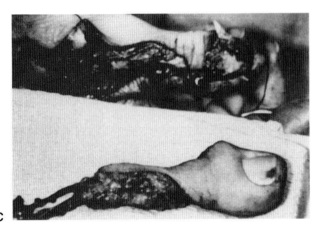
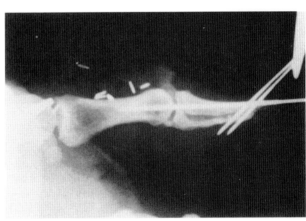

FIG. 3. A: A patient is shown in whom the nail has been destroyed by chemical treatment of a subungual wart. The incisions around the destroyed nailbed are planned to accommodate the larger mass of tissue to be taken from the toe, without discarding any of the normal pulp of the thumb. The straight incisions skirting the nail are labeled *A*, and the back-cuts shown at the corners of the quadrilateral excision are labeled *B*. The length of the back-cut is determined by the fact that *A* + *2B* should equal the skirting incision made in a curvilinear manner around the toenail, which is labeled *C*. **B:** The osteotomy in the distal phalanx is undertaken in such a way as to remove the nail with a significant sliver of bone while maintaining the insertion of the extensor and flexor tendons. This osteotomy is identical in both the thumb and the toe. Reconstruction of the toe is performed by fracturing the plantar sliver and folding it over to close the defect directly. The toe is shortened by half the length of the nailbed. **C:** The dissection is shown here completed on the thumb and the toe. The *V* portion of skin that has been taken from the toe to preserve the dorsal nerves and veins is demonstrated. **D:** The fragment excised from the toe fits well into the defect. Longitudinal and anteroposterior fixation with Kirschner wires, avoiding the nailbed itself, gives secure and extensive cancellous bone contact. *(continued)*

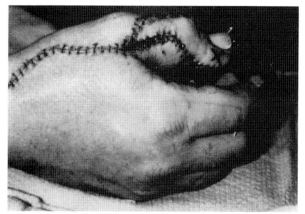

E

FIG. 3. *Continued* **E:** Anastomosis of the dorsalis pedis artery and dorsal vein of the foot to the radial artery and cephalic vein in the thumb has been completed and the wound closed. Good perfusion is seen, and the point marked *X* is that at which subsequent temperature monitoring is performed. **F:** The appearance of the hand is relatively normal. **G:** The healed result, showing normal nail growth and preservation of the normal contact surface of the thumb. The patient was able to return to his profession as a classical guitarist, using the nail as a plectrum.

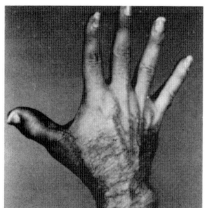

F

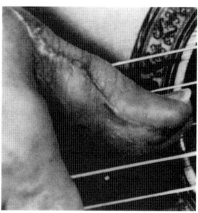

G

References

1. Morrison WA, O'Brien BM, MacLeod AM. Thumb reconstruction with a free neurovascular wraparound flap from the big toe. *J Hand Surg* 1980;5:575.
2. McCash CR. Free nail grafting. *Br J Plast Surg* 1955;8:19.
3. Buncke HJ, Gonzalez RI. Fingernail reconstruction. *Plast Reconstr Surg* 1962;30:452.
4. Flint MH. Some observations on the vascular supply of the nail bed and terminal segments of the finger. *Br J Plast Surg* 1955;8:186.
5. Shrewsbury M, Johnson RK. The fascia of the distal phalanx. *J Bone Joint Surg* 1975;57(A):784.

CHAPTER 272 ■ RADIAL INNERVATED CROSS-FINGER SKIN FLAP TO THE THUMB

J. S. GAUL AND J. E. ADAMSON

The purpose of this procedure is to reconstruct the volar surface of the injured thumb with a cross-finger skin flap containing a sensory nerve supply from the dorsum of the proximal phalanx of the index finger (1–5).

INDICATIONS

This flap is especially suitable for medium (2 cm) or large (3 cm or greater) volar thumb defects, both terminal and intercalary, which preferably retain some deep soft-tissue base. The radial innervated dorsal skin is itself not thick enough to replace all of the pulp. The flap can also be used as a secondary procedure for cases of volar sensory denervation of the thumb from local damage.

The radial innervated cross-finger skin flap should not be used for small thumb defects of 1 cm or less, which can usually be repaired by local or pulp advancement flaps. On the other hand, this is a thin flap and is not indicated for massive thumb avulsion, where there is no soft-tissue covering the skeletal stump.

A diagnostic median nerve block should be done to determine that the dorsal innervation of the superficial radial nerve extends sufficiently distal to the MP joint, to supply the intended flap adequately. In cases where there is an associated severe median nerve sensory defect, in which the superficial radial innervation to the lateral sides of the thumb and to the proximal phalanx of the index finger supports a primitive pinch function, the index should not be used as a donor site.

A relative contraindication may be the presence of a single digit with extensive palmar destruction. Such a useless digit may contribute a valuable neurovascular island flap to the thumb prior to its amputation.

FLAP DESIGN AND DIMENSIONS

A conventional cross-finger flap is designed from the proximal phalanx of the index finger to accommodate the adducted thumb without undue stress. These flaps usually range from 1 to 2 cm in length (which represents the transverse dimension of the donor digit). Flaps can be designed between 1.5 and 4.0 cm in width (which represents the longitudinal dimension of the donor digit).

The flap typically hinges at its base somewhere along the midlateral line of the donor index finger (Fig. 1), and normally it must rotate outward 90° to 150°. Despite this somewhat acute turn, no flaps have been lost.

OPERATIVE TECHNIQUE

First Stage

An incision is made over the radial aspect of the dorsum of the wrist in a Y-shaped configuration. One limb extends distally to the index finger flap and the other limb extends to the ulnar aspect of the thumb defect. That part of the incision over the wrist should be zigzagged as necessary to avoid a straight-line scar.

The superficial radial nerve is identified as it branches to the thumb and to the index finger. The one or two branches to the dorsum of the index finger are carefully traced out to the transverse margin of the flap. A generous layer of subcutaneous tissue around the nerves is preserved, along with a few small vessels if possible.

The distal and ulnar margins of the skin flap (Fig. 1) are incised through skin and subcutaneous tissue. The incision is then made cautiously over the proximal transverse margin of the flap, to avoid damaging the terminal nerve fibers entering that margin of the flap at the subcutaneous level.

The recipient thumb is then brought to the donor index finger. The nerve bundle should pass under the edge of the thumb web and into the thumb volar skin pocket, which has been generously undermined, passing almost directly over the flexor pollicis longus sheath (Fig. 2).

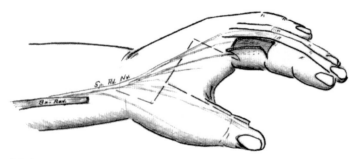

FIG. 1. The basic incision should be Y-shaped, extending from the radial aspect of the wrist where the superficial nerve is identified to both the donor site on the index finger and the ulnar aspect of the defect on the thumb pulp.

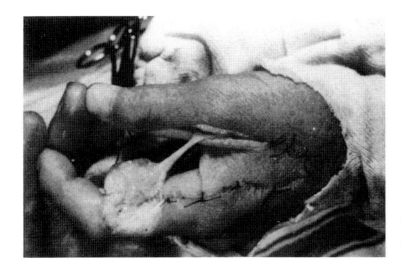

FIG. 2. The flap and its nerve bundle have been mobilized from the index finger and hand. The ulnar volar skin envelope of the thumb has been undermined, and the flap is fitted into the thumb defect as the nerve bundle is simultaneously tucked under the volar ulnar skin margin.

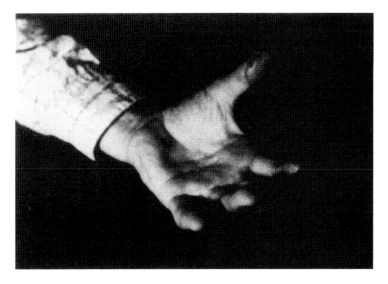

FIG. 3. A radial innervated skin flap now furnishes useful tactile sensation to the thumb pad of a carpenter, whose thumb had been previously denervated by local tissue damage. This patient immediately regained light touch sensation and has used his hand for at least 10 years. The flap "felt like the thumb and the index finger" for several years, but more recently has been interpreted as "thumb," according to the patient.

After the flap is inset, a skin graft is placed over the donor site.

Second Stage

Approximately 3 weeks later the flap is divided. It is apparent at this stage why it is so important to locate the nerve bundle deep under the volar skin flap of the thumb: the nerve then lies deep to the proximal transverse flap suture margin, and should not be at risk when the flap is severed from the index finger.

CLINICAL RESULTS

Twenty-seven cases have been performed with follow-up data by the two authors and their associates working in independent practices in two different communities. No flaps have been lost. Some sensation is almost always restored, usually obvious to the patient the following day (Fig. 3).

Two-point discrimination testing has produced variable, but often good, results. The testing depends very much on the technique of the individual examiner. Many cases have produced good two-point discrimination, frequently in the 6-, 8-, and 10-mm range, while other cases have shown only

consistent light touch. All patients have demonstrated the ability to handle objects effectively with the reconstructed thumb, although one patient complained of persistent numbness even though he had functional use of his thumb.

None of these patients had symptoms of neuroma formation, causalgia, or sympathetic dystrophy. The donor site healed well, although most retained an area of anesthesia in the region of the skin graft.

SUMMARY

The radial innervated cross-finger flap can be used to provide both cover and sensation to volar thumb defects.

References

1. Adamson JE, Horton CE, Crawford HH. Sensory rehabilitation of the injured thumb. *Plast Reconstr Surg* 1967;40:53.
2. Gaul JS. Radial innervated cross-finger flap from index to provide sensory pulp to injured thumb. *J Bone Joint Surg* 1969;51(A): 1257.
3. Brailler F, Horner RH. Sensory cross-finger pedicle graft. *J Bone Joint Surg* 1969;51(A):1264.
4. Wilkinson TS. Reconstruction of the thumb by radial nerve innervated cross-finger flap. *South Med J* 1972;65:992.
5. Miura T. Thumb reconstruction using radial innervated cross-finger pedicle. *J Bone Joint Surg* 1973;55(A):563.

CHAPTER 273 ■ NEUROVASCULAR SKIN KITE FLAP FROM THE INDEX FINGER

G. FOUCHER AND F. VAN GENECHTEN

The skin overlying the dorsal aspect of the proximal phalanx of the index finger can be transferred as a neurovascular island flap (1). Anatomically this flap is an axial pattern skin flap that extends proximally from the level of the metaphalangeal (MP) joint and distally to the level of the proximal interphalangeal (PIP) joint. The neurovascular pedicle contains the first dorsal metacarpal artery, one or two dorsal veins, and the terminal branches of the radial nerve.

INDICATIONS

Advantages of the flap can be summarized as follows. There is a constant and reliable anatomy with ease of dissection. A one-stage procedure provides neurovascular skin cover and it is possible to cover the entire dorsal or palmar aspect of the thumb. The flap can be combined with a radial forearm flap or a neurovascular island flap to cover a complete degloving injury of the thumb. The flap provides sensation. Venous return is so good that it is possible to use the veins to graft a vein defect in cases of replantation with associated skin cover problems (two cases in our series).

ANATOMY

The dorsal metacarpal artery arises from the radial artery at the apex of the first interosseous space, before the radial artery disappears toward the palmar aspect of the hand. The artery runs over the first dorsal interosseous muscle toward the metacarpophalangeal joint of the index finger, giving off at various points the internal dorsal artery of the thumb and a few perforating branches that join the deep palmar arch. The dorsal metacarpal artery was found to be constant in all of 30 specimens dissected (2). Injection studies with methylene blue demonstrate that this artery supplies a skin territory that includes the entire dorsum of the proximal phalanx of the index finger (1).

The sensory branch of the radial nerve and one or two veins are easily found through the same dorsal incision. It is useful to know that in certain cases the sensation to the distal third of the skin flap is provided by the dorsal branch from the neurovascular bundle on the volar aspect of the index finger, the latter coming from the median nerve. This is an important point, particularly when a sensory flap is required. A preoperative local nerve block is mandatory and a selective block of radial or median nerve helps to establish a possible median nerve innervation of the distal third of the skin kite flap.

The two-point discrimination of this area averages 12 to 15 mm (3).

OPERATIVE TECHNIQUE

A reverse S-shaped incision is made over the radial border of the second metacarpal. We dissect the distal part of the radial artery only to identify the origin of the first dorsal metacarpal artery and to avoid confusion with a princeps pollicis artery or a deep muscular branch (Fig. 1). The fascia overlying the interosseous muscle is then cut at its radial side and lifted from the muscle en bloc with the artery. This maneuver will prevent damage to the vascular system. In certain cases a protective cuff of muscle fibers is dissected with the artery.

The dissection then proceeds more superficially toward the ulnar side to free one or two veins and the sensory radial nerve

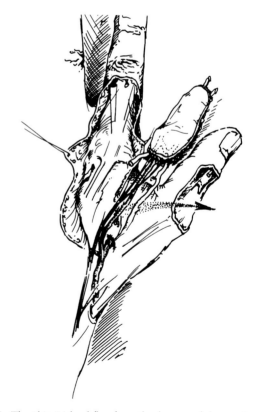

FIG. 1. The "kite" island flap from the dorsum of the proximal phalanx of the index finger transferred to the thumb. Note the neurovascular pedicle composed of the first dorsal metacarpal artery (together with the perivascular fat and the adjacent part of the aponeurosis), one or two superficial veins, and the radial nerve branches to this area of skin. (From Littler, ref. 5, with permission.)

808

branches, leaving some subcutaneous tissue around these neurovascular elements. The axial skin artery anastomoses with a deep interosseous artery at the radial neck of the second metacarpal bone. The dissection at this key point is usually facilitated by first raising the skin flap just before the neurovascular bundle is completely liberated. The sensory axial pattern flap is then ready for transfer. For the transfer of the flap to the thumb, one can tunnel the pedicle underneath the skin of the first web space.

CLINICAL RESULTS

We used this flap in 27 cases between 1976 and 1982, with only partial loss of skin in one case where a small scar crossed the distal part of the skin flap. Our series included 23 cases of injuries to the thumb. Eight cases required skin cover for complex loss of tissue over the dorsal aspect and nine cases required cover of proximal palmar or proximal lateral skin defects. Only in six cases was the flap used to cover the entire palmar aspect of the thumb, with a two-point discrimination averaging 11 mm (a minimum of 9 and a maximum of 14 mm) after 3 months of sensory reeducation (4). Although this two-point discrimination is less than in Littler's experience with the neurovascular island flap (5), a larger area of skin can be transferred with the skin kite flap.

There are only a few disadvantages with this flap. The donor site obviously requires a graft. A full-thickness graft

provides a better cosmetic result with minimal hyperpigmentation. The dorsum of the index finger has hair-bearing skin matching the normal dorsal skin of the thumb, but not the palmar skin. A similar problem exists in the conventional cross-finger flap. Finally, the index finger requires splinting to avoid any loss of extension or flexion.

SUMMARY

The skin kite flap is a reliable and versatile island flap and provides a large and well-vascularized skin area with some sensory discrimination. The length of the neurovascular pedicle provides a wide arc of rotation and allows the flap to reach even the tip of the thumb.

References

1. Foucher G, Braun JB. A new island flap transfer from the dorsum of the index to the thumb. *Plast Reconstr Surg* 1979;63:344.
2. Braun JB. *Les Arteres de la Main.* Thesis, University of Nancy, 1977.
3. Gellis M, Pool R. Two point discrimination distances in the normal hand and forearm: application to various methods of fingertip reconstruction. *Plast Reconstr Surg* 1977;59:57.
4. Dellon AL. *Evaluation of sensibility and re-education of sensation in the hand.* Baltimore: Williams & Wilkins, 1981.
5. Littler JW. Neurovascular pedicle transfer of tissue in reconstructive surgery of the hand. *J Bone Joint Surg* 1956;38(A):917.

CHAPTER 274 ■ INNERVATED DORSAL INDEX FINGER SKIN FLAPS TO THE THUMB

F. J. RYBKA AND F. E. PRATT

In lengthening or reconstructing the thumb, local sensory flaps are favored over distant nonsensory flaps. Among neurovascular island flaps, one adjacent to the thumb, as described below, is generally preferred over a more remote hand flap, e.g., from the ulnar side of the ring finger (1–3). This is because the dorsal index flap is less risky and time-consuming in dissection, and because it can offer a greater paddle of sensory skin (4–7). Although it can be argued that dorsal skin is not as refined in sensation as the more specialized volar skin, this does not appear to be of great clinical importance.

INDICATIONS

Sensory skin from the second metacarpophalangeal dorsal surface has been examined as a possible source for thumb reconstruction for some time (4), but the procedure was originally in

two stages. Used as a rotation flap, it is very useful for (1) reconstructing a denuded thumb or lengthening a foreshortened one, or (2) expanding a contracted first web space (8), a situation that can frequently occur after an otherwise successful replantation of an amputated thumb.

Since 1977 (5) it has been demonstrated that an island flap could reliably be derived from the covering over the proximal phalanx of the index finger, divided from its metacarpal skin yet retaining the nutrient vessels and sensory nerves. This can be used for resurfacing more distal cutaneous defects of the thumb in one stage (6,7).

ANATOMY

The external dorsal branch of the first dorsal metacarpal artery supplies the dorsum of the index proximal phalanx, and this branch is constant (1,6). Two veins usually drain the flap, and the dorsal branch of the radial nerve runs close to these veins on either side of the dorsum (3). The neurovascular elements are not fixed to dermis, but are carried in their own perivascular areolar plane and can be separated from proximal skin without compromise.

FLAP DESIGN AND DIMENSIONS

Prior to the procedure, the dorsal branch of the radial nerve may be blocked, to ascertain its pattern of sensory distribution. If used as a *rotation flap,* as for expansion of the first web space, an S-shaped incision is planned between the defect and the second metacarpophalangeal joint, lateral to the dorsal veins that are usually included in the flap. The flap may be extended without any delay, to include skin over the proximal phalanx of the index finger, depending on the need for length. When this is done, the longitudinal incisions are volar to each of the dorsal veins that are again included in the flap.

OPERATIVE TECHNIQUE

If used as a neurovascular *island flap,* dissection is begun from distal to proximal. Under a high-intensity light, the neurovascular elements are identified and are carefully dissected in their perivascular areolar tissue, away from the overlying dermis back toward the midmetacarpal level. The flap can then be rotated subcutaneously over and onto the thumb. Depending on the case, dog-ears in the flap may be accepted at this point, rather than risking flap refinement. A full-thickness skin graft is used to cover the index donor area (Fig. 1).

CLINICAL RESULTS

Our series of 14 cases is cited as evidence for the dependability of the dorsal flap in thumb reconstruction. Use of the flap as an island resulted in success in six out of seven cases. In the last case, partial necrosis of the flap occurred in a hand crushed by a machine press. Not only was the thumb devascularized,

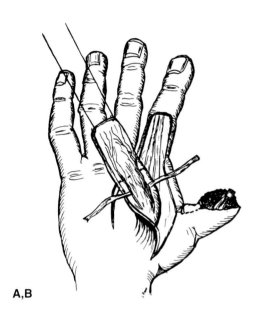

A,B

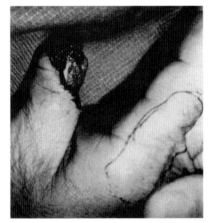

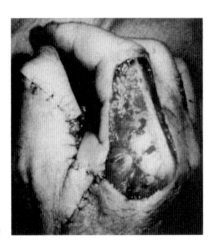

C,D

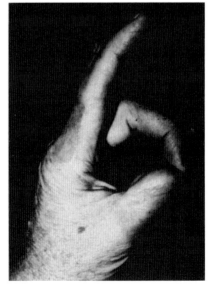

FIG. 1. Use of the dorsal index flap as a neurovascular island. **A:** Diagram of the flap. An umbilical tape is passed beneath the neurovascular bundles to the skin paddle as they are separated from the overlying dermis. **B:** A 45-year-old man, victim of a water ski rope avulsion of his thumb. **C:** Immediate reconstruction, with transfer of the island flap. **D:** Late results at 3 months. (From Rybka and Pratt, ref. 7, with permission.)

but the dorsum of the hand was edematous from the impact. The failure was thought to be the result of this soft-tissue trauma in the donor area.

In all cases the reconstructed thumbs were used actively and painlessly and sensation was retained, although "relearning" was not accomplished. No neuromas developed and there was no loss of function to the donor finger.

SUMMARY

The thumb can be reconstructed with a sensory dorsal index finger skin flap. If elevated with its neurovascular elements intact, it can be extended over the proximal phalanx without delay.

References

1. Tubiana R, Duparc J. Restoration of sensibility in the hand by neurovascular skin island transfer. *J Bone Joint Surg* 1961;43(B):474.
2. Chase R. An alternative to pollicization in subtotal thumb reconstruction. *Plast Reconstr Surg* 1969;44:421.
3. McGregor I. Less than satisfactory experience with neurovascular island flaps. *Hand* 1969;1:1.
4. Adamson JE, Horton C, Crawford H. Sensory rehabilitation of the injured thumb. *Plast Reconstr Surg* 1967;40:53.
5. Rybka FJ, Pratt FE. Thumb reconstruction using a sensory flap from the dorsal index finger. Presented at the Annual Meeting of the American Association of Hand Surgery, San Francisco, Calif., Oct. 29, 1977.
6. Foucher G, Braun J. A new island flap transfer from the dorsum of the index to the thumb. *Plast Reconstr Surg* 1979;63:344.
7. Rybka FJ, Pratt FE. Thumb reconstruction with a sensory flap from the dorsum of the index finger. *Plast Reconstr Surg* 1979;64:141.
8. Flatt A, Wood V. Multiple dorsal rotation flaps from the hand for thumb web contractures. *Plast Reconstr Surg* 1970;45:258.

CHAPTER 275 ■ INFRACLAVICULAR SKIN FLAP TO THE HAND AND FINGERS

V. R. HENTZ

An ideal flap for hand and digital coverage would incorporate the following characteristics: First, the skin and subcutaneous tissue should be thin and pliable, with a minimum of subcutaneous fat (1,2). The tissues of the hand, especially on the volar aspect, are well fixed to the underlying skeleton, permitting more stable grasp. The placement of a thick or bulky flap to reconstruct the prime contact surfaces would seriously diminish the stability of grasp. Second, the skin should be hairless. Except for the dorsum, the hand is relatively hairless. Full-thickness losses, particularly on the glabrous surfaces of the hand, should be replaced by hairless tissue.

INDICATIONS

From very few parts of the body do the skin and subcutaneous tissue meet these special requirements for soft-tissue coverage of the hand and digit. Several alternatives for coverage include the volar aspect of the forearm, the internal surface of the upper arm, the dorsum of the foot, and the infraclavicular area. Of these the infraclavicular area has probably been used the longest, for replacement of full-thickness loss of the hand and digits that is not reconstructable by split-thickness or full-thickness skin grafts or local rotation flaps.

The infraclavicular area usually remains free of thick subcutaneous fat, even in somewhat obese people, and it is usually hairless or relatively hairless, even in the most hirsute individuals.

Fashioned with its pedicle based along the clavicle and with adaptability in positioning the arm and hand, the flap can be used to cover almost any area of the hand and digits. The arm lies comfortably across the chest and the hand is in an elevated position, promoting venous drainage and reducing edema formation. The donor site is reasonably well hidden by shirt or dress, and a surprising amount of skin can be removed, with the donor site still closed primarily.

ANATOMY

The skin and subcutaneous tissue of the infraclavicular area are supplied by several independent vascular systems (Fig. 1). Medially the principal vascular supply is through the intercostal perforating branches from the internal mammary artery. These branches are direct cutaneous arteries arising

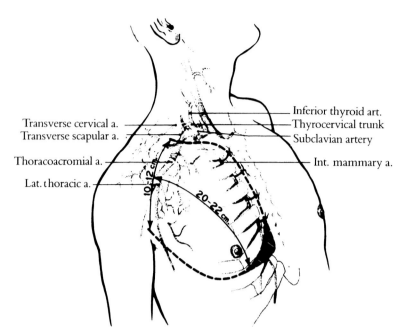

FIG. 1. Sources of cutaneous circulation to the infra-clavicular and anterior chest wall are illustrated. There are three distinct arterial pedicles supplying this area: perforators from the internal mammary artery medially, branches from the transverse cervical and scapular arteries of the thyrocervical axis superiorly, and contributions from the thoracoacromial trunk laterally. (From Conley, ref. 1, with permission.)

from each intercostal space, beginning with the second rib, and they are well described in the chapter on the deltopectoral flap (Chap. 124). Superiorly the skin receives some circulation via branches of the thyrocervical trunk, principally the transverse cervical and transverse scapular arteries. Lateral to this area the infraclavicular skin is supplied by branches of the thoracoacromial trunk, another direct cutaneous artery. Blood supply is also derived from muscular perforators via the pectoralis major muscle and its principal vascular contributions of the medial and lateral pectoral arteries.

FLAP DESIGN AND DIMENSIONS

When used to provide cover for the hand or digit, the flap is usually based superiorly and somewhat laterally. The area will

accommodate a flap of 7 to 8 cm in width and 14 to 15 cm in length, when the distal portion of the flap is directed toward the subaxillary region. Frequently this length allows the pedicle portion of the flap to be tubed. A technical error that frequently accompanies its use for thumb reconstruction is designing the flap with insufficient width to cover the complete circumference of the reconstructed thumb, particularly once a bone graft has been placed inside the skin envelope. The flap needs to be at least 8 cm in width.

Because the skin is thin, pliable, and hairless, it has also been used to resurface digits after degloving injuries, and is particularly well suited for replacing skin deficits in the first web space following release of adduction contractures. Typically the tissues of the first web space comprise a tetrahedron, and replacement involves covering two adjacent sides of the tetrahedron. The flap is designed, therefore, with a

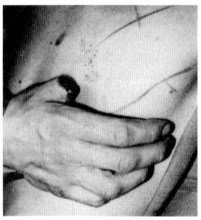 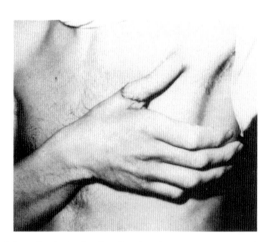 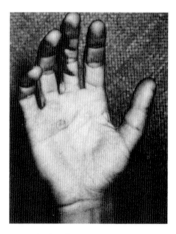

A–C

FIG. 2. An application of the infraclavicular flap for thumb reconstruction is demonstrated. A: The thumb has been amputated just distal to the metacarpophalangeal joint. The proposed flap, based proximally, is outlined along the lateral border of the pectoralis major muscle. The pedicle is tubed and the donor site is closed by advancing the margins of the defect. B: A dorsal V-shaped extension of the flap avoids a circular scar and broadens the area of inset. This improves the rate of neovascularization of the flap from the recipient site, and increases the length of flap supportable by recipient site circulation once the pedicle is divided. C: The reconstruction is completed by placement of a bone graft within the tubed pedicle and by replacement of the insensible skin of the volar surface of the flap by a neurovascular island pedicle taken from the ulnar border of the middle finger. (From Chase, ref. 2, with permission.)

triangular paddle that is inset initially into the dorsal defect, and the pedicle is tubed. At the time of flap takedown, the pedicle is unfolded and trimmed to fit the volar triangle.

OPERATIVE TECHNIQUE

Because this is a random flap, there are no particular technical difficulties encountered in elevating the flap. The underlying muscular fascia is probably best included with the flap.

The flap has been particularly useful in reconstruction of the thumb by osteoplastic pollicization (Fig. 2).

Other technical considerations include methods to immobilize the arm and hand to the donor site. Except in small children I have not had to resort to plaster immobilization. I have found immobilization with strips of adhesive tape satisfactory, with additional padding in the axilla to maintain the arm in abduction.

If the area of inset of the flap is small as in osteoplastic pollicization, the flap should be detached from the chest in increments of a third, performed commonly under local anesthesia, 3 to 5 days apart. Typically the pedicle of the flap may be safely divided sometime in the second or third week. The fact that the pedicle can be tubed allows a non-crushing clamp to be placed across the pedicle base, and the fluorescein technique is used to confirm flap viability based on the new blood supply from the recipient site.

CLINICAL RESULTS

Because scars on the anterior chest wall tend to stretch and hypertrophy, the donor site may be unacceptable to some patients, especially to women who wish to wear "off the shoulder" clothing. This is a hardy flap, however, and complications secondary to inadequate circulation are uncommon.

SUMMARY

For many years the infraclavicular flap has been a reliable source of tissue for hand and digit reconstruction.

References

1. Conley J. *Regional flaps of the head and neck*. Philadelphia: Saunders, 1976;189.
2. Chase RA. *Atlas of hand surgery*. Philadelphia: Saunders, 1973.

 CHAPTER 276. Cross-Forearm Neurocutaneous Flap *B. H. Dolich*
www.encyclopediaofflaps.com

CHAPTER 277 ■ DYNAMIC ABDUCTOR DIGITI MINIMI MUSCULOCUTANEOUS FLAP FOR THE THUMB

V. R. HENTZ

EDITORIAL COMMENT

The use of the ulnar border of the hand, in an otherwise compromised hand, for coverage with muscle flaps is an excellent employment of local flaps. (See Chap. 286.)

Of the many transfers available to restore opposition movements of the thumb, one of the earliest described was transfer of the abductor digiti minimi (1). Its value as a dynamic transfer is widely acknowledged (2). As is the case with many muscle units, it can be transferred as a musculocutaneous flap (3).

INDICATIONS

See Fig. 2 for demonstrations of the ability of the flap simultaneously to restore deficits in both function and skin cover.

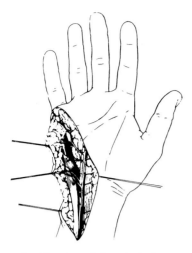

FIG. 1. The proximal location of the principal neurovascular hilum arising from the ulnar artery and nerve is illustrated.

ANATOMY

Vascular injection studies in cadavers have demonstrated the presence of musculocutaneous vessels that perforate the muscle and then supply the overlying skin and subcutaneous tissue. This occurs either directly or indirectly through the palmaris brevis muscle that lies between a portion of the abductor digiti minimi and the overlying skin. The vascular anatomy is shown in Fig. 1 (see also Fig. 1 in Chap. 286).

FLAP DESIGN AND DIMENSIONS

Since the skin can be carried as an "island," the arc of rotation is similar to that illustrated in Fig. 2 in Chap. 286.

OPERATIVE TECHNIQUE

Surgical dissection of the musculocutaneous unit is similar to that described for transfer of the muscle alone (see Chap. 286). As in any musculocutaneous flap, care must be exercised

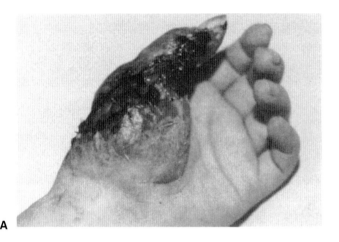

A

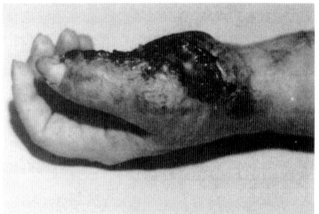

B

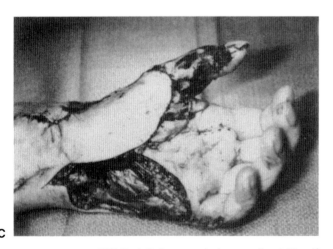

C

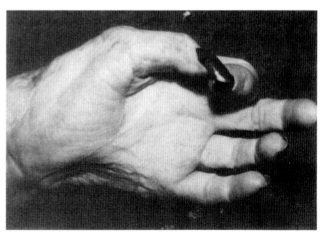

D

FIG. 2. A,B: A progressively expanding A-V malformation has resulted in infection and ulceration of the thenar skin. An arteriogram demonstrated diffuse involvement of the thenar muscles. **C:** The tumor mass and overlying skin were resected and the defect covered with an abductor digiti minimi musculocutaneous flap. The muscle was attached to the tendon of the abductor pollicis brevis. **D:** Fifteen months after surgery, the flap has provided durable skin cover and functional opposition. The donor defect is acceptable and is hidden when the hands are in most functional positions.

so that the skin is not sheared off the underlying muscle during elevation (Fig. 2).

The donor defect may be closed directly if the skin element is small. More likely, a thick split-thickness skin graft will serve as permanent cover.

When the muscle alone is used for functional restoration of thumb opposition, the muscle can be folded over as one would turn over the page of a book. If skin is included, the musculocutaneous unit must be rotated about its neurovascular pedicle to a greater degree.

CLINICAL RESULTS

The functional deficit resulting from transfer of the abductor digiti minimi is negligible.

SUMMARY

The abductor digiti minimi can be used as a dynamic musculocutaneous flap for restoration of thumb opposition.

References

1. Huber E. Hilfsoperation der Medianuslahmung. *Dtsch Z Chir* 1921; 162:271.
2. Littler JW, Cooley SGE. Opposition of the thumb and its restoration by abductor digiti quinti transfer. *J Bone Joint Surg* 1963;45(A):1389.
3. Chase RA, Hentz VR, Apfelberg D. A dynamic myocutaneous flap for hand reconstruction. *J Hand Surg* 1980;5:594.

CHAPTER 278 ■ MICRONEUROVASCULAR FREE TRANSFER OF THE BIG TOE

J. W. MAY, JR., AND R. C. SAVAGE

EDITORIAL COMMENT

Over the past decade, the pendulum has swung to the use of toe parts for reconstruction of the missing thumb. This has allowed for a five-digit hand with a nail on each of the digits. Each of the modifications has added to the success of these procedures. We direct the reader's attention particularly to Chapter 282 on the trimmed toe technique, which allows for a toe transplant that, in addition to its functional aspects, also provides the appearance of a normal thumb. See also Chapter 279–281.

Over the past 25 years, thumb reconstruction by microvascular toe-to-hand transfer has taken an important place in the armamentarium of the reconstructive hand surgeon (1–10). During this period microvascular toe transfer has emerged through the early phase of declaration (1) into a period of application, and recently into a period of refinement (10). This procedure is the piece de resistance of complex free-tissue transfers, in that it involves transfer to the hand of skin-nail, subcutaneous tissue, tendons, bone, joint, nerve, and vessels.

INDICATIONS

In general, we believe that toe-to-hand reconstruction can be useful in cases of subtotal or total thumb traumatic loss where four normal fingers are present or where three or fewer digits remain (7,10). In a hand with a damaged index finger and three remaining normal fingers, index finger pollicization may be indicated (11).

It has been said that the thumb in a normal hand comprises between 40% and 50% of the functional capability in that hand (12). In the mutilated hand the restoration of a strong, sensate, and mobile thumb of normal length can amount to far more than 50% of function in the assisting hand. In some cases the reconstructed thumb may be the most useful digit in the hand.

After injury, it is best to maximize the rehabilitation potential of the remaining element of the hand through a combination of reconstructive surgical procedures and therapy, prior to thumb reconstruction. In a severely mutilated hand these preliminary procedures may involve joint capsulectomy, fusion, or joint replacement, in addition to tendon lysis or graft and nerve reconstruction.

If there is soft-tissue shortage or significant damage to the radial side of the hand, with scarring that will ultimately limit motion, it is often better to transfer a distant flap to this area, prior to toe transfer. This has the advantage of providing ample soft tissue to the damaged area and avoids taking extensive flap tissue from the foot (7,10). The standard groin flap is a useful source of flap tissue, since the tip of the flap can be thinned at initial application (13) and the base of the flap can be sculpted at the time of toe transfer, providing thin and extensive flap coverage. The donor site is inconspicuous.

ANATOMY AND FLAP DESIGN

Knowledge of the similarities and differences between the anatomy of the big toe and that of the thumb is essential (7) in performing a successful reconstruction. The object of thumb metacarpophalangeal joint reconstruction is first, to create stability and second, to provide motion without hyperextension. If hyperextension is allowed to develop, the interphalangeal joint will droop into a compensatory flexed position that detracts from pulp-to-pulp pinch. If a significant flexion contracture exists (fixed Froment's sign), thumbnail-to-digital pulp pinch can result. If the metatarsophalangeal joint is taken with the toe, an angled osteotomy (Fig. 1) of the toe metatarsal must be completed, to hyperextend the metatarsophalangeal joint as it is placed on the hand in a neutral position. This helps avoid further hyperextension of the metacarpophalangeal joint replacement and thus helps prevent a compensatory flexion deformity of the new thumb interphalangeal joint.

The angled osteotomy can be placed in such a way that the volar extent enters the joint. Here the volar plate is divided just distal to the sesamoids, which allows the proximal volar plate and sesamoids to stay with the big toe metatarsal. After transfer, the volar plate is anchored in such a way as to avoid metacarpophalangeal hyperextension in the thumb position. When the metacarpophalangeal joint is reconstructed as outlined, 30° to 60° of active motion can be seen after transfer. This may be particularly useful in the mutilated hand, since metacarpophalangeal joint motion will help vary the range of the first web space. Preservation of the sesamoids with the proximal volar plate on the foot metatarsal may prevent descent of the metatarsal and create a durable pushoff surface in the foot.

Amputation of the big toe through the metatarsophalangeal joint with reconstruction of a new metacarpophalangeal joint is ideal, if articular cartilage is present in the remaining distal thumb metacarpal in the hand. Although the fit is not identical, the curvature between the thumb metacarpal head and the toe

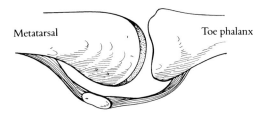

Metatarsal phalangeal joint

Metatarsal　Toe phalanx

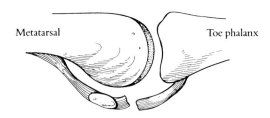

Metatarsal with sesamoid

Metatarsal　Toe phalanx

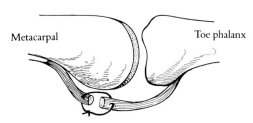

Volar plate capsuloplasty

Metacarpal　Toe phalanx

New metacarpal–phalangeal joint

FIG. 2. Recession of volar plate to avoid hyperextension when a new metacarpophalangeal joint is made, leaving thumb metacarpal articular cartilage intact.

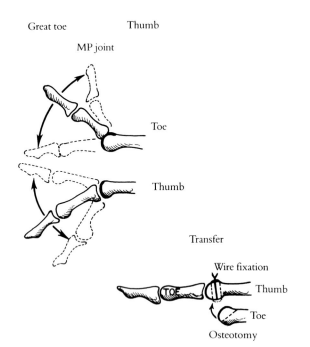

FIG. 1. Angled osteotomy of big toe metatarsal to prevent hyperextension of thumb metacarpophalangeal joint in transferred position. (From Buncke, ref. 3, with permission.)

proximal phalangeal base provides an adequate match, with excellent potential motion. Here again the volar plate is shortened and advanced proximally, to provide stability in extension (Fig. 2).

When the big toe is transferred to the hand with the metatarsophalangeal joint, the reconstructed thumb can provide excellent motion and power, as long as appropriate hand extrinsic and intrinsic tendon counterparts are reconstructed. One can help prevent thumb interphalangeal joint mallet positioning by reconstruction of the intrinsic slips to the extensor pollicis longus (adductor and abductor brevis tendons).

The vascular anatomy of the first web space has been well described (14,15). The inflow of the transfer is most commonly based on the dorsalis pedis artery. The goal, in general, should be to isolate the toe carefully on as large an artery and vein as possible, thus making the repair safer.

As it branches into the first dorsal metatarsal artery, the dorsalis pedis is followed dorsal to the transverse intermetatarsal ligament into the distal communicating artery, into the junction with the plantar supply, and out into the dominant plantar system. No two toes are identical, and care must be taken not to assume any preconceived vascular pattern. We find it helpful to obtain preoperative anteroposterior and lateral arteriograms of the foot and hand (16). This helps in the selection of appropriate recipient vessels in the damaged hand, and helps identify the location of the first dorsal metatarsal artery (78% dorsal, 22% more deeply). Using preoperative arteriography with identification of the largest vessels possible for anastomoses, no tissue has been lost in foot-to-hand transfer procedures.

Because the branching blood supply of the dominant plantar digital artery to the big toe is intact, the entire joint capsule and bony skeleton maintains perfusion after transfer. This perfusion allows prompt capsule healing and early primary bone osteosynthesis. When early primary healing is achieved, early motion after tendon healing can be initiated. If primary osteosynthesis is not achieved, and a bony collapse or avascular dissolution (17) or nonunion is threatened, then prolonged immobilization may be necessary. This awkward situation, seen when nonvascularized bone grafts are transferred to the thumb position, is obviated by primary vascular perfusion of all bony tissues transferred with the toe.

The fact that the big toe is somewhat larger than a normal thumb, even after atrophy, may be an advantage in a mutilated hand, because the larger pulp and increased relative strength may be a welcome assistant to the pinch mechanism against impaired remaining digits. Despite its larger size (Fig. 3D), the big toe, several years after transfer, atrophies to a significant degree, when compared with its initial state (Fig. 3C).

In the mutilated hand the normal extensor and flexor tendons to the thumb may be missing. Here the intrinsic and extrinsic tendons of the thumb need to be motored by tendons previously residing in the remaining or partially remaining digits of the hand. The flexor digitorum superficialis tendons can substitute for the flexor pollicis longus and can be attached at the wrist level, where optimal glide should be achieved. The donor flexor digitorum superficialis tendon should have 2 to 3 cm of excursion for ideal thumb function. This degree of excursion is usually found, if the superficialis tendon resides in a relatively normal digit, or even an abnormal digit, as long as full wrist motion has been maintained.

A,B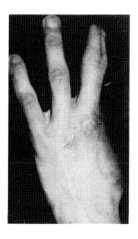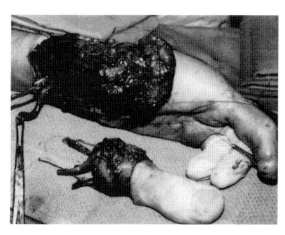

C,D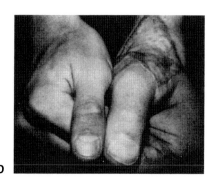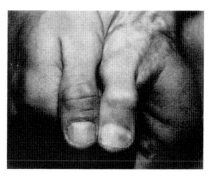

E,F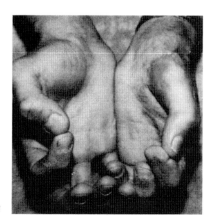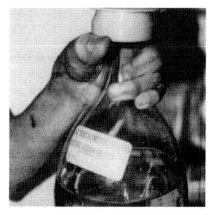

FIG. 3. **A:** A 16-year-old boy 2 years after a bomb blast injury to his left, nondominant hand. An abdominal flap had been placed on the radial side of his hand prior to referral. The thumb was amputated through the distal trapezium and the index ray was amputated at the base of the index metacarpal. **B:** Transferred toe ready for attachment to hand. Note dorsal toe proximal subcutaneous tissues that will be covered by skin graft. The distal metatarsal was fixed to the trapezium using compression wire fixation technique, because the original amputation injury had removed the entire carpometacarpal joint. In addition to standard extensor and flexor tendon repairs, the extensor carpi radialis brevis was repaired via a palmaris longus tendon graft at the primary toe transfer procedure to the proximal phalanx of the toe, thus completing an adductor transfer, as no adductor pollicis remained within the hand. **C:** Comparison of left and right thumbs, 6 months postoperatively. **D:** Comparison of left and right thumbs, 3½ years postoperatively. **E:** Comparison of left and right thumbs in tip pinch, with absence of left metacarpal. He has two-point discrimination of 8 mm, with excellent spatial orientation within the thumb and return of sudomotor activity. Metacarpophalangeal joint active motion is 30° with 55° of active interphalangeal joint motion and adduction key pinch of 7 pounds, adequate for carrying large objects. Preoperative and postoperative gait analysis comparisons at 6 months, 1 year, and 2 years have suggested no significant gait disturbances and the patient has returned to avocational baseball and jogging. **F:** Adequate adductor function to act as assisting hand.

The extensor indicis proprius tendon can substitute nicely for the extensor hallucis longus or extensor hallucis brevis.

If an adductor-opposition plasty is needed, the extensor carpi radialis brevis prolonged by a palmaris longus tendon graft can be used at a second stage. Here we prefer to inset the transfer into bone of the proximal phalanx of the toe and splint for 6 weeks to avoid disruption. If more than one tendon transfer is anticipated, only those that are maximized by a single position of immobilization postoperatively are done (10). Secondary transfers are done at later procedures, which require other positions of immobilization. One can avoid redissection in an area of vessel or nerve repair by leaving behind at the initial procedure a silicone rod that with minimal dissection at a later procedure can be replaced with the desired tendon transfer or graft. If the thumb intrinsic muscles are deficient, intrinsic extension of the thumb interphalangeal joint should be augmented via a split-tendon slip at the time of adductor-opposition plasty.

OPERATIVE TECHNIQUE

Recipient Site

In the hand, incisions must be placed so that palmar and radial flap coverage will remain to cover the plantar digital nerve repairs to the branches of the median nerve, and to cover the flexor hallucis longus tendon in a region where the pulley system of the big toe does not cover this tendon. If flap tissues have not been added prior to toe transfer, we prefer to correct any skin deficiency by thick split-thickness skin grafts added over the dorsal subcutaneous tissue and veins taken with the big toe. In the foot, this triangle of tissue is bordered distally by the cut edge of the dorsal toe skin and medially and laterally by two large draining veins, as they converge proximally to form the greater saphenous vein.

The dissection over the dorsal radial surface of the hand is carried to the region of the anatomic snuff box, where remnants of the extensor pollicis longus and brevis are seen, in addition to the proximal radial artery and a large branch of the cephalic vein. These two vascular structures are used as the recipient vessels for microvascular repair. The extensor and flexor tendons are mobilized, so that the repair to the extensor hallucis longus and the flexor hallucis longus can be done as proximal as possible to the zone of trauma and at a distance from any extensive scarring. In general, on the palmar surface, this means that the flexor tendon repair will be done proximal to the wrist and that the extensor tendon repair will be done distal to Lister's tubercle. The proximal stump of the thumb metacarpal is identified and osteotomized, to freshen the bony segment and to avoid repair of toe metacarpal to scarred soft tissues. If no carpometacarpal joint exists, the trapezium is freshened, to allow osteosynthesis between the toe metatarsal and the trapezium. The hand dissection is frequently started after the foot dissection, because this may take somewhat less time.

Donor Site

The ipsilateral big toe is usually used, because normally the big toe deviates laterally toward the next most radial digit. In addition the dorsal vascular pedicle more easily reaches the recipient vessels if the ipsilateral toe is used. In the foot, under tourniquet control, one must be careful to take only the amount of skin required with toe transfer to cover the new thumb. We prefer to place the toe circumferential skin incision at the plantar proximal toe flexion crease or several millimeters proximal to the

crease (Fig. 3B). This allows an abundance of plantar pushoff callused skin to remain on the foot, and it has prevented any significant donor site problems in the foot.

The incision is then made circumferentially around the big toe and carried in a curvilinear fashion over the dorsum of the foot, located equally between the great saphenous vein and the dorsalis pedis artery. Dissection of the first web area is designed to identify several large branches draining the first web and medial big toe regions. The soft tissues between these two large venous branches are included with the transfer (Fig. 3B), as mentioned previously, to act as a recipient bed for a thick skin graft, if soft-tissue reconstruction is needed in the dorsal first web region. The dorsal venous branches are identified and the extensor hallucis brevis is divided at its muscle tendon junction and turned proximally and distally to expose the dorsalis pedis artery and its dorsal extension, the first dorsal metatarsal artery. Adjacent to the first dorsal metatarsal artery, the deep peroneal nerve is found, half of which will supply the dorsal sensibility of the big toe.

Communication between the hand dissection team and the foot dissection team is imperative, to avoid dividing the toe structures at a point that will be insufficient for reconstruction in the hand. Great care must be taken in tracing the first dorsal metatarsal artery over the distal transverse intermetatarsal ligament. Here the vessel comes close to the ligament and may be damaged in its pathway to join the dominant plantar digital vessels of the big toe. Vessels supplying the second toe must be divided at this point.

The plantar dissection is then undertaken, identifying the lateral plantar digital nerve that runs sufficiently deep to the plantar fascia. This nerve will be found near the mid-axis of the big toe laterally. The flexor hallucis longus tendon will be identified in the midline of the big toe in its plantar location, and the pulley overlying the proximal big toe phalanx should be left intact. The medial digital nerve to the big toe is identified and, through a small longitudinal plantar incision, both of these nerves can be traced well back into the foot.

With this exposure, the nerves can be divided 4 to 7 cm proximal to the metatarsophalangeal joint of the toe; this usually provides ample nerve length to allow a tension-free repair in the hand. If this is not adequate, further exposure for these nerves can be achieved through extension of the plantar incision. The flexor hallucis longus tendon is usually divided by a separate midplantar incision in the foot, as division of this tendon behind the malleolus frequently is accompanied by requirement for an additional incision. All the structures of the big toe are divided, except for the perfusing artery and vein. The tourniquet is released to allow the big toe to have a final drink before reelevation and toe amputation. The toe dissection usually requires a full tourniquet run of 2 to 2½ hours. The big toe is allowed to perfuse for 20 minutes prior to completion of the amputation and transfer of the toe to the hand.

Microvascular Free Tissue Transfer

The big toe metatarsal donor site is narrowed by removing the medial cortical bone projection from the big toe metatarsal, to avoid undue pressure on the foot flap closure. In addition, the sesamoids are left with the big toe metatarsal where possible, and are attached through a small drill hole in the metatarsal, to maintain their position during the healing phase. Intrinsic muscles (abductors and adductors) of the toe should be sutured into position, to maintain soft-tissue bulk in the region of the distal end of the toe metatarsal. When the metatarsal head itself is left with the foot, the narrowing procedure is still carried out, to allow the remaining skin envelope to be closed in a tension-free manner.

In the hand, bony fixation is initially completed, using an internal wire compression twist-down fixation technique (18). If a new metacarpophalangeal joint is being created in the hand, and the toe has been disarticulated, then capsular repair and volar plate plasty are carried out at this point (Fig. 2). Flexor and extensor tendon repairs are completed, and slips of the adductor and abductor brevis are repaired, if present, to the extrinsic extensor mechanism. We usually prefer to repair the dorsalis pedis artery to the dorsal branch of the radial artery end-to-end or end-to-side. The greater saphenous vein is repaired to a branch of the cephalic vein, as the single venous drainage of the big toe. Prior to release of the clamps, all vessels are bathed in a topical 2% xylocaine solution to relieve any vascular spasm. Capillary filling to the big toe should be appreciated, although this may sometimes require several minutes that can seem like hours! Vessel patency tests should always be done to confirm anastomosis patency (19).

Dorsal and palmar nerve repairs are finally completed, using microneural technique, after hemostasis is carefully achieved. All skin and soft tissues are carefully approximated, and the dorsal thick skin graft is placed, if needed, and is treated open as it lies directly over the venous drainage.

A full and noncompressive supporting plaster dressing is made for the foot, ankle, and lower leg, as well as for the hand and forearm. Both the foot and the hand are elevated, and the distal big toe is monitored with surface thermocouple monitoring.

Hand active range of motion exercises are begun 3 weeks postoperatively. Significant passive exercises are not done for 6 weeks, and no dynamic splinting, other than first web space static night splinting, is allowed for 8 to 10 weeks. As the Tinel's sign progresses distally, the patient is begun on a sensory reeducation program and is encouraged to use the thumb actively in small object grasp, despite incomplete reinnervation.

CLINICAL RESULTS

Although none of the 30 toe-to-hand transfer operations done on our service at the Massachusetts General Hospital has failed, a vascular problem has been corrected successfully in two cases to allow full tissue survival. Ultimate sensibility has ranged in our series from two-point discrimination of 5 mm in the young to protective sensibility in the older adult.

Preoperative and postoperative gait analyses in all patients undergoing thumb reconstruction by toe-to-hand transfer have been performed (20). In our studies the patients' follow-up examinations have suggested no significant adverse gait effects. In the foot, the normal weight-bearing balance shifts from the medial big toe metatarsal region preoperatively laterally to the

second ray postoperatively, but has had no adverse effect on gait (20–22).

SUMMARY

In the carefully selected patient, big toe-to-hand transfer for major thumb reconstruction in the mutilated hand can play an important role in upgrading overall hand function.

References

1. Cobbett JR. Free digital transfer. *J Bone Joint Surg [Br]* 1969;518:677.
2. Buncke HJ, McLean DM, George PT, et al. Thumb replacement: great toe transposition by microvascular anastomosis. *Br J Plast Surg* 1973;26:194.
3. Buncke HJ. Toe digital transfer. *Clin Plast Surg* 1976;3:49.
4. O'Brien BM, MacLeod AM, Sykes PJ, Donahoe S. Hallux-to-hand transfer. *Hand* 1975;7:128.
5. Tamai S, Hori Y, Tatsumi Y, Okuda H. Hallux-to-thumb transfer with microsurgical technique: a case report in a 45-year-old woman. *J Hand Surg* 1977;2:152.
6. O'Brien BM, Brennen MD, MacLeod AM. Microvascular free tissue transfer. *Clin Plast Surg* 1978;5:223.
7. May JW, Jr, Daniel RK. Great toe-to-hand free tissue transfer. *Clin Orthop* 1978;133:140.
8. Gilbert A, Tubiana R. Reconstruction of the mutilated hand using microsurgery. In: Reid DAL, Gosset J, eds. *Mutilating injuries of the hand.* Edinburgh: Churchill Livingstone, 1979.
9. Kutz JE, Thompson CB, Klein HW. Toe-to-hand transfer. In: Urbaniak J, ed. *AAOS symposium on microsurgery.* St. Louis: Mosby, 1979.
10. May JW Jr. Aesthetic and functional thumb reconstruction: great toe-to-hand transfer. *Clin Plast Surg* 1981;8:357.
11. Littler JW. Neurovascular pedicle method of digital transposition for reconstruction of the thumb. *Plast Reconstr Surg* 1953;12:203.
12. Campbell R. Reconstruction of the thumb. *J Bone Joint Surg [Br]* 1960; 42:444.
13. May JW Jr, Bartlett S. Staged groin flap in reconstruction of the pediatric hand. *J Hand Surg* 1981;6:163.
14. Gilbert A. Composite tissue transfers from the foot: anatomic basis and surgical technique. In: Strauch B, Daniller AI, eds. *Symposium on microsurgery.* St. Louis: Mosby, 1976.
15. May JW, Chait LA, Cohen BE, O'Brien BM. Free neurovascular flap from the first web of the foot in hand reconstruction. *J Hand Surg* 1977;2:387.
16. May JW Jr, Smith RJ, Peimer C. Toe-to-hand free tissue transfer for thumb construction with multiple digit aplasia. *Plast Reconstr Surg* 1981;67:205.
17. Leung PC, Ma FY. Distal reconstruction using the toe flap: Report of 10 cases. *J Hand Surg* 1982;7:366.
18. Daniel RK, Terzis JK, eds. Replantation of upper extremity amputations. In: Daniel RK Terzis JK, eds., *Reconstructive microsurgery.* Boston: Little, Brown, 1977. Fig. 5-14A-D, p. 147, Fig. 5-10C (x-ray), p. 141.
19. Acland RD. Signs of patency in small vessel anastomosis. *Surgery* 1972;72:744.
20. Clarkson P. Reconstruction of hand digits by toe transfers. *J Bone Joint Surg* 1955;37(A):270.
21. Clarkson P. Toe-to-hand transfers. In: Flynn JE, ed. *Hand surgery.* Baltimore: Williams & Wilkins, 1966.
22. O'Brien BM, Black MJM, Morrison WA, MacLeod AM. Microvascular great toe transfer for congenital absence of the thumb. *Hand* 1978;10:113.

CHAPTER 279 ■ MICRONEUROVASCULAR FREE TRANSFER OF THE SECOND TOE

B. STRAUCH AND E. J. HALL-FINDLAY

The second toe has potential in the reconstruction of both thumb and finger losses. Advantages over the big toe can exist in both minimized donor site morbidity and better recipient site appearance (1–4).

INDICATIONS

The second toe is smaller than the big toe for thumb replacement, but size varies so much from individual to individual that the second toe may have a more pleasing cosmetic effect. In societies where sandals are standard footwear, surgeons

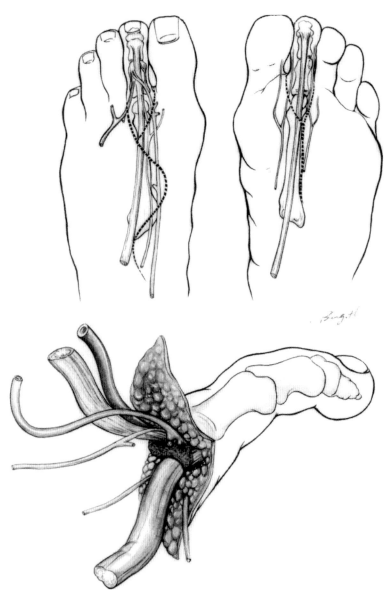

FIG. 1. Preparation of the donor site. A curvilinear incision is made over the dorsum of the foot to harvest adequate vessel, nerve, and tendon lengths.

have been reluctant to sacrifice the big toe and have often preferred the second toe for thumb reconstruction. The extra joint of the second toe and the flexion attitude of the interphalangeal joints usually are not a problem in the thumb.

The second toe has been used less frequently for finger loss, except when all four fingers have been amputated. For salvage of a "metacarpal" hand, the second toe has provided excellent function. It tends to be short and the interphalangeal joints are continually flexed, both of which characteristics would be inappropriate if normally functioning fingers remained on the hand.

The second toe filleted has been used to replace pulp loss of the finger. In contrast to standard insensitive flaps and neurovascular island flaps from other fingers, the toe transfer provides skin of texture and structure similar to those of the finger, with the correct cortical representation.

ANATOMY

The second toe has three phalanges. Both interphalangeal joints are maintained in varying degrees of flexion, while the metatarsophalangeal joint is almost always held in a considerable degree of extension.

The arterial supply to the foot is by way of an interconnected two-arch system. The plantar arch is formed from the posterior tibial artery, and the dorsal arch is formed from the dorsalis pedis artery. The second toe is supplied by two dorsal digital arteries, one from the first dorsal metatarsal artery and one from the second dorsal metatarsal artery. However, it is mainly supplied by two larger plantar arteries that receive contributions both from the plantar arch and from the metatarsal arteries.

The second toe can easily survive if one uses the first dorsal metatarsal artery as the donor artery. The first dorsal metatarsal artery is a branch of the dorsalis pedis artery, usually arising at a superficial level but occasionally branching from a deeper location of the dorsalis pedis artery as it descends between the first and second metatarsals. The first dorsal metatarsal artery can be found either superficial to or at varying levels within the first dorsal interosseous muscle.

Venous drainage occurs by the venae comitantes of the arterial system, but mainly by way of the superficial veins that drain into the dorsal venous arch and then into the saphenous system.

The second toe is innervated by two plantar digital nerves (branches of the medial plantar nerve) and by the lateral portion of the deep peroneal nerve that supplies both sides of the first web space of the foot. The plantar digital nerves can be found with their accompanying digital arteries, and the deep peroneal nerve can be found lying adjacent to the first dorsal metatarsal artery.

Extra skin and subcutaneous tissue can be taken from both plantar and dorsal aspects of the foot, including all the skin of the first web space, depending on recipient site requirements.

The second toe has both long and short extensors and flexors, as well as intrinsic tendon contributions. The tendons used for the transfer of the toe to the hand are usually the long extensor and the long flexor.

FLAP DESIGN AND DIMENSIONS

The arterial anatomy of the foot should be outlined preoperatively by palpation, by Doppler, and by lateral arteriograms. Recipient site requirements are determined and mapped out at the donor site, always weighing the potential benefits to the recipient site against the possible morbidity at the donor site. This refers mainly to extra dorsal foot skin beyond what would allow primary donor site closure. Skin grafts over the

dorsum of the foot have a bad reputation. However, skin grafts on the hand may be perfectly acceptable, except in areas requiring padding or sensation or where required for coverage of the vascular pedicle.

OPERATIVE TECHNIQUE

Donor Site

A curvilinear incision is made over the dorsalis pedis artery. A straight-line incision is avoided, to minimize skin contracture at both donor and recipient sites and to allow wider exposure (Fig. 1).

The veins are quite superficial and care must be taken to preserve them. Once the dissection has progressed, the best donor vein can be chosen and the remainder can be ligated.

The dissection is kept medial to the dorsalis pedis artery, to avoid injuring branches to the second toe. The first dorsal

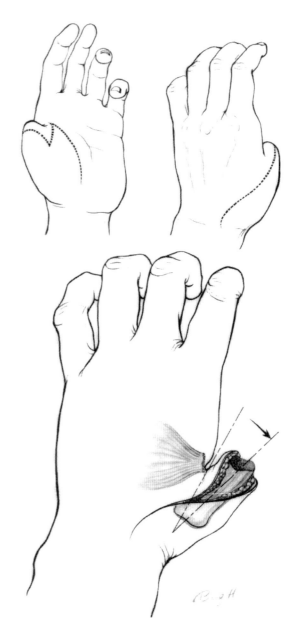

FIG. 2. Preparation of the recipient site for a second toe to thumb transfer. Note that the web space contracture has been released.

metatarsal artery and the deep peroneal nerve are identified either superficial to or within the substance of the first dorsal interosseous muscle. The intermetatarsal ligament is carefully divided to allow better exposure. Both dorsal and plantar arteries on the medial side of the toe are identified, and the connection of the latter to the first plantar metatarsal artery is divided and ligated. The arcuate artery supplying the remaining dorsal metatarsal arteries can be ligated as it passes laterally from the dorsalis pedis artery, as can the descending branch of the dorsalis pedis artery as it passes to join the plantar arch.

The deep peroneal nerve and the plantar digital nerve may need to be separated proximally under magnification, from those branches to the big toe. Both plantar digital nerves are best identified through the racquet-shaped incisions on the plantar aspect of the toe. The plantar digital artery to the lateral aspect of the toe can be identified and traced back (with the nerve) as far proximally as necessary. This can be used for a separate arterial anastomosis, if required. Again, the digital nerve may need to be split proximally, to allow adequate length, always taking more than was indicated by recipient site measurements.

Both the long flexor and the long extensor are divided proximally in the foot or at the ankle. The toe may be either disarticulated at the metatarsophalangeal joint or divided more proximally in the metatarsal. Some of the metatarsal must nevertheless be removed to allow primary donor site closure. Some attempt should also be made to repair the intermetatarsal ligament between the third and big toes, to prevent splaying of the foot.

Recipient Site

The recipient site will determine the structures available for anastomoses (Fig. 2). These will depend on whether the sec-

ond toe is being used for thumb or finger replacement. At least one flexor and one extensor, and one or two arteries and veins, will be needed. Bony fixation can be accomplished with peg fixation, Kirschner wires, or 90°/90° interosseous wiring. Care must be taken to evaluate the position of the toe joint, to place it in appropriate angulation at the recipient site.

Both plantar digital nerves should be anastomosed to the corresponding digital nerves (or more proximal counterparts). The branch of the deep peroneal nerve should be anastomosed to the appropriate radial or ulnar dorsal sensory branches of the hand (Fig. 3).

CLINICAL RESULTS

The donor site can be closed primarily after removing some of the metatarsal. This leaves an almost normal-looking foot that often deceives the casual observer. Some patients have complained of temporary discomfort, perhaps from the partial loss of the plantar arch. If skin grafts are used, especially if extensions of skin into the web space or onto the dorsum of the foot have been made, some patients have had trouble with hyperkeratotic irregularities.

The functional and cosmetic results depend on careful preoperative and intraoperative planning but also on the anatomy of the transferred toe. Some toes are unacceptable for transfer because of the extreme amount of interphalangeal joint flexion. Again, more flexion is probably acceptable for thumb replacement rather than for finger replacement.

Return of function is the ultimate goal, and this depends on the development of adequate sensation. Reported two-point discrimination has varied from 7 to 15 mm. Actual functional correlation often depends more on patient attitude than on two-point testing.

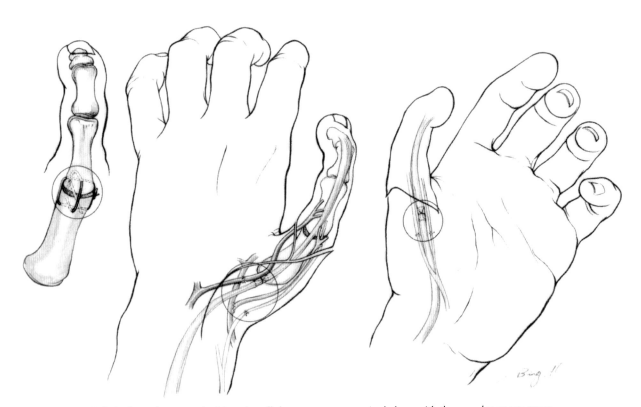

FIG. 3. Second toe transfer. Note that all three nerves are repaired along with the vascular anastomoses. Note that the toe has three phalanges where a thumb usually has two phalanges.

SUMMARY

The second toe can be used to reconstruct thumb or finger loss. It can also be filleted and used for volar soft-tissue loss of a finger. It has the advantage over all other techniques of being a neurovascular transfer with appropriate cortical representation.

References

1. Buncke HJ, Schulz WP. Immediate Nicoladoni procedure in the rhesus monkey, a hallux-to-hand transplantation, utilizing microminiature vascular anastomoses. *Br J Plast Surg* 1966;19:332.
2. O'Brien B McC, MacLeod AM, Sykes PJ, Donahoe S. Hallux-to-hand transfer. *Hand* 1975;7:128.
3. Ohmori K, Harii K. Transplantation of a toe to an amputated finger. *Hand* 1975;7:134.
4. Strauch B. Microsurgical approach to thumb reconstruction. *Orthop Clin North Am* 1977;8:319.

CHAPTER 280 ■ WRAPAROUND TOE FLAP

W. A. MORRISON

The hallux has all the characteristics of a thumb, including nail, pulp, and glabrous skin; but it is usually too large and after such a total transfer the secondary defect in the foot is cosmetically unacceptable. The uniquely thumb-like properties of the big toe can be transferred and wrapped around either a degloved thumb or a bone graft while the hallux is reconstructed (1,2).

INDICATIONS

The wraparound toe sleeve is optimally indicated to resurface traumatically or surgically degloved thumbs, where skeleton and tendon anatomy remain intact. Combined with a bone graft, it is the method of choice for thumb reconstructions distal to the metacarpophalangeal joint, as it achieves the best compromise between function, aesthetics, and secondary morbidity. In these cases, restoration of articular function is not essential.

ANATOMY

Approximately three-quarters of the integument of the hallux, including the nail, is transferred by vascular anastomosis of the dorsalis pedis system of the toe, to the radial artery system at the wrist. This macro type of microvascular anastomosis ensures survival on the order of 100%.

FLAP DESIGN AND DIMENSIONS

The ipsilateral toe is chosen, because the scar seam will lie on the nondominant radial aspect of the reconstructed thumb, and the dominant lateral plantar digital nerve will become the dominant ulnar digital nerve in the thumb.

The circumference and length of the opposite normal thumb are measured, and a template is made for marking the donor toe. A medial skin bridge extending around the tip is preserved, the width being the difference between the circumference of the thumb and the circumference of the toe (Fig. 1A,B). Dorsal veins and the dorsalis pedis artery are identified proximally on the dorsum of the foot and traced into the toe flap.

OPERATIVE TECHNIQUE

Donor Site

The dorsal metatarsal artery becomes continuous with the plantar system as it passes plantarward around the intermetatarsal ligament. The plantar system is ligated, as is the branch to the second toe. The toe flap is then elevated (Fig. 1C), including the terminal one-third of the distal phalanx of the hallux, which is preserved with the flap still attached to the nongerminal nailbed (Fig. 1D). The nailbed proximal to this level is raised subperiosteally, using a flat elevator to avoid damage to its undersurface. This provides a vascularized bone segment and nailbed support to the reconstructed thumb. Paratenon is preserved over the extensor and flexor tendons, and the digital nerves are located in the pulp and sectioned as far proximally as is required for repair with proximal thumb nerves.

The flap is now totally freed, except for its arterial and venous attachments dorsally. If the nail is wider than the corresponding thumbnail, then the flap can be turned upside down and the proximal lateral limits of the nailbed easily defined. The proximal corners of the nailbed are excised obliquely, so that the outgrowing nail will be appropriately narrowed.

A bone graft from the iliac crest or the subcutaneous border of the tibia is removed and shaped for the skeleton. No matter what the sculptured shape, all bone grafts under stress will mold themselves straight, so that excessive

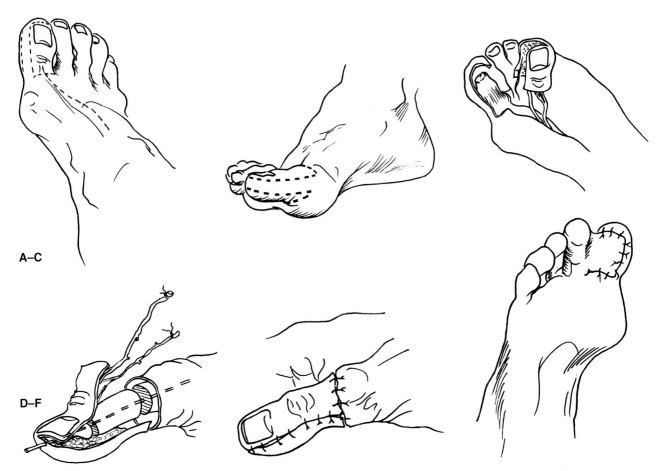

FIG. 1. **A:** Toe markings, dorsal view, showing retained medial and tip flap and dorsal foot incision. **B:** Toe markings, medial view. **C:** Toe flap dissection, with dorsal vasculature. **D:** Toe flap wrapped around the interposition bone graft and transfixed with a longitudinal Kirschner wire. **E:** Toe flap sutured into position. **F:** Toe defect reconstructed on plantar surface with a cross-toe flap.

contouring is naive. The graft should be made as large as can be accommodated within the toe flap, to allow for some possible resorption.

Simultaneous with the thumb revascularization, the toe defect is closed. A further one-third of the distal phalanx is removed, leaving only the proximal one-third intact. The tip flap is folded around the tip and any portion of doubtful viability is excised. A large cross-toe flap from the dorsum of the second toe is raised based medially, and is used to close the plantar defect of the hallux (Fig. 1F). The dorsum of the big and second toes is covered with a split-thickness skin graft. The cross-toe flap is divided at 2 months; at that time some cosmetic revision of the thumb pulp may be undertaken, because there is considerable variance in the aesthetics of the hallux pulp from one person to another.

Recipient Site

The dorsal radial artery and cephalic vein are located just proximal to the wrist crease, and the nerves to the thumb are isolated and trimmed. The bone graft is measured for inter-

position between the thumb stump proximally and the hallux segment distally, where it will be fixed with Kirschner wires.

The toe flap is then detached from the foot and transferred to the thumb, where it is wrapped around the bone graft and sutured loosely into position. A longitudinal Kirschner wire transfixes the bony segments (Fig. 1D). The vascular pedicle is tunneled through a widely undermined dorsal skin bridge to the snuffbox and the anastomoses performed, the flap artery end-to-side of the radial artery, and the flap vein end-to-end to the cephalic vein (Fig. 2C). The digital nerves are finally repaired and the skin closed (Fig. 1E).

Great care is required to monitor the tension at the suture line, particularly distally at the nail area, where in many cases some sutures will require release to restore circulation.

SUMMARY

The wraparound toe flap is an excellent method to reconstruct thumb degloving injuries and is indicated for total thumb reconstruction when sacrifice of the toe is not desired.

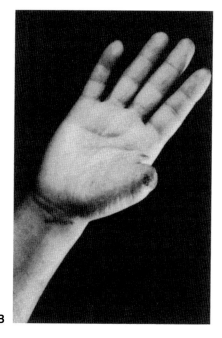
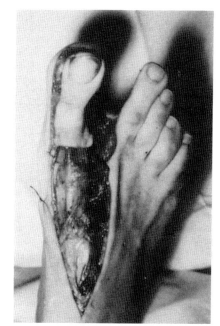

A,B

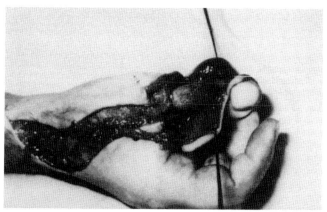
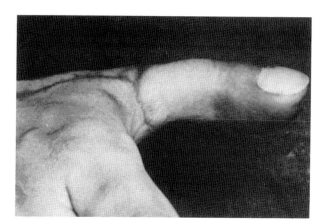

C,D

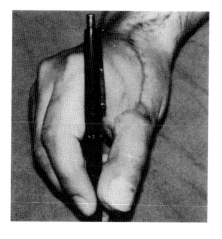
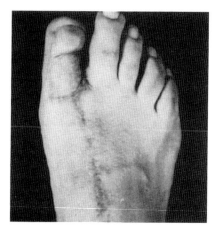

E,F

FIG. 2. A: Complete traumatic amputation of the thumb just distal to the metacarpophalangeal joint in a 33-year-old man. **B:** Toe flap raised, including the distal one-third of the distal phalanx. **C:** Toe flap wrapped around the bone graft and the vascular pedicle transferred to the snuff box. **D,E:** Twelve months following reconstruction by the "wraparound" method of thumb reconstruction. **F:** Toe defect reconstructed with a cross-toe flap to the dorsal surface. (This differs from current policy where the toe flap is now routinely taken from the dorsum of the second toe and applied to the plantar surface of the hallux. The dorsal defect is grafted.)

References

1. Morrison WA, O'Brien BM, MacLeod AM. Surgical repair of amputations of the thumb. *Aust N Z J Surg* 1980;50:237.

2. Morrison WA, O'Brien BM, MacLeod AM. Thumb reconstruction with a free neurovascular wraparound flap from the big toe. *J Hand Surg* 1980;5:575.

CHAPTER 281 ■ MICRONEUROVASCULAR PARTIAL TOE TRANSFER

G. FOUCHER AND F. VAN GENECHTEN

Since the first successful experimental toe-to-hand transfer in 1965 (1), numerous techniques have been described, including partial toe transfer either as a single-tissue transfer (pulp) or as a combination-of-composite-tissue transfer (pulp, nail, bone, joint, epiphysis, tendons).

INDICATIONS

Transfers can be separated into six groups, according to the parts transferred. Different methods of partial transfer can be used, whether from the first toe, the second toe, or both toes: free toe pulp; composite transfer with pulp; nailbed; pulp and nail-complex combination of pulp, nail, and bone fragment; nail complex on its own; double composite toe transfer; and free joint transfer.

Free Pulp Transfer

This technique can replace a traumatic or surgical loss of tissue (tumor), an insensitive pulp (abdominal flap), or an atrophic or painful pulp. It can also provide sensation at the radial aspect of a mitten hand that has been covered with an insensitive abdominal flap.

Indications for transfer appear when it seems impossible or inadequate to use local heterodigital or distant flaps (2–14). This situation can occur in cases with extensive tissue loss or when it is not possible to obtain good quality skin cover for the thumb or index finger, especially as regards skin texture or skin sensation. Another good indication is the hand with multiple injured digits. The free toe pulp transfer avoids the cold intolerance at the donor site frequently noted after a heterodigital island flap. But the island flap still remains useful in the reconstruction of a moderate loss of skin on a thumb.

Tailor-Made Composite Pulp Transfer

Sometimes it is desirable to transfer toe pulp together with other necessary structures at the same time, e.g., with nailbed, with nailbed and chip of bone, or with nailbed, nail matrix, and bone. It is thus possible to avoid a nail horn deformity in certain complicated amputations by lengthening the nailbed support with a fragment of bone.

Filleted Toe Transfer (3)

There are only a few indications for this technique. One category is the transfer of a filleted toe cap, transferring the nailbed and the pulp. This technique is comparable to the wraparound procedure (see Chap. 280). The filleted transfer is used to cover a digit that is not to be amputated, either for aesthetic or functional reasons. (This second technique was used in only one case of skin avulsion of second and third fingers.)

Transfer of the Nail Complex

We have done such a procedure once on a dominant thumb of a child. It has been well proven that the nail plays an important role in grip precision and in the quality of sensation.

Double Composite Transfer

In cases of amputation of the thumb at the interphalangeal joint or at the proximal phalanx, transfer of the big or second toe is rather unaesthetic. The big toe is too voluminous and the second toe too thin. Sometimes it is possible to use only partial composite tissue transfer of the big toe, but this technique is often insufficient, particularly in male patients. Therefore, a more elaborate vascularized double transfer is possible: a tailor-made skin pulp with nail is dissected from the big toe in continuity with the adjoining pulp of the second toe and part of its bony structure and neighboring joint (see Fig. 5).

Free Joint Transfer (4)

The majority of experimental studies have shown that in the absence of vascularization, the transferred joints show progressive changes in the cartilage and growth plate. However, a few successful clinical results have been reported (5,6) where the epiphysis remained active after nonvascularized transfer. Experimentally, only vascularized joints have shown both little histologic alteration and that the epiphysis remains open (7,8) (see Fig. 6).

Indications for a microsurgical joint transfer must be weighed against the use of a nonvascularized transfer, Swanson spacers, or even arthrodesis. Whichever technique is used, the results are usually not above merely average. The microsurgical transfer, in our opinion, finds its strongest indication in multiple proximal interphalangeal joint trauma of index and middle fingers with loss of skin, joint, bone, or tendon elements, in young patients. It has the great advantage of providing composite tissues with growth potential and will result in a useful range of motion.

ANATOMY

Anatomic studies (9,10) have clearly shown the double arterial vascularization of the toes. The vascular supply comes

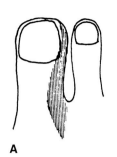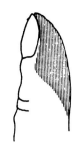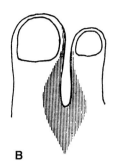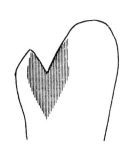

A   B

FIG. 1. A: Pulp transfer (seven cases). B: Web transfer (one case).

from the dorsal arch (dorsal metatarsal artery) and from the plantar arch, anastomosing with each other at the distal level of the first intermetatarsal space. This distal communicating artery is important, as it will make it possible to dissect the dorsal artery in continuity with the collateral plantar arteries when necessary.

DESIGN AND DIMENSIONS

Free Pulp Transfer

This procedure allows the transfer of pulp from the first or second toes, with its neurovascular bundle, to an important finger such as the thumb or index. The ipsilateral foot is used for thumb and the contralateral for index reconstruction.

We prefer to use a transfer from the big toe (Fig. 1A). Although in our experience sequelae at the level of the second toe are rare, the discrepancy in the size of the plantar nerves forces a Y-shaped anastomosis to only one recipient digital nerve. Sensory discrimination at the donor site is also of some importance. It has been established that the second toe has a two-point discrimination of less than 10 to 25 mm, compared with 7 to 18 mm for the first toe pulp (11). Furthermore, there is an important advantage to the large surface area available at the big toe. Since the description of an advancement island

flap (12), we have seen no further indications for second toe pulp transfer.

In cases of complex amputation, it is sometimes useful to cover the thumb and the radial lateral side of the hand by a first web transfer (9,13,14). After such transfers, a sensory reeducation program is necessary. The best two-point discrimination we obtained was in the range of 3 to 4.5 mm after a 6-month reeducation program (Fig. 1B).

Tailor-Made Composite Pulp Transfer

A bone chip attached to the pulp is dissected from the big toe and the distal nail flap is turned over 90° in contact with the bone fragment. In cases of trauma of the nail matrix, it is desirable to replace the matrix as well. In these cases, either the distal part of the second toe or part of the nail matrix of the big toe can be used (Fig. 2).

Free Filleted Toe Transfer

When the avulsed finger skeleton is still intact, with well-vascularized flexor tendon structures, it is feasible to cover more than two-thirds of the whole finger. The remaining one-third is usually covered with skin grafts. The result is cosmetically

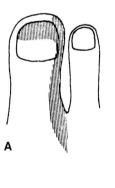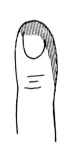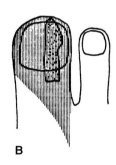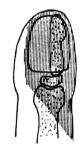

A   B

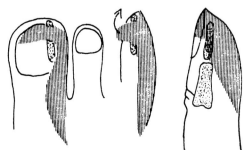

C

FIG. 2. A: Pulp + nailbed (one case). B: Pulp + nail + bone (four cases). C: Pulp + nailbed + bone (six cases).

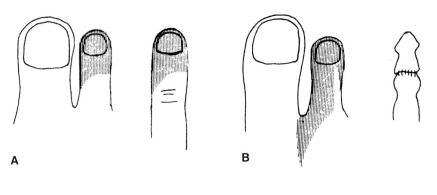

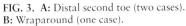

FIG. 3. A: Distal second toe (two cases). **B:** Wraparound (one case).

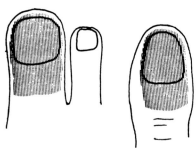

FIG. 4. Nail complex (one case).

acceptable because of the presence of the nail, and functionally acceptable because of distal sensibility and the well-maintained vascularization of the flexor tendon (Fig. 3).

Transfer of the Nail Complex

It is possible to transfer only the nail (with the nail root and the nailbed) from the big toe, as a free transfer with its arterial and venous elements (Fig. 4).

Double Composite Transfer

In one case we used the vascularized total skeleton of the second toe, wrapped in a skin envelope coming only from the big toe. When necessary, even the flexor and extensor tendons can be left attached to the skeleton of the second toe. After turning the two elements 180°, the skeleton of the second toe can be wrapped in the composite skin nail flap of the big toe. The recipient thumb will be functional, with an acceptable aes-

thetic result. The immediate vascularization of the bone graft will avoid the risk of absorption of the iliac bone graft used in the wraparound procedure (3). In the foot the denuded bone of the big toe is then covered with the filleted remaining skin and nail of the second toe, after the secondary ray is removed more proximally (Fig. 5).

Vascularized Joint Transfer

Between 1975 and 1982, six cases of free vascularized joint transfers were done. It is difficult to compare these transfers with more conventional techniques, as indications differ. The advantage of a vascularized transfer lies in the very fact that it is possible to use it as a composite transfer, allowing restoration in a single stage of skin, bone, joint, and tendon loss. If growth is desirable, a vascularized transfer is strongly indicated (Fig. 6).

The transfer of the proximal interphalangeal joint of the second toe, rather than of the metatarsophalangeal joint, is chosen because of its better range of motion. The metatarsophalangeal joint represents limited flexion and hyperextension of 35° to 45°, necessitating a reverse inset and thereby losing the advantage of a composite transfer to provide skin cover and tendon reconstruction. The size of this metatarsophalangeal joint is disproportionate to the proximal interphalangeal joints of the fingers. The proximal interphalangeal joint of the second toe, although smaller in size, can easily be accommodated as a transfer with the skin and tendon space at the level of the proximal interphalangeal joint of the fingers. Flexion will reach 90° after regular night splinting, although the extension deficit will range from 20° to 30°.

The bone requires sufficiently stable fixation to allow early mobilization. An endomedullary osteosynthesis, "corkscrew" type with a simple screw or screw plus cement, is our preferred technique. There is often an important deficit in extension that

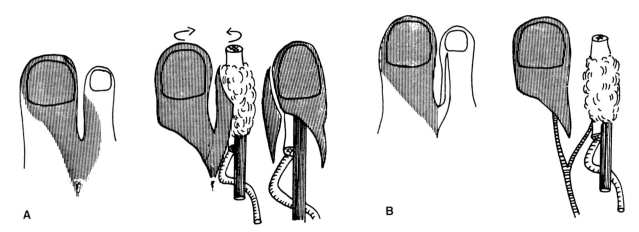

FIG. 5. Double composite (twisted two toes) (four cases). **A:** Type I. **B:** Type II.

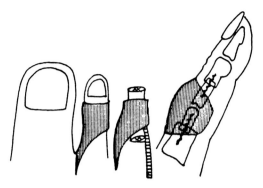

FIG. 6. Joint transfer (six cases).

is difficult to explain, but possible explanations include preexisting flexion of the toe, difficult tension adjustment of the extensor tendon, too long interposed bony segments, the effect of bowstringing of the flexor tendon over the transferred joint, or shifting of the lateral extensor slips of the recipient finger.

OPERATIVE TECHNIQUE

Donor Site

Complete dissection of the vascular supply to the toe could be achieved from the dorsal aspect of the foot in the majority of cases. When the skeleton of the second ray is used, a high division of the second metatarsal bone will not only permit access to the plantar vascular system and the flexor tendons, but will also improve closure of the donor site in the foot after the suturing of the intermetatarsal ligament. The absence of a scar on the sole of the foot will allow earlier walking by the fifth day postoperatively. This approach also permits exploration of the plantar metatarsal artery in the second intermetatarsal space in those cases where the dorsal or plantar network of the first intermetatarsal space appears to be inadequate.

A study of foot pressure prints has shown that resection of the second ray in the foot does not alter the weight-bearing pattern in any important way. Only in some cases did we notice a tendency to hallux valgus.

The veins are selected out of the dorsal venous network, usually at the side of the greater saphenous vein. The nerves are chosen according to the type of transfer and the size of the recipient nerve ends. The size of the plantar nerves of the big toe corresponds, in most cases, to that of the recipient volar digital nerves. However, there is a discrepancy in size between the nerves of the second toe and the nerves at the recipient site.

Recipient Site

The material used for bone fixation can be introduced at the level of the donor site, before dividing the vascular pedicle. Kirschner wires are usually sufficient in partial transfer. In certain cases, however, we recommend an intramedullary type of osteosynthesis, such as with intramedullary screws, a "block nail," or a "bilboquet." This type of osteosynthesis, sometimes cemented, will allow burying all the material in the medullary canal with stable fixation of the bone, and it facilitates the manipulation of tissues later in the procedure. Sometimes it is possible to telescope the toe phalanx into the phalanx of the recipient digit and fix it with an axial Kirschner wire. We use this latter technique in many cases involving children.

Meticulous nerve anastomoses are important, because the functional result will often depend on the quality of sensation

regained. The anastomosis must be placed as distal as possible on the recipient nerve. In cases of partial second toe transfer, there will often be a marked discrepancy between size in the donor and the recipient nerves. In these cases we join both donor nerve ends as a Y to one recipient nerve. In selected cases it is advisable to suture some branches of the musculocutaneous nerve of the foot to the radial nerve of the hand.

The extensor tendons are sutured with overlap of both ends; the flexor tendons are sutured in the classic way, staggering the position of the suture lines of the flexor profundus and flexor superficialis tendons. Discrepancy in size between the flexor tendons of the second toe and the hand flexors is managed by wrapping the larger tendon around the smaller one. Only the flexor profundus has to be repaired in the thumb, but resecting the superficial flexor tendon slips of the foot too distally must be avoided.

We then deal with the arterial anastomosis. In cases of thumb reconstruction we use the radial artery as the recipient vessel, with an end-to-side or end-to-end anastomosis. In the end-to-end anastomosis we shift the radial artery from underneath the extensor pollicis longus. In a few cases we used the pollicis princeps artery as recipient with an end-to-end anastomosis. In other cases it was feasible to dissect the proximal end of a donor artery in a T shape at the level of the dorsal or plantar arch in the first intermetatarsal space. This T shape can be interposed as an arterial graft with end-to-end anastomosis, thereby preserving the continuity of the radial artery at the donor site. But this depends on the length of the vascular pedicle and is not always possible.

In reconstruction of a long finger, we also use an end-to-end anastomosis between the division of the common digital artery and a dorsal or plantar intermetatarsal artery of the same diameter. This has the advantage of not excessively disturbing the digital vascular supply through the contralateral digital artery and the transverse retrotendinous vessels.

Finally, after tunneling the vein under a dorsal skin bridge, the anastomosis is performed through a small transverse incision on the dorsum of the hand, to keep external scarring to a minimum. The donor vein is preferably drained through a side branch, to avoid venous congestion.

CLINICAL RESULTS

In our unit at Strasbourg, of 65 toe transfers with a 7.7% rate of failure, 33 were partial transfers. The average age of the patients was 31 years; the youngest was 11 years old and the oldest 46.

SUMMARY

Toe transfer adds a variety of new techniques and alternatives to reconstructive surgery of the hand. It allows a tailor-made finger reconstruction in an elegant one-stage repair for certain otherwise difficult or impossible mutilations.

References

1. Buncke HJ, Schulz WP. Immediate Nicoladoni procedure in the rhesus monkey, a hallux-to-hand transplantation, utilizing microminiature vascular anastomoses. Br J Plast Surg 1966;19:332.
2. Buncke HJ. Toe digital transfer. Clin Plast Surg 1976;3:49.
3. Morrison WA, O'Brien BM, MacLeod AM. Thumb reconstruction with a free neurovascular wrap-around flap from the big toe. J Hand Surg 1980;5:575.
4. Buncke HJ, Daniller Al, Schulz WP, Chase RA. The fate of autogenous whole joints transplanted by microvascular anastomoses. Plast Reconstr Surg 1967;39:333.

5. Foucher G, Hoang P, Citron N, et al. Joint reconstruction following trauma: comparison of microsurgical transfer and conventional methods: a report of 61 cases. *J Hand Surg [Br]* 1986;11-B:388.
6. Tsai TM, Jupiter J, Kutz JE, Kleinert HE. Vascularized autogenous whole joint transfer: a clinical study. *J Hand Surg* 1982;7:335.
7. Hurwitz PH. Experimental transplantation of small joints by microvascular anastomoses. *Plast Reconstr Surg* 1979;64:221.
8. Tsai TM, Ogden L, Jaeger SH, Okubo K. Experimental vascularized total joint autografts: a primate study. *J Hand Surg* 1982;7:140.
9. Gilbert A. Composite tissue transfers from the foot: anatomic basis and surgical technique. In: Daniller AT, Strauch B, eds. *Symposium on microsurgery.* St. Louis: Mosby, 1976.
10. May JW, Chait LA, Cohen BE, O'Brien BM. Free neurovascular flap from the first web of the foot in hand reconstruction. *J Hand Surg* 1977;2:387.
11. May JW, Daniel RK. Great toe-to-hand free tissue transfer. *Clin Orthop* 1978;133:140.
12. Venkataswami R, Subramanian N. Oblique triangular flap: a new method of repair for oblique amputations of the fingertip and thumb. *Plast Reconstr Surg* 1980;66:296.
13. May JW, Chait LA, Cohen BE, O'Brien BM. Free neurovascular flap from the first web of the foot in hand reconstruction. *J Hand Surg* 1977;2:387.
14. Strauch B, Tsur H. Restoration of sensation to the hand by a free neurovascular island flap from the first web space of the foot. *Plast Reconstr Surg* 1978;62:361.

CHAPTER 282 ■ TRIMMED BIG-TOE TRANSFER FOR THUMB RECONSTRUCTION

N. CARVER AND F.-C. WEI

EDITORIAL COMMENT

This is an excellent technique for reconstruction of the thumb, which relies on some of the older methods but advances them to a new height. By reducing the bone stock, a thumb of normal caliber closely equal to that on the opposite hand can be reconstructed.

The trimmed big-toe transfer for thumb reconstruction (1) is a combination of the wraparound (2) and total big-toe transfer methods (3,4). This technique involves reduction of both bony and soft-tissue elements along the medial aspect of the transferred big toe, to produce a more normal-sized thumb.

INDICATIONS

Total big-toe transfer would be appropriate when toe size is comparable to that of the normal thumb, and in cases where there is associated severe injury to the remainder of the hand and optimal hand function is the main concern. Second-toe transfer would be more appropriate for patients unable to tolerate the loss of the big toe; when the second toe is comparable in size to the normal thumb; and when less than optimal function and appearance of the reconstructed thumb are required. The big-toe wraparound flap is more appropriate for thumb amputation distal to the interphalangeal joint, or for thumb-skin avulsion distal to the metacarpophalangeal joint, with intact interphalangeal joint function.

The trimmed big-toe transfer is for thumb reconstruction at or distal to the metacarpophalangeal joint. This technique is indicated when the big toe is much larger than the normal thumb, and when the motion of the interphalangeal joint and

the appearance of the thumb are equally important (5). Patients should expect and accept the cosmetic deformity and possible functional impairment in the absence of the big toe; however, these are generally relatively mild.

Among the major techniques for thumb reconstruction, the total big-toe, big-toe wraparound, and trimmed big-toe transfers provide greater strength and a more stable surface for pinch and grasp than any second-toe transfer (6), and are more suitable for some types of manual workers. Because of its relatively small size and the possible claw appearance, the second-toe transfer generally provides an obviously inferior thumb replacement.

ANATOMY

Although the big toe has most of the features of a thumb, it has a greater circumference (transverse diameter), nail width, and phalangeal and joint size (1). The widest transverse diameter can be up to 12 mm larger than that of the thumb, and the nail width 4 mm larger. The difference in the size of the bony elements is approximately 2 mm for the distal phalanx, 4 to 6 mm for the interphalangeal joint, and 4 mm for the proximal phalanx. These measurements are guidelines for the trimming procedure.

Anatomic variations relating to this flap and other toe transfers primarily concern the anatomy of the vascular pedicle (7–9). In most cases, the dominant vessel entering the first web space is the first dorsal metatarsal artery, which divides to supply the lateral digital artery of the big toe and the medial digital artery of the second toe. Proximally, this vessel (which is a continuation of the dorsalis pedis artery) can be either superficial or deep in relation to the first dorsal interosseous muscle, but it always passes dorsally over the transverse

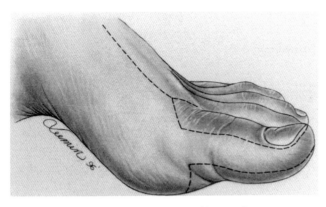

FIG. 1. Design of the trimmed big-toe flap.

metatarsal ligament. In a minority of cases, a plantar metatarsal artery is the dominant vessel that courses deep to the transverse metatarsal ligament.

To avoid confusion during pedicle dissection, proceeding in a distal-to-proximal direction is recommended, starting with identification of the common digital artery and its branches in the first web space (10). The dissection continues 1 to 2 cm proximally, to determine whether the dorsal or plantar metatarsal artery is dominant. If both vessels are of similar caliber, the dorsal vessel is preferred, since its dissection is easier and the pedicle longer. If the plantar vessel is significantly larger, it should be dissected proximally. However, plantar dissection to obtain a long pedicle can be tedious and more destructive to the foot; the use of a vein graft should be considered.

Venous drainage proceeds from the dorsal veins of the big toe to join with others to form the greater saphenous system.

FLAP DESIGN AND DIMENSIONS

The circumference of the normal thumb is measured at three points: (1) at the nail eponychium; (2) at the widest point (the interphalangeal joint); and (3) at the middle of the proximal phalanx. A longitudinal line is drawn from the distal edge of the big toe along the medial side of the nail to the base of the proximal phalanx, preserving the nail fold. Measurements from the normal thumb are then transposed to corresponding

points on the big toe, starting at the longitudinal line and leaving a medial strip of skin representing the difference between toe and thumb dimensions (Fig. 1). The toenail is not reduced in size, to avoid deformity of the nail fold. To each circumferential measurement, 2 to 3 mm are added to allow a tension-free closure. The medial skin strip usually measures 0.8 to 1.5 cm in width, and is tapered to a point around the tip of the toe 2 mm beneath the nail, to facilitate skin closure.

The proximal circumferential skin-incision line and level of proximal bone division are determined by the level of thumb amputation.

OPERATIVE TECHNIQUE

Dissection is performed under tourniquet control. The vascular pedicle is dissected from distal to proximal, to avoid the possible anatomic confusion described above. The medial skin strip is elevated from distal to proximal (Fig. 2A). The skin incision is deepened to the periosteum at the tip of the distal phalanx, and includes only soft tissue and skin on the medial side of the toe above the medial collateral ligament. A second dorsal longitudinal incision is then made through the periosteum along the dorsal margin of the medial collateral ligament and joint capsule. This tissue is then elevated in a subperiosteal plane to the midplantar surface of the proximal and distal phalanges, creating a periosteum-medial collateral ligament–joint capsule flap (Fig. 2B). This also exposes the medial bony excess of the proximal and distal phalanges, which is to be removed.

A longitudinal osteotomy is then performed with an oscillating saw, to remove 4 to 6 mm of the medial proximal interphalangeal joint prominence, and 2 to 4 mm of the shafts of the distal and proximal phalanges. Rasping of the bone edges will ensure a smooth contour (Fig. 2C).

The periosteum-medial collateral ligament-joint capsule flap is then redraped over the raw bony surfaces and closed tightly with interrupted sutures, after trimming any excessive bulk (Fig. 2D). The medial skin incision is closed, and the level of proximal bone division is selected (Fig. 2E). At least 1 cm of proximal phalanx should be left, to preserve the important weight-bearing area. The lengths of the vascular pedicle, plantar digital nerves, and flexor and extensor tendons are selected from the recipient-site dissection performed by a second team.

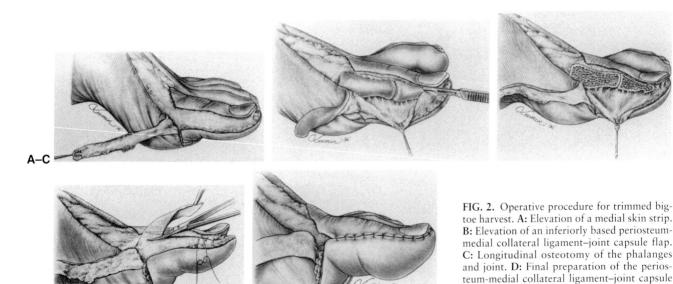

A–C

D,E

FIG. 2. Operative procedure for trimmed big-toe harvest. **A:** Elevation of a medial skin strip. **B:** Elevation of an inferiorly based periosteum-medial collateral ligament–joint capsule flap. **C:** Longitudinal osteotomy of the phalanges and joint. **D:** Final preparation of the periosteum-medial collateral ligament–joint capsule flap. **E:** Closure of the trimmed-toe wound before transfer.

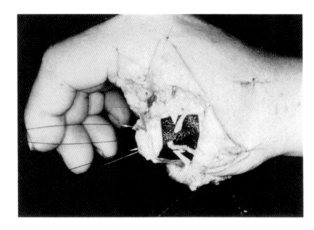

FIG. 3. Traumatic thumb amputation at the level of the interphalangeal joint.

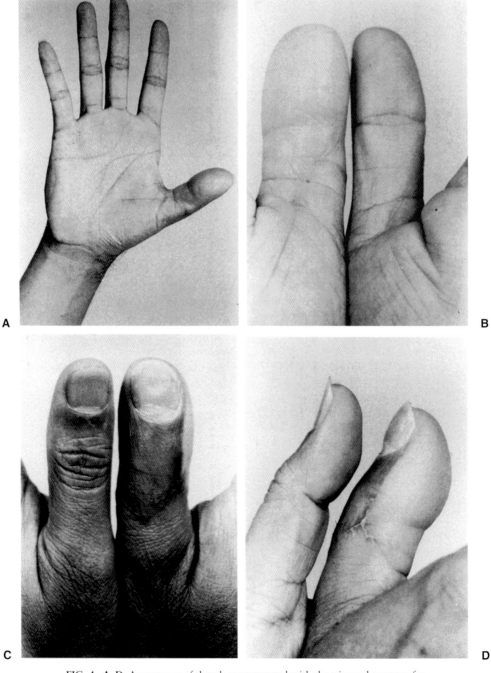

FIG. 4. A–D: Appearance of thumb reconstructed with the trimmed-toe transfer.

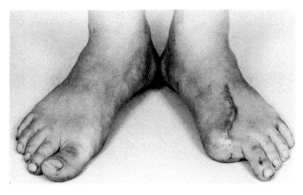

FIG. 5. Appearance of the donor site following the transfer.

Following flap harvest, the donor site is closed primarily. If necessary, the proximal part of the medial skin strip is used to achieve tension-free closure.

Transfer of the trimmed big toe is then performed with osteosynthesis, tendon repair, nerve suture, skin closure, and microvascular anastomoses. Loss of first metacarpal bone length and inadequate soft tissue can be made up by means of an iliac-crest bone graft and a pedicled groin flap in a pre–toe-transfer procedure. Reconstruction at the interphalangeal joint level includes the functional interphalangeal joint of the toe transfer. Distal to the interphalangeal joint, a modified big-toe wraparound flap can be harvested and trimmed of soft tissue and distal phalanx in a similar manner.

If the pulp is still excessive after thumb reconstruction, it can be reduced at a second stage. Pulp debulking involves excision of a midline elipse of skin and soft tissue from the interphalangeal crease to the thumb tip.

CLINICAL RESULTS

A review of patients following trimmed big-toe transfer (1) has found no patient complaints regarding the size of properly trimmed toes (Figs. 3 and 4). Solid, stable, and painless pinch, grip, and movement have been maintained in all patients. Interphalangeal joint movement averaged 20°, compared with 29° after total big-toe transfers (11). Maintenance of interphalangeal joint movement facilitates the nail pinch needed for fine manipulation. In those with isolated thumb injury reconstructed with trimmed big-toe transfer, grip strength averaged 65% of the normal contralateral hand and key pinch averaged 75%.

Tight repair of the periosteum-medial collateral ligament-joint capsule flap ensures the stability of the interphalangeal joint. Development of degenerative arthritis has not occurred. Biomechanical analysis and clinical observation of foot function has shown no significant donor-foot deficits (Fig. 5). Preservation of 1 cm of the proximal phalanx improves the appearance and push-off function of the donor foot (12).

SUMMARY

The trimmed big-toe transfer is a useful technique of thumb reconstruction, providing the most normal aesthetic appearance, as well as stable and mobile interphalangeal joint movement for grip and fine pinch.

References

1. Wei F-C, Chen HC, Chuang CC, Noordhoff MS. Reconstruction of the thumb with a trimmed toe transfer technique. *Plast Reconstr Surg* 1988;82:506.
2. Morrison WA, O'Brien BMcC, Mcleod A. Thumb reconstruction with a free neurovascular wrap-around flap from the big toe. *J Hand Surg* 1980;5:575.
3. Cobbett JR. Free digital transfer: report of a case of transfer of a great toe to replace an amputated thumb. *J Boint Joint Surg* 1969;51B:677.
4. Buncke HJ, McLean DH, George PT, et al. Thumb reconstruction: great toe transplantation by microvascular anastomosis. *Br J Plast Surg* 1973;26:194.
5. Wei F-C, Chen HC, Chuang CC, Chen SHT. Microsurgical thumb reconstruction with toe transfer techniques: selection of various techniques. *Plast Reconstr Surg* 1994;93:345.
6. Leung PC. Thumb reconstruction using second toe transfer. *Hand Clin* 1985;1:285.
7. Gilbert A. Vascular anatomy of the first web space of the foot. In: Landi A, ed. *Reconstruction of the thumb.* London: Chapman and Hall, 1989;199.
8. May JW Jr. Microvascular great toe to hand transfer for reconstruction of the amputated thumb. In: McCarthy JG, ed. *Plastic surgery,* vol. 8. Philadelphia: Saunders, 1990;5153.
9. Leung PC. Thumb reconstruction using the second toe. In: Landi A, ed. *Reconstruction of the thumb.* London: Chapman and Hall, 1989;199.
10. Wei FC, Silverman RT, Hsu WM. Retrograde dissection of the vascular pedicle in toe harvest. *Plast Reconstr Surg* 1995;96:1211.
11. Poppen NK, Norris TR, Buncke HJ. Evaluation of sensibility and function with microsurgical free transfer of the great toe to the hand for thumb reconstruction. *J Hand Surg* 1983;8:516.
12. Wei F-C, El-Gammal TA, Ma HS, et al. Biomechanical analysis of foot function following big toe transfer with preservation of the proximal phalangeal base. *Plast Reconstr Surg* in press.

CHAPTER 283. Rhomboid-to-W Flap *H. Becker*

www.encyclopediaofflaps.com

CHAPTER 284 ■ PALMAR AND THENAR INNERVATED SKIN FLAPS TO THE HAND

B. B. JOSHI

In degloved, mutilated hands where skin for transfer is very scarce, palmar flaps have been used following the principles of sliding and rotation, with later conversion into island flaps for further distal migration and adjustment. These flaps can provide sensation to the areas of contact needed in pinch and grasp (1,2).

INDICATIONS

The main indications for these flaps are in transverse amputations of the hand with degloved phalangeal remnants that have been covered with skin grafts but are anesthetic, or in a metacarpal hand in which either the thumb or the ulnar post is to be reconstructed by osteoplastic technique, using a tube pedicle and bone graft.

ANATOMY

The hand is richly supplied by blood vessels. The radial and ulnar arteries anastomose freely in the palm as superficial and deep palmar arches. Common volar digital vessels arise from the superficial arch and run toward the respective web spaces, to divide into volar digital vessels for the fingers. The branches from the median and ulnar nerves accompany the common volar digital vessels in the palm and are deep to the palmar fascia, continuing to give twigs to it as perforating branches for the overlying skin. If dissection is made in the deeper plane to the vessels and nerves, arterialized flaps of palmar skin can be raised.

The area supplied by the median and ulnar nerves is well known, although some variations are not uncommon. In addition, there is sensory overlap provided by the diffuse plexus formed in the palm by cutaneous branches of the terminal part of the radial nerve, the lateral cutaneous nerve of the forearm, the medial cutaneous nerve of the forearm, and palmar cutaneous branches of the median and ulnar nerves.

FLAP DESIGN AND DIMENSIONS

The various flaps included in this group are essentially neurovascular and are based on known volar digital vessels and nerves. They can be converted into island flaps on their specific neurovascular connections.

The initial advancement is by rotation along with the nerves and vessels ensheathed in the flaps, and additional advancement is achieved by flexing the metacarpophalangeal joints.

The flaps may be designed as Z-plasties, taking advantage of the loose skin over the stumps that is then used to fit into the defect created at the donor site. Where this is not possible, split-thickness skin grafts are used to cover the donor defect.

The flaps have limited advancement, from 2.5 to a maximum of 3 cm, because of restrictions imposed by neurovascular connections and palmar fascia. Tension on the neurovascular bundles is minimized by mobilizing them proximally and sectioning the palmar fascia and its septal connections down to the wrist. When one is undermining the flap, the nerves and vessels entering it are kept clinging to its deeper surface, since the neurovascular supply is from perforating twigs arising from these structures.

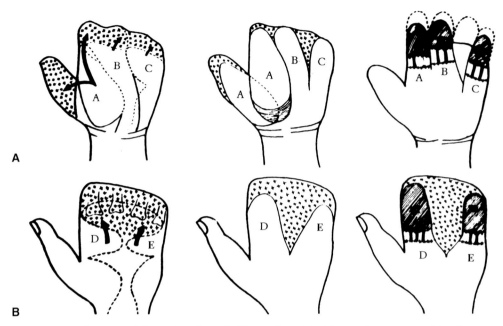

FIG. 1. Line drawings of the various flaps. **A:** Thenar flap. *A* is either used as a transposition flap to cover a thumb defect or as a sliding flap to cover the distal end of an index amputation stump. Flaps *B* and *D* are transposed to cover the remaining distal stumps. **B:** Flap *D* is radially based and can be used to cover a radial hand amputation stump. Flap *E* is similar to that shown in **A** and is ulnarly based. (From Joshi, ref. 1, with permission.)

OPERATIVE TECHNIQUE

Palmar Skin from the Thenar Region and Base of the Index Finger (Fig. 1A)

The flap *A* is based mainly on the palmar cutaneous branch of the median nerve and the cutaneous twigs from the digital branches to the index finger that enter its central portion along with the twigs from common volar digital vessels. Marking of flap *A* is shown in Fig. 1. The thenar

crease line is extended to the base of the index finger and includes the common palmar digital branch of the median nerve.

The thenar flap in Fig. 2 is used to provide sensation over the palmar aspect of a thumb that has been reconstructed using a tube pedicle in a radial hemiamputated hand.

The flap can also be used in the form of a sliding island flap, as the nerve and vessels enter it as in an umbrella (Fig. 3A,B). It can easily be shifted distally for about 2.5 cm or so as an island flap, and can later be converted into a creeping flap for further migration (Fig. 3C,D).

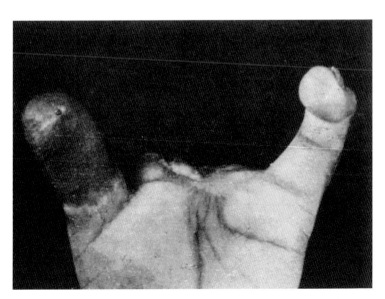
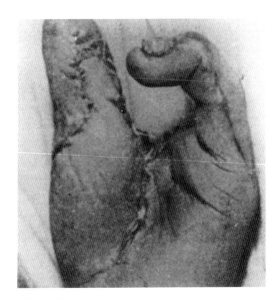

FIG. 2. Thenar flap transferred to thumb. (From Joshi, ref. 1, with permission.)

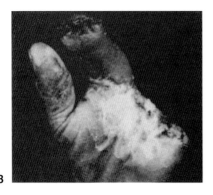
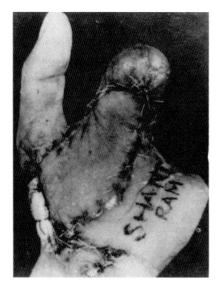

A,B

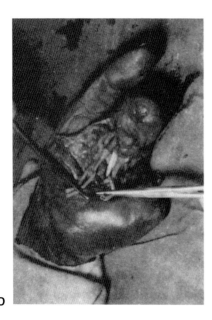
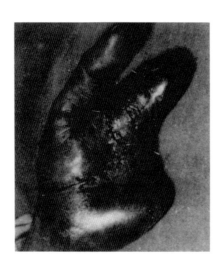

C,D

FIG. 3. **A,B:** Thenar flap as sliding island flap for index finger remnant. **C,D:** Later conversion of thenar sliding island flap into sensory island for further migration on neurovascular attachments. (From Joshi, ref. 2, with permission.)

Ulnar Flap from the Base of the Index and Middle Fingers (Fig. 1A)

This is a rotation flap *B* developed from the skin over the bases of the middle and index fingers. It incorporates the digital branches of the median nerve. The flap can be used to provide sensation over the middle finger stump or the central area of the degloved metacarpal hand (Fig. 4). Sensation over the radial aspect of the index finger can be preserved by sparing the most radial common digital branch in this region and not including it in the flap.

Radial Flap from the Base of the Middle and Ring Fingers (Fig. 1B)

This flap *D* is based on a neurovascular bundle and is raised from the base of the index and middle fingers. The flap will supply the innervated skin over the strategic area on the volar and radial aspects of the index finger stump.

The three common digital branches of the median nerve are retained and migrated along with the flap after dissection, to release them proximally in the palm (Fig. 5). The distal part of this flap can again be converted into a creeping type of island flap for further advancement over the longer amputation stump.

Flap from the Ulnar Innervated Segment of the Palm (Fig. 1B)

The flap *E* is raised from the ulnar aspect and has digital nerves and vessels of the little finger and the ulnar neurovascular bundles of the ring finger supplying the ulnar aspect of the palm. The flap is usually mapped distal to the proximal palmar crease and is suitable for migration to the little finger stump (Fig. 5). It can also be used to provide sensation to a reconstructed ulnar post in a metacarpal hand (Fig. 4).

CLINICAL RESULTS

Following the transfer of these flaps, sensation may be diminished because of nerve stretching, but recovery is rapid; sensation is regained within 10 to 12 weeks.

Marginal necrosis of the tip of the Z-plasty flap may occur if it is sharply angled, but this can be avoided by rounding. No case of circulatory embarrassment has been noted.

A salvaged prehensile hand unit can stand positive comparison with an artificial limb because of the added advantage of having sensation. The flaps described here can be used advantageously to provide a signal area for the servomotor mechanism. The advancement of these flaps is a limited one, from 2.5 to 3 cm, and the flaps can be helpful only in providing

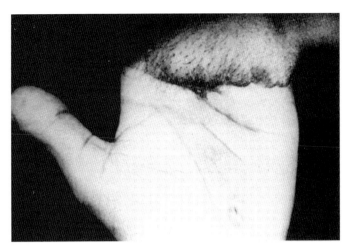
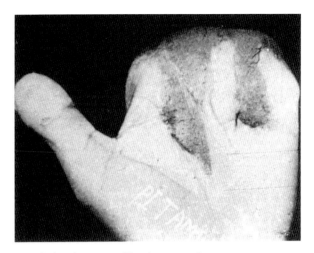

FIG. 4. Possible use of palmar skin at the strategic area of grasp in a degloved metacarpal hand. (From Joshi, ref. 1, with permission.)

A–C

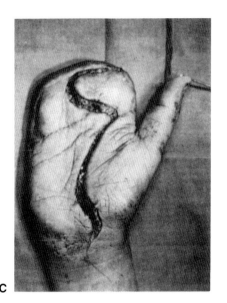
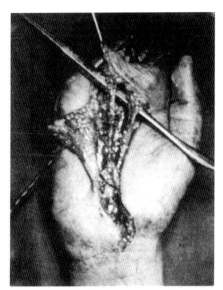
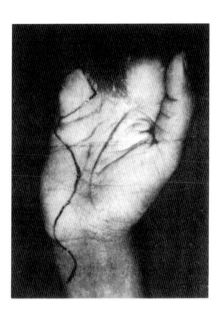

D,E

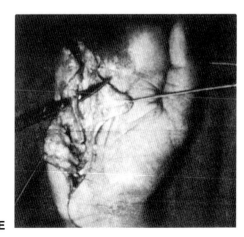
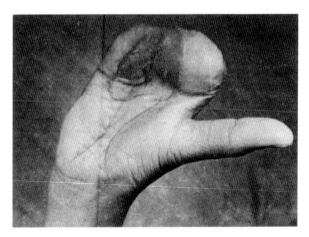

FIG. 5. A,B: Rotational advancement of radially based median flap for index finger stump. **C,D:** Ulnar innervated flap for little finger. **E:** Postoperative result. (From Joshi, ref. 1, with permission.)

sensation over remnants of the proximal phalanx in degloved hands or to a limited area of volar contact in reconstructed radial or ulnar posts in mutilated hands. The grade of sensation achieved is tactile gnosis. The procedures are well appreciated by patients, as can be judged by their agreement to surgery in multiple stages.

For sensory rehabilitation of the degloved, mutilated hand, slow advancement by multistage operations is unavoidable, as failure will add further insult. The creeping method of advancement ensures safety in conditions of scarcity. If we show a little ingenuity, many of these flaps can find their way into osteoplastic reconstructive surgery of the mutilated hand.

SUMMARY

Various palmar and thenar innervated flaps can be used to provide some sensation to the injured hand.

References

1. Joshi BB. Sensory flaps for the degloved mutilated hand. *Hand* 1974;6:247.
2. Joshi BB. Sensory flaps for the degloved mutilated hand. In: Campbell Reid JA, Gosset J, eds. *Mutilating injuries of the hand*, G.E.M. Monograph No. 3. New York: Churchill Livingstone, 1979;12–21.

CHAPTER 285 ■ FIRST DORSAL INTEROSSEOUS MUSCLE FLAP

V. R. HENTZ

Use of the first dorsal interosseous muscle is possible in particular clinical instances when a small but strategically located hand defect may be best covered by one of several muscle or musculocutaneous flaps available in the hand, although the use of muscle or musculocutaneous flap procedures generally has only limited application for defects in the upper limb.

INDICATIONS

The particular placement of the first dorsal interosseous muscle allows its use for small defects around the metacarpophalangeal joint of the thumb, such as might occur with deep avulsion injuries or small electrical burns with potential or definite joint exposure. Other indications might include small full-thickness injuries to the dorsum of the hand in circumstances where rotation flaps might be less indicated, such as in ulcers resulting from extravasation of chemotherapeutic substances, especially those that expose extensor tendons devoid of paratenon.

Further indications hinge on the fact that the muscle can be transferred in such a way as to minimize the functional deficit that accompanies complete paralysis of this muscle—as, for example, in an ulnar nerve palsy with its sequelae of weak pinch and lateral instability of the index finger.

ANATOMY

The abundant blood supply to the upper limb allows the safe transfer of a great variety of intrinsic random flaps whose use in the lower limb, for example, would fail. Although there are duplicate muscles to perform certain functions in the upper limb and therefore potential sources for muscle or musculocutaneous flaps, very few exist in the hand. When necessary, the

mobility of the arm allows the hand to be brought easily to other potential donor sites where, again, safe random flaps (such as the subclavicular or cross-arm flap) or so-called direct arterial flaps (such as the groin flap) have been used routinely for coverage of both large and small hand defects.

The first dorsal interosseous muscle is a source for one of the several muscle or musculocutaneous flaps available in the hand that can be used in particular clinical instances when a small but strategically located hand defect may be best covered by flaps of this type. The muscle is located on the radial border of the index metacarpal. It can potentially be transferred as either a muscle flap or a musculocutaneous flap, although its location in the important first web space significantly limits its usefulness as a musculocutaneous flap because the skin of that area is relatively privileged. It is a functionally important muscle, abducting the index finger at the metacarpophalangeal joint and participating in stabilizing this digit against the considerable force of the thumb in pinch, especially lateral or key pinch.

The muscle originates from the bases of the first and second metacarpals and inserts principally into the base of the proximal phalanx of the index finger (1). There is a somewhat inconstant attachment to the radial lateral band of the extensor mechanism over the proximal phalanx.

Innervation of the muscle is by way of the deep motor branch of the ulnar nerve that enters the muscle on its deep surface in its proximal third. The principal blood supply comes from contributions from the dorsal branch of the radial artery as it dives ulnarward in the first web space to contribute to the deep palmar arch (Fig. 1). There are usually two or three specific branches to the muscle, either separately or as branches from the princeps pollicis artery or the princeps indicis branch. These vessels supply the muscle in its proximal third, as well. Therefore, the vascular

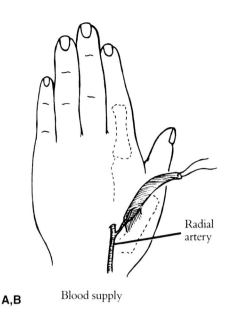
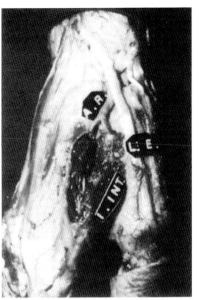

Radial artery

A,B   Blood supply

FIG. 1. **A:** The principal vascular pedicle arises from the dorsal branch of the radial artery as it dives palmarward between the bases of the first and second metacarpals. **B:** In this dissection the two "heads" of the muscle have been separated to demonstrate the multiple branches of the radial artery (*AR*) to each portion of the muscle.

anatomy of the muscle permits its transfer as a proximally based rotation flap.

In most instances, the muscle is divisible into two discrete masses, a dorsal radial and an ulnar portion (Fig. 2). The dorsal radial portion is more superficial, arises from the first metacarpal, and inserts primarily into the extensor expansion at the proximal phalanx. The more volar and ulnar portion of the muscle, located closer to the metacarpal, arises from the second metacarpal and has a bony insertion into the base of the proximal phalanx. These two portions can be separated quite far proximally, and the more superficial portion used as a transfer, leaving behind sufficient first dorsal interosseous muscle to provide some stability to the radial side of the index finger, particularly in pinch functions.

FLAP DESIGN AND DIMENSIONS

The potential arc of rotation of the superficial portion of the muscle is demonstrated in Fig. 3 (2). The principal vascular pedicle arises from the dorsal branch of the radial artery as it dives palmarward between the bases of the first and second metacarpals (Fig. 4).

CLINICAL RESULTS

A significant functional deficit would result from transfer of the entire muscle. This would be particularly noticeable as

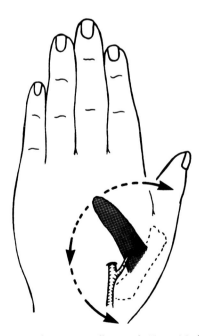

FIG. 2. The dorsal radial (superficial) portion of the muscle is generally larger than the volar-ulnar portion of muscle. It has been detached at its insertion to demonstrate the vascular intercommunications between the two "heads."

FIG. 3. The arc of rotation is illustrated. (From Mathes and Nahai, ref. 1, with permission.)

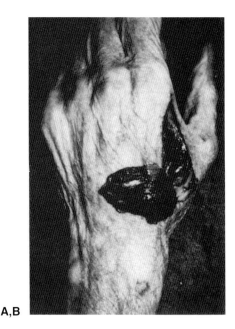
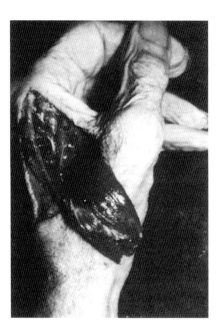

A,B

FIG. 4. **A,B:** The dissected specimens illustrate potential sites of application for this flap.

weakness in key pinch; for this reason the muscle is seldom used as a total transfer.

SUMMARY

The dorsal radial portion of the first dorsal interosseous muscle can be used in a few instances to cover various defects, particularly around the metacarpophalangeal joint of the thumb (3).

References

1. Mathes SJ, Nahai F, eds. *Clinical atlas of muscle and musculocutaneous flaps.* St. Louis: Mosby, 1979.
2. Kaplan EB, ed. *Functional and surgical anatomy of the hand.* Philadelphia: Lippincott, 1953.
3. Stern P. Personal communication.

CHAPTER 286 ■ ABDUCTOR DIGITI MINIMI MUSCLE FLAP

V. R. HENTZ

The abductor digiti minimi is a relatively expendable muscle, serving only to abduct the little finger—a function performed somewhat by the extrinsic extensors to the little finger. For many years it has been used as a functional transfer to replace loss of opposition of the thumb. In fact, it was among the first opponens transfers described (1).

INDICATIONS

The abductor digiti minimi has been used clinically to cover small defects about the fifth metacarpal (2) and the dorsal-ulnar aspect of the hand or carpus (3). It is particularly useful either to assist in the revascularization of the median nerve

at the wrist following neurolysis or nerve grafts, or as padding over the median nerve following operations for recurrent carpal tunnel syndrome. Except for an inability to widely abduct the little finger, the functional deficit resulting from its transfer is minimal.

ANATOMY

The abductor digiti minimi takes its origin from the pisiform, the tendinous attachment of the flexor carpi ulnaris and the base of the fifth metacarpal. It inserts into the base of the proximal phalanx of the little finger and contributes to the formation of the ulnar lateral band.

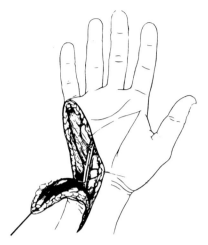

FIG. 1. The neurovascular hilum enters the muscle on its deep surface. The motor nerve usually arises from the ulnar nerve, just as it divides into superficial sensory and deep motor components. The muscle also receives additional blood supply via more distally located vessels, although the entire muscle can survive on only its proximal vascular pedicle.

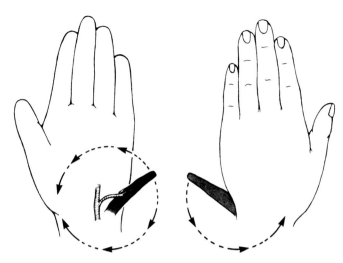

FIG. 2. The volar and dorsal arcs of rotation are illustrated. (From Mathes and Nahai, ref. 4, with permission.)

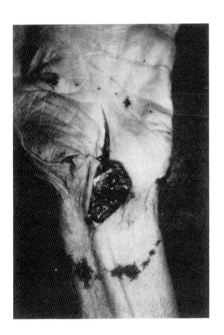
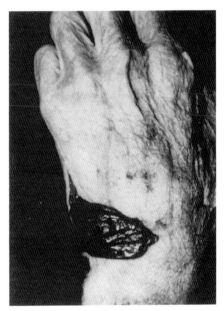

FIG. 3. Cadaver dissections illustrate several potential sites of use, for example, over a scarred median nerve at the wrist or to cover a small defect on the dorsal ulnar aspect of the hand.

The neurovascular anatomy is very constant (Fig. 1). Branches from the ulnar nerve and artery enter the muscle on its deep surface near its origin.

FLAP DESIGN AND DIMENSIONS

The superficial location of the abductor digiti minimi on the ulnar aspect of the hand, and its very proximal neurovascular arrangement, permit great mobility in transfer. The flap axis of rotation is depicted in Fig. 2 (4). Several cadaver dissections (Fig. 3) demonstrate potential uses.

OPERATIVE TECHNIQUE

The muscle is easily exposed through an incision along the ulnar border of the hand. After detaching the tendinous insertion, dissection proceeds proximally. Proximal dissection, and particularly separation from the adjacent flexor digiti minimi,

is sometimes difficult, although transfer of the flexor, in addition to the abductor digiti minimi, seems to result in no greater functional deficit.

SUMMARY

The abductor digiti minimi muscle can be transferred to cover small defects about the dorsal-ulnar aspect of the hand. Its use results in a minimal functional deficit.

References

1. Huber E. Hilfsoperation der Medianuslahmung. *Dtsch Z Chir* 1921;162: 271.
2. McCraw J. Personal communication.
3. Reisman N, Dellon AL. The abductor digiti minimi muscle flap: a salvage technique for palmar wrist pain. *Plast Reconstr Surg* 1983;72:859.
4. Mathes SJ, Nahai F. *Clinical atlas of muscle and musculocutaneous flaps.* St. Louis: Mosby, 1979;617.

CHAPTER 287 ■ PALMARIS BREVIS TURNOVER FLAP AS AN ADJUNCT TO INTERNAL NEUROLYSIS OF THE CHRONICALLY SCARRED MEDIAN NERVE IN RECURRENT CARPAL TUNNEL SYNDROME

E. H. ROSE

EDITORIAL COMMENT

This is a useful flap for secondary, tertiary, and quaternary carpal tunnels.

The palmaris brevis "turnover" flap as an adjunct to internal neurolysis, following failed primary carpal tunnel release, can provide some degree of subjective and objective improvement. This local muscle flap is recommended as a valuable adjunct in secondary surgery of the scarred median nerve.

INDICATIONS

Treatment failures occur in 3.2% to 19% of patients in large clinical series of carpal tunnel release (1–4). In large series of reexploration, the most common pathologic findings are tenosynovitis or fibrous proliferation within the carpal tunnel, compressing the nerve (5,6). Symptoms return, on average, 1 to 1.5 years after the first surgery (6). In cases of severe epineural fibrosis or interstitial scar, internal neurolysis has been suggested as an effective means of enhancing axonal regeneration of the chronically compressed nerve (7–9).

Local transposition muscle flaps have been used to provide a nutritive interface between the neurolysed median nerve and the adherent dysesthetic scar (10–13). Several criticisms of this technique, using the abductor digiti minimi muscle, have been offered (10). A new flap of palmaris brevis muscle has been used as an adjunct to internal neurolysis in 11 patients (13 hands) with secondary decompression of the median nerve in recurrent carpal tunnel syndrome. This broad, thin, vestigial sheet of muscle, immediately adjacent to the carpal tunnel, is easily rotated over the dissected nerve, with no significant dynamic functional deficit. The procedure affords additional cushioning superficial to the median nerve, and apparently enhances neovascularization of ischemic fascicular surfaces.

The palmaris brevis flap affords additional blood supply to the "raw" nerve surface. Although it cannot be proved that direct inosculation from the palmaris flap occurs at a fascicular level, an improved nutrient bed is suggested by the indirect means of microangiogram, methylene blue studies, and latex injection. Magnetic resonance imaging (MRI) demonstrates apposition of the nutrient muscle to the median nerve at 6 months' follow-up. In addition, the literature offers evidence for the efficacy of interposing muscle between an injured nerve and dysesthetic scar tissue of the skin (10–15). Improved grip strength following the procedures is probably related to less tenderness of the palmar scar from aberrant nerve endings; in addition to enhancing vascularity, the palmaris muscle flap may suppress the growth of nerve sprouts into overlying skin.

A major advantage of the palmaris turnover flap is the proximity of innervated muscle to the surgical field, obviating the need for a distant donor site and more lengthy operative procedure. No motor loss is created by using the muscle; the "unroofed" ulnar neurovascular bundle is still well padded by thick hypothenar skin and subcutaneous fat.

ANATOMY

The bifascicular, trapezoid-shaped palmaris brevis muscle is of variable size and thickness, but is absent in only 2% of cases (16,17). The muscle arises from the flexor retinaculum in the midpalm and inserts in the fibrofatty tissue along the ulnar margin of the hypothenar eminence and the pisiform. It lies palmar to the ulnar nerve and artery, forming the "roof" of the ulnar tunnel of the wrist (Guyon's canal) (15,16). Length averages 2.7 cm on the radial border and 3.6 cm on the ulnar border. The average width is 2.6 cm.

There are two fascicular muscle groups or "heads," each of which has its own neural and vascular supply. In microfilm injection studies, both nutrient arteries usually arise from the deep palmar branch of the ulnar artery distal to its bifurcation (Fig. 1). In one cadaver dissection, the proximal branch arose from the ulnar artery slightly before the takeoff of the superficial arch. In another, the distal branch arose from the common digital artery to the fourth cleft. In all dissections, the proximal nerve pedicle originated from the ulnar nerve trunk, and the distal pedicle from either the common sensory

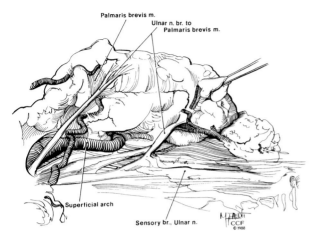

FIG. 1. Dual arterial blood supply to the palmaris brevis muscle. These arteries usually arise from the deep palmar branch of the ulnar artery distal to its bifurcation. (From Rose et al., ref. 19, with permission.)

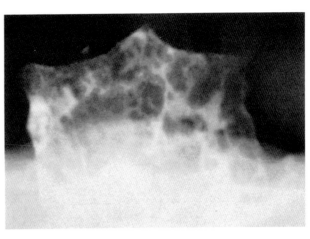

FIG. 3. Microangiogram of elevated palmaris flap. Note brisk vascular arcade within muscle. (From Rose et al., ref. 19, with permission.)

to the fourth cleft or the ulnar sensory branch to the little finger (Fig. 2). In one specimen, three motor branches to the palmaris brevis were noted.

Microangiograms show a brisk vascular arcade within the palmaris brevis muscle mass (Fig. 3). Methylene blue injections demonstrate the punctate capillary perforators on the surface of the muscle. The dorsal fascia, where the vascular network enters the muscle, was consistently present in all dissections and clinical cases, regardless of the thinness of the muscle.

Radially, the dorsal fascia blends with the palmar aponeurosis and ulnarly with the hypothenar fascia. Proximally, the dorsal fascia merges with the fibrofatty tissue over the antebrachial fascia, and distally with similar tissues in the palm. The function of the palmaris brevis is "mysterious" (18); it contracts when the adjacent abductor or flexor digiti minimi contracts, cupping the palm.

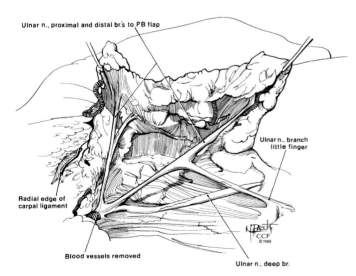

FIG. 2. Motor branches of ulnar nerve to palmaris muscle. The proximal nerve pedicle arises from the trunk of the ulnar nerve. The distal originates either from the common sensory nerve to the fourth cleft or the ulnar sensory branch to the little finger. (From Rose et al., ref. 19, with permission.)

OPERATIVE TECHNIQUE (19)

The incision parallels the thenar wrist crease and extends transversely across the distal flexion crease of the wrist (Fig. 4A). The tip of the skin flap is elevated subdermally to avoid injury to the palmar cutaneous branch of the median nerve (20). The hypothenar flap is raised superficial to the palmaris brevis muscle fibers. Sharp scissors or a knife is needed to section the numerous fibrous septa between the muscle and skin. Some fat usually remains on the muscle.

After division of the transverse carpal ligament and microneurolysis of the median nerve, the palmaris flap is elevated by dividing the attachments of the muscle from the dermal skin at its ulnar border, carefully avoiding injury to the deeper ulnar nerve and artery (Fig. 4B).

The dorsal fascia is teased from the fascia of the hypothenar intrinsic muscles, to transpose in a "book leaf" fashion across the carpal tunnel (Fig. 4C). The free edge is secured with sutures to the cut radial remnant of the transverse carpal ligament (Fig. 4D). The vascular surface of the flap convolutes into the dead space of the tunnel and apposes the "raw" fascicular surfaces of the neurolysed median nerve. Cosmetic closure is within crease lines (Fig. 4E). Postsurgical cross-sectional wrist MRI evaluations demonstrate a cushion of palmaris muscle between the nerve trunk and the dermal skin surface.

CLINICAL RESULTS

In a series of 13 hands of 11 patients, at surgical exploration the nerves were encased in dense restrictive scar tissue and often adherent to the radial wall of the carpal canal. The nerve trunk was diffusely narrowed by epineural fibrosis. Insterstitial scarring was severe and, in most patients, the fine longitudinal perineural vasa nervorum were obliterated on microscope inspection. No incomplete division of the transverse carpal ligament was found in any explorations.

Subjective assessment of pain relief ranged postoperatively from 25% to 100%. All hands with abnormal preoperative two-point discrimination showed numerical improvement. Grip strength improved in 11 of 13 hands (average: 15.2%). Thenar atrophy grossly improved at least one grade in all hands. Pulp pinch improved in 10 hands (average: 31.9%). Mean key pinch improved by 5.5%.

In one patient, increased numbness of the long finger developed, with worsening of two-point discrimination at 6 months

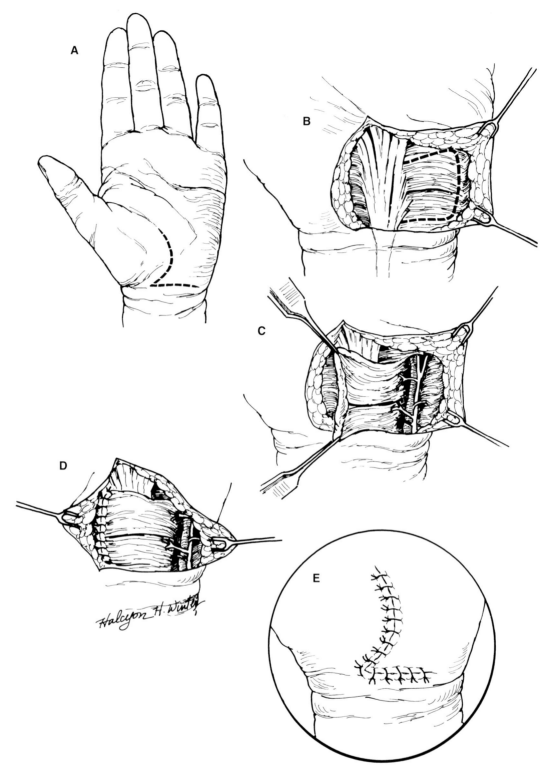

FIG. 4. Operative technique. A: Incision in thenar and wrist creases. B: Design of palmaris flap. Muscle insertions to dermis divided. C: Flap transposed as "book leaf" over carpal tunnel. D: Turnover flap inset into radial edge of retinaculum. E: Incisions closed. (From Rose et al., ref. 19, with permission.)

postoperatively; sensory parameters returned to normal by 1 year. The more complex operative procedure extended disability time to an average of 4.8 months (longer than the usual 1.5 to 3 months for simple carpal tunnel release). Six patients returned to previous employment, and four were retrained to less strenuous occupations. One patient retired after surgery.

No infections occurred in this series. Blistering was noted at the tip of the palmar skin flap in one patient, but represented only superficial slough and healed by re-epithelialization. Hypothenar tenderness lasted at least 4 months, also increasing the duration of morbidity over routine carpal tunnel release.

SUMMARY

Although postoperative donor morbidity is lengthened and rehabilitation time prolonged by the procedure (compared with routine carpal tunnel release), subjective assessment of "pain relief" and clinical measurements of grip strength, pinch strength, and sensory parameters, appear to justify the usage of the palmaris brevis turnover flap as an adjunct to internal neurolysis in difficult recurrent carpal tunnel cases.

References

1. Phalen GS. The carpal tunnel syndrome: seventeen years experience in diagnosis and treatment of six hundred fifty-four hands. *J Bone Joint Surg* 1986; 48A:211.
2. Phalen GS. Reflections on 21 years experience with the carpal tunnel syndrome. *JAMA* 1970;212:1365.
3. Macdonald RI, Lichtman DM, Hanlon J, Wilson JN. Complications of surgical release for carpal tunnel syndrome. *J Hand Surg* 1978;3:70.
4. Kulick MI, Gordiuo G, Javidi T, et al. Long term analysis of patients having surgical treatment for carpal tunnel syndrome. *J Hand Surg* 1986;11A:59.
5. Langloh ND, Linsheid RL. Recurrent and unrelieved carpal tunnel syndrome. *Clin Orthop* 1972;83:41.
6. Wadstroen J, Nigst H. Reoperation for carpal tunnel syndrome. *Ann Chir Main* 1986;5:54.
7. Curtis RM, Eversmann WW. Internal neurolysis as an adjunct to the treatment of the carpal tunnel syndrome. *J Bone Joint Surg* 1973;55A:733.
8. Rhoades CE, Mowery CA, Gelberman RN. Results of internal neurolysis of the median nerve for severe carpal tunnel syndrome. *J Bone Joint Surg* 1985; 67A:253.
9. Mackinnon SE, O'Brien JP, Dellon AL, et al. An assessment of the effects of internal neurolysis on a chronically compressed rat sciatic nerve. *Plast Reconstr Surg* 1988;81:251.
10. Milward TM, Scott WG, Kleinert HE. The abductor digiti minimi muscle flap. *Hand* 1977;9:82.
11. Reisman NR, Dellon AL. The abductor digiti minimi muscle flap: a salvage technique for palmar wrist pain. *Plast Reconstr Surg* 1983;72:859.
12. Wilgis EFS. Local muscle flaps in the hand. Anatomy as related to reconstructive surgery. *Bull Hosp Jt Dis Orthop Inst* 1984;44:552.
13. Leslie BM, Ruby LK. Coverage of a carpal tunnel wound dehiscence with the abductor digiti minimi muscle flap. *J Hand Surg* 1988;13A:36.
14. Mackinnon SE, Dellon AL, Hudson AR, Hunter DA. Alteration of neuroma formation by manipulation of its microenvironment. *Plast Reconstr Surg* 1985;76:345.
15. Dellon AL, Mackinnon SE. Treatment of the painful neuroma by neuroma resection and muscle implantation. *Plast Reconstr Surg* 1986;77:427.
16. Le Double AF. *Traité des variations du systeme musculaire del'homme et leur signification au point de vue de l'anthropologie zoologique.* Paris: Reinwald, 1897;170–171.
17. Shrewsbury MM, Johnson RK, Osterhout DK. The palmaris brevis—a reconsideration of its anatomy and possible function. *J Bone Joint Surg* 1972;54A:344.
18. Kaplan EB, Smith RJ. Kinesiology of the hand and wrist and muscular variations of the hand and forearm. In: Spinner M, ed. *Kaplan's functional and surgical anatomy of the hand.* Philadelphia: Lippincott, 1944.
19. Rose EH, Norris MS, Kowalski TA, et al. Palmaris brevis turnover flap as an adjunct to internal neurolysis of the chronically scarred median nerve in recurrent carpal tunnel syndrome. *J Hand Surg* 1991;16A:191.
20. Talesnik J. The palmar cutaneous branch of the median nerve and the approach to the carpal tunnel: an anatomical study. *J Bone Joint Surg* 1973; 55A:1212.

CHAPTER 288 ■ PRONATOR QUADRATUS MUSCLE FLAP

A. L. DELLON AND S. E. MACKINNON

The pronator quadratus muscle can be elevated on a single, well-defined neurovascular pedicle and transposed within a wide arc to provide a well-vascularized pad of muscle for a variety of clinical needs in the distal forearm (1). Although the muscle supplies only a small area of soft-tissue coverage, this is often all that is necessary for reconstructive purposes in this region. For example, recent reports have demonstrated the clinical usefulness of small muscle flaps for skin and nerve (2) problems in this area. The flap may thus serve as an alternative to larger distant and more extensive reconstructive flap procedures (3,4).

subcutaneous tissue. There is therefore limited musculocutaneous flap potential. The groin flap has been the most frequently used flap for coverage in the distal forearm (3,5). The distal flexor aspect of the forearm would thus benefit from the availability of a local muscle flap to provide a bed for skin grafting over exposed vital structures, or to provide a well-vascularized bed for a nerve graft, for implantation of sensory nerves after neuroma resection (6,7) or elective amputation. Such a flap could provide a nutritive interface between an internally lysed nerve and overlying dysesthetic or adherent skin (2).

INDICATIONS

The distal forearm is devoid of superficial muscles, and vital structures in this area are protected only by skin and

ANATOMY

Cadaver dissections were performed on 16 upper extremities in eight specimens. The muscle was found to average 5 cm in

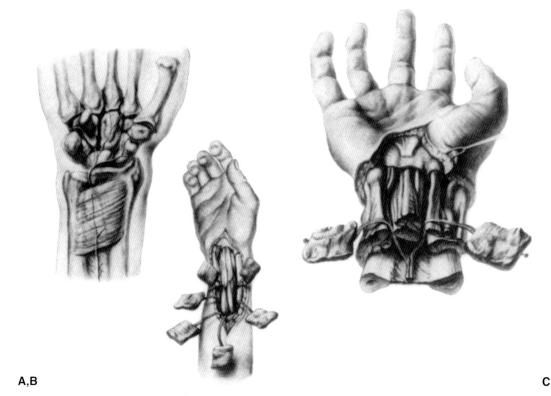

A,B   **C**

FIG. 1. **A:** The pronator quadratus muscle shown schematically. The muscle is supplied by the anterior interosseous neurovascular bundle with vessels perforating the interosseous membrane. **B:** The arc of rotation of the pronator quadratus muscle flap allows coverage of the median and lateral aspects of the forearm and distally to the proximal wrist crease. **C:** The flap may be transferred superficially by either a radial or an ulnar route. (From Dellon and Mackinnon, ref. 1, with permission.)

length and 4 cm in width (with the forearm supinated). There was no significant variation between right and left or male and female extremities.

The neurovascular bundle uniformly consisted of the anterior interosseous artery and nerve lying on the flexor surface of the interosseous membrane and entering the muscle on its dorsal surface. The neurovascular bundle lies on the midlongitudinal axis of the limb and enters the muscle between 1 and 2 cm distal to its proximal edge. At this point the dorsal branch of the artery pierces the interosseous membrane.

A series of perforating vessels are found at 2-cm intervals proximal to the leading edge of the muscle. These vessels branch from the anterior interosseous vessels and pierce the interosseous membrane.

FLAP DESIGN AND DIMENSIONS

If the dissection of the neurovascular bundle is carried proximally as far as the first branch of the anterior interosseous nerve to the flexor pollicis longus, the muscle can be raised on a neurovascular pedicle that is 5 to 6 cm in length. This provides an arc of rotation that will allow coverage of the distal forearm and the medial and lateral aspects of the wrist (Fig. 1).

It is emphasized further that the flap can provide coverage no further distally than the proximal wrist flexion crease, and the skin must be mobilized to cover the muscle without tension. Muscle coverage more distal than this can be provided by the abductor digiti minimi muscle flap (2).

OPERATIVE TECHNIQUE

The pronator quadratus muscle may be approached through any preexisting palmar wrist scar or longitudinal incision. The proximal limit of the incision must be extended, usually to 12 cm proximal to the wrist crease, to permit dissection of the neurovascular pedicle.

The necessary exploration and dissection are carried out before dissection of the pronator muscle. The majority of the required procedures can be performed then, leaving only the more delicate operative procedures (such as nerve grafting) until after the pronator quadratus muscle is elevated.

Elevation of the muscle flap is facilitated by approaching the muscle radially between the flexor profundus muscle group and the flexor pollicis longus tendon (Figs. 2 and 3). The distal edge of the muscle is divided sharply from the radius and ulna (Fig. 2A), and the terminal branches of the anterior interosseous artery and nerve (8) are divided (Fig. 2B). The insertion of the pronator onto the radius is next divided by an incision at the most radial border with a scalpel, and then by elevation more medially to the interosseous membrane with an elevator.

There are deep muscle fibers on the ulnar border of the interosseous membrane. Although the origin of the pronator from the ulna may be reached through this approach, the next step is facilitated by development of a plane between the profundus muscle and the flexor carpi ulnaris. Here the ulnar border of the muscle is incised and the medial dissection is performed with the elevator. The muscle may now be dissected from distal to proximal aspects by gentle traction,

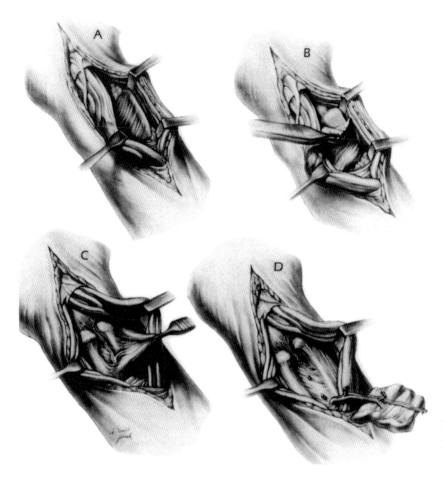

FIG. 2. A–D: Technique of pronator quadratus muscle flap elevation (see text for description). (From Dellon and Mackinnon, ref. 1, with permission.)

elevating it from the interosseous membrane until the dorsal branch of the anterior interosseous artery tethers the elevation (Fig. 2C).

Next, the anterior interosseous neurovascular bundle is identified proximally and dissected to this same tethering point. The membrane is incised on its ulnar border to facilitate

ligation of these dorsal branches, thereby freeing the entire muscle flap. More length is gained on the pedicle by proximal dissection. The proximal perforating branches are ligated and the flap is elevated on its neurovascular bundle (Figs. 2D and 3). The flap may then be transferred superficially to provide soft-tissue coverage.

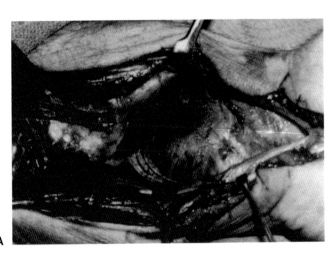

A

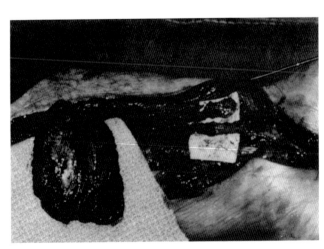

B

FIG. 3. Intraoperative views. **A:** Pronator quadratus muscle exposed. Note proximal neurovascular bundle (*left*). Pronator quadratus muscle elevated to show neurovascular bundle entering its deep side (*vessel loop top right*). **B:** Pronator quadratus muscle elevated. Note neurolysed median nerve and palmar cutaneous neuroma (*overlying background*). *(continued)*

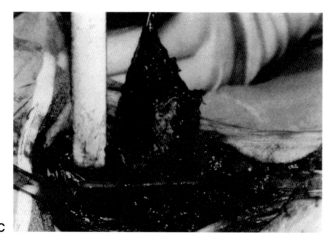
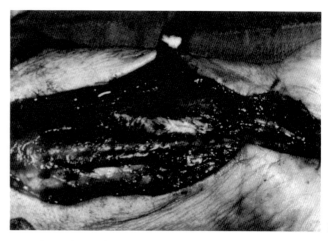

C   D

FIG. 3. *Continued.* C: Muscle flap being interposed between skin and neurolysed median nerve. D: Flap in place. Palmar cutaneous neuroma has been resected and nerve implanted into the muscle. (From Dellon and Mackinnon, ref. 1, with permission.)

CLINICAL RESULTS

This flap has been elevated surgically without technical complications in nine patients (1). There has been one immediate postoperative complication, a hematoma that drained spontaneously. Flap viability has been assessed intraoperatively by deflation of the pneumatic tourniquet and observation of bleeding from the muscle edges.

Viability of the flap postoperatively has been suggested by the palpable bulge beneath the skin flap and occasionally by a palpable contraction or wrinkling of the skin overlying the muscle, with the patient attempting resisted pronation. In three patients evaluated at 10, 13, and 14 months after operation, electromyography with the needle inserted into the pronator quadratus muscle and recording proximal from the median nerve demonstrated silence at rest and normal potential and recruitment as the patient attempted pronation, thus demonstrating a viable muscle.

One more way to prove that this pronator muscle flap is viable would be to use it as a bed for a skin graft. Although we have not yet had the clinical opportunity, skin-grafting this muscle is possible and should prove to be as successful in the upper extremity as similar procedures have proved to be in the lower extremity (3).

Clinically, six of the seven patients treated for pain have had either good or excellent results at a mean of 32 months after operation. The seventh patient had a wooden beam fall on the wrist 6 months after the operation, causing the previously palpable muscle mass to flatten, and this patient has had recurrent pain. This patient's early good result is considered a poor long-term result. No patient's condition was made worse. The remaining six patients have returned to work or are able to carry out their household activities, although two of the six are working at reduced capacity. (This includes all three patients involved in Workmen's Compensation cases.)

Two patients in whom the pronator quadratus muscle flap was used to provide a vascularized bed for a nerve graft demonstrated excellent rates of recovery of sensibility.

Loss of function of the pronator quadratus muscle has not been a problem to any of the nine patients. All can still pronate with some resistance, even with the elbow flexed. This action may be provided by the deep head of the pronator teres (4,9).

SUMMARY

The degree of technical difficulty in the use of the pronator quadratus muscle flap suggests that its clinical use should be more in "salvage" type procedures than in primary procedures, and in conjunction with neurolysis and tendolysis.

References

1. Dellon AL, Mackinnon SE. The pronator quadratus muscle flap. *J Hand Surg* 1984;9A:423.
2. Reisman N, Dellon AL. The abductor digiti minimi muscle flap: a salvage technique for palmar wrist pain. *Plast Reconstr Surg* 1983;72:859.
3. McGregor IA. Flap reconstruction in hand surgery: the evolution of presently used methods. *J Hand Surg* 1979;4:1.
4. Mackinnon SE, Weiland AJ, Godina M. Immediate forearm reconstruction with a functional latissimus dorsi island pedicle myocutaneous flap. *Plast Reconstr Surg* 1983;71:706.
5. Wray CR, Wise DM, Young VI. The groin flap in severe hand injuries. *Ann Plast Surg* 1982;9:459.
6. Dellon AL, Mackinnon SE, Pestronk A. Implantation of sensory nerve into muscle: preliminary clinical and experimental observations on neuroma formation. *Ann Plast Surg* 1984;12:30.
7. Mackinnon SE, Dellon AL, Hunter D, Hudson A. Alteration of neuroma formation produced by manipulation of neural environment in primates. Presented at the Annual Meeting of the American Society of Plastic and Reconstructive Surgery, Dallas, TX, 1983.
8. Dellon AL, Mackinnon SE. Terminal branch of anterior interosseous nerve as source of wrist pain. *J Hand Surg* 1984;9B:316.
9. Lister GD. Personal communication, 1983.

CHAPTER 289 ■ RADIAL FOREARM FASCIAL FLAP

P. H. GROSSMAN, A. M. MAJIDIAN, M. BRONES, M. YOUNG, AND A. R. GROSSMAN

The radial forearm flap is a workhorse for coverage of soft-tissue defects of the hand, when distally based; it can be based proximally to cover defects in the elbow region. A dis-advantage of the fasciocutaneous flap is the aesthetically dis-pleasing donor site. The radial forearm *fascial* flap, without inclusion of overlying skin, avoids donor-site morbidity and provides a pliable and thin coverage for the recipient defect (1–4).

INDICATIONS

The radial forearm fascial flap is ideally suited for recon-struction of soft-tissue defects of the hand, when thin, pliable coverage is needed and long periods of immobilization are contraindicated. The flap is thin enough to have proven very satisfactory for resurfacing the thumb. A complete palmar arch with good retrograde flow into the radial artery is a prerequisite for the distally based flap. If necessary, bone and tendon repairs may be performed at the same sitting.

The proximally based flap can be used for coverage of exposed bone or tendon in the elbow territory. Both radial and ulnar arteries must be patent, and the hand must be well per-fused by the ulnar artery alone.

ANATOMY

The radial artery and its accompanying veins lie deep within the volar forearm between the flexor carpi radialis and the brachioradialis. The vessels run within the lateral intermuscu-lar septum, which is continuous with the investing fascia of the forearm musculature. Venous drainage of the fascial flap is entirely via the venae comitantes.

FLAP DESIGN AND DIMENSIONS

The flap is designed over the volar aspect of the forearm and, if necessary, may extend over the radial and ulnar aspects of the forearm. In general, it is prudent to avoid the radial edge of the forearm, when possible, to minimize injury to the radial cutaneous nerve branches. The flap may be easily and reliably elevated; the distal forearm need not be avoided, as with the fasciocutaneous flap, since the underlying tendons will not require skin grafting (Figs. 1 and 2).

OPERATIVE TECHNIQUE

When planning a proximally based flap, a preoperative Allen's test is performed to establish patency in both arteries,

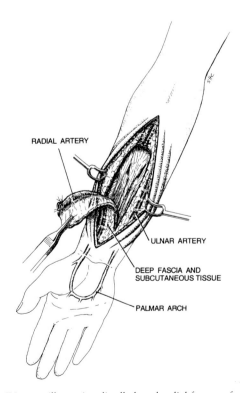

FIG. 1. Diagram illustrating distally based radial forearm fascial flap for coverage of hands and digits.

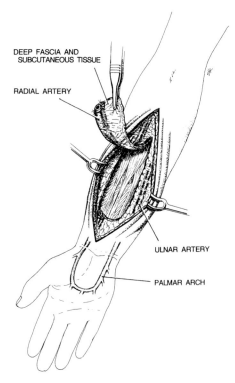

FIG. 2. Diagram illustrating proximally based flap for coverage of elbow.

and to ensure good perfusion of the hand by the ulnar artery alone. For a distally based flap, a safe and easy method of ensuring a complete arch and adequate retrograde flow through the radial artery is the following: With a Doppler flowmeter, the radial artery is located at the wrist. Next, the radial artery is occluded proximal to the probe, and the ulnar artery is occluded at the wrist. There should then be no Doppler signal distal to the occlusion. The ulnar artery occlusion is released, and a signal should then be heard over the radial artery, just distal to the point of continued radial-

artery occlusion. If there is no signal, reevaluation of the surgical options may be indicated.

The skin incision may be straight, curvilinear, or zigzag. The skin flaps are elevated, with care taken to leave some subcutaneous tissue on the underlying fascia investing the superficial musculotendinous layer of the forearm. The fascia is sharply incised in the shape and with the dimensions desired for the particular defect. The fascia is then elevated directly off the underlying muscles from the radial and ulnar directions, until the osseocutaneous septum is reached. Here, the radial artery and its accompanying veins run between the flexor carpi radialis and the brachioradialis. Sensory nerves are spared whenever possible.

The vessels are ligated and appropriately divided (distally for elbow coverage, proximally for hand coverage), and elevated along with the overlying fascia and subcutaneous tissue. For the distally based flap in particular, it is important to avoid skeletonizing the venae comitantes, as bridging vessels within the surrounding cuff of tissue contribute to retrograde venous flow (5).

The flap is skin-grafted after insetting. The donor site is closed directly (Figs. 3 and 4).

CLINICAL RESULTS

This flap has proved clinically reliable and useful for coverage of upper-extremity defects, as described. The most serious complications of hand ischemia or flap loss can be avoided entirely by careful preoperative evaluation of the arterial supply and appropriate dissection of the flap vessels. Inclusion of a thin layer of subcutaneous tissue with the fascia adds some padding—especially important for the elbow—and provides a good bed for skin-graft application. Injury to significant segments of the radial sensory nerve may lead to neuroma or dysesthesia.

SUMMARY

The radial forearm fascial flap can be used with minimal donor defect for upper-extremity defects, when thin tissue is desirable. The flap is reliable and can be elevated relatively rapidly, avoiding the need for microvascular anastomoses. The flap is versatile enough to be used as a free flap, as well (6,7).

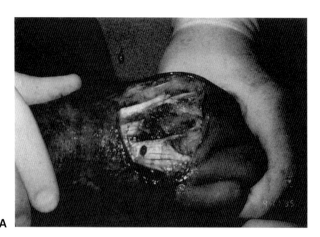

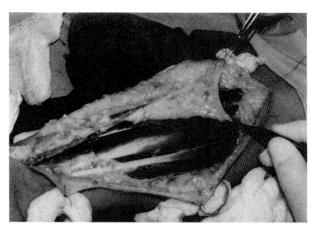

FIG. 3. Case 1. A: Patient with defect on dorsal aspect of hand with exposed tendon. B: Distally based fascial flap elevated with radial artery and accompanying veins. *(continued)*

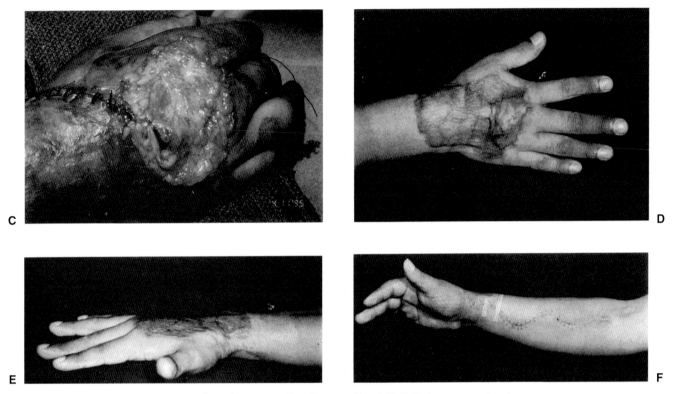

FIG. 3. *Continued.* **C:** Flap inset on dorsal aspect of hand. **D–F:** Early postoperative views.

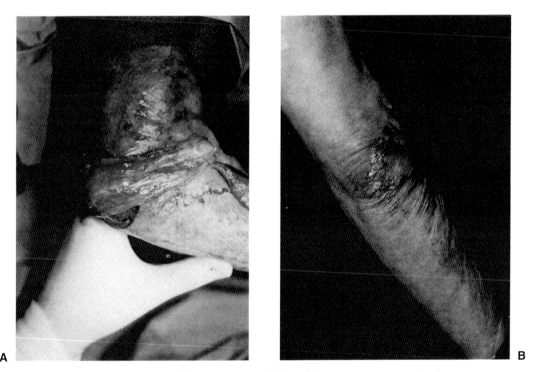

FIG. 4. Case 2. **A:** Insetting of flap for coverage of elbow defect. **B:** Late postoperative view.

References

1. Jin Y, Guan W, Shi T, et al. Reversed island forearm fascial flap in hand surgery. *Ann Plast Surg* 1985;15:340.
2. Reyes FA, Burkhalter WE. The fascial radial arm flap. *J Hand Surg* 1988; 13A:432.
3. Cheruup LL, Zachary LS, Gottlieb II, Petti CA. The radial forearm skin graft-fascial flap. *Plast Reconstr Surg* 1990;85:898.
4. Weinzweig N, Chen L, Chen Z. The distally based radial forearm fasciosubcutaneous flap with preservation of the radial artery: an anatomic and clinical approach. *Plast Reconstr Surg* 1994;94:675.
5. Lin S, Lai C, Chiu C. Venous drainage in the reverse forearm flap. *Plast Reconstr Surg* 1984;74:508.
6. Batchelor AG, Palmer JH. A novel method of closing a palatal fistula: the free fascial flap. *Br J Plast Surg* 1990;43:359.
7. Khouri RK, Ozbek MR, Hruza GJ, Young VL. Facial reconstruction with prefabricated induced expanded (PIE) supraclavicular skin flaps. *Plast Reconstr Surg* 1995;95:1007.

CHAPTER 290 ■ PEDICLED RADIAL FOREARM FASCIOSUBCUTANEOUS FLAP FOR HAND RECONSTRUCTION

N. WEINZWEIG

EDITORIAL COMMENT

This is an extremely clever variation of the radial forearm flap, utilizing perforating vessels alone. This allows for salvage of the radial artery itself. In a single-vessel forearm, this would be very critical.

The distally based radial forearm fasciosubcutaneous flap with preservation of the radial artery is a useful and reliable method for repairing soft-tissue defects of the hand. This flap avoids sacrificing a major artery, and militates against morbidity and a poor cosmetic appearance at the donor site (1–10). The flap is especially useful in traumatized and thermally injured hands, as well as in cases in which only the radial artery is functioning.

INDICATIONS

This flap is a safe, simple, and effective one-stage procedure that incorporates the thin, pliable, richly vascularized subcutaneous tissue and fascia of the forearm, vital to preserve exposed and/or damaged structures such as bone, joint, or tendon. It can be readily employed for coverage of the thumb-index web space, the palm, and the dorsum of the hand. The flap is easy to contour, making it an excellent choice for the tetrahedral first web space. It can also be used in the situation following tendon grafting or tenolysis, providing a smooth gliding surface. Previous burns to the forearm, with injury to the superficial venous system, do not prohibit use of the flap; instead, it is often the primary option in reconstructive surgery of the burned hand. In cases where bone is required, in addition to soft tissue, the classic osteofasciocutaneous flap should be employed.

Both donor and recipient sites are located within the same operative field. The donor-site skin is closed primarily, surviving on its dermal vascular network, with no underlying subcutaneous support, thus minimizing the cosmetic deformity. There is minimal discomfort postoperatively, facilitating early mobilization and rehabilitation.

ANATOMY

The pedicled radial forearm flap for hand reconstruction has been widely described in its many forms (2–5,11–20), based on the radial artery and its venae comitantes or with preservation of these vessels. The pedicled radial forearm fasciosubcutaneous flap described here is based on the perforating vessels of the distal radial artery. The blood supply emanates from 6 to 10 septocutaneous perforators in the vicinity of the anatomic "snuff box." These vessels fan out at the level of the deep fascia to form a rich plexus supplying the forearm fascia and subcutaneous tissue.

Perforators originate approximately 1.5 cm proximal to the radial styloid and recur proximally at 0.4- to 1.5-cm intervals, arising from both the radial and ulnar aspects of the radial artery, and measuring between 0.3 and 0.8 mm in external diameter (Fig. 1). There appears to be a definite directional component, with the arterioles running longitudinally along the intermuscular septum, and the fascial perforators passing transversely from these arterioles. Multiple transverse anastomoses occur between these vessels.

Venous drainage is from both the superficial and deep systems. There are multiple anastomoses between these venous channels. One or both venae comitantes ordinarily follow each of the fascial arterial perforators, with communicating branches between the venae comitantes allowing reverse flow via both crossover and bypass patterns. Sufficient reverse flow venous drainage occurs to ensure flap survival.

The reverse-flow fasciocutaneous flap is pedicled on the distal fascia and subcutaneous tissue and the fasciosubcutaneous vascular network described. It is a random-pattern flap, as there is no axial artery in the pedicle. However, incorporation of sizable perforating vessels and a well-developed longitudinal vascular network within the subcutaneous tissue provide significant vascularity to the flap.

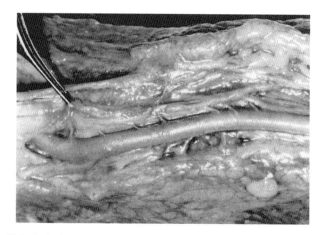

FIG. 1. At least seven septocutaneous perforators emanate from the radial aspect of the distal radial artery at 0.4- to 1.5-cm intervals, to nourish the forearm fascia.

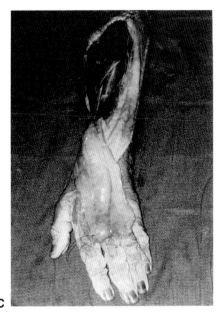
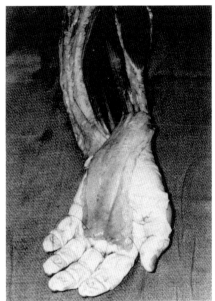
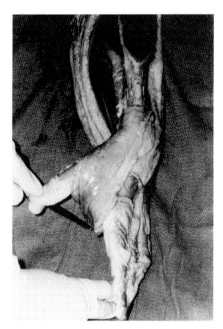

A–C

FIG. 2. **A–C:** Cadaver dissection. The radial forearm fascial flap is based solely on the distal perforators of the radial artery. The pivot point is located 5 to 8 cm above the radial styloid along the dorsoradial aspect of the hand. Care must be taken to identify and preserve the superficial radial nerve as it emerges between the brachioradialis and extensor carpi radialis longus tendons 8 to 11 cm above the radial styloid. The arc of rotation of this flap facilitates coverage of the dorsum of the hand (**A**), the palm (**B**), and the thumb-index web space (**C**).

FLAP DESIGN AND DIMENSIONS

The flap can be utilized for coverage of the dorsum of the hand, the palm, and the thumb-index web space (Fig. 2). It is designed based on the distal perforating vessels of the radial artery and its venae comitantes. The flap should measure at least 6 cm in width, so as to include as much of the longitudinal plexus of vessels as possible; its longitudinal axis is centralized directly over the radial vessels. The pivot point is situated at least 5 to 8 cm above the radial styloid. This is the usual site of the most proximal perforating vessel of the distal zone of perforators of the radial artery.

The flap is planned in reverse using a template, with its distal edge placed at the pivot point. The maximal dimensions are not yet known. Flaps with surface areas of up to 96 cm^2 have been reliably harvested; however, larger flaps, incorporating much of the forearm fasciosubcutaneous tissue, can probably be safely elevated and transferred. The flap is designed slightly larger than the measured defect, including as many of the distal perforating vessels as possible, and accounting for variation in the location of the most proximal of the distal perforating vessels. This will ensure maximum flap vascularity.

OPERATIVE TECHNIQUE

Following elevation exsanguination of the upper extremity, dissection proceeds under tourniquet control. A curvilinear or S-shaped incision, oriented along the central axis of the proposed flap directly over the radial vessels, is carried through skin and down to the relatively avascular plane just beneath the hair follicles and dermis.

Using loupe magnification, skin undermining proceeds radially and ulnarly in this plane to the margins of the proposed flap. The lateral antebrachial cutaneous nerve is identified coursing superficially through the subcutaneous tissue. The superficial radial nerve is identified as it emerges between

the brachioradialis and extensor carpi radialis longus tendons, and preserved.

The incision is deepened along the margins of the flap, to incorporate the deep fascia overlying the muscle bellies of the flexor carpi ulnaris, palmaris longus, flexor digitorum superficialis, and flexor carpi radialis. Subfascial dissection then proceeds expeditiously over the muscle bellies proximally and the tendons distally. Sparse proximal and middle zone perforators are serially ligated. Flap transfer should be attempted before the first distal zone perforator is visualized, if possible. Sacrifice of the distal perforating vessels should be avoided, unless absolutely necessary to cover the defect. The fasciosubcutaneous flap can be transferred to cover the defect either through a subcutaneous tunnel or turned over distally 180°.

The redundant edges of the forearm cutaneous flaps, supplied by the dermal vascular plexus, can be conservatively trimmed back for several millimeters, so as to maximize their vascularity; however, closure must be accomplished without any tension whatsoever. Suction drains are placed beneath the flap and the donor skin flaps. Biobrane, a sterile dressing, and a short-arm plaster splint are applied. Delayed skin grafting is performed on the third or fourth postoperative day, after flap edema has subsided.

CLINICAL RESULTS

During the past 4 years, eight flaps were utilized in seven patients. Flaps were employed for coverage of the thumb-index web space (three cases), the dorsum of the hand (four cases) (Fig. 3), and both the palm and dorsum of the hand (one case). Soft-tissue coverage was undertaken following reconstructive procedures such as tendon grafting, tenolysis, and bone grafting, in patients sustaining crush-avulsion injuries, severe infections, shotgun blasts, and thermal insults. Flap sizes ranged from 30 cm^2 to 286 cm^2 (mean: 106.2 cm^2).

Flap survival was excellent in seven of the eight cases. Minor flap loss was limited to the peripheral margin and

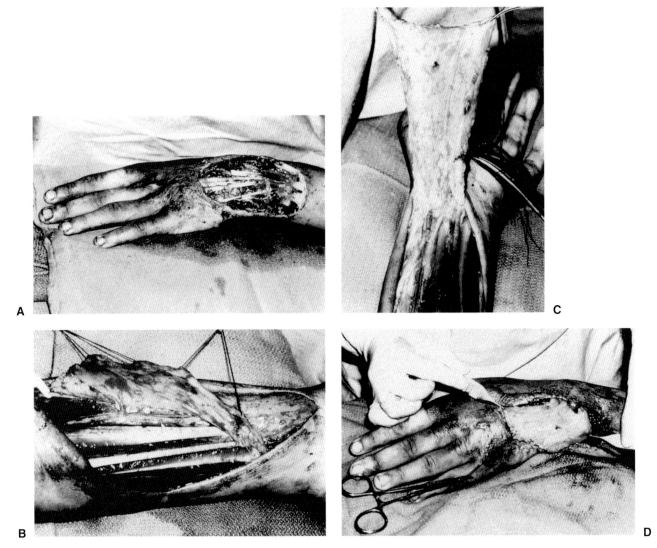

FIG. 3. A 15-year-old male patient who sustained a severe crush-avulsion injury to the dorsum of the hand. **A:** Following debridement, a retinacular flap is used to cover the exposed carpus, and the extensor tendons are repaired. **B:** During elevation of the fasciosubcutaneous flap in a proximal-to-distal fashion, the sparse middle-zone perforators (*on background*) of the radial artery (*arrow*) are identified and serially ligated. The superficial branch of the radial nerve is encircled with a vessel loop and protected as it is carefully dissected away from the flap. **C:** The radial forearm fasciosubcutaneous flap is elevated. Note that the radial artery and venae comitantes are left intact. **D:** The flap is tunneled subcutaneously to cover the dorsal defect.

most distal portion of the flap. Only the largest flap in the series, incorporating virtually the entire forearm fasciosubcutaneous tissue and measuring 286 cm^2, suffered significant loss. This was most likely due to the intricate method of flap transfer, which folded the flap upon itself several times in order to achieve coverage of both the palm and dorsum of the hand.

Despite the excellent vascularity observed following release of the tourniquet, several flaps in the series suffered minor skin-graft loss for unexplained reasons. Moderate flap edema, with an apparent decrease in flap vascularity, was observed for 3 to 4 days postoperatively, followed by dramatic spontaneous improvement in flap perfusion, probably related to gradual flap accommodation to the reverse-pattern venous flow. Of interest, others have observed this same phenomenon following the immediate skin grafting of fascial flaps, with no obvious explanation. Skin grafting is now delayed until flap edema subsides, to avoid this potential problem.

Donor sites healed uneventfully, except for a narrow margin of the forearm skin edges in two cases, which healed secondarily without problem. Functionally, results were related to the extent of the original injury and to the patient's compliance with occupational therapy. Even in the one patient who had previously sustained a thermal burn to his midvolar forearm, there were no problems with the vascularity of either the fasciosubcutaneous or donor skin flaps.

SUMMARY

The distally based radial forearm fasciosubcutaneous flap, based on the perforating vessels of the distal radial artery, can be a very useful and reliable procedure in hand reconstruction, and obviates the need for the classic fasciocutaneous flap or even a free flap. Not only is the radial artery preserved, which is essential in cases where only this vessel is functioning after severe trauma, but a more acceptable donor site is also provided.

References

1. Weinzweig N, Chen L, Chen Z-W. The distally based radial forearm fascio-subcutaneous flap with preservation of the radial artery: an anatomic and clinical approach. *Plast Reconstr Surg* 1994;94:675.
2. Stock W, Muhlhauer W, Biemer E. Der neurovaskulare Unterarm-Insel-Lappen. *Z Plast Chir* 1981;5:158.
3. Lu KH, Zhong DC, Chen B, Luo JW. The clinical applications of the reverse forearm island flap. *Chin J Surg* 1982;20:695.
4. Reid D, Moss ALH. One-stage repair with vascularized tendon grafts in a dorsal hand injury using the "Chinese" forearm flap. *Br J Plast Surg* 1983;36:473.
5. Soutar DS, Tanner NSB. The radial forearm flap in the management of soft tissue injuries of the hand. *Br J Plast Surg* 1984;37:18.
6. Yang G, Yang C, Chen B, et al. Forearm free skin flap transplantation. *Natl Med J China* 1978;61:139.
7. Song R, Gao Y, Song Y, et al. The forearm flap. *Clin Plast Surg* 1982;9:21.
8. Timmons MJ, Missotten FEM, Poole MD, Davies DM. Complications of radial forearm flap donor sites. *Br J Plast Surg* 1986;39:176.
9. Boorman G, Brown JA, Sykes PJ. Morbidity in the forearm flap donor arm. *Br J Plast Surg* 1987;40:207.
10. Brenner P, Berger A, Caspary L. Angiologic observations following autologous vein grafting and free radial artery flap elevation. *J Reconstr Microsurg* 1988;4:297.
11. Biemer E, Stock W. Total thumb reconstruction: a one-stage reconstruction using an osteocutaneous forearm flap. *Br J Plast Surg* 1983;36:52.
12. Foucher B, van Genechten F, Merle N, Michon J. A compound radial artery forearm flap in hand surgery: an original modification of the Chinese forearm flap. *Br J Plast Surg* 1984;37:139.
13. Jin Y-T, Guan W-X, Shi T-M, et al. Reversed island forearm fascial flap in hand surgery. *Ann Plast Surg* 1985;15:340.
14. Reyes FA, Burkhalter WE. The fascial radial flap. *J Hand Surg* 1988;13A:432.
15. Chang YT, Wang XF, et al. The reversed forearm fasciocutaneous flap in hand reconstruction: ten successful cases. *Chin J Plast Surg Burns* 1988;4:41.
16. Marty FM, Montandon D, Gumener R, Zbrodowski A. The use of subcutaneous tissue flaps in the repair of soft tissue defects of the forearm and hand: an experimental and clinical study of a new technique. *Br J Plast Surg* 1984;37:95.
17. Lai C-S, Lin S-D, Chou C-K, Tsai C-W. Clinical application of adipofascial turn-over flaps for burn wounds. *Burns* 1993;19:73.
18. Yang J-Y, Noordhoff MS. Early adipofascial flap coverage of deep electrical burn wounds of upper extremities. *Plast Reconstr Surg* 1993;91:819.
19. Lamberty BGH, Cormack GC. The forearm angiotomes. *Br J Plast Surg* 1982;35:420.
20. Timmons MJ. The vascular basis of the radial forearm flap. *Plast Reconstr Surg* 1986;77:80.

CHAPTER 291 ■ POSTERIOR INTEROSSEOUS ARTERY FLAP

C. R. GSCHWIND AND M. A. TONKIN

EDITORIAL COMMENT

This can serve as a very useful flap for resurfacing defects in the hand. Dissection is not easy, but once mastered, a good and serviceable flap can be provided.

The posterior interosseous artery (PIA) flap does not compromise the two principal arteries of the forearm (1). It is generally raised as a distally based pedicle flap with reversed blood flow, to cover small to medium-sized defects on the dorsum of the hand and proximal phalanges, or defects in the first web space and on the thumb.

INDICATIONS

Defects on the dorsum of the hand require coverage with a thin, pliable flap, and flap sensation is usually not of primary importance. If flap sensation is required, the posterior antebrachial cutaneous nerve can be identified and connected with an appropriate recipient nerve (2,3). Using a distally based pedicle PIA flap, even when the pedicle is raised to its maximal length, the flap cannot be extended beyond the proximal interphalangeal joint of the fingers. It is therefore most suitable for small or medium-sized dorsal hand or thumb web defects. Hair growth and pedicle length make the PIA flap less optimal for coverage of palmar defects.

Small or moderate-sized defects around the elbow can be covered by a proximally based PIA flap with anterograde blood flow (2–8). Use as a fasciocutaneous flap, a fascial flap, an osteomyocutaneous flap (9), and a free flap (10) has been reported. To avoid an unsightly donor area and possible donor-site morbidity, direct closure of the defect is desirable; however, this limits the width of a fasciocutaneous flap to 4 to 5 cm.

ANATOMY

At the level of the radial tuberosity, the common interosseous artery arises from the ulnar artery and divides into posterior and anterior interosseous branches. The PIA passes through the chorda obliqua and the interosseous membrane deep to the supinator, and enters the posterior compartment of the forearm (Fig. 1). The artery lies ulnar-dorsal to the posterior interosseous nerve. The surface marking for the point of entry into the posterior compartment is located at the junction of the middle and proximal thirds on a line drawn between the lateral epicondyle and the inferior radioulnar joint (Fig. 2). The artery and nerve then pass under the fibrous arcade of the extensor

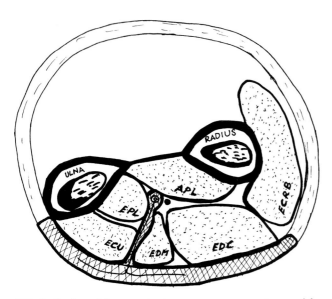

FIG. 1. Outline of the posterior interosseous artery, septum, and fasciocutaneous territory.

muscles of the fingers, to enter the septum between the extensor digiti minimi laterally and the extensor carpi ulnaris medially.

Further distally, the artery lies between the long abductor and long extensor muscles of the thumb, and then under the extensor indicis muscle. Along its course within the septum, the artery gives off between 7 and 13 cutaneous branches and 13 to 22 muscular and periosteal branches. The septocutaneous branches anastomose in the superficial layer of the deep fascia, and form arcades with longitudinal anastomoses. Three patterns of distribution have been described for the fasciocutaneous perforators (5). Most commonly, there is a perforator every 1 to 2 cm. The largest one is the most proximal perforator, which often originates from the common interosseous artery or the recurrent branch of the PIA. The constancy of a large cutaneous perforator, 1 to 2 cm distal to the midpoint of the epicondylar-ulnar line, has been demonstrated (8). Cadaver studies have shown that the PIA narrows in the middle third of the forearm. In 5% of clinical cases and anatomic dissections, the PIA terminates at mid-forearm level.

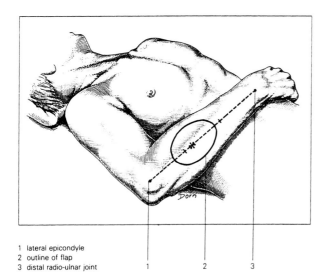

1 lateral epicondyle
2 outline of flap
3 distal radio-ulnar joint

FIG. 2. Surface markings and flap design. (From Tubiana et al., ref. 12, with permission.)

Near the wrist joint, the artery communicates with the anterior interosseous artery, the dorsal carpal network, and the ulnar artery. Absence of any distal communication is rare, but well described (1,3,7,11). The transverse branch between the PIA and the dorsal branch of the anterior interosseous artery is the most consistent and important anastomosis, and lies under the extensor indicis proprius tendon, about 1 to 2 cm proximal to the inferior radioulnar joint. This represents the pivot point of the distally based PIA pedicle flap.

At the point of entry into the dorsal compartment, the caliber of the artery varies from 0.9 to 2.7 mm. At the level of the communication with the anterior interosseous artery, the caliber varies between 0.2 and 1.2 mm. A small caliber of the vessel can be responsible for flap failure, when retrograde flow through the pedicle cannot perfuse the proximally based flap adequately. Venous drainage of the distally based flap depends on reversed blood flow through the venae comitantes.

The relationship between the PIA and the posterior interosseous nerve may pose significant problems in flap dissection. At the entrance into the dorsal compartment, the nerve gives off branches to the epicondylar muscles, i.e., the extensor carpi ulnaris, extensor digiti minimi, and extensor digitorum communis. The artery is commonly crossed over by the posterior interosseous nerve branch to the extensor carpi ulnaris. In some cases, the branch crosses over the PIA and the most proximal significant septocutaneous perforator. In the septum, the posterior interosseous nerve is found deep and radial to the artery, but often within a distance of only 1 to 3 mm. The nerve gives off five branches to the abductor pollicis longus, extensor pollicis brevis, extensor pollicis longus, and extensor indicis proprius, from proximal to distal. After supplying the extensor indicis proprius muscle, the nerve is sensory for the wrist capsule.

The dorsal ulnar skin of the forearm is innervated proximally by the posterior antebrachial cutaneous nerve, and distally by branches of the medial and lateral antebrachial cutaneous nerves. The posterior antebrachial cutaneous nerve can be identified and used to make the flap sensate.

The cutaneous territory of the PIA flap extends from 2 to 3 cm below the elbow crease to the wrist. The ulnar margin is defined by the subcutaneous border of the ulna. Medially, the territory extends to the radial border of the radius, i.e., a line drawn from the lateral epicondyle to the radial styloid.

FLAP DESIGN AND DIMENSIONS

Classically, the flap is centered on the emergence of the artery in the posterior compartment in the proximal forearm. Small flaps should be designed distally to the point of emergence of the PIA, in order to include the septocutaneous perforator in the lower two-thirds of the forearm. In a large series (8), the authors recommend keeping the flap design distal to the proximal quarter of the epicondylar-ulnar line, in order to avoid proximal flap necrosis. More proximal extension of the flap depends on random-pattern perfusion, which may be variable, according to the distance to the most proximal septocutaneous perforator.

Distally, the cutaneous radial nerve and dorsal cutaneous branch of the ulnar nerve can be damaged in flap dissection. The distal limit should be about 3 to 4 cm above the wrist joint. Medially, the flap should not extend beyond the subcutaneous border of the ulna. The radial margin should not extend more than 3 to 4 cm from the epicondylar-ulnar line. It is possible to raise a flap of 10 cm in width; however, skin grafting is necessary for defects greater than 4 to 5 cm.

The pivot point of the pedicle is just proximal to the level of the inferior radioulnar joint, i.e., the anastomosis with the anterior interosseous artery. As this connection is occasionally absent, a preoperative Doppler evaluation is recommended.

For a proximally based flap, the skin territory is designed on the lower third of the forearm. The first medium-sized

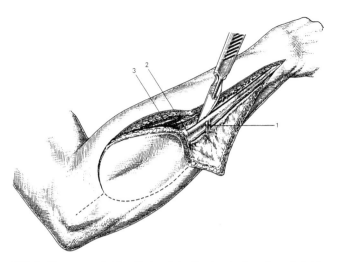

FIG. 3. The septum is identified and the flap is raised on the radial side first. *1:* cutaneous pedicle within the septum. *2:* aponeurosis. *3:* extensor digitorum communis. (From Tubiana et al., ref. 12, with permission.)

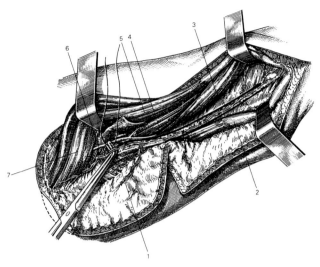

FIG. 5. The posterior interosseous artery is dissected proximally and ligated distal to the nerve branch to the extensor carpi ulnaris. *1:* proximal ligature of the posterior interosseous artery. *2:* extensor carpi ulnaris. *3:* extensor indicis proprius. *4:* abductor pollicis longus. *5:* extensor digiti minimi. *6:* posterior interosseous nerve. *7:* supinator. (From Tubiana et al., ref. 12, with permission.)

perforator is placed about 7.5 cm above the wrist joint. Flap design should not go more distally, in order to avoid damage to the radial and ulnar sensory nerve branches. The pivot point of the pedicle is at the emergence of the PIA, at the junction of the upper and mid-third of the forearm. A fibrous band deep to the extensor digiti minimi indicates a level at which the pedicle is long enough to reach the anterior aspect of the elbow or the olecranon.

OPERATIVE TECHNIQUE

Distally Based Pedicle Flap

The elbow is positioned in full pronation and 90° of flexion. Surface markings indicate the lateral epicondyle and inferior radioulnar joint. The point at the junction between the proximal and middle third marks the emergence of the PIA in the

dorsal extensor compartment; this is 7.5 to 9.5 cm distal to the lateral epicondyle. Flap design should not extend more than 3 cm proximal to this point. Small flaps should be centered on the midpoint of the epicondylar-ulnar line.

The flap is outlined, depending on the size of the defect (Fig. 2). For flap siting, it is wise to continue the distal margin of the design beyond the midpoint of the epicondylar-ulnar line, to include the constant perforator previously described (8). The distal incision is extended just to the level of the deep fascia (Fig. 3). The septum between the extensor carpi ulnaris and the extensor digiti minimi is identified, and the fascia incised on either side of the septum. The PIA is identified, and the communication with the anterior interosseous artery, after retraction of the extensor indicis proprius tendon, is verified (Figs. 4 and 5).

The septum containing the artery and its perforators is dissected proximally to the skin paddle, by retracting the extensor carpi ulnaris medially and the extensor digiti minimi and extensor indicis proprius to the radial side (Fig. 6). The skin-

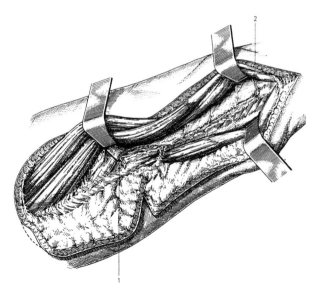

FIG. 4. The deep arch of the extensor digitorum communis is incised to obtain a view of the artery emerging from underneath the supinator muscle. *1:* extensor carpi ulnaris. *2:* posterior interosseous artery with venae comitantes. (From Tubiana et al., ref. 12, with permission.)

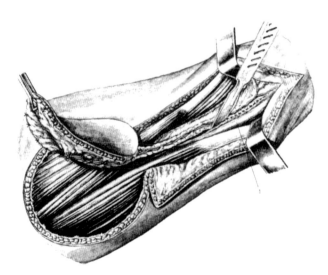

FIG. 6. After raising the ulnar side of the skin paddle, the pedicle is dissected off the ulnar shaft. *1:* ulnar shaft. (From Tubiana et al., ref. 12, with permission.)

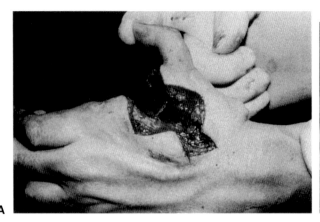 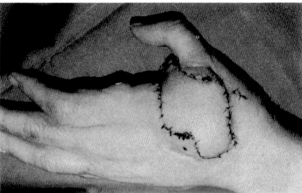

A   B

FIG. 7. A,B: Posterior interosseous artery flap after release of first web contracture. Retrograde flow was insufficient, and the flap was transferred as a free flap. (From Tonkin and Stern, ref. 10, with permission.)

paddle incision is carried through the level of the fascia, and an extra 1 cm of fascia is included circumferentially. To avoid shearing forces between the skin and the fascia, fine absorbable stitches are used to fix the fascia to the skin. The skin paddle itself is then raised with the fascia, beginning with dissection on the radial side over the wrist extensors, and more ulnarly over the common finger extensors.

The deep arch of the extensor digitorum communis has to be incised to obtain a clear view of the artery as it emerges from underneath the supinator. At this point, the posterior artery gives off its recurrent branch, which runs toward the elbow and gives off several musculocutaneous branches. This recurrent branch of the PIA can occasionally also give origin to the first significant fasciocutaneous perforator, in which case part of it may be included in the dissection. Inclusion of this perforator is mandatory only when there is no main perforator present farther distally.

Under magnification, the PIA is also isolated from the branches of the posterior interosseous nerve. The motor branch to the extensor carpi ulnaris crosses superficial to the interosseous recurrent artery when it arises proximally, or crosses the PIA when it arises distal to the supinator. When this motor branch is found to cross the posterior interosseous vessel, the vessel should be ligated distal to the nerve (Fig. 5). The ulnar side of the skin paddle is then raised, and the pedicle itself is dissected off the ulnar shaft (Fig. 6).

If there is any doubt about the presence or size of the distal anastomosis between the PIA and the anterior interosseous artery, the PIA is temporarily occluded with a small artery clamp at its most proximal point. The tourniquet is let down, and the adequacy of the retrograde flow is verified. It is at this point that

a decision may be made to resort to a free-flap transfer (Fig. 7), if the distal anastomosis is too small and the retrograde flow insufficient for flap survival. The PIA may be dissected proximally and the flap transferred as a free flap, or the dissection is abandoned and the flap returned to its original site.

After mobilization of the pedicle, the flap can then be inset on the dorsum or the palm of the hand (Figs. 7 and 8). The donor defect can be closed primarily, when flap width does not exceed 4 to 5 cm. Otherwise, a split-thickness skin graft is necessary.

Proximally Based Pedicle Flap

The skin flap is outlined on the distal aspect of the forearm. The distal flap limit should be at least 3 cm above the inferior radioulnar joint. The tendons of the extensor digiti minimi and extensor carpi ulnaris are retracted after their fascia has been incised, and raised *en bloc* with the septum. The pedicle is followed proximally, and care is taken to separate the nerve from the artery. The artery is followed as far as the fibrous band deep to the extensor digiti minimi. This usually provides sufficient length to cover defects on the anterior aspect of the elbow or over the olecranon.

ALTERNATIVE TECHNIQUES

Elevation as a Fascial Flap

The technique is the same as previously described, but after the skin incision only the fascia is raised. It is important to leave a

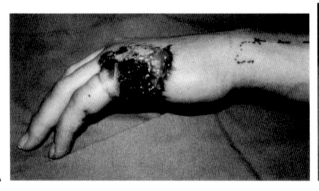 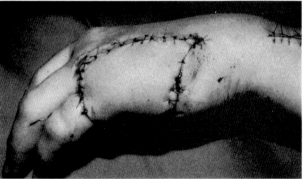

A   B

FIG. 8. A,B: Distally pedicled flap used for coverage of a defect on the lateral aspect of the hand, after traumatic amputation of the little finger and revascularization of the ring finger.

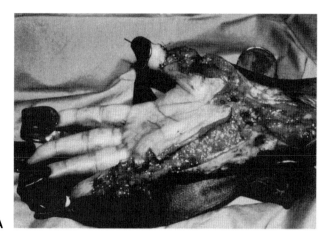

A

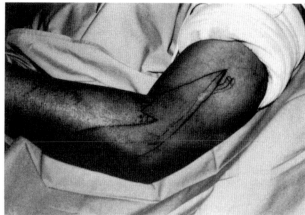

B

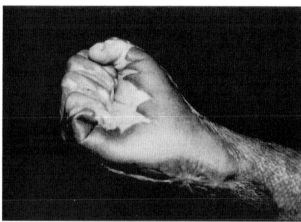

C

FIG. 2. Clinical case. **A:** Complex palmar defect following release of severe burn contracture. **B:** Design of the bilobed proximal forearm flap. **C:** Final outcome, flexion.

the septa attach to the lateral epicondyle, the dissection is just superficial to the periosteum.

The posterior cutaneous nerve of the forearm is preserved within the flap, and enough length is retained to allow repair to a sensory nerve at the recipient site. Above the lateral epicondyle, the dissection continues, as described for the lateral arm flap (4). If only the forearm skin is to be utilized, a proximal extension of skin overlying the pedicle is included, resembling a tennis racket, to aid in a tensionless skin closure at the recipient site. For additional length and pedicle size, the profunda brachii can be traced back to its origin by a separate medial approach (6).

CLINICAL RESULTS

We have performed 31 proximal forearm flaps on 29 patients. Twenty were for upper-extremity reconstruction, seven for lower-extremity reconstruction, and four for penile construction. The sizes of the flaps ranged from 35 × 12 cm to 14 × 5 cm (average: 24 × 10 cm). The flaps extended beyond the lateral condyle for a distance of 7 to 15 cm (average: 10 cm). The reach of the flap from proximal pedicle to flap tip ranged from 35 to 14 cm (average: 22 cm). Follow-up ranged from 6 months to 2 years. Results have been quite acceptable (Fig. 2).

SUMMARY

By including the rich vascular plexus that terminates the posterior radial collateral artery and extends well into the forearm, the pedicle of the lateral arm flap can perfuse the entire posterior proximal half of the forearm, capturing the cutaneous territory of the posterior interosseous artery. The posterior cutaneous nerve of the forearm provides constant direct innervation to the proximal forearm flap. The flap can be used as a pedicled or free flap, depending on the recipient site, and it provides very thin sensate skin, with minimal donor-site morbidity.

References

1. Kuek LB, Chuan TL. The extended lateral arm flap: a new modification. *J Reconstr Microsurg* 1991;7:167.
2. Rivet D, Buffet M, Martin D, et al. The lateral arm flap: an anatomical study. *J Reconstr Microsurg* 1987;3:121.
3. Brand KE, Khouri RK. The lateral arm/proximal forearm flap. *Plast Reconstr Surg* 1993;92:1137.
4. Katsaros J, Schusterman M, Beppu M, et al. The lateral upper arm flap: anatomy and clinical applications. *Ann Plast Surg* 1984;12:489.
5. Schusterman M, Katsaros J, Beppu M. The lateral arm flap: an experimental and clinical study. In: Williams HB, ed. *Transactions of the VIII International Congress of Plastic Surgery.* 1983;132.
6. Acland RD, Madison S, Moffet TR, et al. A long-pedicled extension of the lateral upper arm flap. Presented at the VIth Annual Meeting of the American Society of Reconstructive Microsurgery, Toronto, Canada, 1990.

CHAPTER 293. Paired Abdominal Skin Flaps for the Hand *T. Miura*

www.encyclopediaofflaps.com

CHAPTER 294 ■ ANTERIOR CHEST WALL SKIN FLAPS TO THE FOREARM AND HAND

R. G. KATZ AND W. L. WHITE*

The application of a skin flap to the forearm or hand may be indicated as part of the initial treatment of an acute wound involving a loss of skin, or as the first step in later reconstruction of a disabled upper extremity (1). At the current time in the era of axial pattern flaps and free flaps, random pattern flaps originating from the anterior chest wall remain an infrequently needed but useful tool in the hand surgeon's armamentarium (2,3).

INDICATIONS

Cutaneous defects of the upper limb can usually be repaired with skin grafts or with local skin flaps. When these two modalities are not satisfactory, flaps from a distance are indicated. Chest wall flaps have the advantage of permitting elevation of the hand at the time of initial application, in distinction to flaps originating on the abdomen or in the groin that require placement of the extremity in a dependent position.

FLAP DESIGN AND DIMENSIONS

A skin flap from the anterior chest wall originates in the area bounded by the nipple line superiorly, the umbilicus inferiorly, and the midaxillary line laterally. Considerations in the selection of a flap donor site include the location and size of the recipient site, the ease of application of the flap to the extremity, the patient's comfort while the extremity is immobilized, the availability and quality of skin at the tentative donor site, and the resultant cosmetic deformity at the flap donor site.

Anterolateral Chest Wall Skin Flap

Flaps based laterally on the lower anterolateral chest derive their blood supply from the intercostal and the thoracoepigastric vessels. The skin in this area has great mobility, as it normally must move over the flare of the lower ribs during movements of the thorax (Fig. 1). In comparison with the lower abdomen, this skin is more pliable, the subcutaneous fat layer is thinner, and the surrounding skin is more elastic. These characteristics usually permit elevation and application of the flap in one stage and closure of the donor defect without resorting to a skin graft. In addition, the thinner tissue in the anterolateral chest resembles that of the hand and forearm and allows accurate fitting of the flap, minimizing the need for a secondary defatting of the flap. The fact that there is generally scant growth of hair in this area is an additional benefit (4).

Contralateral Anterolateral Chest Wall Flap

The anterolateral chest opposite to the side of the injured upper extremity is an ideal source of skin flaps not exceeding approximately 7 to 8 cm in width and approximately 10 to 12 cm in length (length to width ratio of approximately 1.5:1) for application to the digits, palm, dorsum of the hand, and occasionally to the wrist. These transversely oriented flaps should not extend across the ventral midline, since the collateral blood supply of the skin across the midline in this region is poor (Fig. 4).

Ipsilateral Anterior Chest Wall Flap

Flaps based on the lower anterolateral chest on the same side as the involved upper extremity are best suited for coverage about the elbow, forearm, and proximal wrist (4). These flaps may be based laterally, superiorly, or inferiorly, and if need be, can be extended to the upper abdomen. These flaps have a length to width ratio of approximately 1.5:1.

Anteromedial Chest Wall Flap

Flaps originating on the anterior chest wall can also be based medially. The blood supply to these flaps is provided by perforating vessels from the internal thoracic artery and/or the superior epigastric artery. By placing the base of the flap approximately 5 to 6 cm from the midline, the important vascular system nourishing the flap is maintained. If a flap is of appropriate width, it can extend in length to the region of the anterior axillary line. Such flaps have previously been

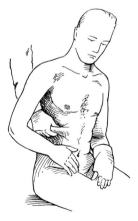

FIG. 1. The tissue over the flare of the lower ribs is thin, pliable, generally hairless, and well vascularized. The tissue laxity is such as generally to allow direct closure of the donor defect. (From White, ref. 2, with permission.)

* Deceased.

862

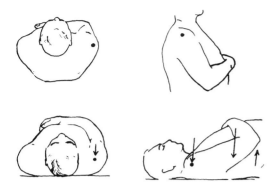

FIG. 2. The cross-chest position of the forearm in an obese or emphysematous patient is easily obtained with the body upright. On reclining, however, the thorax is thrust anteriorly and the shoulders fall posteriorly. This produces tension on the attached flap. (*Upper left and right*) Views of the upper extremity position with the patient standing. (*Lower left and right*) Views of the upper extremity position with the patient supine. (From White, ref. 2, with permission.)

described for use in breast reconstruction (5,6). These flaps are suitable for application to the hand or distal forearm and are based on the ipsilateral or contralateral side of the chest, depending on the location of the recipient site (Fig. 2).

Epigastric Skin Flap

When the recipient defect is large and is located on the distal forearm and/or the hand, an apron flap based inferiorly just above the umbilicus provides a great expanse of skin (Fig. 3). This flap is most useful in male patients and makes use of the cross-chest position. The width of these flaps is limited only by the width and convexity of the torso. The upper border of these flaps may be placed from the fifth intercostal space to the xyphoid tip. They may be 18 to 20 cm in width and 15 to 18 cm in length. If these flaps are divided and inset in stages, it is possible to resurface the distal forearm circumferentially. Delay procedures are more often required if the skin is not supple. Occasionally it is preferable to base these epigastric flaps superiorly in the region of the xyphoid. However, application of the flap may be technically difficult, as the skin of the upper abdomen is somewhat thicker and less pliable than that of the lower chest.

Infraclavicular Flap

When small skin flaps are needed for digital cover or for extension of the digits, the area just below the clavicle on the contralateral side is an excellent source of tissue (7). The skin

is thin, the blood supply is excellent, and the position the patient must maintain is both stable and comfortable. This area is not suitable for larger flaps and is contraindicated in women because of the unsightly scar. In men there may be a heavy growth of hair present in this area. With an obese or emphysematous patient, a flap suitable for the extremity without tension on the flap will be difficult to maintain (Fig. 2).

OPERATIVE TECHNIQUE

When applying a flap to the upper extremity, consideration should be given to attempting to obtain a closed wound in the flap donor site, the flap pedicle, as well as in the recipient site. A closed wound may be achieved by combining tubing of the flap pedicle, direct closure of the donor site, and skin-grafting open areas of the donor site and/or pedicle, as appropriate for the specific situation. This will avoid the undesirable inflammatory effects of an open wound on the hand and flap, and drainage from such a wound. Still, closure of the open area of a flap pedicle frequently is not practical and the open wound can be well managed with petrolatum-impregnated fine mesh gauze dressings.

Contralateral Anterolateral Flap

Closure of the defect may be facilitated and a dog-ear avoided by giving the flap a temporary extension (tapered to a point) across the midline. After the flap is elevated, the tissue that was beyond the midline should be discarded (Fig. 4). The ability to close the donor defect directly provides the potential for rotation of the flap through a range of 180° (Fig. 5). Rotation is accomplished by extending the superior or inferior limb of the initial incision. If the superior incision is extended laterally for a distance equal to the width of the flap, the flap will be rotated superiorly on closure of the donor site. Conversely, if the inferior limb of the initial incision is extended laterally, the flap will be rotated inferiorly. In general, the situation where the flap is ultimately based inferiorly (as shown in Fig. 3A) is the preferred orientation, inasmuch as it minimizes venous congestion and edema formation in the flap by permitting dependent drainage.

If the chest wall skin flap is to be tubed (as in application to a degloved thumb), the base of the flap is not rotated as discussed above. The margins of the donor defect are simply approximated and the flap is tubed. Since there is relatively little fat present about the lower chest, this flap may be tubed with minimal thinning. In addition, because of the excellent vascularity of the area, this flap seldom needs to be delayed.

Using the area above the umbilicus as a donor site for flaps to be applied to the hand and wrist permits the recipient forearm to be positioned across the lower chest and upper

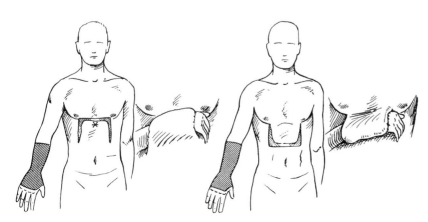

FIG. 3. Flaps from the epigastric area may be quite large. If they are based inferiorly, a delay procedure may be necessary. Because of the poor blood supply in the midline, tissue loss is frequently encountered in this area (*). The donor site defect should be closed by means of skin grafts. (From White, ref. 2, with permission.)

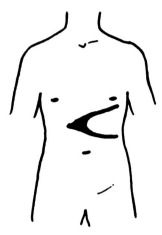

FIG. 4. The point of the flap reaching across the midline should be removed, as the blood supply across the midline in this area is poor. (From White, ref. 2, with permission.)

abdomen with the elbow flexed at approximately 90°. This cross-chest position of the forearm permits the patient significant comfort and mobility (Fig. 6). The arm is held flush with the trunk, preferable to having the elbow protrude, which would occur if the flap were raised from the ipsilateral chest area. The patient with his forearm fixed in a cross-chest position can wear street clothes and may be managed as an outpatient approximately 5 to 7 days after flap application.

Early in the postoperative period, with adult patients of slender or average habitus, the operated extremity is immobilized by dressings and elastic bandages. A light plaster covering added over the bandages ensures more secure mobilization and is recommended for children and some adults of heavy build.

Ipsilateral Anterior Chest Wall Flap

Depending on the size of the donor defect, direct closure of the donor site may not be possible and a skin graft may be required to close the donor defect and to cover the open area of the bridging portion of the flap pedicle. In the case of defects about the proximal forearm, there is usually little choice in regard to other skin flap donor sites. These flaps offer the same advantages of excellent tissue and ease of forearm positioning as described above.

Epigastric Skin Flaps

A split-thickness graft is necessary to close the flap donor site. The graft should cover the bridging portion of the flap as well.

In female patients, small donor defects located in the inframammary region can be closed with minimal deformity. However, the closure of large donor sites in this area may displace the breasts inferiorly. In those instances in female patients where a large flap is required, it is preferable to use the lower abdomen as the flap donor site.

Separation of Flaps: Delay Procedures

If the flap has a relatively large area of inset relative to the total area of the flap that is to be transferred, if there is no compromise of flap viability, and if the area of flap inset is well healed, then the flap may be divided 2 weeks after its application. Occasionally the division of a large flap may need to be undertaken in stages, particularly if an extension of the flap is needed to obtain tissue to wrap around the extremity. A trial clamping of the base of the flap may be done. The adequacy of the blood supply can be judged clinically by inspection or by fluorescence.

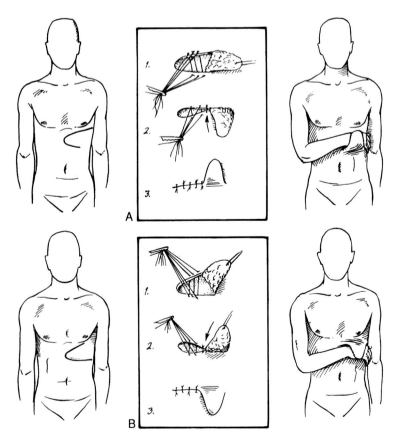

FIG. 5. Demonstrating the rotation of the flap which occurs when the superior (A) or inferior (B) limb of the donor site incision is extended and the donor site is closed. (From White, ref. 2, with permission.)

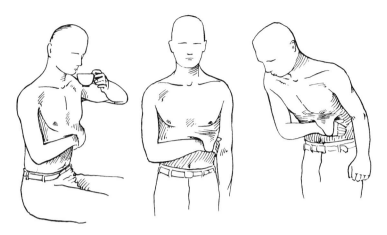

FIG. 6. The cross-chest position permits comfortable movement and independence of the patient. (From White, ref. 2, with permission.)

Occasionally after elevation, a flap will be noted to have poor color and circulation, necessitating returning it to the donor site and postponing its transfer. Although a delay procedure will improve flap circulation, it will cause some induration and fibrosis of the flap, making later fitting of the flap to the recipient site somewhat more difficult.

CLINICAL RESULTS

The application of an anterior chest wall flap to the upper extremity has the disadvantages of requiring significant immobilization of the shoulder and of producing scarring that is exposed when the patient is clothed in swimwear or similar attire.

The difficulty most frequently encountered in applying flaps from the anterior chest wall to the upper extremity is an increased anteroposterior diameter of the chest. This may be secondary to obesity but is more often caused by pulmonary emphysema. In these barrel-chested individuals, it is relatively easy to place the forearm across the trunk if the patient is standing or sitting. When the patient is supine, however, the rib cage is pushed anteriorly and the shoulders fall posteriorly. If this change of relative position of the chest and shoulders is not considered when the flap is planned, there will be difficulty achiev-

ing satisfactory immobilization of the extremity and this may result in tension on the flap base (Fig. 2). Placing the patient in a semi-sitting position in bed somewhat alleviates this problem.

SUMMARY

The chest wall can be a good source of skin flap coverage for hand and forearm defects, especially when other flaps are not available.

References

1. Gillies H. Design of direct pedicle flaps. *Br Med J* 1932;2:1008.
2. White WL. Cross-chest flap grafts. *Am J Surg* 1960;99:804.
3. White WL. Anterior chest wall skin flaps for the arm and hand. In: Grabb W, Myers B, eds. *Skin flaps.* Boston: Little, Brown, 1975;397.
4. Greeley PW. Practical procedures for correction of scar contractures of hand. *Am J Surg* 1947;74:622.
5. Cronin TD, Upton J, McDonough TM. Reconstruction of the breast after mastectomy. *Plast Reconstr Surg* 1977;59:1.
6. Davis WM, McCraw JM, Carraway JH. Use of a direct transverse, thoracoabdominal flap to close difficult wounds of the thorax and upper extremity. *Plast Reconstr Surg* 1977;60:526.
7. Chase RA. *Atlas of hand surgery.* Philadelphia: Saunders, 1973.

CHAPTER 295 ■ HAND SANDWICH

D. W. FURNAS

EDITORIAL COMMENT

As with all major reconstructive efforts, the possibility of amputation combined with a good working prosthesis should always be considered.

Major tissue losses involving both the volar and the dorsal surfaces of the upper limb present a formidable reconstructive problem. Paired flaps, forming a hand sandwich, have proved to be a satisfactory solution to this problem (1,2).

INDICATIONS

An earlier technique was designed at a time when the only axial flaps described were the deltopectoral flap, the groin flap, the epigastric flap, and the temporal artery flap. A trial with plastic patterns showed that the distance between a pair of groin flaps would have been too great for the flaps to reach the hand defect simultaneously. Thus, random pattern flaps were designed that satisfied the goal of immediate coverage of the exposed tendons, nerves, and bone.

FLAP DESIGN AND DIMENSIONS

In the original design (1), paired flaps on two separate opposing body surfaces, the chest and the upper arm, were used to envelop the raw hand (Fig. 1). Serial delay incisions on the arm and the chest were used to outline the tissue destined to resur-

face the distal parts of the hand. In the final stage, the flaps were elevated, the arm and chest were separated, and the flaps were closed over the hand. The raw surfaces of the hand and forearm were repaired with split-thickness skin grafts (Fig. 2).

The potential donor sites for "sandwich" coverage of the hand multiplied dramatically with the advent of musculocutaneous flaps, muscle flaps, and other useful axial flaps. The use of paired axial flaps was developed for the repair of a degloved hand (2). Ipsilateral groin and tensor fasciae latae flaps were used in an ingenious design (Figs. 3 and 4). This flap greatly improved on the original sandwich design by obviating delay incisions and improving mobility of the shoulder. Other musculocutaneous, muscle, and axial flaps would appear to have similar applicability.

Among possible candidates as hand sandwiches are (1) groin flap plus epigastric flap, (2) posterior trapezius musculocutaneous flap plus pectoralis major musculocutaneous flap, (3) latissimus dorsi musculocutaneous flap plus pectoralis musculocutaneous flap, and (4) paired gracilis flaps.

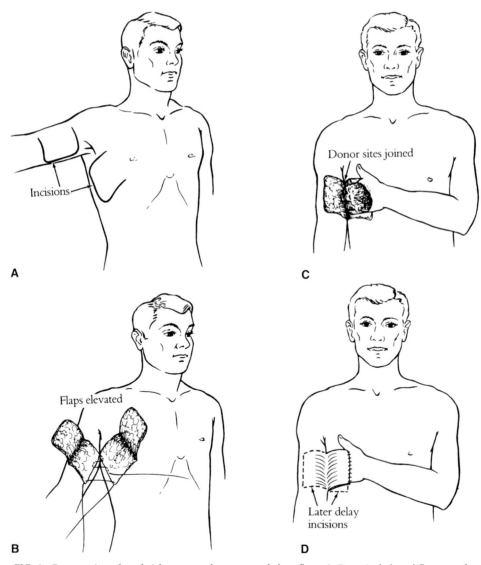

FIG. 1. Construction of sandwich coverage from arm and chest flaps. **A:** Posteriorly based flaps are plotted. (The entire axilla could be included in the flaps, but the axillary skin may have a less dependable blood supply.) **B:** The donor area of the arm is joined to the donor area of the chest, making an extended pocket. **C:** The raw hand is placed between the flaps. **D:** The flaps are sutured together, enveloping the hand. Additional skin can be gained by delay incisions (*dashed lines*). (From Smith and Furnas, ref. 1, with permission.)

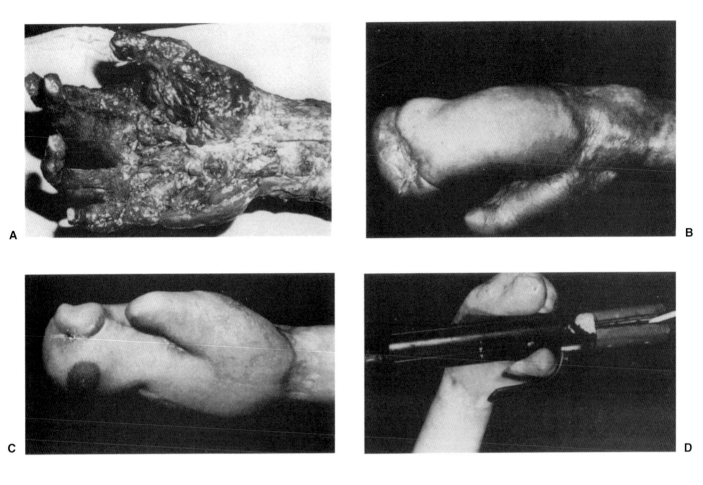

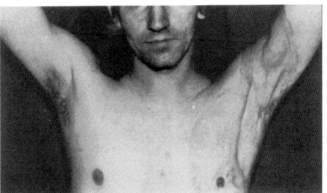

FIG. 2. **A:** A degloving injury of the entire wrist, the entire hand, and all five digits with extensive fascial, nerve, and tendon losses and injuries. **B:** The early appearance after repair with sandwich flaps that included the axilla and were extended by delay incisions to include the skin of the chest. **C:** The early appearance of the sandwich flaps, with the nipple transferred to the hand. **D:** One-and-a-half years after the injury, the patient has sufficient grip to hold a welding rod while he controls a torch with his normal hand. **E:** The donor sites encompassed the entire axilla, but he now has a normal range of motion and function of the shoulder. (The nipple was transplanted back to the chest as a free graft.) (From Smith and Furnas, ref. 1, with permission.)

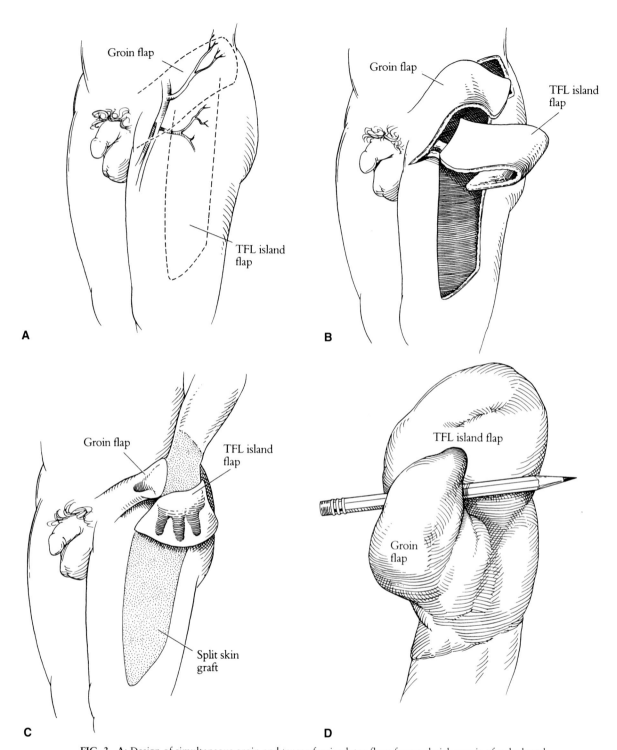

FIG. 3. **A:** Design of simultaneous groin and tensor fasciae latae flaps for sandwich repair of a degloved hand. **B:** Simultaneous elevation of a tensor fasciae latae island flap and a groin flap. (The territory of the groin flap overlies the base of the tensor fasciae latae flap.) **C:** Flaps in position, enveloping a degloved hand. The groin flap envelops the thumb and thenar area. The tensor fasciae latae flap envelops the hand and palm. Split-thickness skin grafts cover the remaining dorsum. **D:** Functioning mitten that results from this repair. (After Watson and McGregor, ref. 2, with permission.)

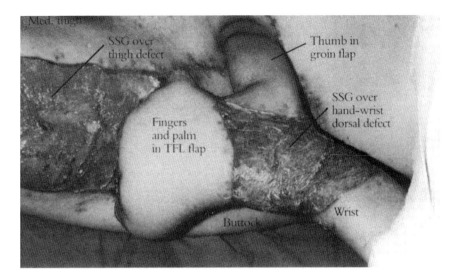

FIG. 4. Photograph of a patient with a degloved hand enveloped in a groin flap and a tensor fasciae latae flap as noted in Fig. 3. (From Watson and McGregor, ref. 2, with permission.)

Certain *single* flaps could be considered as material for a hand sandwich (more a bun than a sandwich): (1) A single latissimus dorsi muscle flap, surfaced with a skin graft, could sandwich an entire hand. It could be based on the thoracodorsal artery or on the collateral arteries (reverse latissimus). It could even be transferred as a microvascular flap to save the intervening stage and to maintain a permanent arterial pattern. A skin graft would be needed only on the hand, as the donor site would be closed primarily. (2) The omentum could be used in similar fashion, and would have the potential of sandwiching each digit individually. The patient could have the independent use of each finger from the start.

SUMMARY

The "hand sandwich" idea can thus be invoked in any of a multitude of current forms when the urgent need arises for coverage of the degloved hand.

References

1. Smith RC, Furnas DW. The hand sandwich: adjacent flaps from opposing body surfaces. *Plast Reconstr Surg* 1976;57:351.
2. Watson ACH, McGregor JC. The simultaneous use of a groin flap and a tensor fasciae latae myocutaneous flap to provide tissue cover for a completely degloved hand. *Br J Plast Surg* 1981;34:349.

CHAPTER 296 ■ DERMO-EPIDERMAL FLAP TO THE HAND

P. COLSON AND H. JANVIER

EDITORIAL COMMENT

The design of the bipedicle demoepidermal flap should avoid crossing the antecubital fosse to prevent flexion contractures across the elbow joint.

Defatting gave birth to the dermo-epidermal flap (1–4). Initially it was used to cover small defects of the fingers and then it was expanded to cover large defects of the hand (3).

The dermo-epidermal flap can be raised with a single pedicle or bipedicle from various parts of the body including the abdomen, thorax, and arm.

INDICATIONS

We have used the dermo-epidermal bipedicle brachial flap mainly for the repair of burned hands, and we use the classic "crossed arms" position (5,6). Our choice is explained, in part, by the quality of the tissues (hairless skin, well suited to

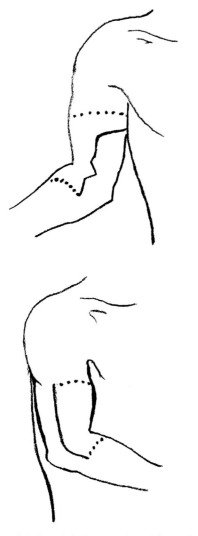

reinnervation) and also by the possibility of maintaining the hand and all its fingers in a good functional position without the use of an apparatus.

FLAP DESIGN AND DIMENSIONS

A pattern of the same dimensions and shape as the defect is used to design the dermo-epidermal flap. It is essential to design a flap that is larger than the defect.

Before the operation, the patient should be examined standing and asked to hold the donor arm with the burned hand, with the fingers on the anterior surface of the arm, while the thumb is extended on the posterior surface of the arm. The elbow of the donor arm is flexed at a right angle, so that the ulnar aspect of the hand rests on the forearm. It will then be possible to design the line of incision and to locate the two flap pedicles, one based on the arm and the other based on the forearm (Figs. 1 and 2; also see Fig. 7).

OPERATIVE TECHNIQUE

Bipedicle Flap: General Procedures

The skin is incised with a scalpel, stopping when the lobules of fat begin to herniate. We have totally abandoned rapid and imprecise blunt dissection. We feel it is preferable to be able to control the progression of the blade and, at the same time, both to visualize and to feel our way.

In this plane, the subdermal plexus is visualized, the veins are bulging with blood, and they deflate on section. Total defatting must be limited to only the surface necessary to cover the defect, and this technical point is very important.

The base of the flap is raised at a deeper level to include the blood vessels that nourish the pedicle.

For the mobilization and fixation of the dermo-epidermal flap, it is useful to take precautions, as the blood circulation on the dermal capillary plexus is susceptible to mechanical and other problems. The flap possesses extensibility and spontaneous retraction much greater than certain of the

FIG. 1. Design of the bipedicle dermoepidermal flap with one pedicle based on the arm and the other based on the forearm.

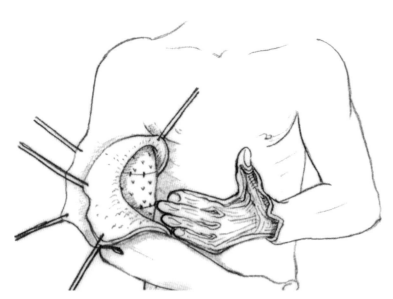

FIG. 2. After the flap is elevated, the donor site is covered with a moderately thick split-thickness skin graft.

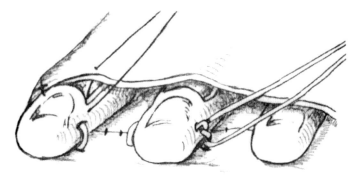

FIG. 3. The flap is sutured to the fingers, and the fingers are sutured to the arm to keep the flap well immobilized. This is essential since the flap survives on the dermal-subdermal plexus in some areas, but in others "takes" as a graft.

classic flaps. This is why the prudent surgeon does not exploit the elasticity of the flap by excessive stretching with a tight closure. Rather, he makes the flap pedicle a little longer. The surgeon should also fix the flap carefully to the defect edge, and should avoid applying the flap on a finger flexed at an acute angle. Knuckle prominence on the deep surface is enough to produce an area of compromised circulation.

Dermo-Epidermal Bipedicle Brachial Flap

First Stage

On the operating table, the appropriate position of the hand on the donor arm is verified, and the initial flap design is modified if necessary (Fig. 1).

Because of the pliability of the flap, separation can be achieved under visualization, while a full-thickness flap requires more laborious tunneling. After preparing the dermo-epidermal flap, the donor surface is covered with a split-thickness skin graft of moderate thickness (Fig. 2).

All burned tissue is widely excised and the procedure is completed by tenolysis of the extensors and sometimes by arthrolysis. We stress placing the fingers in optimal position, i.e., in a state of mild flexion, allowing them to rest on the curvature of the donor arm. In cases of positional malalignment, where fingers are not easily movable, the joints should be pinned with two small Kirschner wires. The hand is slid under the dermo-epidermal flap and it traverses the tunnel. If the pedicles have been well designed (one on the arm, the other on the forearm), and if the elbow is held in flexion at a right angle, the hand is easily introduced without overly distending the flaccid flap.

The hand is then firmly fixed to the arm, positioning the thumb and fingers by hooks glued to the nails, or even by nonabsorbable good-sized sutures, going through the finger pulp and deeply into the arm skin, to ensure firm fixation (Fig. 3). The fingers are separated from each other and

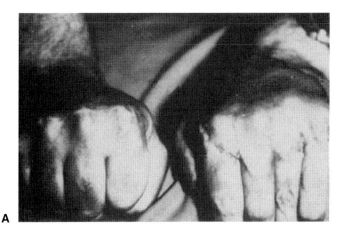

A

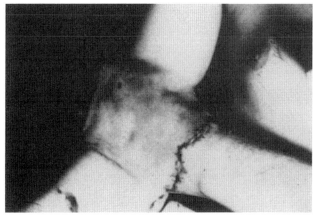

B

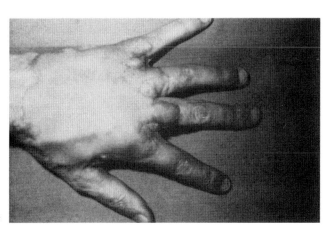

C

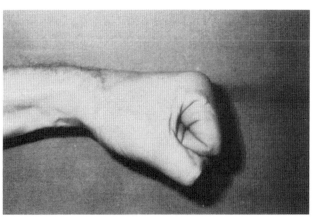

D

FIG. 4. A: Despite two attempts at skin grafting, this burn patient could not completely flex his fingers. **B:** Flap in place. Note that one pedicle is from the arm and the other is from the forearm. Note also the discoloration that occurs in the flap. **C,D:** Postoperative extension and flexion.

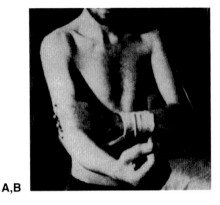 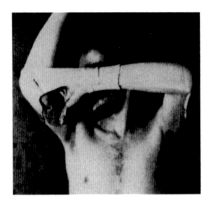

A,B

FIG. 5. **A,B:** Even with the forearms taped, there is enough mobility for shoulder exercises.

fanned out, not only to maintain open commissures, but also to increase the surface of the flap that will be available for covering the lateral surfaces of the fingers. Immobility of the hand is important for adhesion formation and for "take" of the flap, which behaves like a free graft (7). After the hand is fixed, the flap itself is sutured to the wrist skin, using an undulating or zigzag pattern, and fine sutures are placed in each of the fingers to cover the growth plate of the nail and the nailbed (Fig. 3).

The two elbows are attached to each other by nonextendable adhesive bandages, to prevent separation of the arms and to alleviate pain in the digital pulps, which have been fixed with sutures. Small compresses impregnated with a solution of cortisone are applied on all the raw surfaces and are slid under the flap between the fingers. We do not risk compressive dressings.

The patient is placed in bed on his back, with arms resting horizontally on the bed and the forearm suspended vertically.

By now the dermo-epidermal flap, originally of a nice red color, has become violaceous across its width and has multiple areas of beads of serosanguineous fluid (Fig. 4). This is a transitory state that disappears in a few days. On the third postoperative day, the patient leaves bed and begins to use his fingers actively and the donor arm for self-feeding. The degree of immobilization is reduced each day (Fig. 5).

Second Stage

Fifteen to 20 days after the first procedure, pedicle division frees the hand. If sizeable raw surfaces remain in the deep surface of the flap and on the lateral surfaces of the fingers, in spite of cortisone application, they may be debrided. The finger webs are then bisected, stopping the incision 2 to 3 cm above the web, i.e., the commissure. The little flaps thus created are sutured to the skin of the lateral edges of the fingers, following an undulating line (Fig. 6). When the lateral

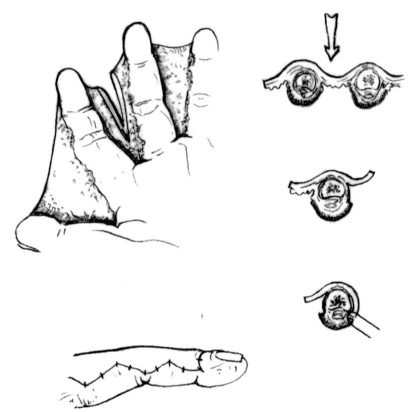

FIG. 6. After the flap is divided, the areas between the fingers are debrided. The flap is then inset as necessary, taking care to avoid straight line scars.

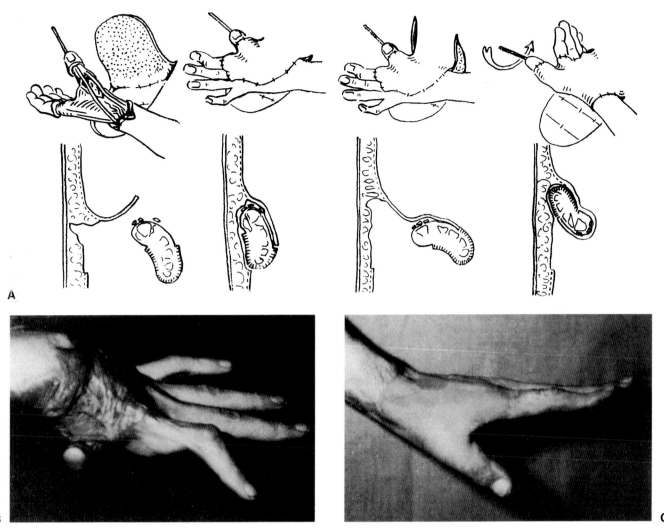

FIG. 7. **A:** Unipedicle dermo-epidermal flap from the abdomen used in two stages to cover the dorsal, radial, and palmar surfaces of the hand. **B:** Preoperative appearance. **C:** Postoperative result.

surfaces of the fingers are completely denuded (quite rare, in our experience), the distal ends of the little flaps reach the palmar surface. It is then advised to make a small Z-plasty at the base of the digit, a preventive procedure to avoid retraction of the palmar suture line (see Chap. 314).

The surgeon has a certain amount of leeway in tailoring the free edge of the flap, since capillary circulation is well supported at all the flap extremities. Between the thumb and the index finger we routinely rotate two triangular flaps, one on the dermo-epidermal flap, the other on the palm, to ensure a large aperture for the first commissure, i.e., the web space of the hand.

Over a period of several months, the flap changes its appearance, becoming supple and thin, and allowing for decompression of the contracture on the surface of the hand.

Dermo-Epidermal Unipedicle Flap from the Abdomen

Since a dermo-epidermal flap can be taken from different parts of the body, it is possible to use the flap on two surfaces of the hand at two separate times, employing the principles of pronation and supination (Fig. 7).

Dermo-Epidermal Unipedicle Flap from the Arm

We have adopted this technique for severe contractures of the thumb-index web space, to maintain a large space between them without an apparatus.

CLINICAL RESULTS

Most often, negligence or error in the choice of patient or of operative technique has been responsible for necrosis. Surgeons who have been trained to depend on flap thickness or on the existence of a deep arterial-venous circuit appear hesitant to use the dermo-epidermal flap. When total defatting is proposed, they also must change their habitual opinions.

Although there are multiple difficulties in using the flap, which vary from case to case, in our first published series of 18 cases using bipedicle and cross-arm dermo-epidermal flaps, we had 15 cases yielding good results without any necrosis; two cases with minimal necrosis at the margin along the suture line, which scarred in after secondary resection of the necrotic border; and one case of necrosis appearing in the center of a 6 × 2-cm dermo-epidermal flap, which was treated by excision and grafting and which caused delayed healing, but without functional impairment. In respect to the donor arm, the appearance of the free graft was quite acceptable, and the motion of the elbow was totally conserved.

SUMMARY

The dermo-epidermal flap can be used to provide thin, pliable, yet durable coverage for the hand.

References

1. Morel-Fatio D, Lagrot F. Les réparations des pertes de substance cutanées. *Proceedings of the 56th annual meeting of the French Surgical Society.* Paris: Hasson, 1954;76,130—131.
2. Baux S, Isclin F. Brûlure et écrasement de la main et des doigts: empochement immediat. *Ann Chir Plast* 1965;10:41.
3. Colson P, Houot R, Gangolphe M, et al. Utilisation des lambeaux degraissés en chirurgie réparatrice de la main. *Ann Chir Plast* 1967;12:298.
4. Kelleher JC, Sullivan JG, Dean RK. Use of a tailored abdominal pedicle for surgical reconstruction of the hand. *J Bone Joint Surg* 1970;52A:1552.
5. Bunnell S. Redundant fat. In: *Surgery of the hand,* 2d ed. Philadelphia: Lippincott, 1948;170–171,178; Fig. 138.
6. Iselin L, Iselin F. *Trade de chirurgie de la main.* Paris: Flammarion, 1967;248.
7. Smahel J. Biology of the stages of plasmatic imbibition. *Br J Plast Surg* 1971;24:133.

 CHAPTER 297. Abdominal Bipedicle Flap for Dorsal Defects of the Hand *N. H. Antia*
www.encyclopediaofflaps.com

CHAPTER 298 ■ FIRST DORSAL METACARPAL ARTERY FLAP

M. M. SHERIF

EDITORIAL COMMENT

This is a useful source of local donor tissue. The blood supply is reasonably reliable and good sensibility can be provided within the flap.

The first dorsal metacarpal artery (FDMA) flap is an axial flap based on the first dorsal metacarpal artery and its terminal dorsal digital branches, and it is harvested from the skin of the dorsal surface of the hand, index finger, and thumb. It can be raised as a proximally or distally based fascial or fasciocutaneous flap; vascularized tendon, periosteum, or bone can be included.

INDICATIONS

This flap is used mainly as a sensory flap for coverage of skin defects over the palmar surface of the thumb (1–8); for reconstruction of dorsal thumb skin defects (9); and for the reconstruction of the first web space, especially in cases of severe contracture (10,11). The flap can be raised from the dorsal

surface of either the thumb or index finger. A reversed-flow flap allows the coverage of skin defects up to the distal phalanx of the index finger (12).

The FDMA flap is especially indicated in severe first web-space contractures with irregular surfaces and exposed blood vessels and nerves. Release of contracted fascia and muscles can thus be provided. As a sensory flap, it can be used for reconstruction of the volar skin of the thumb (Fig. 1), and it is able to cover the whole volar surface up to the thumb tip (10,11). Despite a less than optimal restoration of thumb sensation (9) and some question as to durability for thumb coverage, the skin displays an excellent ability to withstand the wear and tear on the working surface of the hand (11), and flap sensibility is comparable to that of Littler's flap (10).

An FDMA can also be taken from the dorsal aspect of the thumb, to provide sensation to an index stump (13). A reversed-flow fascial flap can be used to provide sensation to an index stump by neurotization of the radial nerve to one of the severed digital nerves of the index finger (11–13).

The flap has commonly been used to replace the dorsal skin of the thumb and is considered by some (9) to be irreplaceable for this indication. An extended version of the flap has been used to cover the proximal phalanx of the thumb, both from its volar and dorsal surfaces (15).

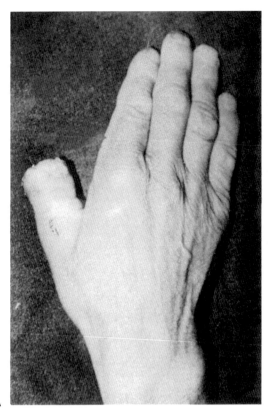
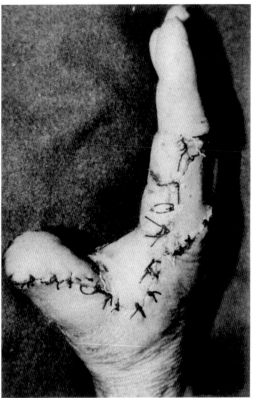

A

B

FIG. 1. **A:** Amputated thumb distal to the interphalangeal joint. **B:** One week after thumb reconstruction with an island sensory FDMA flap. The flap is tapered proximally, and the skin on the lateral side of the thumb is released to avoid compression of the pedicle in the interphalangeal area.

An island flap can cover the dorsal surface of the carpus, the wrist, and the metacarpophalangeal (MCP) joint of the little finger. It can reach most areas in the palm, either through the space between the two heads of the first dorsal interosseous muscle, or around the free margin of this muscle and the adductor pollicis (10).

An extensor tendon has been included in the flap as a vascularized tendon to bridge a defect in the thumb or middle finger (11). In addition, a reversed-flow fasciocutaneous flap has been used to cover defects on the index finger, with the ability to reach the distal phalanx of this finger (12). A reversed-flow fascial flap can cover an exposed extensor tendon around the MCP joint or an exposed joint, after capsulotomy in a postburn hand. The flap provides a suitable bed for skin grafting, instead of shifting to a distant flap. The deep fascia on the dorsum of the hand, proximal to the level of the wrist, has been included with the flap; this coverage can reach the proximal phalanx of the ring finger and the index distal interphalangeal (DIP) joint.

Other uses have included vein-carrier flaps in cases of thumb replantation, to correct the loss of dorsal veins; anastomoses are done between the distal veins of the flap and the dorsal veins of the replanted thumb. The flap can also enhance arterial flow after insufficient restoration of circulation to the thumb (8). The FDMA flap has also been used in pollicization of the index finger, as a single vascular supply to the index finger after injury to both palmar digital arteries (16). As a bone flap from the neck of the second metacarpal, the FDMA flap has been used in treating nonunion of the scaphoid (17).

Double FDMA flaps can be raised based on the double vascular supply of this area, one cutaneous and the other fascial (11); they can be used for coverage and lining of exposed extensor tendons.

ANATOMY (FIG. 2)

The FDMA is a constant branch (8,14,18–23) that arises from the radial artery (RA) distal to the extensor pollicis longus tendon, just before the artery dips between the two heads of the first dorsal interosseous (DIO) muscle. The FDMA runs either over or within the DIO fascia. As the artery is completely fixed to this fascia, the first DIO muscle is always exposed during dissection of the pedicle.

Some authors (9,18) describe the presence of a second FDMA deep to the DIO fascia (the muscular or deep fascial FDMA). Although the double system was detected in only 10% to 12% of their dissected hands, meticulous dissection of this area has shown the presence of these two systems in all cases (14). However, it appears that both systems are completely separate, except at the MCP joint area, where they end at the anastomosis around this joint. As in other dorsal metacarpal arteries, when the main branch of this dorsal system is small, it is usually replaced by a large perforator connecting the palmar and dorsal systems of the hand (19).

In about 10% of dissected cadaver hands (14), the FDMA gives off a small direct cutaneous branch that follows the course of the superficial branch of the radial nerve. More commonly, this vessel arises from the radial artery itself (14,20). It rapidly divides into ascending and descending branches supplying the radial nerve and the skin overlying it. Due to its small size, this vessel is very difficult to isolate and dissect. However, its size is inversely proportional to the FDMA itself. When the descending branch is large, it anastomoses with branches of the FDMA at the level of the MCP joint of the index finger.

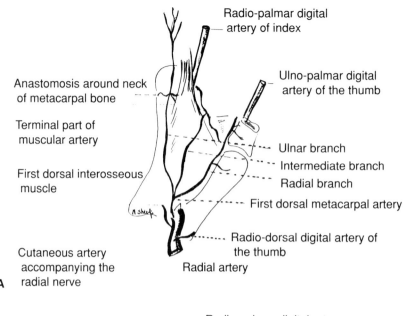

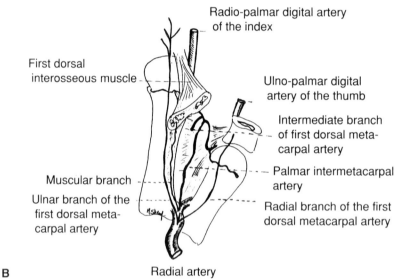

FIG. 2. Diagrams illustrating the anatomy of the FDMA and its anastomosis in the first web area. **A:** FDMA embedded in the fascia of the first dorsal interosseous muscle with its three branches (radial, ulnar, intermediate). Cutaneous nerve accompanying the radial nerve has been cut. **B:** First dorsal interosseous muscle and intermediate branch of FDMA have been removed to expose the muscular branch inside the ulnar head of the muscle and the anastomosis at the metacarpal neck area.

The FDMA itself divides into three branches: a radial, an intermediate, and an ulnar branch (14,21). They run close to the first metacarpal bone, in the middle of the first interosseous space or close to the second metacarpal bone, respectively. The size of these branches is variable, and one or more may arise separately from the RA. The intermediate branch ends by anastomosing in continuity with the first palmar metacarpal artery. This branch is well developed in only 15% to 18% of cases (14,18,19,21). The radial and ulnar branches may continue as the dorsal digital artery of the thumb or index fingers. More commonly, they terminate as a plexus dorsal to the extensor tendon (8,14,18,20). At the level of the neck of the second metacarpal bone, they anastomose with the palmar and intermuscular vessels. Two other anastomoses are present at the level of the proximal phalanx—one at the dermal level (20) and the other deep to the extensor tendon (9,23). A reverse-flow flap is supplied through these anastomoses.

Branches arise from the FDMA or its divisions to supply the nearby tendons (9) and periosteum (9,17). The presence of multiple anastomotic channels in the area of the neck of the second metacarpal bone (9,22) makes it the most favorable donor site for a fascioperiosteal flap (17).

Two venae comitantes are present around the artery. They drain the flap and anastomose freely with the superficial venous system. The flap is also drained by the superficial veins over the dorsal surface of the hand.

FLAP DESIGN AND DIMENSIONS

The FDMA flap can be raised as a proximally based fasciocutaneous flap. In cadaveric injection studies, the skin overlying the dorsum of the hand from the radial side of the thumb to the third metacarpal bone is usually stained (14). However, in

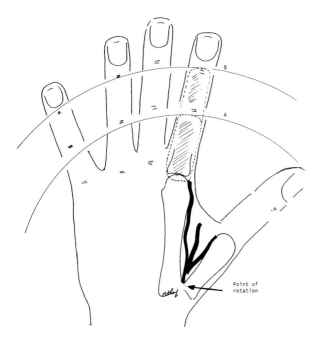

FIG. 3. Arc of rotation of the proximally based FDMA flap.
A: Conventional version. B: Extended version.

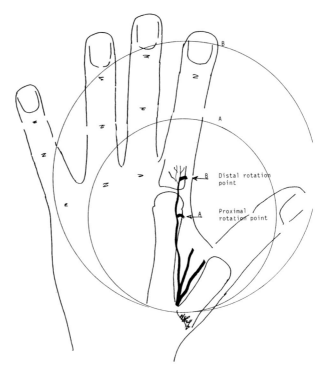

FIG. 4. Arc of rotation of the distally based FDMA fasciocutaneous
flap. A: Based on the perforator situated at the level of the neck of the
metacarpal bone of the index finger. B: Based on the anastomosis distal to the metacarpophalangeal joint and the subdermal anastomosis.

clinical practice, the cutaneous territory of skin flaps is usually
larger than in the injection study. Similarly, the dorsal surface
of the index and thumb are faintly stained (14), while, in
clinical cases, the skin overlying the index finger up to the
DIP joint can be raised completely (22). The flap rotates
around the point of origin of the artery at the base of the first
interosseous space (Fig. 3).

When utilized as a distally based fasciocutaneous flap, the
flap is raised on the distal perforator at the level of the
metacarpal neck (9), or on the rich dermal plexus at the base
of the index finger (12). The skin territory is usually limited by
the proximal boundary of the first metacarpal space. The flap
can reach the proximal interphalangeal (PIP) joint and the
middle phalanx (Fig. 4).

The flap can also be raised as a distally based fascial flap.
This flap is based at the MCP joint area on the perforator connecting the palmar and dorsal metacarpal arteries. The fascia
raised can include the deep fascia of the hand up to the extensor retinaculum of the wrist.

OPERATIVE TECHNIQUE

Although the vessel is constantly present in all cases, it is safer
to check the pulsation of the FDMA against the metacarpal
bones before starting the operation. An ultrasonographic
examination has been recommended (24) before embarking
on raising any dorsal metacarpal flap. This may not always be
necessary in the first web space, except in cases of congenital
deformities or trauma to the area.

The dissection technique should take account of the
anatomic variations in the location and the variable dominance
of the vessels. The pedicle should contain the interosseous
aponeurosis to include the three branches of the FDMA. The
superficial dorsal veins should be preserved in the pedicle.

Pedicled Flap

The flap is drawn on the dorsum of the hand, index finger, or
thumb, according to the position of the skin defect. The flap is

elevated from distal to proximal, starting superficial to the
extensor tendon paratenon. At the level of the metacarpal neck,
a perforator is always present; this should be coagulated or ligated. To avoid first web-space contracture, the skin over this
space should not be included in the flap. If this skin is necessary
to cover the skin defect, the flap is extended ulnarly toward the
third metacarpal, so that the web is again covered by a flap and
is not grafted. To rotate the flap, the dorsal interosseous fascia
is incised from the metacarpal bones as far as necessary.

Island Flap

This flap is drawn on the dorsum of the index proximal phalanx from the PIP to the MCP joint. The pedicle is dissected to
include the interosseous fascia with the three branches of the
FDMA, as well as the superficial veins, the superficial radial
nerve, and its accompanying artery. The latter is exposed
through a dorsal S-shaped incision starting from the base of
the first interosseous space, and ending at the proximal edge
of the flap. The skin over the interosseous space is dissected
just deep to the dermis, to include the dorsal veins and terminal branches of the radial nerve in the flap pedicle. The flap is
raised from distal to proximal at a plane superficial to the
extensor tendon paratenon. A constant perforator is coagulated at the neck of the metacarpal bone, and the interosseous
fascia is released from the metacarpal bones. The pedicle
length can reach 7 cm in an adult (10), thus allowing a wide
arc of rotation. A wide subcutaneous tunnel is dissected, and
the flap is rotated without twisting the pedicle.

If the flap is used for reconstruction of the palmar skin of
the thumb, the pedicle will cross the side of the interphalangeal joint where the skin is tight and the flap pedicle can be
easily compressed; it is better to open the lateral side of the
finger proximally and elongate the skin island of the flap
proximally (10,11).

Care should be taken when including a tendon with the flap, to avoid disruption of the fine vessels supplying the tendon.

Reversed-Flow Flap

The proximal part of the flap is incised first, and the FDMA is dissected. The artery is then ligated from its origin from the radial artery. The incision around the flap is completed, and the dissection is taken down to the interosseous fascia. The flap is raised from proximal to distal. The perforator can be ligated at the neck of the second metacarpal, and the flap is thus nourished only by the dermal anastomosis (12). In these cases, the pedicle should be freed with a large portion of dermal and subcutaneous tissue. The donor area is either closed directly or skin grafted.

Reversed-Flow Fascial Flap

The interosseous fascia is exposed, as in the island flap. The FDMA is ligated at its origin from the radial artery, and the interosseous fascia is dissected from the underlying muscle and both metacarpals. At the level of the metacarpal neck, the anastomosis between the dorsal and palmar systems can be easily seen. One of these perforators should be preserved, to allow the flap to rotate freely. The fascia can then be covered with a skin graft, and the donor area closed directly.

CLINICAL RESULTS

Flap necrosis due to arterial or venous complications is rare. In 29 cases reported (25), there were only three failures; two of them were due to technical error. Although venous congestion may be common in reversed-flow flaps, only one case was reported in the literature of reversed-flow FDMAs (9). In this case, about half the flap was lost due to excessive tension on the pedicle.

The donor area is usually covered by a split-thickness skin graft, although a full-thickness graft can be used in females, so that a better color match with the dorsum of the hand is achieved. To avoid skin grafting, an aponeurotic flap can be raised, taking the interosseous fascia and subcutaneous tissue of the index finger, while leaving the skin intact. However, the defect left after raising the FDMA flap is minimal, and grafting on the dorsal surface of the index finger is aesthetically satisfactory to both patient and observers (11); this type of flap is rarely indicated (9).

Neuroma and sensory deficit in the radial-nerve area is liable to occur, especially in cases of neurotization; however, this has not been reported in the literature. Hair growth in the palm was noted in one case after thumb palmar-surface reconstruction. This was treated by electrical epilation (11).

SUMMARY

The FDMA flap is reliable and versatile, with rapid and easy dissection, and with a constant anatomy and expendable artery. Use of the flap in hand reconstruction can decrease the need for many of the distant pedicled or free flaps previously used in this area.

References

1. Hilgenfeldt O. *Operativer Daumenersatz.* Stuttgart: Enke Verlag, 1950.
2. Gaul JS. Radial innervated cross finger flap from the index finger to provide sensory pulp to injured thumb. *J Bone Joint Surg* 1969;51A:1257.
3. Kuhn H. Reconstruction du pouce par le lambeau de Hilgenfeldt. *Ann Chir Plast* 1961;6:620.
4. Holevich J. A new method of restoring sensibility to the thumb. *J Bone Joint Surg* 1963;45B:496.
5. Adamson JE, Horton C, Crawford H. Sensory rehabilitation of the injured thumb. *Plast Reconstr Surg* 1967;40:53.
6. Rybka FJ, Pratt FE. Thumb reconstruction with a sensory flap from the dorsum of the index finger. *Plast Reconstr Surg* 1979;64:141.
7. Lesavoy M. The dorsal index finger neurovascular island flap. *Orthop Rev* 1980;9:91.
8. Foucher G, Braun JB. A new island flap transfer from the dorsum of the index finger to the thumb. *Plast Reconstr Surg* 1979;63:344.
9. Dautel G, Merle M. Direct and reverse dorsal metacarpal flap. *Br J Plast Surg* 1992;45:123.
10. Small JO, Bennen MD. The first dorsal metacarpal artery neurovascular island flap. *J Hand Surg* 1988;13B:136.
11. Sherif MM. First dorsal metacarpal artery flap in hand reconstruction. II. Clinical application. *J Hand Surg* 1994;19A:32.
12. Schoofs M, Chambon E, Leps P, et al. The reverse dorsal metacarpal flap from the first web. *Eur J Plast Surg* 1993;16:26.
13. Lie KK, Posch JL. Island flap innervated by radial nerve for restoration of sensation in an index stump. *Plast Reconstr Surg* 1971;47:386.
14. Sherif MM. First dorsal metacarpal artery flap in hand reconstruction. I. Anatomical study. *J Hand Surg* 1994;19A:26.
15. Gebhard B, Meissl G. An extended first dorsal metacarpal artery neurovascular island flap. *J Hand Surg* 1995;20B:529.
16. Germann G, Hornung R, Raff T. Two new applications for the first dorsal metacarpal artery pedicle in the treatment of severe hand injuries. *J Hand Surg* 1995;20B:525.
17. Burnelli F, Matboulin C, Saffar P. Greffon pedicule d'origine metacarpienne dans les pseudoarthroses du scaphoid carpien. Communication au Symposium sur le Poignet, Paris, France, April 6–8, 1995.
18. Earley MJ. The arterial supply of the thumb, first web and index finger and its surgical application. *J Hand Surg* 1986;11B:123.
19. Coleman SS, Anson BJ. Arterial patterns in the hand based upon a study of 650 specimens. *Surg Gynecol Obstet* 1961;113:409.
20. Dautel G, Merle M, Borrelly J, Michon J. Variation anatomique du reseau vasculaire de la premiere commissure dorsal. Applications au lambeau cerf-volant. *Ann Chir Main* 1989;8:53.
21. Murakami T, Tayaka K, Outi H. The origin, course and distribution of arteries of the thumb with special reference to the so-called artery princeps pollicis. *Okajimas Folia Anat Jpn* 1969;46:177.
22. Earley MJ, Milner RH. Dorsal metacarpal artery flaps. *Br J Plast Surg* 1987;40:333.
23. Bonnel F, Teissier J, Allieu Y, et al. Arterial supply of ligaments of the metacarpophalangeal joints. *J Hand Surg* 1982;7A:445.
24. Healy G, Mercer NSG, Earley MJ, Woodcock J. Focusable Doppler ultrasound in mapping dorsal hand flaps. *Br J Plast Surg* 1990;3:296.
25. Braun MF, Merle M, Foucher G. Le lambeau cerf-volant. *Ann Chir Main* 1988;7:147.

CHAPTER 299 ■ LUMBRICAL MUSCLE FLAP OF THE PALM

H. KONCILIA, R. KUZBARI, A. WORSEG, M. TSCHABITSCHER, AND J. HOLLE

EDITORIAL COMMENT

These flaps have been used to successfully treat painful neuromas in continuity.

The coverage of the scarred and devascularized median nerve and its branches poses a challenging problem, as it is often a sequel of multiple surgical procedures and causes disabling pain and numbness. We describe the anatomy and clinical applications of the lumbrical muscle flap. Only the two radial lumbrical muscles are suitable for flap transposition. Pedicled on branches originating in the superficial palmar arch (SPA) and from the common palmar digital artery (CPDA), the lumbrical muscles can be transposed to reach the entire palm up to the proximal flexion crease. Clinical use of the first and second lumbrical muscle flaps demonstrates the value of these flaps for coverage of the median nerve and its branches in the palm.

INDICATIONS

To date, the blood supply of the lumbrical muscles has not been described and the muscles have not been used surgically as pedicled flaps. The present study describes the blood and nerve supply of the lumbrical muscles and demonstrates that the two radial lumbricals can be transposed as proximal-based vascular island flaps. These flaps have a wide arc of rotation and a favorable shape, enabling coverage of the median nerve and its branches in the palm.

ANATOMY

The lumbrical muscles, usually four in number, are cylindrical muscles located in the midpalmar dorsal to the palmar aponeurosis. The muscles have a moveable origin, arising from the tendons of the flexor digitorum profundus (FDP) muscles; the ulnar two are bipennate. Each lumbrical muscle passes to the radial side of the corresponding finger and inserts into the radial lateral band of the extensor expansion (1–4).

According to biomechanical and electromyographic studies (5–8), the main function of the lumbrical muscles is interphalangeal joint extension. Although the direct contribution to interphalangeal joint extension is small or even nonexistent in flexed fingers, their indirect contribution to interphalangeal joint extension, by decreasing the force of the flexor profundus, is pronounced (5,6). The lumbrical muscles are minor metacarpophalangeal joint flexors. However, in all their functions, the lumbrical muscles assist the much stronger synergistic interosseus muscles (7).

The vascular and nerve supplies of the lumbrical muscles were investigated in 20 fresh human cadaver hands of both sexes (12 to 20 hours postmortem). In all cadaver hands, the brachial artery was injected with a colored latex–lead oxide solution, and the ulnar artery and superficial palmar branch of the radial artery were dissected at the distal forearm and traced distally, carefully preserving all arterial branches. All vessels entering the lumbrical muscles were dissected with the aid of an operating microscope (×10 magnification). The points of entry of the vessels into the muscle bellies, and the diameter and length of the entering vessels, were measured using a caliper. To visualize the filling of the internal muscle vasculature, the lumbrical muscles were isolated and then examined radiologically after the arterial injection with the lead oxide solution. In addition, the nerves that entered the muscles were dissected, and the points of nerve entry into the muscle bellies were marked and measured.

The origin and insertion of the lumbrical muscles were also investigated. Muscle length and width were measured before and after removal of the epimysium. The arc of rotation of a proximal-based lumbrical muscle island flap was determined after division of the minor vascular branches and complete detachment of the muscle origin and insertion.

First and Second Lumbrical Muscles

The vascular supply of the first and second lumbrical muscles was consistent in all examined hands. The first lumbrical was consistently supplied by one or two dominant arterial branches originating from the superficial SPA and several nondominant minor branches from the radialis indicis artery (Fig. 1). The second lumbrical muscle was consistently supplied by one or two dominant arterial branches, arising either from the SPA (67%) or from the first CPDA (33%), and minor nondominant branches from the first CPDA (Fig. 2). In both lumbricals, the dominant vessels typically entered the muscles on their radial-palmar surface at the junction of the proximal and middle thirds of the muscle. The diameters of the dominant branches ranged from 0.45 mm to 1.92 mm (mean: 1.22 mm); the length ranged from 15 to 22 mm (mean: 19 mm).

As previously reported (9), a single branch of the radial digital nerve to the index finger supplied the first lumbrical muscle in all examined hands. A single branch of the common digital nerve to the second web supplied the second lumbrical muscle in 18 of the 20 hands. In two cadaver hands, the second lumbrical muscle was supplied by two or more branches of the same nerve. In all hands, the motor nerves entered the muscle bellies, together with the dominant vessels, at the junction of the proximal and middle thirds of the lumbricals. A common neurovascular hilus was present in 90% of the first

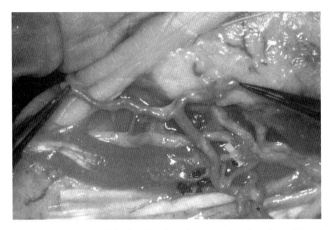

FIG. 1. Dissection of the first lumbrical muscle showing the origin of the dominant pedicle, which consists of two adjacent branches of the superficial palmar arch (SPA) (*two vertical arrows* and dark rubber). Note the accompanying nerve branch (*oblique arrow* and light rubber) arising from the radial digital nerve to the index finger. The SPA is marked by an *asterisk*.

lumbrical muscles and in 40% of the second lumbricals. In the remaining muscles, the nerve and vessels entered the muscles at different locations.

FLAP DESIGN AND DIMENSIONS

The anatomic findings demonstrate that the first and second lumbrical muscles have a "type II" vascular pattern according to the classification of Mathes and Nahai (10), with one or two dominant vessels entering and supplying each muscle at the junction of its proximal and middle thirds, and two minor pedicles entering the distal part of the muscles. The first two lumbricals can, thus, be transposed as proximally pedicled island muscle flaps based on their dominant vascular pedicles. The arc of rotation of such proximally pedicled muscles reaches the proximal palm to the level of the proximal flexion crease (Fig. 3). The first and second lumbrical muscles may be raised together, in order to increase the width of the transposed muscle tissue.

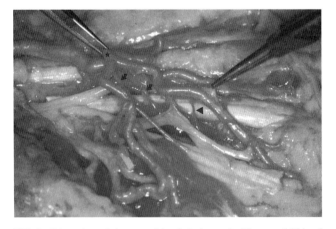

FIG. 2. Dissection of the second lumbrical muscle. The arterial blood supply is from one or two dominant vessels (*two oblique arrows*) originating from the SPA (67%) and the first common palmar digital artery (CPDA) (33%), respectively. Note the nondominant minor branch from CPDA (*horizontal arrows*). The SPA is marked by an *asterisk*.

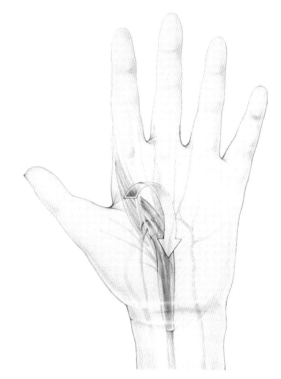

FIG. 3. The first lumbrical muscle is shown schematically supplied by one or two dominant branches arising from the SPA. The arc of rotation allows a 180-degree transposition of the flap for coverage of the median nerve proximally to the wrist flexion crease.

The use of the third and fourth lumbrical muscles as pedicled flaps appears impractical, in view of the multiple variations in length, width, and vascular supply of these muscles.

OPERATIVE TECHNIQUE

The surgical technique for the elevation of the first and second lumbrical muscle flaps is similar. Under tourniquet control, the lumbrical muscle flap is elevated through a standard carpal-tunnel incision, which is extended to the second interdigital web in a zig-zag pattern. The palmar aponeurosis is incised and elevated, and the lumbrical muscle is identified, protecting the digital nerve to the index finger (it is superficial to the first lumbrical muscle). The SPA is exposed proximally, and its branches that supply the lumbrical muscle are preserved. To facilitate the separation of the lumbrical muscle from the FDP tendon, the lumbrical tendon is first identified distally, and the muscle flap is dissected in a distal-to-proximal direction.

The dominant vascular pedicle is identified at the junction of the proximal and middle thirds of the muscle and preserved. The minor pedicles entering the distal part of the muscle are ligated. The tendon of the lumbrical muscle is then divided, raising a piece of tendon with the flap to facilitate the fixation of the lumbrical at the recipient site. Finally, the muscle origin is sharply separated from the FDP tendon, to increase the arc of rotation of the flap. The muscle island flap is allowed to perfuse before transposition. If needed, the epimysium is removed, to increase muscle width and to allow the lumbrical muscle to fan out over the median nerve. When the flap is used for defects in the palm, the muscle is covered with a skin graft. Postoperatively, a splint is applied for 10 days, maintaining the finger joints in intrinsic-plus position of metacarpophalangeal flexion and interphalangeal extension. Elevation and transposition of the muscle flaps can be carried out in about 30 minutes of tourniquet time.

SUMMARY

This study demonstrates that the first and second lumbrical muscles can be transposed as proximally pedicled flaps. The constant and reliable vascular supply of these flaps originates from the SPA and the CPDA, respectively (11). The lumbrical muscles are thin and easily accessible, and have a longitudinal shape and an arc of rotation that easily reaches to the distal flexion crease of the wrist. To increase flap width, the first and second lumbrical muscles may be transposed simultaneously, although this was not needed in our clinical cases.

References

1. Basu SS, Hazary S. Variations of the lumbrical muscles of the hand. *Anat Record* 1960;136:501.

2. Schmidt R, Heinrichs HJ, Reissig D. Die Mm. Lumbricales an der Hand des Menschen, ihre Variation in Ursprung und Ansatz. *Anat Ariz* 1963;113:414.
3. Metha HJ, Gardner WU. Study of lumbrical muscles in the human hand. *Am J Anat* 1961;109:227.
4. Braithwaite F, Channel GD, Moore FT, Whillis, J. The applied anatomy of the lumbrical and interosseus muscles of the hand. *Guy's Hospital Reports* 1948;97:185.
5. Backhouse KM, Catton WT. An experimental study of the functions of the lumbrical muscles in the human hand. *J Anat* 1954;88:133.
6. Eyler DL, Markee JE. The anatomy and function of the intrinsic musculature of the fingers. *J Bone Joint Surg (Am)* 1954;36A:1.
7. Ranney D, Wells R. Lumbrical muscle function as revealed by a new and physiological approach. *Anat Record* 1988;222:110.
8. Basmajian JV. Electromyography-dynamic gross anatomy: a review. *Am J Anat* 1980;159:245.
9. Lauritzen R, Szabo RM, Lauritzen DB. Innervation of the lumbrical muscles. *Br J Hand Surg* 1996;2113:57.
10. Mathes SJ, Nahai F. *Clinical applications for muscle and musculocutaneous flaps.* St. Louis: Mosby, 1982.
11. Koncilia H, Kuzbari R, Worseg A, Tschabitscher M, Holle J. The lumbrical muscle flap: anatomic study and clinical application. *J Hand Surg (Am)* 1998;23:111.

CHAPTER 300 ■ GROIN SKIN FLAP

I. A. MCGREGOR AND D. SOUTAR

EDITORIAL COMMENT

This is the classic description that gave rise to the whole field of axial-type flaps. The use of fluorescein intraarterially to demarcate the extent of the primary territory was very helpful in determining the extent of the flap, although it always underestimated it.

Until the early 1970s, it was generally accepted that strict rules governing length-to-width ratio had to be acknowledged when raising a single pedicled flap on the trunk or limbs without prior delay. The deltopectoral flap (1) with a length-to-width ratio in excess of 2:1 appeared to break these rules. To explain this anomaly, it was postulated (2) that the flap contained an anatomically recognizable arteriovenous system running in its long axis.

On the basis of this hypothesis, a search was instituted for comparable axial arteriovenous systems in other sites on which skin flaps could be based, with characteristics similar to those of the deltopectoral flap. The search resulted in description of the groin flap. This concept of raising a flap based on a specific vascular pattern is, in fact, a rediscovery (3–7).

Flaps with such an arteriovenous system were termed axial pattern flaps (8), and the concept not only revolutionized pedicle flap design in general (9) but opened up the whole field of free tissue transfer using microvascular anastomosis (10).

INDICATIONS

The standard groin skin flap has been used to resurface the hand and forearm, to substitute for the standard abdominal tubed pedicle flap, and as a local transposition flap. Resurfacing the hand and forearm is probably the main use of the flap (11). Defects of the elbow cannot readily be reconstructed because the length of the flap required is not entirely safe.

The abdominal tube pedicle is now rarely used. The 6-week period of maturation of the classically designed tube can be eliminated by using the groin flap. This can be raised, tubed, and attached to a wrist carrier in a single stage. Transfer to the wrist in a single stage not only saves time, but has the advantage of being technically easier because of the absence of previous surgery in the vicinity of the flap. The long pedicle allows the flap to be attached to either the radial or the ulnar side of the wrist, whichever is appropriate for the next stage.

ANATOMY

The skin of the groin and hypogastrium is supplied by a cartwheel of arteries arising from the femoral artery, just below the inguinal ligament, and it is drained by a corresponding cartwheel of veins draining into the saphenous opening (Fig. 1). It seems likely that any flap based on this arteriovenous cartwheel will survive, its safe length depending on the length of the particular "spoke of the cartwheel" (12). Intraarterial fluorescein studies of this cartwheel demonstrate it to be an ellipse rather

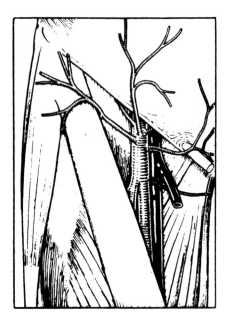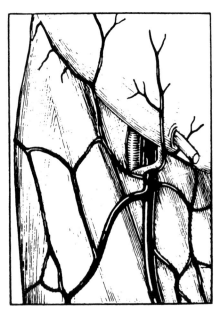

FIG. 1. Vascular anatomy of the groin showing the "cartwheel" of arteries and veins.

than a circle, with its long axis in the line of the groin flap and its short axis in the line of the hypogastric flap (Fig. 2). This suggests that the length of the "cartwheel spoke" in the axis of the groin flap is considerably longer than that in the axis of the hypogastric flap.

The anatomy of the superficial circumflex iliac artery was initially thought to be fairly constant (12), and in practice its constancy is certainly adequate for the flap as originally described and used. The variations (Fig. 3) that have been reported (10) following studies on 100 cadaveric dissections become relevant when the flap is used as a free flap. Similar variations have been reported by other authors (13,14) who, in fact, found four instances, in a series of 86 flaps, in which no trace of vessels large enough to nourish the flap were found.

When the groin flap is used as a standard single pedicled axial pattern skin flap, the takeoff point of its vascular axis, i.e., the center of the "cartwheel," is the most important point of reference, and this point is 2 to 3 cm below the midinguinal point. From there the axial artery, the superficial circumflex iliac, passes laterally parallel to the inguinal ligament as far as a point below the anterior superior iliac spine (Fig. 4). There it divides into three branches that anastomose with branches of

the deep circumflex iliac artery, the superior gluteal artery, and the ascending branch of the lateral circumflex femoral artery.

At its origin from the femoral artery, the vessel lies deep to the deep fascia; and it pierces this structure near the medial border of the sartorius muscle, coming then to lie in the subcutaneous tissue. As it passes laterally, it becomes more superficial. The medial border of the sartorius is a key point in raising the flap and isolating its vascular pedicle. There it is tethered by branches that pass deep to the sartorius and also by the lateral cutaneous nerve of the thigh that crosses the vessel at this point.

The flap has a rich venous drainage; witness its extreme pallor when raised and transferred and the absence of significant edema immediately following its transfer. It has, in fact, two venous systems, deep and superficial. The dominant system is superficial and comprises the superficial circumflex iliac vein, either as a single vessel or as a group of veins, and the superficial epigastric vein. Together, the superficial system has a total diameter of some 3 to 6 mm and it terminates in the saphenous bulb. The deep system comprises the venae comitantes that accompany the artery and drain into the femoral vein. In some cases both systems terminate in the saphenous

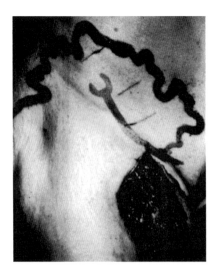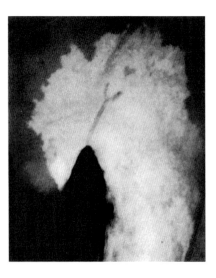

FIG. 2. Shape of the territory of the arterial "cartwheel" of the groin in two patients, showing the outline to be elliptical rather than circular, with the long axis in the line of the groin flap and the short axis in the line of the hypogastric flap.

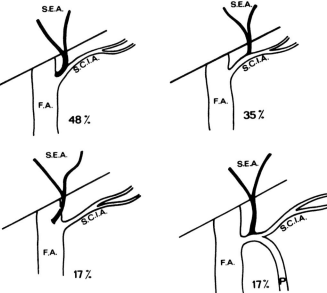

FIG. 3. Variations in the arterial anatomy in the groin, based on the findings in 100 cadaver dissections. (From Taylor and Daniel, ref. 10, with permission.)

bulb, but in our experience both have invariably been present, although separated by a layer of subcutaneous fat.

FLAP DESIGN AND DIMENSIONS

The line of the inguinal ligament is marked on the skin, the femoral artery is identified, and the point of origin of the superficial circumflex iliac artery is marked on it 2.5 to 3 cm below the line of the inguinal ligament. From this point, a line drawn laterally parallel to the inguinal ligament marks the course of the axial vessel of the flap. The sartorius, curving downward from the anterior superior iliac spine, is drawn on the skin, with particular attention to its medial border that is a key line in mobilizing the flap. The flap is designed around the axial vessel (Fig. 5) and, although an attempt is usually made to keep this axis in a central position, failure to do this accurately appears to make little difference.

The width of the flap is dependent on the clinical problem; it has varied between 5 and 19 cm. Although a wider flap is theoretically possible, it has not yet been required in our experience. Most commonly, a flap of approximately 10-cm width is sufficient and allows easy tubing of the pedicle, if this is required.

The maximum length of the flap that can be raised is more difficult to define, depending as it does on the lateral extent of the territory of the axial artery. Dissection has shown that the vessels lateral to the anterior superior iliac spine rapidly "disappear" as they anastomose with the arteries in the vicinity. When the length of the territory as established by intraarterial fluorescein studies is compared with the length of flap that has been found empirically to be safe, the latter exceeds the former. By trial and error, it has been found safe to add a 1:1 flap to the end of the truly axial component. It would appear that this addition is in the nature of a random flap. In clinical practice the flap can safely be extended beyond the anterior superior iliac spine by a distance equal to the width of the flap.

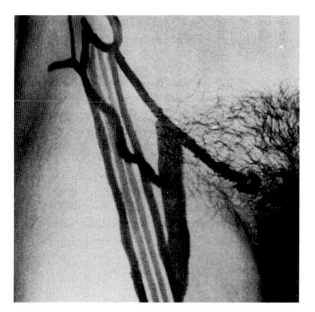

FIG. 4. Course of the superficial circumflex iliac artery in relation to the underlying structures of the groin.

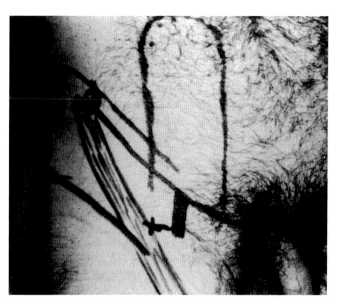

FIG. 5. Outlines of groin and hypogastric flaps, with the relevant anatomic landmarks marked on the skin.

When used for resurfacing of the hand and forearm, the flap has the considerable advantage that reverse planning is not necessary, since the pliable pedicle can be manipulated readily. The flap can be applied to either surface of the hand or forearm and, in practice, the pedicle of the flap is usually tubed to eliminate all raw surfaces.

OPERATIVE TECHNIQUE

Donor Site

The technique for raising a groin flap depends on whether it is being used as a standard skin flap or as a free flap transfer. In raising it as a standard skin flap, it is rarely if ever necessary to visualize the vascular pedicle. In a free groin flap transfer, it is this vascular pedicle and venous drainage system that are of paramount importance, and they must consequently be visualized at an early stage in the dissection.

The flap is raised in its entirety with no delay of any kind. The correct dissection plane, ensuring that the flap contains its axial vessels, is most easily found if the upper skin incision is made first. This incision divides the superficial epigastric artery and its branches; if the flap is raised in a plane deep to these vessels, it will certainly include the superficial circumflex iliac arteriovenous systems, since both it and the superficial epigastric system lie in the same plane. The flap is raised until the lateral border of the sartorius is reached.

At this point the fascia covering the muscle is incised and included in the flap, dissection thereafter proceeding directly over the muscle. At the medial border of the sartorius, the flap will be found to be tethered by branches passing into the underlying muscles and by the lateral femoral cutaneous nerve of the thigh that crosses the arterial pedicle. Elevation of the flap should stop along this line. Although the deep branch of the artery can be ligated at this point to allow mobilization of the pedicle further, it is safer to leave it undisturbed. If greater length of flap is required, it is wiser to add the necessary centimeters at the distal end of the flap.

How safe it is to thin the flap remains a difficult problem. Increasing experience indicates that it is probably safe to thin it quite radically toward its distal end. It has been shown (15) that surprisingly large flaps raised with virtually no subcutaneous fat can survive, apparently entirely on a subdermal plexus. Provided that care is taken to avoid damaging recognizable axial vessels, thinning of the flap is reasonably safe. However, if there is the least doubt, it is certainly wiser to postpone thinning until transfer is complete.

The secondary defect of most groin flaps can be closed directly, although it may be necessary to flex the hip to reduce tension on the wound during suture. Only defects of exceptional width require split-thickness skin grafting. It is certainly preferable, where possible, to use direct closure. Not only does it simplify the whole operative procedure and postoperative management, but it leaves virtually no functional loss and the scar is hidden within the bikini area.

Recipient Site

In practice, the pedicle of the flap is usually tubed to eliminate all raw surfaces. Continuous suction, using a large bore catheter with extra holes cut along its length, is provided by introducing the catheter along the length of the tube. The ability both to tube the pedicle and to close the donor defect provides a long pedicle that permits freedom of movement without embarrassing the blood supply.

Movement should be restricted during the immediate postoperative period, particularly during recovery from the anes-

thetic, and the use of elastic adhesive strapping is generally sufficient. Thereafter there is no need for elaborate immobilization. The extent of immobilization depends on the state of the wound but can usually be quickly discarded.

The position taken by the arm is a relatively comfortable one and has been termed "the hand in pocket" position. The patient is actively encouraged to move the joints of the upper limb through as wide a range as possible. In particular, the length of the pedicle allows adequate mobility of the wrist and fingers.

The ability to mobilize the upper limb early appears to be of considerable importance in preventing the development of edema fluid that might otherwise collect in the dependent hand; it more than adequately offsets the effect of gravity.

Subsequent Stages

When cover of the defect by the flap is virtually complete, the flap is divided in its entirety at the end of 3 weeks, but is not inset (Fig. 6). Final insetting is postponed for a further week. The handling is basically similar to that of an ordinary direct flap. It is well recognized that rim necrosis, often following division and immediate insetting of a flap (17), can be avoided by postponing insetting for a week.

When the flap is being transferred on a wrist carrier, the situation calls for greater care, because of the need to be certain that there is enough blood flow through the attachment to sustain the flap. The presence in the flap of a preexisting, efficient arteriovenous system through its groin attachment means that there is little to encourage the development of an effective vascular flow through the wrist carrier attachment.

The way to encourage the development of adequate vascular flow through the wrist attachment is to reduce the efficiency of the already present arteriovenous system by formally ligating and dividing the feeding artery (18,19). Because of this, a delay stage should be made a formal part of the procedure, with careful search for, and division of, the superficial circumflex iliac artery (Fig. 7).

It is important also to appreciate that once the axial vessel is divided, the flap loses the characteristics it previously possessed by being an axial pattern flap. After delay, therefore, it must be managed in the same way as a standard abdominal tubed pedicle.

CLINICAL RESULTS

Used as a conventional axial pattern skin flap, the groin flap has proved safe and reliable. Necrosis has generally been

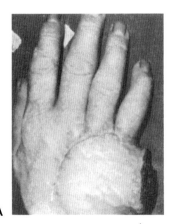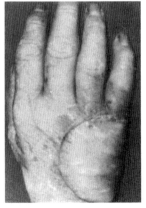

FIG. 6. Division of a groin flap applied to the hand 3 weeks following application (**A**), completion of insetting 1 week later (**B**). (From McGregor, ref. 16, with permission.)

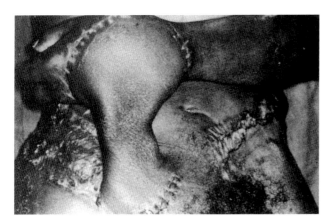

FIG. 7. Use of a delay stage 3 weeks after transfer, to ensure survival of the bridge segment prior to final division, and the use of the bridge segment to resurface the palm of the hand. (From McGregor, ref. 16, with permission.)

References

1. Bakamjian VY. A two stage method for pharyngo-esophageal reconstruction with a primary pectoral skin flap. *Plast Reconstr Surg* 1965;36:173.
2. McGregor IA, Jackson IT. The groin flap. *Br J Plast Surg* 1972;25:3.
3. Wood J. Case of extreme deformity of the neck and forearm from the cicatrices of a burn, cured by extension, excision and transplantation of skin, adjacent and remote. *Med Chir Trans* 1863;46:149.
4. Aymard JL. Nasal reconstruction. *Lancet* 1917;2:888.
5. Joseph J. *Nasenplastik and sonstige Gesichtsplastik nebst einem. Anhang ueber Mammaplastik und einige weitere Operationen aus dem Gebiete der aeusseren Koerperplastik.* Leipzig: Curt Kabitzsch, 1931.
6. Shaw DT, Payne RL. One stage tubed abdominal flaps. *Surg Gynecol Obstet* 1946;83:205.
7. Khoo BC. John Wood and his contribution to plastic surgery: the first groin flap. *Br J Plast Surg* 1977;30:9.
8. McGregor IA, Morgan RG. Axial and random pattern flaps. *Br J Plast Surg* 1973;26:202.
9. Smith PJ. The vascular basis of axial pattern flaps. *Br J Plast Surg* 1973;26:150.
10. Taylor GI, Daniel RK. The anatomy of several free flap donor sites. *Plast Reconstr Surg* 1975;56:243.
11. Lister GD, McGregor IA, Jackson IT. The groin flap in hand injuries. *Injury* 1973;4:229.
12. Smith PJ, Foley B, McGregor IA, Jackson IT. The anatomical basis of the groin flap. *Plast Reconstr Surg* 1972;40:41.
13. Harii K, Ohmori K, Torii S, et al. Free groin skin flaps. *Br J Plast Surg* 1975;28:225.
14. Ohmori K, Harii K. Free groin flaps: their vascular basis. *Br J Plast Surg* 1975;28:238.
15. Colson P, Houot R, Gangolphe M, et al. Use of thinned flaps (flap grafts) in reparative hand surgery. *Ann Chir Plast* 1967;12:298.
16. McGregor IA. The groin flap. In: Grabb WC, Myers MB, eds. *Skin flaps.* Boston: Little Brown, 1975.
17. Stark RB, Kernahan DA. Reconstructive surgery of the leg and foot. *Surg Clin North Am* 1959;39:469.
18. Stranc WE. The delay procedure and its effect on blood now in tubed pedicle flaps. In: Sanvenero-Rosselli G, Boggio-Robutti G, eds. *Transactions of the Fourth International Congress of Plastic and Reconstructive Surgery.* Amsterdam: Excerpta Medica, 1969:1190.
19. Stranc MF, Labandter H, Roy A. A review of 196 tubed pedicles. *Br J Plast Surg* 1975;28:54.

the result of obvious technical error or the use of a flap that extended too far beyond the territory of the axial artery. This happened mainly during the period of initial exploration of the flap potential and before the need to observe the 1:1 ratio of its terminal random segment was fully appreciated.

SUMMARY

The groin flap is a reliable, efficient flap for covering hand and forearm defects.

CHAPTER 301 ■ HYPOGASTRIC (SHAW) SKIN FLAP

T. BARFRED

Since 1973, when a choice between the groin flap and the hypogastric flap became possible, I have used the hypogastric flap in about half of my cases (1). When both flaps seem equally comfortable, the groin flap is chosen because of the texture of the flap and the position of the donor site (2–8).

INDICATIONS

The flap is suitable for any defect of the hand, either palmar or dorsal, but especially for the latter (Fig. 6). If several fingers are to be covered, an artificial syndactyly is created for one regular defect (Fig. 6B). In subsequent syndactyly operations, the flap is defatted and the cosmetic result is satisfactory.

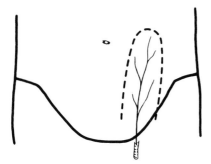

FIG. 1. The hypogastric (Shaw) flap.

The flap has been used for primary or secondary defects or for defects created in reconstructive procedures, with equally good results. The tube itself has even been used as a flap for another defect on the same hand or on the opposite hand.

Secondary reconstructive procedures (Fig. 5) can be performed easily under the flap at a later stage.

ANATOMY

In a study of 100 dissections of the iliofemoral region (9), the superficial circumflex iliac and superficial inferior epigastric arteries had a common origin from the femoral artery in 48%. In 17% the two vessels had a separate origin, and in the remaining 35%, the superficial inferior epigastric artery was absent and was replaced by smaller branches from the superficial circumflex iliac artery. They found that the superficial inferior epigastric artery, when present, covered a fan-shaped area from the border of the rectus abdominus muscle to the iliac crest.

FLAP DESIGN AND DIMENSIONS

The hypogastric flap should be based just proximal to the ipsilateral inguinal ligament, centered over the femoral artery and vein (Fig. 1). The flap should be directed slightly lateral and designed to the defect in the proximal part. Distally, a width of 7 to 8 cm is generally necessary to tube this fairly abundant part of the flap. Most flaps are 16 to 18 cm long. There has been no verified use of extraordinarily long flaps of this type, but the anatomic studies indicate that a groin flap should be chosen for coverage of very large defects.

A preoperative positioning test is most important, to decide which flap will give the best possibilities for positioning and moving the hand and arm, when attached to the trunk.

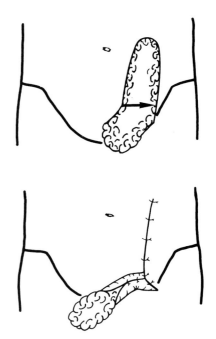

FIG. 2. The raw area of the flap can be directed laterally by staggering the incision at the base of the tube.

OPERATIVE TECHNIQUE

Proximally, the flap is raised at the level of the deep fascia, but it may be thinned in its peripheral random pattern part. Distally, the flap is raised just superficial to Scarpa's fascia. The donor defect is closed primarily. When tubing the base of the flap, it is important to decide the best direction for the raw area of the flap (Fig. 2). It can be easily directed medially, laterally, or facing upward, depending on the most relaxed position of the hand. Transition between the tube and flap is facilitated if a reverse flap from the hand can be created (Fig. 3).

Until the tube is divided, every effort must be made to maintain movement in the shoulder, elbow, wrist, and fingers (Fig. 4). If a contralateral flap is used, shoulder movement is difficult, but this may be the primary choice if an ipsilateral hypogastric flap or groin flap is contraindicated.

Ten to 12 days after the first stage, the tube is clamped with a pliable intestinal forceps for 5 to 30 minutes, to observe the vascular reaction in the flap. It is possible that some "training effect" is obtained at the same time. The flap is routinely divided after 3 weeks. If part of the tube must be used, a delay operation to divide the axial vessels is advised.

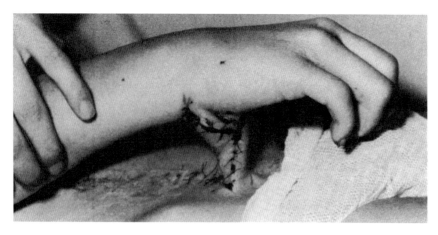

FIG. 3. The transition from the tube to the hand is facilitated by a reverse flap from the hand.

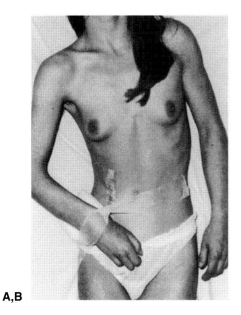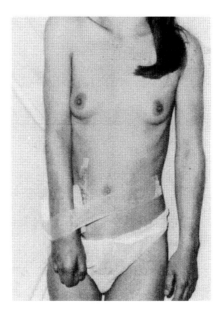

A,B

FIG. 4. A,B: The range of movement possible with a hypogastric flap in place in a short-armed patient.

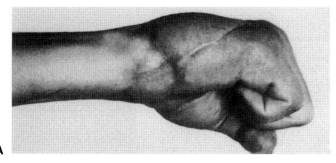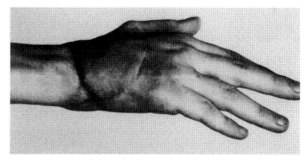

A

B

FIG. 5. Flexion and extension after a hypogastric flap and secondary reconstruction of all the extensor tendons to the fingers.

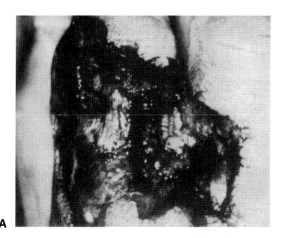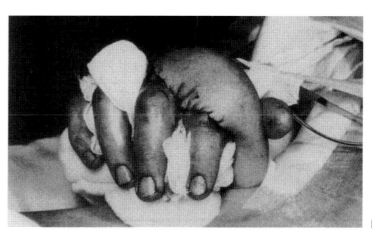

A

B

FIG. 6. A: Defect of the index and long fingers with bone and tendon injuries. B: The hypogastric flap applied after artificial syndactyly to create one defect.

CLINICAL RESULTS

Thirty-three flaps have been performed on 31 patients between 1956 and 1981. One flap was totally lost because of severe hemorrhage from the flap, simultaneous with severe hematemesis. One flap included an appendectomy scar and was partially lost, resulting in reamputation of the thumb. One flap had only a partial loss, but the severely burned hand had to be amputated because of increasing necrosis.

Ten cases had partial necrosis of the flap. Six of these healed spontaneously. In two cases, the flap was detached, the necrosis excised, and the flap reapplied, without further complications. One patient had minor necrosis, and a large tear had to be grafted later. One patient had a total skin loss, but the subcutaneous flap tissue survived and allowed coverage of the defect with a full-thickness skin graft, using the crane principle (10). Thus, in only two of 33 flaps did the intended result not occur.

The skin color of the flap is generally somewhat darker than normal skin, and the hair growth more ample. Quite a few patients developed a slight sensation for touch. One patient gained weight after the operation, to almost double his original, without increasing the subcutaneous tissue of the flap. No complications were found in 14 subsequent reconstructions and eight defatting procedures.

SUMMARY

The hypogastric flap remains an alternative procedure to the groin flap for hand reconstruction. The needs of the individual patient will determine which flap is the more appropriate.

References

1. Barfred T. The Shaw abdominal flap. *Scand J Plast Reconstr Surg* 1976; 10:56.
2. Wood J. Case of extreme deformity of the neck and forearm from the cicatrices of a burn, cured by extension, excision, and transplantation of skin, adjacent and remote. *Med Chir Trans* 1863;46:149.
3. Shaw DT, Payne RL. One stage tubed abdominal flaps. *Surg Gynecol Obstet* 1946;83:205.
4. Bunnell S. *Surgery of the hand,* 2d Ed. Philadelphia: Lippincott, 1948; 194–195.
5. McGregor IA, Jackson IT. The groin flap. *Br J Plast Surg* 1972;25:3.
6. Li CS, Nahigian SH, Richey DWG, Shaw DT. Primary application of the one stage abdominal tubed pedicle. *Hand* 1972;4:184.
7. Kojima T. One stage tubed abdominal flap for the hand. *Jpn J Plast Reconstr Surg* 1973;16:300.
8. Baudet J, Lemaire JM. Le lambeau abdominal en chirurgie de la main. *Ann Chir Plast* 1975;20:215.
9. Taylor GI, Daniel RK. The anatomy of several free flap donor sites. *Plast Reconstr Surg* 1975;56:243.
10. Millard DR, Cooley SGE. A solution to coverage in severe compound dorsal hand injuries. *Plast Reconstr Surg* 1972;49:215.

 CHAPTER 302. Microvascular Free Transfer of the Groin Skin Flap *K. Harii*
www.encyclopediaofflaps.com

CHAPTER 303 ■ MICROVASCULAR FREE TRANSFER OF A DORSALIS PEDIS SKIN FLAP WITH EXTENSOR TENDONS

G. I. TAYLOR AND R. J. CORLETT

The combined loss of skin and tendon on the dorsum of the hand, seen especially after avulsion or degloving injuries, is a challenging problem. When the defect is large, the conventional repair of such a wound usually requires a distant abdominal flap, with tendon grafting or transfer done as a secondary procedure. These multistage procedures impose a protracted convalescence and difficult assessment of accurate tendon graft length, due to retraction of the involved muscle bellies.

INDICATIONS

In carefully selected cases, a composite free flap with attached vascularized tendon grafts offers an immediate one-stage solution to this problem as a primary procedure (1). Several donor sites are now available, including the radial or ulnar forearm flaps with attached segments of the forearm flexor tendons, the groin flap and the tensor fasciae latae flap with vascularized strips of the external oblique aponeurosis and the fascia

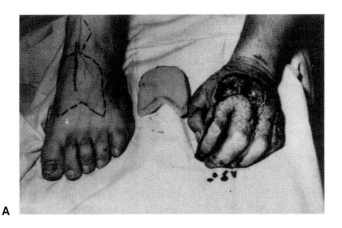

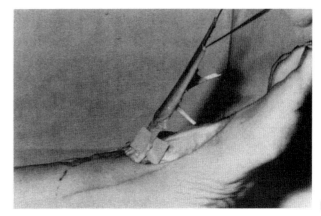

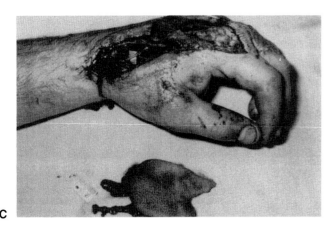

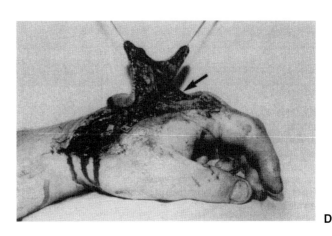

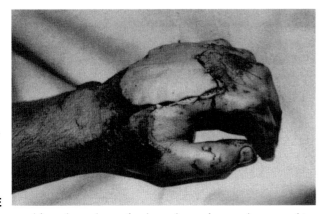

FIG. 1. A: A 19-year-old salesman sustained a heavily contaminated degloving abrading injury to the dorsum of his dominant left hand when his automobile overturned. An 8 × 5-cm area of skin was missing, together with 4-cm defects in the extensor tendons of the index and middle fingers. The dorsal cortices of the second and third metacarpals were also missing. The wound was debrided and then reconstructed as a delayed primary procedure 48 hours later. A pattern of the defect was outlined on the dorsum of his ipsilateral foot. **B:** A composite free flap, with attached vascularized segments of the extensor hallucis brevis to the big toe and the extensor digitorum longus to the second toe, was isolated on the dorsalis pedis vessels. The dissection commenced distally, and a long vascular pedicle was obtained by a dissection of the vessels to the level of the ankle joint. **C:** The flap was detached and revascularized by anastomosis to the radial vessels and the cephalic vein on the dorsum of the wrist joint. **D:** The revascularized flap with tendon grafts in position. The vascular paratenon is marked with an *arrow*. **E:** Bright red bleeding was noted from the tendon grafts; the tendon grafts were then sutured in position and the skin defect was closed. The donor site on the dorsum of the foot was covered with a split-thickness skin graft. The hand was immobilized in a volar slab with the wrist in extension and the metacarpophalangeal joints in flexion. Three weeks later, the plaster was removed and mobilization of the fingers commenced. After a further 3 weeks, the patient returned to work, at which time the range of movement of the fingers was almost normal. *(continued)*

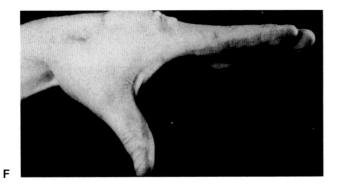

F

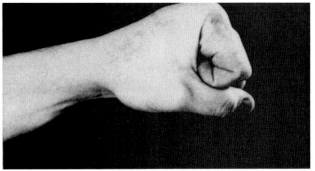

G

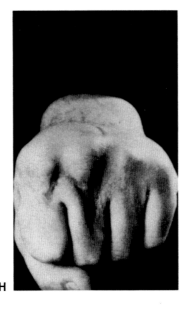

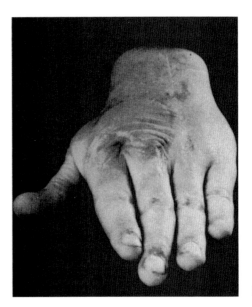

FIG. 1. *Continued.* F–I. By 2 months, a full range of flexion and extension was evident, and no further surgery has been required. The follow-up period has been 6 years and, to date, the donor site has presented no problems. (From Taylor and Townsend, ref. 1, with permission.)

H

I

lata, respectively, and the dorsalis pedis flap with attached extensor tendons. The latter flap is ideally suited for the repair of skin and tendon defects on the dorsum of the hand, as the anatomy of these two areas bears a close resemblance.

ANATOMY

The dorsalis pedis artery has been shown to nourish the extensor hallucis longus and brevis tendons, together with the long and short extensors of the other toes as they fan across the dorsum of the foot. When combined with the overlying dorsal skin, this unit provides a very thin skin flap with a mobile complex of one or more extensor tendons. The effectiveness of this composite flap as a free transfer is well shown in the illustrations.

OPERATIVE TECHNIQUE

Fig. 1; see Chapter 518.

CLINICAL RESULTS

In the patient shown, the dominant hand was involved and the composite free flap provided an excellent result. Not only was

there a deficiency of skin and tendon, but the metacarpal bones were also involved—a situation where conventional tendon grafts would have been prone to adhesion. This was not the case with the vascularized tendon grafts. Presumably, they did not adhere along their length, because of an intact intrinsic and extrinsic blood supply and the gliding paratenon, which was transferred with the tendons.

The composite dorsalis pedis free flap with attached tendon grafts can be expanded to include a nerve supply and the second metatarsal bone. However, in general, the dorsum of the foot cannot be regarded as a donor site without problems. Hypertrophic unstable scars are not uncommon, and it is therefore essential that cases be carefully selected.

SUMMARY

The free dorsalis pedis skin flap with attached vascularized tendons can be used effectively to provide coverage for hand defects that include segmental tendon loss.

Reference

1. Taylor GI, Townsend PLG. Composite free flap and tendon transfer: an anatomical study and a clinical technique. *Br J Plast Surg* 1979;32:170.

CHAPTER 304 ■ MICROVASCULAR AND MICRONEUROVASCULAR FREE TRANSFER OF A DORSALIS PEDIS FLAP

R. K. DANIEL

The dorsalis pedis free flap, when first developed (1), had several advantages when used in covering hand defects. It was much thinner than the groin flap (2). Although there were some minor problems with donor site morbidity, it was extended and expanded to provide an innervated free flap as well (3,4).

INDICATIONS

The first web space free flap (see Chap. 323) (5–7) and various toe free flaps (see Chaps. 233, 234, 236, 237, and 257) can be used instead of or in addition to the dorsalis pedis free flap.

The dorsalis pedis free flap, although somewhat tedious to dissect, has a reliable arterial supply and venous drainage. It is innervated by an expendable cutaneous sensory nerve. It has an acceptable two-point discrimination, approaching 10 mm in its most medial distribution. The addition of a first web space or toe flap can provide improved sensibility. It is an extremely thin flap, having a minimal amount of subcutaneous tissue. A long neurovascular stalk can be adapted to various recipient site requirements. The donor site, although causing some minor problems, is inconspicuous.

ANATOMY

When used as a neurovascular free flap, the innervation of the superficial peroneal nerve must be carefully documented. This can be done preoperatively by using selective local anesthetic blocks. By anesthetizing the sural, the saphenous, and medial and lateral plantar nerves, one is left with the maximum area of sensory distribution for the superficial branch of the peroneal nerve. The quality of two-point discrimination ranges from 10 to 20 mm, being lowest in the area medial to the extensor hallucis longus.

FLAP DESIGN AND DIMENSIONS

Initially the flap was felt to be restricted to 10 × 8 cm. With the addition of the first web space and toe flaps, the size of the flap can be expanded significantly. This consequently increases the amount of donor site morbidity.

OPERATIVE TECHNIQUE

The innervation of the dorsalis pedis flap can be mapped out intraoperatively using electrophysiologic techniques (Fig. 1). The superficial peroneal nerve is carefully dissected proximally for about 10 cm, to ensure fusion of its medial and intermediate branches. It is then transected. Under high magnification, the cross-sectional anatomic topography of the nerve is outlined. There are usually nine fascicles that can be isolated. After assessing the viability of each fascicle by electrical stimulation, the area of skin innervated by each fascicle can be determined. Using electrophysiologic techniques, the skin on the dorsum of the foot is mechanically stimulated and the corresponding fascicle determined. The appropriate fascicles can then be sutured to the appropriate branches of the median and/or ulnar nerves in the recipient site (Fig. 2). For details of flap elevation see Chapter 518.

SUMMARY

The dorsalis pedis free flap dramatically altered the approach to reconstructive surgery of the hand. It was further expanded into

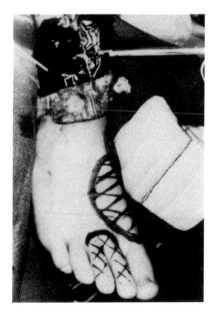

FIG. 1. Sensory skin mapping completed on the donor site with the electrophysiologic recording setup shown at the level of the ankle.

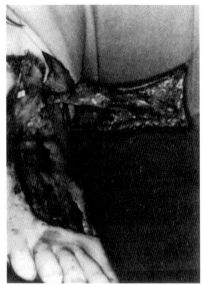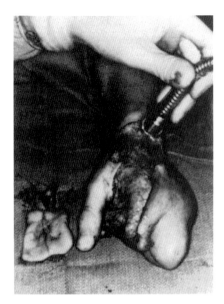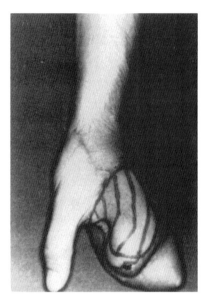

A–C

FIG. 2. **A:** Isolation of the dorsalis pedis neurovascular free flap. **B:** The neurovascular free flap ready for microsurgical anastomoses in the recipient hand. **C:** The flap at 5 months. The extent of reinnervation at this time is indicated by hatch marks.

a neurovascular free flap, which improved both function and cover. Electrophysiologic techniques refined the approach to restoring sensation. These techniques are mandatory when the nerve distribution far exceeds the size of the flap required, or when mixed nerves of sensorimotor composition are used.

References

1. McCraw JB, Furlow LT. The dorsalis pedis arterialized flap: a clinical study. *Plast Reconstr Surg* 1975;55:177.
2. Daniel RK, Taylor GI. Distant transfer of an island flap by microvascular anastomoses. *Plast Reconstr Surg* 1973;52:111.
3. Daniel RK, Terzis J, Schwartz G. Neurovascular free flaps: a preliminary report. *Plast Reconstr Surg* 1975;56:13.
4. Gilbert A. Composite tissue transfers from the foot: anatomic basis and surgical technique. In: Daniller AT, Strauch B, eds. *Symposium on microsurgery.* St. Louis: Mosby, 1976.
5. May JW Jr, Chait LA, Cohen BE, O'Brien BM. Free neurovascular flap from the first web of the foot in hand reconstruction. *J Hand Surg* 1977;2:387.
6. Morrison WA, O'Brien BM, MacLeod AM, Gilbert A. Neurovascular free flaps from the foot for innervation of the hand. *J Hand Surg* 1978;3:235.
7. Strauch B, Tsur H. Restoration of sensation to the hand by free neurovascular flap from the first web space of the foot. *Plast Reconstr Surg* 1978;62:361.

CHAPTER 305 ■ BICEPS FEMORIS PERFORATOR FREE FLAP FOR UPPER-EXTREMITY RECONSTRUCTION

P. C. CAVADAS, J. R. RAMÓN SANZ, AND L. LANDIN

EDITORIAL COMMENT

A useful flap but not first choice.

Perforator flaps are now being widely recognized as useful adjuncts to reduce donor morbidity in reconstructive micro-surgery. The anatomy of the musculocutaneous perforating vessels of the short head of the biceps femoris muscle is described as a source for free-tissue transfer for upper-extremity reconstruction. The vascular anatomy is relatively constant. Flap dissection is straightforward under tourniquet control; donor morbidity is low, if primary closure is possible; and pedicle size is appropriate for repair. When a moderately sized (up to 20 × 7 cm), moderately thick, medium-sized pedicle, far from the recipient area (double-team approach) free flap is needed, the biceps femoris perforator (BiFeP) flap can be considered among possible alternatives.

INDICATIONS

The BiFeP flap can be harvested as a fasciocutaneous flap for soft-tissue coverage of medium-sized defects of the upper extremity. If it is harvested as a fasciosubcutaneous flap, BiFeP flap size matches that of small defects and first web-space contracture release. As with other perforator flaps of the thigh, the BiFeP flap can be used for postoncologic head and neck reconstruction (1–6). A few publications have reported the use of lateral thigh flaps in the reconstruction of the Achilles tendon (7).

The BiFeP flap should be preferably used in thin patients; otherwise, debulking procedures will be necessary. Color matching will be much better if the flap is used to reconstruct the lower extremity, rather than the upper extremity, and this issue should be stressed before surgery in dark-skinned patients.

ANATOMY

The posterolateral region of the thigh was described as a donor area for free-tissue transfer by Baek in 1983, in a paper reporting an anatomic study and a single clinical case (8). The BiFeP flap is closely related to the "lower posterolateral thigh flap" described by Laitung (9) in 1989 and clearly different from the lateral-posterolateral flap described by Baek and later widely reported in the head and neck literature (1–6). Reports by Hayashi and Maruyama (10) have focused on describing the superior lateral genicular artery (SLGA) flap, and more recently, they have reported on an anatomic study of the lateral intermuscular septum of the thigh and the short head of the biceps femoris muscle (BFsh) (11), in which the importance of the SLGA in the vascularization of the distal BFsh was stressed. An attempt at clarifying the anatomic confusion regarding lateral-thigh skin vascularization is also made in the present chapter.

The skin of the lateral thigh is vascularized by different vessels. The profunda femoris artery provides the classic "perforating" branches that run along the septum between the vastus lateralis muscle and the BFsh, named the lateral intermuscular septum, to emerge through the fascia lata and to irrigate the proximal two thirds of the lateral thigh. The distal third of the thigh skin may vary in its vascular nourishment.

We studied the distal-third vascularization of the thigh. In our cadaver study, three sizable BFsh perforators (more than 0.5 mm external diameter) were consistently found in all specimens (Fig. 1). Their location was also constant. The lower perforator was located at 6 cm from the knee-joint line (range: 5 to 6.5 cm), and was a branch off the SLGA in all cases. This artery was a branch from the popliteal artery that runs close to the bone and sends out several muscular branches and one musculocutaneous branch. The middle perforator was located at 11.6 cm from the joint line (range: 10 to 14 cm). It was a direct branch off the first portion of the popliteal artery in 60% of the cases (Fig. 2), and off the "classic" perforating branch of the profunda femoris artery (probably the third) in 40% of the cases (Fig. 2). The upper perforator was located at 15.3 cm from the joint line (range: 14 to 17 cm) and was usually the least substantial of the three vessels. Its course was variable, it being a true perforator in 80% of the cases and piercing the lateral intermuscular septum in the remaining 20%. In all cases, it had a common intramuscular origin with the middle perforating vessel. Other less substantial musculocutaneous perforators were distributed over the BFsh.

The flap described herein as the BiFeP flap is more distally located than the "posterolateral thigh flap" based on the third perforator of the profunda femoris artery, described by Baek (8) and widely reported by other authors for head and neck cancer surgery. The branch of these previously reported flaps is located about the midpoint of the line connecting the greater trochanter and the lateral femoral condyle, septal or musculocutaneous, depending on the description, whereas the BiFeP flap is based on a BFsh perforator located well below this point, 11 cm above the knee joint. The flap described by Laitung (9) as the "lower posterolateral thigh flap" is closely related to the BiFeP flap and could well be the same flap, although Laitung only suggested the possibility of freely transferring this flap. The lateral genicular flap of Hayashi and Maruyama (10) is based on the SLGA, the distal BFsh perforator in our anatomic study.

OPERATIVE TECHNIQUE

The BiFeP flap can be elevated in supine, midlateral, or lateral position, although supine is preferred. The knee is flexed, the hip is flexed and internally rotated, and a sandbag is placed below the ipsilateral buttock. The interval between the vastus lateralis-iliotibial tract and the long head of biceps femoris muscle is easily palpated in the lower half of the thigh. (Knee extension for tensioning the iliotibial tract may be necessary for accurate palpation in overweight patients.) The predicted positions of perforating vessels are plotted with a directional Doppler probe, although they can reliably be found at 10 to 14 cm from the knee joint line. A flap up to 20 × 7 cm can be elevated under tourniquet control with partial exsanguination.

The anterior edge of the flap is elevated first, proceeding in the loose areolar plane above the iliotibial tract and the thick fascia lata posteriorly. Once the BFsh is reached, the exact position of the perforators is determined. There are usually three sizable vessels and some additional minor ones. The branch located 11.6 cm (10 to 14 cm) proximal to the knee-joint line (middle perforator) is selected as the pedicle of the flap, although any of the perforating vessels could be. This vessel is traced back intramuscularly for several centimeters to meet the required length and caliber of the particular case. The skin island is best oriented proximally so that the perforator enters its distal end. In this way, the thinner upper portion of the skin is used, and the scar is kept away from the knee joint.

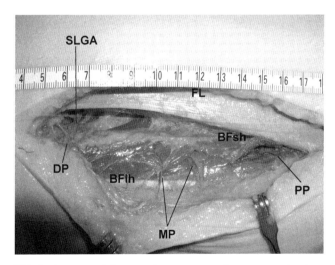

FIG. 1. Anatomy of the musculocutaneous perforators over the short head of the biceps femoris in a fresh human specimen. Left thigh, supine position, ruler indicating the distance in centimeters from the knee-joint line. Left margin is distal, up is ventral in the figure. There are three main perforators located about 6, 12, and 25 cm, respectively, from the joint line. DP, distal perforator; MP, middle perforator; PP, proximal perforator; FL, fascia lata overlying the vastus lateralis muscle; BFsh, biceps femoris short head; SLGA, superior lateral genicular artery.

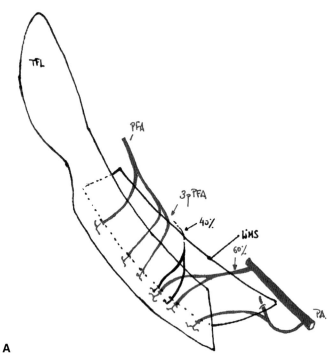

A

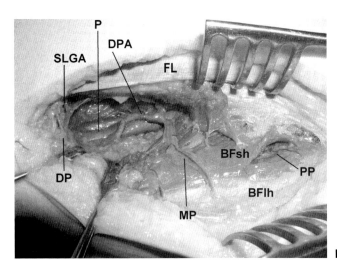

B

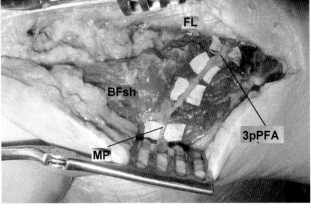

C

FIG. 2. Anatomic origin of the musculocutaneous perforators over the short head of the biceps femoris muscle. **A:** PFA, profunda femoris artery; 3pPFA, third classic perforator off the profunda femoris artery; LIMS, lateral intermuscular septum; PA, popliteal artery. (Modified from Hayashi A, Maruyama Y. *Plast Reconstr Surg* 2001;108:1646.) **B:** Left thigh, supine position. Left margin is distal, and up is ventral in the figure. The distal perforator is always a branch from the superior lateral genicular artery. The middle perforator is a direct branch from the popliteal artery in 60% of the cases. The proximal perforator is a branch off the middle perforator. DP, distal perforator; MP, middle perforator; PP, proximal perforator; FL, fascia lata overlying the vastus lateralis muscle; BFsh, biceps femoris short head; BFlh, biceps femoris long head; SLGA, superior lateral genicular artery; P, popliteal vessels; DPA, direct branch from the popliteal artery. **C:** Left margin is distal, up is ventral in the figure. The middle perforator is a branch off the profunda femoris artery in 40% of the cases (presumably its third perforating branch, although not explicitly determined in the present anatomic study). MP, middle perforator; FL, fascia lata overlying the vastus lateralis muscle; BFsh, biceps femoris short head; 3pPFA, third perforator of the profunda femoris artery.

Once the desired pedicle length and size are dissected, the posterior border of the flap is incised and quickly elevated. The maximal length of the pedicle depends on the origin of the middle perforator. When it comes from the popliteal vessels, up to 7 to 8 cm can be obtained. When it is a branch of the profunda femoris, longer pedicles can be obtained, although the dissection below the femur can be very tedious. Donor areas are directly closed.

CLINICAL RESULTS

In our series of 10 patients, there were 7 acute skin losses and 3 delayed reconstructions (releases of adduction retraction of the thumb). All 10 flaps were based on the middle musculocutaneous perforator. Two of the flaps were subcutaneous free flaps. Nine free flaps healed without any complication. One flap developed arterial ischemia on postoperative day 2. The flap was reexplored, but partial distal necrosis developed, probably because of the undue secondary ischemia time. Donor areas were directly closed in every case, although there were two wound dehiscences that

required revision. Four of the flaps required a debulking procedure at a second stage.

The BiFeP flap is based on a constant anatomy and can be elevated under tourniquet control, which are definite advantages over other perforator flaps. The pedicle is of moderate size in terms of length (up to 7 to 8 cm) and caliber (artery up to 2 to 2.5 mm, vein 3 to 4 mm), and it is a rather thick flap, which somewhat limits its applications. When a thin flap with a long or large-caliber pedicle is required, other free flaps are a better choice. The donor area of the BiFeP flap is relatively well hidden and inconspicuous if direct closure is possible. If direct closure is not possible (pinch test), then skin grafting would be necessary, and other options should take preference over a BiFeP flap. The use of the subcutaneous version of this flap partially avoids the donor morbidity of large flaps.

Because the BiFeP flap is a genuine perforator flap, surgical injury to the BFsh should be minimal, and no functional disability is to be expected from its harvest, although this was not specifically addressed in the clinical series presented here. A relatively high incidence of donor-site complications, especially dehiscence, seroma formation, and delayed healing, has been reported in the head and neck literature, and was also found in the present series. More attention to technical detail in wound closure and postoperative knee immobilization might reduce this incidence. The use of quilting sutures can also reduce the incidence of seroma.

In our experience, the flaps were rather small, although a 20 × 7-cm flap survived completely. The maximal dimensions of the BiFeP flap are yet to be defined, but based on the vast clinical experience with the anterolateral thigh flap, larger skin islands are likely to survive completely based on a single perforator. The skin over the distal lateral thigh is thinner anteriorly than it is posteriorly, and a substantial thickness of fat is present at the angle between the vastus lateralis and the BFsh muscles. The skin island is oriented proximally, with the perforating vessel entering about its distal end, to keep the scar far from the knee joint and to take advantage of the thinner, more proximal skin. The distal perforator (SLGA) is not used as the pedicle of the BiFeP flap, to avoid scars in the lateral knee region.

SUMMARY

The BiFeP flap is a low-morbidity, genuine perforator free flap, based on musculocutaneous perforators located distally over the BFsh, that can be quickly elevated under tourniquet control and that should probably be within the group of first-choice flaps when a moderately pedicled and relatively thin free flap is needed. The amount of skin required is within the range that permits direct closure. Its usefulness in upper-extremity reconstruction has been demonstrated, and it would also probably be a good choice in lower-extremity reconstruction as a regional free flap. Attention must be paid to ensure color matching and desired thickness.

References

1. Hayden RE. A new technique in pharyngoesophageal reconstruction. In: Bloom HJG, ed., *Head and neck oncology*. New York: Raven Press, 1986.
2. Hayden RE. Lateral cutaneous thigh flap. In: Baker S, ed., *Microsurgical reconstruction of the head and neck*. New York: Churchill Livingstone, 1989.
3. Hayden RE. Lateral thigh flap. *Otolaryngol Clin North Am* 1994;27:1171.
4. Hayden RE, Deschler DG. Lateral thigh free flap for head and neck reconstruction. *Laryngoscope* 1999;109:1490.
5. Truelson JM, Leach JL. Lateral thigh flap reconstruction in the head and neck. *Otolaryngol Head Neck Surg* 1998;118:203.
6. Miller MJ, Reece GP, Marchi M, Baldwin BJ. Lateral thigh free flaps in head and neck reconstruction. *Plast Reconstr Surg* 1995;96:334.
7. Inoue T, Tanaka K, Imai K, Hatoko M. Reconstruction of Achilles tendon using vascularized fascia lata with free lateral thigh flap. *Br J Plast Surg* 1990;43:727.
8. Baek SM. Two cutaneous free flaps: the medial and lateral thigh flap. *Plast Reconstr Surg* 1983;71:354.
9. Laitung JKG. The lower posterolateral thigh flap. *Br J Plast Surg* 1989; 42:133.
10. Hayashi A, Maruyama Y. The lateral genicular artery flap. *Ann Plast Surg* 1990;24:310.
11. Hayashi A, Maruyama Y. Lateral intermuscular septum of the thigh and short head of the biceps femoris muscle: an anatomical investigation with new clinical applications. *Plast Reconstr Surg* 2001;108:1646.

CHAPTER 306. Free Parietotemporalis Fascial Flap *J. Upton and C. Rodgers*
www.encyclopediaofflaps.com

CHAPTER 307 ■ MICROVASCULAR FREE TRANSFER OF THE LATERAL ARM FASCIOCUTANEOUS FLAP

L. SCHEKER AND G. LISTER

The lateral arm flap is especially useful in hand reconstruction, where the thinness, color, and texture of the flap give not only a good functional result, but also a pleasing cosmetic match.

INDICATIONS

Like any other thin, fasciocutaneous flap, the lateral arm flap can be used for many defects; however, its use for intraoral reconstruction may be limited by the amount of hair that is often present. It is an excellent flap for hand reconstruction in both elective and emergency situations, for it is possible to elevate small areas of skin in almost any orientation. If only a segment of vascularized subcutaneous tissue is required, a fascial flap alone can be harvested.

Because the lateral arm flap, like the radial and ulnar forearm flaps, has through-flow characteristics (1,2), structures distal to the flap can be revascularized with the distal end of the pedicle.

This flap can also be divided transversely so as to cover two defects, for example on the palm and dorsum, provided only that the intermuscular septum is maintained.

ANATOMY

The profunda brachii artery is the first branch of the brachial artery. After giving origin to some muscular branches in the medial aspect of the arm, it winds behind the humerus in company with the radial nerve in the spiral groove. The two terminal branches of the profunda brachii artery, the middle collateral and the radial collateral arteries, originate here.

The middle collateral is usually larger than the radial collateral. It enters the substance of the long and medial heads of the triceps, descends along the posterior aspect of the humerus, and disappears deep to the aconeus. The radial collateral artery, appearing laterally in front of the triceps, divides into two terminal branches, the anterior radial collateral and the posterior radial collateral artery. The anterior radial collateral runs between brachialis and brachioradialis accompanying the radial nerve.

The posterior radial collateral artery—the pedicle of the lateral arm flap—enters the lateral intermuscular septum close to the insertion of the deltoid muscle, between the brachioradialis muscle anteriorly and the triceps muscle posteriorly. The artery remains in the lateral intermuscular septum close to the humerus, giving off several periosteal and muscular branches. It continues close to the lateral epicondyle and ends by supplying the skin of the forearm over the radial head. In its course, the posterior radial collateral artery gives origin to two or three septal branches that pass to the deep fascia and irrigate the skin. The most proximal of these branches is closely related to the posterior cutaneous nerve of the forearm.

The venous return of this flap is through two systems, the superficial veins that are tributaries of the cephalic vein and

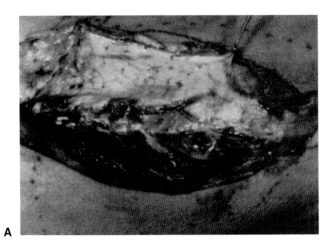

A

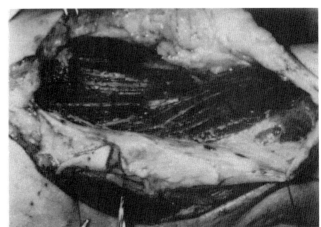

B

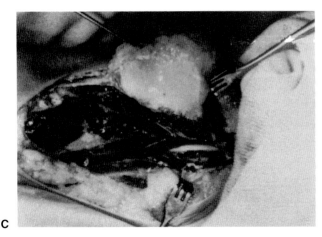

C

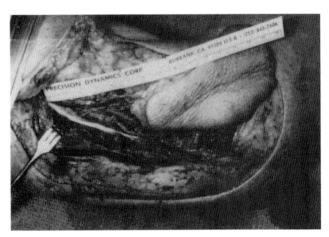

D

FIG. 1. **A:** The dissection of the lateral arm flap has commenced posteriorly. In this clinical photograph, the dotted marks on the skin at the lower side of the photograph represent the extent of the fascia that was taken with the flap. The fascia has been dissected sharply off the underlying triceps muscle, which is shown in the wound. The posterior radial collateral artery can be seen running in the lateral intermuscular septum. The lower vessel of the two at the bifurcation is the one that can be used for through-flow in replantation or revascularization. **B:** The anterior dissection in the same patient shows that fascia has been taken from over the brachialis muscle at the upper left and the brachioradialis muscle at the upper right. **C:** The anterior dissection has been completed, and the flap has been raised by incising the lateral intermuscular septum. The radial nerve is clearly seen passing anteriorly between the brachialis and brachioradialis muscles, and so out of the field of dissection. Its accompanying vessel, the anterior radial collateral artery, can be divided to give greater pedicle length. **D:** The flap has been raised completely. Note that a pedicle of at least 6 cm can be obtained while still working in a bloodless field. The sterile tourniquet is seen at the upper left of the photograph. In this photograph the triceps tendon can be seen running along the lower margin of the wound.

the deep venae comitantes. Either system is satisfactory as a flap pedicle, but in practice we prefer the venae comitantes.

The pedicle is constant and its length varies according to the design of the flap, ranging from 4 to 8 cm. The caliber of the artery in our practice has always been greater than 1.2 mm and the venae comitantes larger than 2.0 mm.

The posterior cutaneous nerve of the arm innervates this flap. The posterior cutaneous nerve of the forearm runs through the deep tissues with the posterior radial collateral artery, and has to be sacrificed in most cases.

FLAP DESIGN AND DIMENSIONS

The lateral arm flap is based on the posterior radial collateral artery, a terminal branch of the profunda brachii system. It may be raised purely as a fascial flap, or with bone, or with overlying skin, with or without innervation.

The flap consists of the skin of the distal half of the lateral aspect of the arm and the proximal fifth of the forearm, centered on a line running from the insertion of the deltoid to the lateral epicondyle, with the extremity extended. The estimated width of skin that can be harvested with this flap varies from 10 to 14 cm (3–6), but this large donor site defect may prove troublesome. We prefer to restrict the width of the skin flap to 6 cm, facilitating primary closure of the donor defect. The area of fascia that may be taken, either alone or with skin is, of course, much larger, to a practical maximum of 20 × 14 cm.

The insertion of the deltoid and the lateral epicondyle is marked with the elbow extended. A dotted line is drawn between these two structures. The pattern of the primary defect is centered on the dotted line that corresponds to the lateral intermuscular septum. A sterile tourniquet is positioned as high as possible on the arm and inflated.

OPERATIVE TECHNIQUE

The skin is incised posteriorly and distally first, and the dissection continues until the deep fascia is encountered. Two additional centimeters of fascia are included in the posterior extent of the flap. The deep fascia is incised and the dissection is continued in a subfascial plane. Elevation can be facilitated by suturing the fascial and skin margins together.

At the anterior border of the triceps, the deep fascia turns down toward the humerus, forming the lateral intermuscular septum. By coagulating the small vessels that enter the triceps, the pedicle can be visualized in its entire course from the insertion of the deltoid to the lateral epicondyle lying within the septum in its distal two-thirds (Fig. 1A).

The skin is then incised at its anterior border, the deep fascia is again found, and two extra centimeters are included.

Elevation of the deep fascia here requires sharp dissection, as the brachioradialis muscle has fibers originating from the lateral septum (Fig. 1B). Once the vascular pedicle is again seen, the lateral septum can be elevated from the humerus starting distally. Because the pedicle is seen from both sides, it can readily be protected during the rest of the dissection.

Care is needed proximally where the pedicle leaves the lateral intermuscular septum. Here the vessel of the flap arises from the common radial collateral artery. Both this vessel and its anterior branch lie very close to the radial nerve (Fig. 1C). The anterior branch must be divided to give a longer pedicle for the flap (Fig. 1D). Up to a point some 4 cm proximal to the division, the dissection can be done in a bloodless field. If a longer pedicle is needed, the tourniquet has to be removed. In most cases we stop at this point and, after separating and ligating the vessels, divide the flap and release the tourniquet.

CLINICAL RESULTS

A longitudinal scar and an area of anesthesia in the posterior aspect of the forearm are the only sequelae of this flap (Fig. 1). Patients have been satisfied with the results when the donor site has been closed directly. If a larger flap is required, and the donor site cannot be closed primarily, every effort should be made to cover the lateral epicondyle with subcutaneous tissue, because a split-thickness skin graft over the epicondyle may produce later problems.

SUMMARY

The lateral arm flap is a fasciocutaneous free flap that can be used, with minimal donor site morbidity, to cover various hand and forearm defects.

References

1. Song R, Gao Y, Song Y, et al. The forearm flap. *Clin Plast Surg* 1982;9:21.
2. Scheker L, Lister G. Variations in the use of the radial flap. In: Williams HB, ed., *Transactions of the VIII International Congress of Plastic and Reconstructive Surgery,* 1983;725.
3. Song R, Song Y, Yu Y, Song Y. The upper arm free flap. *Clin Plast Surg* 1982;9:27.
4. Shusterman M, Acland RD, Banis JC, Beppu M. The lateral arm flap: an experimental and clinical study. In: Williams HB, ed., *Transactions of the VIII International Congress of Plastic and Reconstructive Surgery,* 1983;725.
5. Katsaros J, Schusterman M, Beppu M, et al. The lateral arm flap: anatomy and clinical applications. *Ann Plast Surg* 1984;12:489.
6. Matloub HS, Sanger JR, Godina M. The lateral arm neurosensory flap. In: Williams HB, ed. *Transactions of the VIII International Congress of Plastic and Reconstructive Surgery,* 1983;125.

CHAPTER 308 ■ FREE DELTOID SKIN FLAP

J. D. FRANKLIN AND R. D. GOLDSTEIN

The neurovascular territory designated for the deltoid flap comprises the skin and subcutaneous tissue over the deltoid muscle and the posterior superior aspect of the upper arm. This is a fasciocutaneous neurosensory free flap receiving its blood supply from the cutaneous branch of the posterior circumflex humeral artery, and its innervation from a branch of the axillary nerve, the upper lateral cutaneous nerve of the arm (1,2).

INDICATIONS

Among the advantages of this neurovascular free flap is its ability to provide thin, pliable, fasciocutaneous tissue, with the added provision of sensation. Primary indications would be for those areas where a thin, fasciocutaneous flap would be advantageous and for weight-bearing and pressure areas where protective sensation would be of benefit. Its greatest use has been in head and neck reconstruction, where an excellent color and texture match is provided, and as a sensory flap on the upper extremity and foot.

ANATOMY

The third portion of the axillary artery that extends from the lower border of the pectoralis minor to the distal border of the tendon of the teres major gives off the posterior humeral circumflex artery, just distal to the subscapular artery (3,4). The posterior humeral circumflex artery runs dorsally with the axillary nerve through the quadrilateral space (bounded by the subscapularis and teres minor proximally, the teres major distally, the long head of the triceps medially, and the surgical head of the humerus laterally). The majority of its branches supply the deltoid muscle.

The artery continues to wind around the neck of the humerus and as it exits the quadrilateral space it anastomoses with the anterior humeral circumflex and the profunda brachii. Other branches supply the skin and subcutaneous tissue of the deltoid region and posterior aspect of the arm.

A cutaneous branch of the distal posterior circumflex artery, about 1 mm in diameter at its origin, lies in the areolar tissue underneath the deltoid, overlying the lateral head of the triceps. This artery, accompanied by two venae comitantes, and the sensory nerve, emerge from the deltoid-triceps groove, to swing up over the muscle above the fascia and supply the tissue over the deltoid muscle. Some small branches of the vascular pedicle also supply the skin beneath the deltoid-triceps groove.

The axillary nerve is derived from the posterior cord off the brachial plexus. It passes through the quadrilateral space with the posterior humeral circumflex artery and, after giving off motor branches, sends out a cutaneous branch, the upper lateral cutaneous nerve of the arm. The lateral brachial cutaneous nerve, originating from the inferior division of the axillary nerve, accompanies the cutaneous artery and veins lateral to the pedicle. This sensory nerve innervates the skin over the posterior inferior two-thirds of the deltoid muscle and the upper portion of the triceps, an area ranging from 10 to 15 cm in diameter.

A vessel 2 to 4 mm in diameter is obtained by the division of the posterior circumflex humeral artery proximal to the origin of the cutaneous artery supplying the flap. The accompanying posterior circumflex humeral vein is 1.5 to 2.0 times the size of the artery. A neurovascular pedicle some 6 to 8 cm may be obtained when elevating this flap (Figs. 1 through 4).

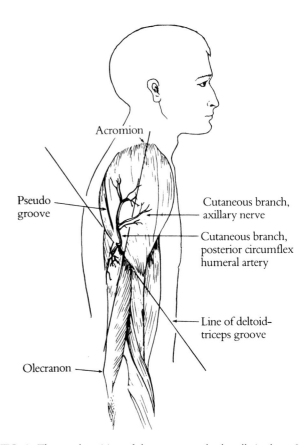

FIG. 1. The usual position of the neurovascular bundle is about 2 to 3 cm posterior to lines intersecting from the acromion to the olecranon and deltoid triceps groove.

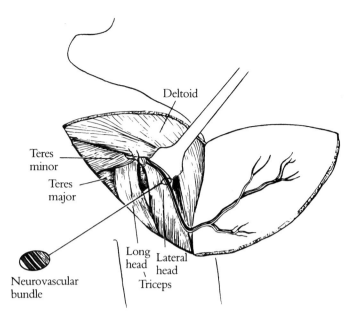

FIG. 2. Elevation of the deltoid flap showing anatomic landmarks.

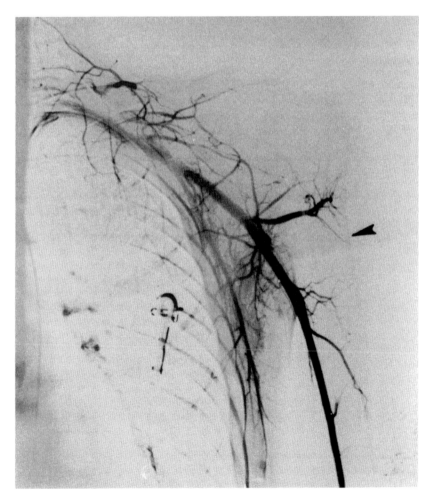

FIG. 3. *Arrow* demonstrates on an angiogram the cutaneous branch of the posterior circumflex humeral artery.

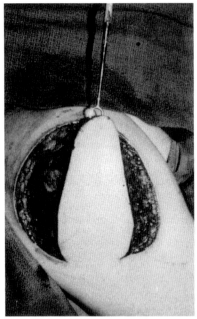
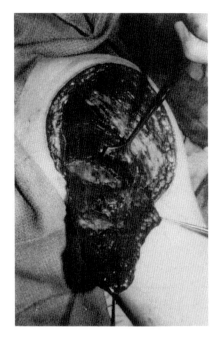
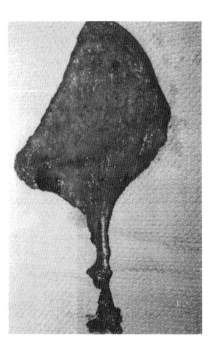

A–C

FIG. 4. **A:** Elevation of the deltoid flap. **B:** Deltoid elevated with the neurovascular bundle lying deep in the areolar tissue on the triceps muscle. **C:** Deltoid flap has been elevated and detached.

FLAP DESIGN AND DIMENSIONS

In designing the deltoid flap, the surgeon must determine the approximate entry of the neurovascular bundle. This is accomplished by drawing a line from the acromion to the medial epicondyle; another line is drawn over the deltoid-triceps groove. The pedicle usually emerges from beneath the deltoid muscle at the point of intersection of the two lines. A more precise entry of the artery may be determined using the Doppler probe.

The flap to be elevated is designed so that the neurovascular bundle, in most instances, enters at one flap end or edge. The pedicle emerges from beneath the deltoid muscle at a point 2 to 4 cm posterior to the intersection of the lines along the deltoid-triceps groove. The flap can extend two-thirds or more its length over the deltoid proximally (can actually go past the deltoid superiorly), and one-third over the triceps distally. It can extend for a variable length along the axis of the arm. Its distal limit is not exactly known. The neurovascular pedicle can be anywhere from 6 to 8 cm in length, with a vessel diameter of 2 to 4 mm possible, by taking the posterior circumflex humeral artery proximal to the origin of the cutaneous artery.

Flaps as large as 15 × 27 cm have been elevated, supplied by the single neurovascular pedicle. The area best supplied by the artery is that portion over the posterior lateral aspect of the deltoid muscle; however, tissue overlying the entire deltoid muscle, as well as a portion overlying the triceps and up onto the shoulder almost to the midline, may be safely elevated.

OPERATIVE TECHNIQUE

After the flap has been outlined, it may be elevated in one of two ways: a dome-shaped incision can be made around the proposed flap, making no incision over the deltoid triceps groove; or an incision may be made along the posterior lateral aspect of the flap and over the deltoid-triceps groove.

If a dome-shaped incision is used, the flap is elevated down to and including the fascia. Dissection proceeds toward the posterior lateral aspect of the deltoid muscle. During this elevation,

the surgeon must observe through the fascia for evidence of the neurovascular pedicle entering the flap. Occasionally, a pseudogroove is encountered in the deltoid muscle that contains no vessels and may be confused with the deltoid-triceps groove; this is easily recognized because the muscle fibers above and below the groove run in the same direction (Fig. 1).

As soon as the groove between the deltoid and triceps muscles is identified, the neurovascular pedicle can be approached from a medial or lateral direction. The deltoid muscle is elevated superiorly. With blunt dissection, the neurovascular bundle, containing one artery, two veins, and the nerve, is easily dissected. On most occasions this is a single structure; however, in approximately 5% to 10% of cases, the pedicle may divide prematurely, resulting in two smaller pedicles supplying the flap.

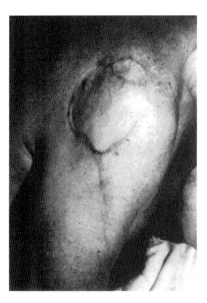

FIG. 5. Deltoid donor site that is closed, a portion of it primarily and the remainder with a skin graft.

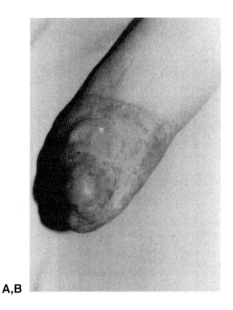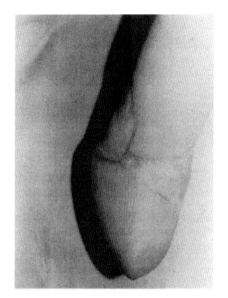

A,B

FIG. 6. **A:** Insensate skin graft amputation stump of an elbow. **B:** Sensate deltoid flap on the elbow stump.

The neurovascular bundle is dissected out in the plane between the deltoid above and the triceps below. The vessels are easily traced to the larger arteries and veins. Arterial and venous branches to the deltoid muscle are doubly clamped and transected. The posterior circumflex artery and vein are divided in the quadrilateral space. While the vessels are still intact, flap viability can be demonstrated by bleeding from the underlying dermis. The artery measures 2 to 4 mm in this area, with an accompanying single vein of adequate diameter. The sensory nerve is divided last, since it lies beneath the vessels.

If the deltoid-triceps groove is opened first, the neurovascular pedicle is identified first, and the flap is then appropriately designed and elevated to meet the particular needs of the reconstruction.

Although the artery can be taken for some distance to its origin from the axillary artery, the nerve pedicle is limited to its point of origin from the axillary nerve, to prevent the sacrifice of motor supply to the deltoid and the teres minor. The donor site is closed either primarily or with a skin graft, as required by the dimensions of the harvested flap.

In men the thinnest flaps are best elevated from the more anterior aspect of the shoulder; the flap tends to be thicker in women. The donor site is more easily closed primarily when the flap is raised more toward the posterior lateral aspect of the deltoid muscle and onto the back. An example of a donor site closed with skin graft and primarily is demonstrated in Fig. 5.

CLINICAL RESULTS

We have had experience with over 40 free deltoid flaps, 20 of which have been used to reconstruct upper extremity, foot, and ankle defects. Only four flaps have been used in the upper extremity (Figs. 6, 7), all of which survived. To date, no functional deficit has been demonstrated, such as denervation of the deltoid muscle or restriction of activity from skin grafting or the tightness of primary closure.

Complications and compromise have been primarily associated with the recipient vessels and the extremities, and

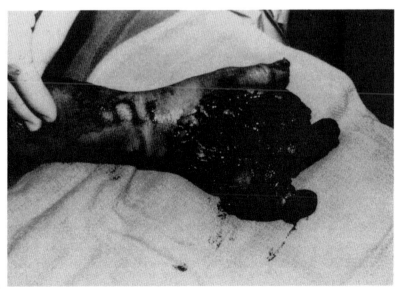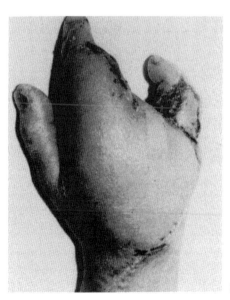

A   **B**

FIG. 7. **A:** A 24–year-old woman with a mangled hand. **B:** The hand reconstructed primarily with a deltoid flap.

not with those vessels supplying the flap. On only one occasion has a deltoid flap been elevated in which no vascular pedicle supplying the area could be demonstrated: the pedicle has indeed been demonstrated to be consistent; it contains a large vein, artery, and sensory nerve supplying the fascia, subcutaneous tissue, and skin overlying the deltoid muscle.

The greatest problems with the flap have been in the donor area. Two patients who had donor sites closed primarily developed a pseudo-bursa that needed to be revised and closed secondarily. If flaps greater than 7 to 9 cm in diameter are used, the defect usually needs to be at least partially closed with a split-thickness skin graft.

Although the donor site may be hidden by clothing, since it is on the posterior lateral aspect of the arm and shoulder, the result is less than ideal. Those donor sites that have been closed primarily tend to form fairly large hypertrophic thickened scars on the shoulder and posterior arm. In selected cases, tissue expanders to close these sites with less tension should be considered.

SUMMARY

The deltoid flap is a fasciocutaneous neurosensory free flap, supplied by the posterior circumflex humeral artery and by a nerve from a branch of the axillary nerve. It is especially useful when a thin fasciocutaneous flap is needed, especially in weight-bearing and pressure areas requiring protective sensibility, and in the head and neck.

References

1. Serafin D, Voci VE. Reconstruction of the lower extremity: microsurgical composite tissue transplantation. *Clin Plast Surg* 1983;10(1):55.
2. Franklin JD. The deltoid flap: anatomy and clinical applications. In: Buncke HJ, Furnas DW, eds. *Symposium on clinical frontiers in reconstructive microsurgery,* Vol. 24. St. Louis: Mosby, 1984;63–70.
3. Goss CM, ed. *Gray's anatomy of the human body,* 29th Ed. Philadelphia: Lea & Febiger, 1973;454–455, 610–614, 960–968.
4. Grant JCB, ed. *An atlas of anatomy,* 6th Ed. Baltimore: Williams and Wilkins, 1972; Figs. 14–34.

CHAPTER 309. Scapular and Parascapular Flaps *J. Baudet, T. Nassif, J. L. Bovet, and B. Panconi*

www.encyclopediaofflaps.com

CHAPTER 310 ■ MEDIAL UPPER ARM FASCIOCUTANEOUS FLAP FOR PALMAR DEFECTS OF THE HAND AND DISTAL FOREARM

S. BHATTACHARYA, S. P. BHAGIA, S. K. BHATNAGAR, S. D. PANDEY, AND R. CHANDRA

EDITORIAL COMMENT

The skin of the medial upper arm can be used, based on any one of the intermuscular branches from the brachial artery. It is most useful if it is based on the most proximal intermuscular branch, in which case the flap can be outlined with greater length.

The medial upper arm fasciocutaneous flap, based either distally or proximally, appears to be a solution for large cutaneous defects on the palmar aspect of the hand and distal forearm, especially in acute injuries where other alternatives are not possible. This flap protects and preserves functional nerves and tendons, and is uniformly dependable and cosmetically acceptable.

INDICATIONS

Palmar defects of the hand and distal forearm, often seen in accident victims, are best covered by split-thickness skin grafts. However, if the recipient area contains tendons without paratenon or exposed bones without periosteum, or if future bone or tendon surgery is contemplated, full-thickness skin coverage is required. Traditional flaps used to cover the dorsum of the hand (1–5) necessitate a painful and poorly tolerated

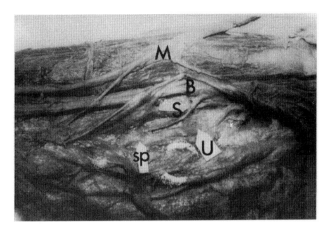

FIG. 1. Anatomic dissection of the medial upper arm showing the medial intermuscular septum *(sp)* into which the superior ulnar collateral artery *(S)* enters. This arises from the brachial artery *(B)*, which, along with the median nerve *(M)*, runs lateral to the intermuscular septum. The ulnar nerve *(U)* is seen running medial to the septum. (From Bhattacharya et al., ref. 6, with permission.)

supination of the recipient arm. The medial surface of the contralateral upper arm remains a site from which a flap will allow the recipient arm to lie comfortably in a midprone position across the chest, leaving the elbow and forearm of the donor limb relatively free (6).

ANATOMY

The flap is a type B fasciocutaneous flap (7) centered along the medial intermuscular septum, which lies between the biceps muscle anteriorly and the triceps muscle posteriorly. According to early cadaveric studies (8), three fasciocutaneous perforators originating in the medial intermuscular septum can be used as the basis for this flap: (1) One of the bicipital arteries gives off a fasciocutaneous perforator lateral to the brachial artery (unnamed, but frequent and large). (2) Infrequent fasciocutaneous perforators go directly from the axillary or brachial artery. (3) There is a not infrequent fasciocutaneous branch of the superior ulnar collateral artery medial to the brachial artery.

The fasciocutaneous branch of the superior ulnar collateral artery has been reported further (9,10). This artery is marked arising from the brachial artery at the middle of the upper arm, where it is accompanied by the ulnar nerve. It pierces the medial intermuscular system to course on its posterior surface, and then descends between the medial epicondyle and olecranon. Keeping this artery along a central axis, a fasciocutaneous flap with a length-to-width ratio of 3:1 can be safely raised.

The medial intermuscular septum is quite thick, tough, and cord-like. The brachial artery and median nerve closely follow the course of the septum anteriorly, while the ulnar nerve does so posteriorly. These structures are identified and preserved while harvesting the flap (Fig. 1).

FLAP DESIGN AND DIMENSIONS

The course of the brachial artery is marked on the skin; it can be palpated in the axilla. From there, it courses along the anterior surface of the medial intermuscular septum, covered by the coracobrachialis and biceps muscles, and then takes a slightly spiral course, to appear at the elbow midway between the humeral epicondyles. The superior ulnar collateral artery is marked arising from the middle of the upper arm and coursing between the biceps anteriorly and triceps posteriorly,

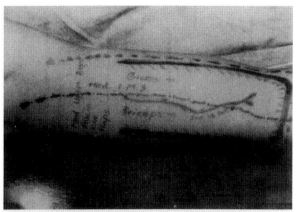

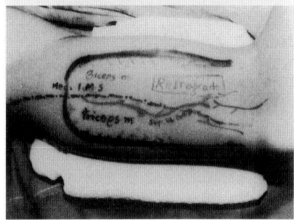

FIG. 2. Flap design. A: Surface markings of proximally based medial upper arm fasciocutaneous flap. B: Surface markings of distally based medial upper arm fasciocutaneous flap.

toward the midpoint between the medial epicondyle and olecranon. Keeping this artery as the axis, both proximally and distally based flaps can be fashioned (Fig. 2A,B).

The proximally based flap should have its base designed as high as the insertion of the pectoralis major, but extension beyond this, although possible, should be avoided. The apex of this flap can descend to the level of the elbow. The flap can be extended anteriorly and posteriorly to the midanterior and midposterior lines of the upper arm. The superior limit of the retrograde flap is at the level of the origin of the superior ulnar collateral artery; its base is slightly above the level of the medial epicondyle. Anterior and posterior limits remain the same.

OPERATIVE TECHNIQUE

The anterior incision is made first, and the deep fascia is divided 0.5 cm from the skin and sutured to the skin with 3–0 catgut. The flap is raised at the subfasical level until the medial intermuscular septum is reached. The brachial artery and median nerve are identified as they run close to the septum, and these structures are gently dissected off the septum (Fig. 3). The posterior incision is now made, and the fascia over the triceps (which is thicker than that over the biceps) is incised 0.5 cm from the skin and sutured to the skin with catgut. The flap is now elevated at the subfascial level until the ulnar nerve is identified running close to the medial intermuscular septum. The nerve is separated from the septum, and the two incisions, anterior and posterior, are joined in an arc.

The flap is elevated both anteriorly and posteriorly, and the media intermuscular septum (now resembling a thick, cord-like

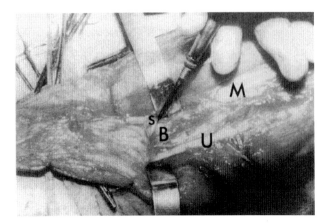

FIG. 3. The superior ulnar collateral artery (*S*) is seen entering the flap from the brachial artery (*B*). The median (*M*) and ulnar (*U*) nerves are also seen.

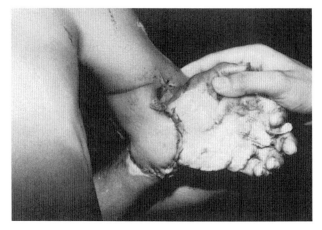

FIG. 5. Proximally based medial upper arm flap used to cover a palmar defect on the distal forearm, postexcision of a desmoid tumor. Note comfortable position for case management.

structure) is divided along with multiple perforators, as close to the bone as possible, to preserve the anastomosis between the perforators (Fig. 4). Flap elevation takes about 30 minutes.

The donor site can be closed primarily with wide undermining up to the lateral intermuscular septum anteriorly, and posteriorly with lateral fasciotomies. The process of flap elevation and donor-site closure may cause edema in the distal arm. When a relatively wide flap has been harvested, the donor area can be reduced in size and a split-thickness skin graft can be utilized.

CLINICAL RESULTS

Ten patients with palmar defects on the distal forearm, hand, and fingers were treated with the medial upper arm fasciocutaneous flap. Two retrograde and eight antegrade type B flaps were used. Of the latter eight, five were based on the main trunk of the superior ulnar collateral artery, and three on its main cutaneous branch. The donor area in four patients was closed primarily after wide undermining and internal fasciotomy. In the remaining six patients, the donor defect was reduced in size and a split-thickness skin graft was applied. Immobilization was achieved with Elastoplast strapping, so that the elbow of the donor arm could be kept free for use, and

the flap could be observed with the patient raising both arms above the head (Figs. 5 and 6). The flap pedicle was divided by a selective delay (palpating the medial intermuscular septum and its vessel) 21 days after flap transfer, and flap division was done 5 to 7 days after the delay.

All flaps survived completely with no evidence of necrosis, infection, or hematoma formation. The donor arm developed edema in three patients, in two of whom the donor area had been closed primarily. This was managed by Elastoplast strapping, limb elevation, and physiotherapy for 3 to 4 days. One patient showed evidence of ulnar-nerve paresis, which subsided within 1 week. The donor area in all patients was cosmetically satisfactory and well concealed. All patients returned to their original work.

The flap provides an excellent color match for the forearm, but not for the palm. It is usually nonhirsute, but in one patient hair growing in the palm proved embarrassing.

SUMMARY

The medial upper arm fasciocutaneous flap has a clinical place in the management of palmar defects. However, the flap is used by necessity, rather than by election, for those defects that cannot support free skin grafting.

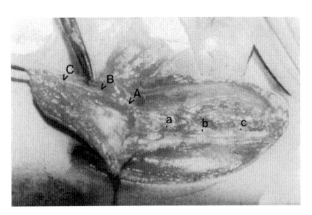

FIG. 4. The flap has been elevated by dividing the medial intermuscular septum close to the bone (*Aa, Bb, Cc*), in order to incorporate the superior ulnar collateral artery.

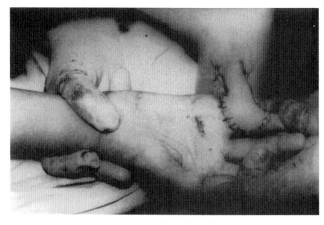

FIG. 6. Distally based medial upper arm flap used to cover a palmar defect on the ulnar two fingers of the contralateral hand, following release of severe postburn contracture.

References

1. McGregor IA, Jackson IT. The groin flap. *Br J Plast Surg* 1972;25:3.
2. Stranc MF, Sanders R. Abdominal wall skin flaps. In: Grabb WC, Myers BM, eds. *Skin flaps*. Boston: Little, Brown, 1968;419–426.
3. Dias AD, Thatte RL, Patil UA, et al. The use of the SEPA flap in the repair of defects in the hands and fingers. *Br J Plast Surg* 1987;40:340.
4. Chandra R, Kumar P, Abdi SHM. The subaxillary pedicled flap. *Br J Plast Surg* 1988;42:169.
5. Bhattacharya S, Pandey SD, Chandra R, Bhatnagar SK. Lateral chest wall fasciocutaneous flaps in the management of burn contractures on the dorsum of the hand. *Eur J Plast Surg* 1988;11:8.
6. Bhattacharya S, Bhagia SP, Bhatnagar SK, et al. The medial upper arm fasciocutaneous flap. *J Hand Surg* 1991;16B:342.
7. Cormack GC, Lamberty BGH. A classification of fasciocutaneous flaps according to their patterns of vascularization. *Br J Plast Surg* 1984; 37:80.
8. Song RY, Song YG, Yu YS, Song YL. The upper arm free flap. *Clin Plast Surg* 1982;9:27.
9. Cormack GC, Lamberty BGH. Fasciocutaneous vessels in the upper arm: application to the design of new fasciocutaneous flaps. *Plast Reconstr Surg* 1984;74:244.
10. Kaplan EN, Pearl RM. An arterial medial arm flap: vascular anatomy and clinical applications. *Ann Plast Surg* 1980;4:205.

CHAPTER 311 ■ ULNAR ARTERY FREE FLAP

D. R. H. CHRISTIE, G. M. DUNCAN, AND D. W. GLASSON

EDITORIAL COMMENT

This is, in essence, a flap similar to the radial artery forearm flap but based on the ulnar artery. It gives the surgeon a wider latitude in choice; otherwise, there is no serious difference in advantages between the two.

The ulnar artery free flap is described for situations in which small to medium amounts of composite tissue are required. This flap is best suited for reconstruction after cancer surgery in the head and neck, especially for oral cancers. It is also an appropriate method of repair of distal limb defects, usually in the ankle, foot, wrist, and hand.

INDICATIONS

Radial and ulnar artery flaps share some important advantages (1–6). Both are relatively thin fasciocutaneous flaps that may include skin, muscle, bone, and tendons for the reconstruction of small to medium-sized tissue defects. Both have sensory potential. In each flap, the large-caliber vessels and long vascular pedicles allow easy inset and anastomosis. The arterial architecture permits flow through, maintaining circulation distal to the flap. The remote donor site enables two surgical teams to work simultaneously, reducing operating time.

The flaps share some significant disadvantages. Fracture of the donor bone is common to both, the risk being similar for the radius and the ulna (7). In our experience, all patients in whom bone is harvested have been immobilized in an above-elbow cast for 6 weeks. The risk of encountering abnormal vascular anatomy is also common to both flaps. Both the radial and ulnar arteries demonstrate anatomic variations in a small percentage of patients. These may render the arm unsuitable for

a safe raising of the flap. However, the presence of a superficial ulnar artery has not been a contraindication to using an ulnar artery free flap and may, in fact, facilitate the raising of this flap.

The ulnar artery free flap confers three important additional advantages. The first of these is ease of donor-site healing and repair. Considerable difficulty has been encountered with repair of the radial donor site; indeed, a method of repairing that donor defect using an ulnar flap has been proposed (8). The ulnar donor site is easily repaired, often by primary closure, and donor-site healing is usually rapid. No long-term complaints or objective disabilities have been noted.

The second advantage is cosmetic acceptability. The scar from the ulnar donor site lies more proximally along the ulnar border, and is therefore less obvious during normal daily activity.

The third advantage, relative hairlessness, is important for those undergoing intraoral reconstruction. Hair on the intraoral surface can be irritating and is difficult to remove. The relative hairlessness of the ulnar side of the forearm makes this site preferable for intraoral reconstruction, particularly in Caucasians, who commonly have hair along the radial side of the forearm.

ANATOMY AND FLAP DESIGN

The flap is based on the ulnar artery distal to the common interosseous branch. Vascular pedicles pass from the artery to adjacent muscles and to the skin of the ulnar border of the forearm, running in the fascial septum between the flexor carpi ulnaris and the flexor digitorum superficialis. Small nutrient vessels also pass directly to the ulnar nerve. The fascia of the flap is continuous with the periosteum of the subcutaneous border of the ulna (Fig. 1).

Dual venous drainage is provided by the superficial forearm veins, usually the basilic and the venae comitantes. The medial cutaneous nerve of the forearm may be taken with the flap, if sensory reconstruction is planned.

SKIN

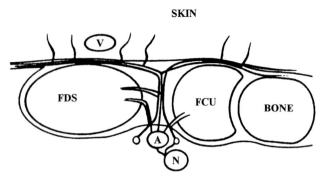

FIG. 1. Diagram showing vascular pedicles passing from the ulnar artery to the adjacent muscles and skin. (From Glasson et al., ref. 3, with permission.)

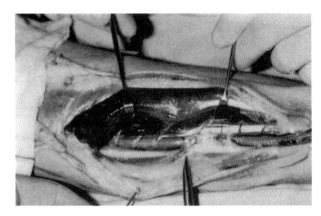

FIG. 2. Initial incision exposing major vessels and nerves. (From Christie et al., ref. 4, with permission.)

The skin island is designed on the ulnar palmar aspect of the forearm. There is a reasonable degree of freedom, providing that fascial continuity is maintained with the septum between the flexor carpi ulnaris and the flexor digitorum superficialis.

The final position of the flap is often determined by the pattern of the superficial veins. Any minor adjustment to the skin island can be made after the radial side of the flap is elevated and the position of the septal pedicles is determined. This adjustment may be reassuring, if a very small flap is used.

OPERATIVE TECHNIQUE

An Allen's test is performed prior to surgery. The operation is begun distal to the flap, where the ulnar artery and vein are identified. Depending on flap design, the artery may be dissected as far as the wrist. This will allow sufficient distal arterial length for revascularization by reverse flow. The incision is continued proximally along the radial border of the flap, which is easily separated from the underlying belly of the flexor digitorum superficialis. This plane is developed, with radial retraction of the flexor digitorum superficialis, allowing clear identification of the ulnar nerve, the ulnar artery, and the vascular pedicles (usually, two or more) passing from it (Fig. 2). Should the planning of the flap not coincide with the position of the pedicles, the ulnar side margin can be altered.

The ulnar margin is then incised, and the flap is raised subfascially from the flexor carpi ulnaris. The draining superficial vein is dissected, and an extended length can be taken by continuing this dissection above the elbow, if required. The medial cutaneous nerve of the forearm accompanying the basilic vein, is easily identified.

The ulnar artery is divided distally, and the flap is dissected free from the ulnar nerve, coagulating or clipping pedicles to other destinations (nerve or muscles).

The palmaris longus may be included in the flap, as may the flexor carpi ulnaris, depending on reconstructive requirements (e.g., extensor tendon reconstruction, muscle to fill a bony cavity, or provision of bulk in the floor of the mouth).

To include a length of hemiulna, a fascial extension is designed in continuity with the bone segment. This can be done by including a large component of the flexor carpi ulnaris, or by dissecting a thin superficial lamina of muscle that is attached to bone. In female nondominant arms, this attachment to the ulna can be flimsy. Limited subperiosteal stripping of extensor compartment muscles allows a clear view for longitudinal osteotomy and preserves the fascioperiosteal attachment on the palmar aspect of the bone. The

bone is thin in the middle and distal portions, and care must be taken to preserve adequate metaphysis. Bone segments of 16 cm are not difficult to harvest.

The surgeon must always be aware of the possible need to reconstruct the ulnar artery; however, this is not routinely required (no cases in our series). The donor sites of smaller flaps may be closed directly. Where primary closure is not possible, a skin graft is applied to the exposed muscle bellies. Tendons are usually not exposed by the forearm defect. If the flexor carpi ulnaris has been included in the flap, exposing the ulnar nerve, the flexor digitorum superficialis should be sutured over the nerve, to prevent the skin graft from being applied directly to it. If bone has been taken, the arm is immobilized in an above-elbow cast for 6 weeks.

CLINICAL RESULTS

All 56 patients treated by the authors were analyzed by retrospective review of the medical records (4). The presenting diagnoses fell into two major categories: neoplasia of the head and neck, usually in the mouth, and trauma, in most cases resulting from motor-vehicle accidents involving tissue loss in the lower limbs. The flap included bone in 21 patients, all of whom had oral cancers.

Direct closure of the donor site was used in 25 patients (45%), with the remaining 31 requiring split-thickness skin grafts applied over exposed muscle bellies; no graft failures occurred. Two significant problems were identified regarding donor-site morbidity. Transient paresthesias of the ulnar nerve occurred in 18 patients (32%), but were always mild and resolved completely within 2 weeks. In 21 patients, bone had been included in the flap, and 6 patients (29%) sustained fractures in the remaining length of hemiulna. One fracture occurred intraoperatively and was fixed internally. Five fractures occurred postoperatively and were managed conservatively. No deformity was evident following any of the fractures, and none of the complications affected the long-term outcome in any of the cases reviewed.

Of the 56 cases, two were abandoned intraoperatively, and two failed following transfer. In two patients, an abnormal vascular pattern was noted during raising of the flap. No perforators from the ulnar artery to the skin could be identified in the fascia, and the skin circulation was noted to be severely compromised prior to flap separation. The procedure was abandoned, and the flap was reset. In one patient, 50% of the flap subsequently necrosed. In the two other patients, the flap necrosed within 48 hours following venous congestion. Both of these cases were early in our series and involved grade IV lower-limb trauma. Limited proximal vascular resection was carried out, and anastomoses were performed within the area of tissue damage. Salvage was not attempted. Both failures were attributed to lack of experience.

SUMMARY

The ulnar artery free flap is highly versatile and reliable in the reconstruction of a variety of defects, where small to medium amounts of composite tissue are required. The main indication has been intraoral reconstruction after ablative cancer surgery. The flap has also been used to repair other head and neck defects and soft-tissue defects of the lower limb.

References

1. Song R, Gao Y, Song Y, et al. The forearm flap. *Clin Plast Surg* 1982;9:21.
2. Lovie MJ, Duncan GM, Glasson DW. The ulnar artery forearm free flap. *Br J Plast Surg* 1984;37:486.
3. Glasson DW, Lovie MJ, Duncan GM. The ulnar forearm free flap in penile reconstruction. *Aust N Z J Surg* 1986;56:477.
4. Christie DRH, Duncan GM, Glasson DW. The ulnar artery free flap: the first seven years. *Plast Reconstr Surg* 1994;93:547.
5. Glasson DW, Lovie MJ. The ulnar island flap in hand and forearm reconstruction. *Br J Plast Surg* 1988;41:349.
6. Soutar DS, McGregor A. The radial forearm flap in intraoral reconstruction: the experience of 60 consecutive cases. *Plast Reconstr Surg* 1986;78:1.
7. Boorman JG, Brown JA, Sykes PJ. Morbidity in the forearm flap donor arm. *Br J Plast Surg* 1987;40:207.
8. Elliot D, Bardsley AF, Batchelor AG, Soutar DS. Direct closure of the radial forearm flap donor defect. *Br J Plast Surg* 1988;41:358.

CHAPTER 312 ■ FIBULAR OSTEOCUTANEOUS FREE FLAP FOR METACARPAL CONSTRUCTION

Y. K. CHUNG

The fibular osteocutaneous flap can be very versatile for composite hand defects involving single or multiple metacarpal losses.

INDICATIONS

The fibula or fibular osteocutaneous free flap has been widely used for reconstruction of long-bone defects of both the upper and lower extremities and the mandible. The fibula has been rarely used in reconstruction of metacarpal defects. A few cases have been reported on metacarpal reconstruction in the form of a nonvascularized strut graft. Rarely has a vascularized fibula flap been used in metacarpal reconstruction (1,2) (Fig. 1).

Composite defects involving metacarpal bone(s) and surrounding soft tissue can result from trauma, chronic infection, and tumor ablation. The classic treatment for such cases is staged, involving healing of the soft tissue first and bone reconstruction later. But this requires a long recovery and

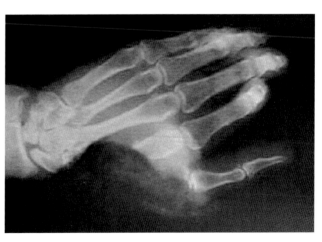

FIG. 1. Hand trauma radiograph shows loss of metacarpal I and II.

increases the period of patient morbidity. For a small defect of the metacarpal bone, a nonvascularized bone graft can be effective. However, extensive and composite injuries of the hand may need a more complex and difficult procedure. The fibula osteocutaneous free flap offers excellent solutions in those cases. It provides both bone and soft tissues simultaneously and can be used in multiple metacarpal defects. Moreover, it also can be used with a flow-through technique to revascularize the injured digits.

ANATOMY

The fibula is triangular, about 1.5 to 2 cm in diameter, and 40 cm in length. It is composed of highly dense cortical bone and a relative paucity of cancellous components. It supports one-sixth of our body weight. It articulates with the tibia proximally and distally, and maintains the stability of the knee and ankle joints. Most muscles that control foot motion originate from the fibula.

The peroneal artery supplies the fibula in two forms—periosteal and endosteal. The nutrient artery from the peroneal artery gives the bone endosteal circulation through the nutrient foramen, which ranges from one to three in number, usually one (69%), and in more than 70% of cases is located in the middle third of the fibula (3,4). The fibula can be used with overlying skin in an osteocutaneous flap. The lateral skin of the lower leg is supplied with cutaneous branches from the peroneal artery, ranging from three to eight in number. There are two types of cutaneous branches, musculocutaneous and septocutaneous (4–6). The musculocutaneous perforators are more numerous and more proximal than the septocutaneous perforators (4,6).

The septocutaneous perforators, which pass through the posterior crural septum between the peroneal muscles and soleus, are found along the posterior margin of the fibula and are distributed from the middle third to the lower third of the fibula (4,5). Although the reliability of the septocutaneous perforators is still controversial, Wei et al. (5) reported excellent survival rates for the osteoseptocutaneous fibular flap. Even if the septocutaneous perforator is absent, the musculocutaneous branch supplies adequate circulation to the same area.

FLAP DESIGN AND DIMENSIONS

Some technical points need to be stressed:

1. Preoperatively, a Doppler probe is used to mark the cutaneous perforator along the posterior margin of the fibula. In thin individuals, the posterior crural septum may be palpable as a cleft in the fibular posterior margin.
2. To harvest the fibula, it is important to place the point between the upper and middle thirds of the fibula in the center of the flap, to maximally contain the nutrient branch of the peroneal vessels; most of the nutrient foramen is located in the upper two thirds of the fibula.
3. Obtaining a longer fibula than measured will allow for a longer pedicle and easier insetting of the flap in cases with a different configuration of skin and bone defect.
4. Six to 8 cm of the proximal and distal fibula is preserved to maintain stability of the knee and ankle joints.
5. In order to obtain an osteocutaneous flap based on the septocutaneous perforators, the center of the skin paddle is placed along the posterior margin of the middle third to distal third of the fibula (4–6).
6. Two or three cutaneous branches to the lateral skin of the leg, which have been marked along the posterior border of the fibula with the Doppler, are included in the skin paddle. It is desirable that the design of the cutaneous portion be larger than the defect size. Wei et al. (5) recommended that the skin paddle can be up to 25 cm in length and 14 cm in width, with one or two sizable septocutaneous branches, and that the dimensions should be minimally 8 to 10 cm in length and 4 cm in width (7).
7. The donor site should never be closed by primary repair under severe tension but rather should be skin-grafted.

OPERATIVE TECHNIQUE

Elevation of Osteocutaneous Fibula—Lateral Approach with Patient in Supine Position

A skin incision to the subcutaneous layer is made. The skin flap is elevated from the peroneal muscle anteriorly and the soleus muscle posteriorly in a subfascial plane. An alternative method involves elevating the skin flap initially in the suprafascial level, and as the dissection approaches the posterior crural septum, the deep fascia investing the peroneal and soleus muscles should be incised and included in the skin flap to prevent accidental tearing of the cutaneous branches. The superficial peroneal nerve should be carefully protected because of its subcutaneous position in the distal third of the lower leg. At this point, inspect the septum for inclusion of the cutaneous perforator(s). Just one or two branches of the septocutaneous perforators secure the viability of the skin paddle. If viability is suspect, dissect and clamp the musculocutaneous branch within the septum, release the tourniquet, and check perfusion. After viability is confirmed, the musculocutaneous branch is cut and ligated.

If the septum contains no vessels, intramuscular dissection is continued to the origin of the musculocutaneous branch to the skin flap. The peroneal muscle is dissected from the lateral border of the fibula, and dissection is continued to the intermuscular septum between the lateral and anterior compartments and extensor digitorum longus and extensor hallucis longus, carefully exposing the interosseous membrane, so as not to injure the anterior tibial vessels and deep peroneal nerve. Also, by keeping the Metzenbaum scissors tight against the bone, a minimal amount of muscle can be left on the fibula. The interosseous membrane is incised, and the tibialis posterior is exposed. After a Gigli saw is used for the proximal and distal osteotomy, posterolateral traction with a bone hook will allow for easy identification of the peroneal artery. At the posterior portion of the flap, the soleus muscle is separated from the posterior crural septum; next, the flexor hallucis longus is dissected from the fibula, exposing the peroneal pedicle between the posterior tibial muscle and flexor hallucis longus. Occasionally, the peroneal vessels are within the flexor hallucis longus, requiring the harvest of a portion of the flexor hallucis longus with the pedicle. The dissection is continued to the peroneal vessel bifurcation (Fig. 2). The elevated osteocutaneous fibula can be osteotomized into a number of segments in situ as necessary.

Recipient Preparation

In case of two metacarpal defects, a small portion of the intervening central segment between either side segments of the fibula can be resected subperiosteally, to snugly place the fibula segments into the missing metacarpals. The osteotomized fibula segment is fixed to the remnant of the missing bone with miniplates or screws. If the metacarpophalangeal joint or carpometacarpal joint is lost, arthrodesis can be performed. To reconstruct the thumb metacarpal, it is extremely important to keep in mind that opposition and pinching action be restored (Figs. 1, 3, and 4).

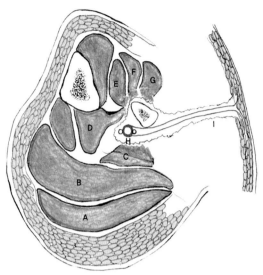

A. Gastrocnemius m., B. Soleus m., C. Flexor hallucis longus m., D. Tibilalis posterior m., E. Extensor hallucis longus m., F. Extensor digitorum longus m., G. Peroneus longus m., H. Peroneus artery, I. Crural fascia.

FIG. 2. Cross-section of dissection of fibula and skin paddle.

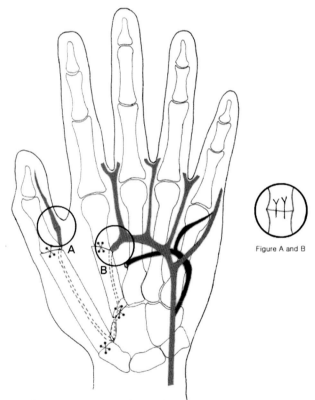

Figure A. Princeps pollicis atrery– distal peroneal artery
Figure B. Superficial palmar arch–proximal peroneal artery

FIG. 3. Drawing of inset of two fibula bone grafts and revascularization by the superficial palmar arch and princeps pollicis and flow-through peroneal artery.

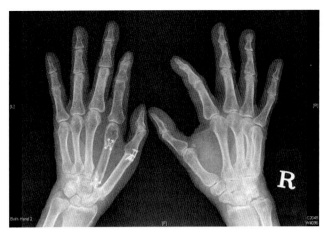

FIG. 4. Postoperative radiograph.

CLINICAL RESULTS

A very satisfactory aesthetic result can be obtained using a fibular osteocutaneous flap for composite metacarpal-defect reconstruction. However, several factors should be considered in terms of functional recovery. The degree of hand-mobility recovery will depend more on the extent of joint, tendon, intrinsic muscle, and soft-tissue damage in the area of the injured metacarpal bone, rather than the missing metacarpal bone defect length (2). Especially in a composite defect, intactness of the joint is a more important prognostic factor than other tissue damage. Thus, an intact thumb carpometacarpal joint, like the metacarpophalangeal joint of the other digits, will allow for a more favorable result.

SUMMARY

The osteocutaneous fibula free flap provides many advantages in metacarpal reconstruction: (a) a good size match for metacarpal bone, (b) multiple segments of the fibular strut for multiple metacarpal defects, (c) more rapid and better bony union than the nonvascularized bone graft, (d) good flexibility of the septocutaneous skin paddle for insetting and contouring the flap, (e) use as a flow-through system to revascularize an injured digit, (f) one-stage reconstruction for composite defect, and (g) an excellent aesthetic result.

References

1. Lee HB, Tark KC, Kang SY, et al. Reconstruction of composite metacarpal defects using a fibula free flap. *Plast Reconstr Surg* 2000;104:1448.
2. Lin CH, Wei FC, Rodriguez ED, et al. Functional reconstruction of traumatic composite metacarpal defects with fibular osteoseptocutaneous free flap. *Plast Reconstr Surg* 2005;116:605.
3. Mckee NH, Haw P, Vettese T. Anatomic study of the nutrient foramen in the shaft of the fibula. *Clin Orthop Rel Res* 1983;184:141.
4. Yoshimura M, Shimada T, Hosokawa M. The vasculature of the peroneal tissue transfer. *Plast Reconstr Surg* 1990;85:917.
5. Wei FC, Chen HC, Chuang CC, Noordhoff MS. Fibular osteocutaneous flap: anatomic study and clinical application. *Plast Reconstr Surg* 1986; 78:191.
6. Schusterman MA, Reece GP, Miller MJ, Harris S. The osteocutaneous free fibula flap: is the skin paddle reliable? *Plast Reconstr Surg* 1992;90:787.
7. Wei FC, Seah CS, Tsai YC, et al. The oteoseptocutaneous flap for reconstruction of composite mandibular defects. *Plast Reconstr Surg* 1994; 93:294.

CHAPTER 313 ■ DORSAL RECTANGULAR SKIN FLAP FOR WEB SPACE RECONSTRUCTION

E. Z. BROWNE, JR.

Although an interdigital web space collapses with adduction, it assumes a rectangular shape with abduction of the fingers. Reconstructive procedures designed to restore the web space must result in a pliable, rectangular structure with maximum distensibility along the volar edge of the web. Although interdigitating flaps can be used to restore the rectangle, it is difficult to create the appropriate slope from dorsal to volar edge, and pliability can be limited by scarring within the rectangle. A single, dorsal proximally based, rectangular skin flap is preferable for total web space reconstruction. This flap is passed between the fingers and set into an inverted T in the palmar skin (Fig. 1).

INDICATIONS

The flap has application in instances where the entire web space has been obliterated, causing a true syndactylism. It is not indicated in situations where only part of the web space is involved, such as a dorsal adduction contracture sparing the volar edge. This may be treated satisfactorily with skin grafts or with various modifications of Z-plasties (1–3).

The dorsal rectangular skin flap can be adapted for use in a number of conditions, such as congenital deformities (4), traumatic defects, and revision after reconstructive procedures such as distant flaps. It is especially useful in the treatment of burn syndactyly (5), and has also been useful in improving prehension by deepening scarred web spaces associated with partial amputation, especially with loss of a thumb (Fig. 2). In general, the flap has not been found to be as useful for release of the first web space as the four-flap Z-plasty (6).

FLAP DESIGN AND DIMENSIONS

This is a random skin flap, and it is elevated midway in a plane between dorsal and volar skin. The volar surface is split longitudinally and the flap is placed into an inverted "T" set into the palmar skin (Fig. 3). The defects created along the sides of the fingers are skin-grafted. The base of the flap must extend proximally to the metacarpal heads for flaps used between the fingers, and may extend back to the level of the middle of the first metacarpal for reconstruction of the first web space. It is important to bring the volar T more proximal into the palm than would be anticipated, in order to avoid a secondary contracture along the volar edge. The length-to-width ratio has

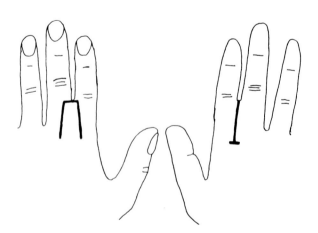

FIG. 1. Dorsal, proximally based rectangular flap, set into inverted volar T.

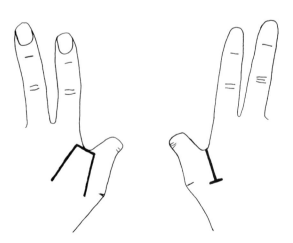

FIG. 2. Use of flap to deepen first web space.

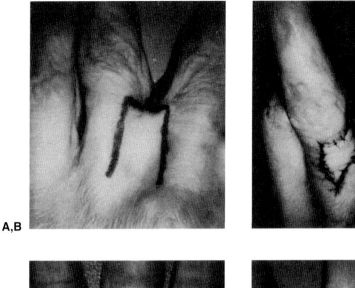

A,B

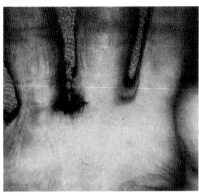

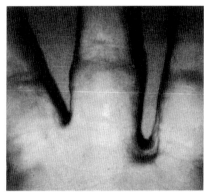

C,D

FIG. 3. **A:** Markings before release. **B:** Flap inset with skin graft on the sides of the fingers. **C:** Volar view of flap inset. **D:** Final result. (From Browne et al., ref. 5, with permission.)

not been found to be critical, in spite of the nature of the scarred skin, and it is appropriate to use the entire length of the skin available for the flap.

OPERATIVE TECHNIQUE

In elevating the flap, care must be exercised to avoid the neurovascular structures, especially in congenital deformities. When the flap is used in the first web space, it is necessary to divide the fascia overlying the first dorsal interosseous muscle, and to release any scar causing contracture of this fascia to the adductor pollicis. It should be kept in mind that the radial artery may be encountered during this procedure. Unless the interval between the interosseous and the abductor is opened widely, the first web space will not be effectively deepened.

It is usually necessary to preserve as much flap length as possible, and marginal areas seem always to survive. By setting the flap into an inverted "T" in the palmar skin, the principle of a double-opposed Z-plasty is used, thus minimizing contracture along the volar edge.

CLINICAL RESULTS

In spite of the apparent disregard for length-to-width ratio, this flap has been very reliable, even in circumstances such as

burn syndactyly where the flap is composed of old skin graft. The flap has been used in well over 70 instances of varying types of traumatic syndactyly, without loss of a single flap. Although there has been loss, on occasion, of some of the skin grafts placed in the defects on the sides of the fingers, it has been possible to regraft these, and there have been no instances of functional deficit associated with the flap.

SUMMARY

The dorsal rectangular skin flap is an excellent means of reconstructing the web space, especially between adjacent fingers.

References

1. Adamson JE, Crawford HH, Horton CE, et al. Treatment of dorsal burn adduction contracture of the hand. *Plast Reconstr Surg* 1968;42:355.
2. Shaw DT, Li CS, Richey DWG, Nahigian SH. Interdigital butterfly flap in the hand: the double-opposing Z-plasty. *J Bone Joint Surg* 1973;55A:1677.
3. Krizek TJ, Robson MC, Flagg SV. Management of burn syndactyly. *J Trauma* 1974;14:587.
4. Bauer TB, Tondra JM, Trusler HM. Technical modifications in repair of syndactylism. *Plast Reconstr Surg* 1956;17:385.
5. Browne EZ Jr, Teague MA, Snyder CC. Burn syndactyly. *Plast Reconstr Surg* 1978;62:92.
6. Woolf RM, Broadbent TR. The four flap Z-plasty. *Plast Reconstr Surg* 1972;49:48.

CHAPTER 314 ■ LATERAL DIGITAL SKIN FLAP FOR WEB SPACE RECONSTRUCTION

P. COLSON AND H. JANVIER

The lateral surface of the finger is often spared in burn injuries. It is therefore available to be used as a flap for web space reconstruction (1). The technique will vary, depending on whether the burned skin is on the dorsal (most frequent) or palmar aspect of the hand.

INDICATIONS

The lateral digital flap may be indicated in different instances: trauma, tumor excision, congenital deformities, Dupuytren's contracture, and burn injuries (2–7). In the latter circumstance, experience shows that, apart from the functional results, the cosmetic appearance is very satisfactory. This is a major psychological factor in early and complete rehabilitation.

FLAP DESIGN AND DIMENSIONS

The technique of reconstruction will depend on the location and severity of the contracture (8,9).

Dorsal Burns

In the patient who can still make a fist in spite of some skin blanching, such moderate interdigital webbing can be satisfactorily dealt with by small lateral digital flaps.

A narrow tongue of unburned skin and subcutaneous tissue is designed on the fingers on each side of the web (1). Both flaps will have the same pedicle at the base (Fig. 1A). The two tongues are detached, rotated 180°, and brought into contact—as two rabbit's ears—and sutured to each other and to the edges of the defect created by the dorsal incision.

If the flaps are small and the burned skin on the rest of the finger is not too extensive, the donor site can be closed primarily.

In the patient who cannot completely flex the metacarpophalangeal joints and in whom there is a severe contracture, a large flap is needed. The defect resulting from such a large flap must be covered with a split-thickness skin graft.

Palmar Burns

In most cases of palmar burns, the contracture not only limits separation of the fingers with transverse retracted webs, but

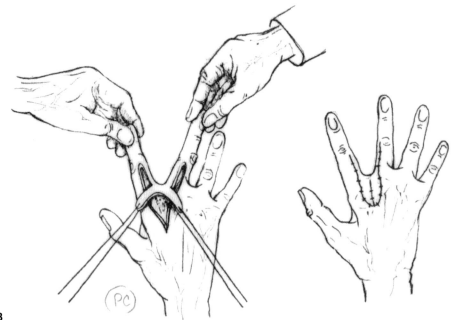

FIG. 1. A: A narrow "lateral digital" skin flap is raised from each side, so that the two flaps share the same pedicle. These two flaps have been compared with two "rabbit's ears" (S. Bunnell). **B:** The two flaps rotated 180° are inset into the dorsal defect. Each donor site is sutured with *slight* tension.

A,B

912

also keeps the proximal phalanges in permanent flexion, with longitudinal contracted bands crossing over the digitopalmar crease. For this reason, repair usually requires two lateral digital flaps cut from each interdigital space and used in two stages. The first flap, rotated 90°, allows for extension of the flexed finger (Fig. 2A), and the second flap, rotated 180°, widens the commissural web (Fig. 2B).

Thenar Web

Web space contractures of the thumb with mild adduction may be corrected by means of two lateral digital flaps raised from the thumb and index finger. Split-thickness skin grafts are usually used to resurface the raw areas.

If the web space contracture is significant, a distant flap such as a brachial dermo-epidermal flap should be used (see Chap. 296).

OPERATIVE TECHNIQUE

Careful attention to detail is most rewarding: the longitudinal incision on the dorsum of the hand must release not only the retracted skin, but also the underlying fibrosed tissue, sometimes including the strong transverse intermetacarpal ligament. The flap is cut as wide as good skin will permit, and the tip is designed to extend as close to the distal interphalangeal joint as possible.

To free the flap, the neurovascular bundle is first identified under Cleland's ligament. The ligament is severed along its entire length. The flap then carries with it some subdermal tissue and a few small vessels and nerves issuing directly from the palm.

The flap is then rotated 180° and the tip is inserted into the proximal end of the dorsal longitudinal incision. Sutured into the defect of the incised web, the flap will fit well if it is supple. Such a flap has very good viability, even if cut long—less

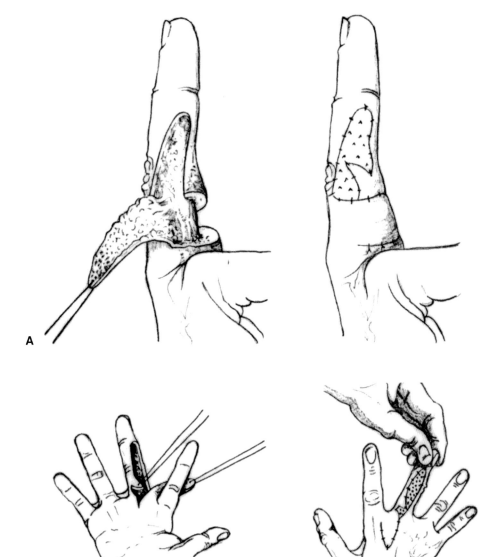

A

B

FIG. 2. A: First stage in release of palmar burn contracture: the palmar longitudinal retracted scar is entirely severed and the finger is extended. Thereafter, the laterodigital flap can be satisfactorily designed. One flap is required to maintain release of the flexion contracture, as shown here. B: A second flap is designed at a later stage, to release the web space contracture. Note the technical details to avoid both the shortening of the interdigital space and the retraction of the palmar suture line.

than 2% distal necrosis in our experience—provided it is not sutured into place under tension. This is an important technical point, because the flap grows thinner from its base to its extremity. Its blood supply moves mainly through the subdermal vascular plexus.

To avoid a straight line contracture along the flap donor site, the digital incision is prolonged to penetrate the palm for a few millimeters, and a small triangular extension of the palmar skin is cut, rotated, and fitted into the raw area near the digitopalmar crease (Fig. 2B).

SUMMARY

The lateral digital flap, when used with the proper indications, can successfully release interdigital and thenar web space contractures in both dorsal and palmar burns.

References

1. Boyes JH. *Bunnell's surgery of the hand,* 4th ed. Philadelphia: Lippincott, 1964;190; Figs. 223, 224.
2. Colson P, Janvier H, Gangolphe M. Un procédé de S. Bunnell pour la refection de commissures digitales par rotation de lambeaux. *Ann Chir Plast* 1960;5:205.
3. Tubiana R, Baux S, Kenesi C. À propos de trois cents brûlures thermiques récentes des mains. *Ann Chir* 1967;23:1387.
4. Vilain R, Michon J. *Chirurgie plastique cutanée de la main.* Paris: Masson, 1968;93.
5. Iselin M, Iselin F. *Traité de chirurgie de la main.* Brussels: Flammarion, 1967; 266–267.
6. Colson P, Janvier H. Brûlures du dos de la main: problèmes posés par la réparation secondaire de la région des commissures. *Ann Chir Plast* 1970;15:14.
7. Morel-Fatio D. Chirurgie des pertes de substance cutanées. In: *Encyclopédie médico-chirurgicale.* Paris: Editions Techniques; 8–10; Figs. 399, 400, 403.
8. Lister G. The theory of the transposition flap and its practical application in the hand. *Clin Plast Surg* 1981;8:115.
9. Beasley RW. Secondary repair of burned hands. *Clin Plast Surg* 1981;8:141.

CHAPTER 315 ■ FIVE-SKIN FLAP FOR RECONSTRUCTION OF WEB SPACE CONTRACTURE

M. ROUSSO, M. R. WEXLER, AND I. J. PELED

EDITORIAL COMMENT

This technique probably provides the widest first web space, compared with any other of the reconstructions.

Web space contractures are most frequently caused by burns. Usually, one surface is spared. The clinical features of web space contractures are distortion of the normal web concavity and the appearance of a transverse interdigital scar that limits abduction. Sometimes, a dorsal or volar digitopalmar skin contracture is present hyperextending or, on the contrary, flexing, metacarpophalangeal joints and proximal interphalangeal joints.

Congenital, posttraumatic (including burns), and spastic contractures are amenable to release by the five-skin flap technique (1–5).

INDICATIONS

Reconstruction can achieve several goals: (1) interdigital abduction, especially in the first web space; (2) deepening of the web spaces, restoring them to their normal symmetric concavity and dihedral shape; and (3) lengthening of the dorsal or volar digitopalmar skin, releasing longitudinal metacarpophalangeal or proximal interphalangeal associated deformities.

The five-skin flap technique can achieve all three objectives. Different combinations and modifications can be used, depending on the degree of severity.

FLAP DESIGN AND DIMENSIONS

The five–skin-flap technique involves two balanced opposed Z-plasties along the line of contracture, with a transverse V-Y-plasty advancing deep into the middle of the reconstruction (Figs. 1B and 2).

If the skin contracture is not linear but occurs in two dimensions, the flap is modified as shown in Fig. 3A. This is especially useful for congenital, posttraumatic, or spastic contractures.

If the transverse dorsal scar is linear and neatly protruding, the dangers of transposing scarred flaps can be completely avoided by a simplified technique that advances all flaps with minimal transposition or undermining (Fig. 4A).

The final result of the three variations is similar from a geometric point of view to that of Mustardé's method for repair of congenital contractures of the inner palpebral angle (6).

If the results are incomplete, they can be improved 6 months later by multiple V-Y-plasties (Fig. 5A).

The five-flap principle can be applied to various locations and combinations of contractures. (Fig. 6).

Text continues on page 918.

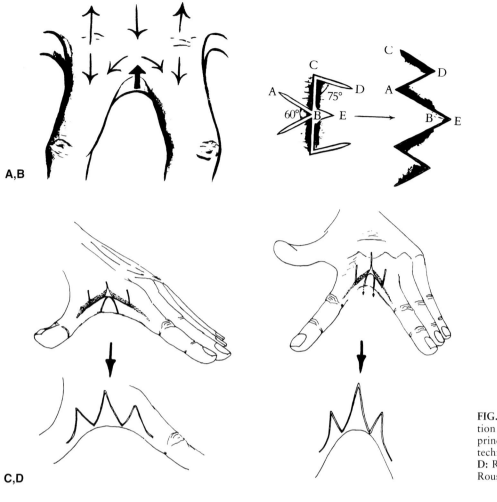

A,B

C,D

FIG. 1. A: The objectives of redistribution of skin tension. B: The geometric principles involved in the five-skin flap technique. C: Release of the first web. D: Release of an interdigital web. (From Rousso, ref. 2, with permission.)

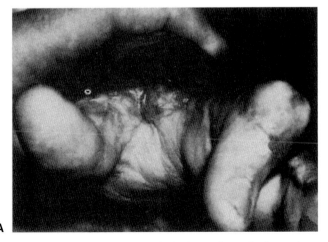
A

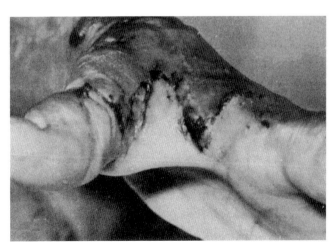
B

FIG. 2. A,B: Release of a first web space contracture using the standard technique.

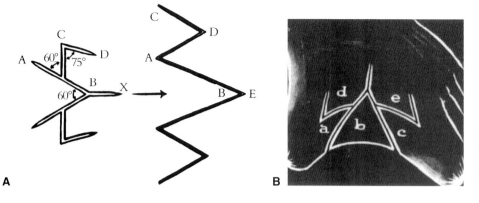

FIG. 3. Modification of the standard five-skin flap technique. **A:** Geometric principles of the modification. **B:** Application to a first web space contracture. (From Rousso, ref. 2, with permission.)

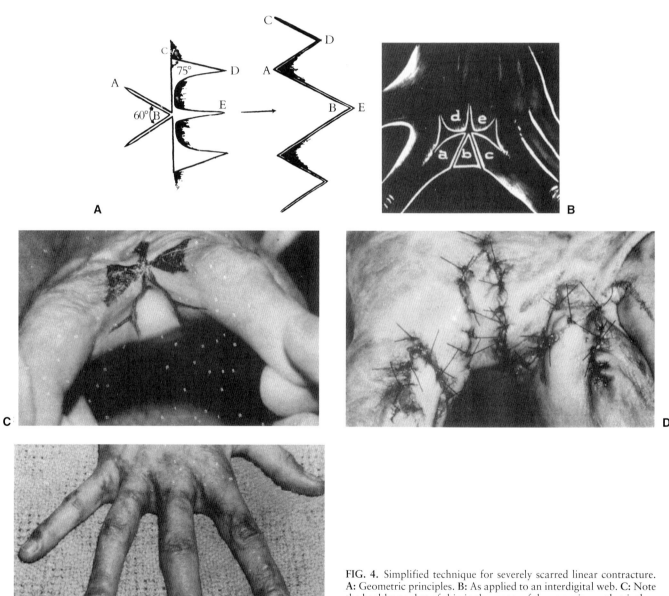

FIG. 4. Simplified technique for severely scarred linear contracture. **A:** Geometric principles. **B:** As applied to an interdigital web. **C:** Note the healthy pocket of skin in the center of the commissure that is then shaped into a V-Y-plasty and advanced without undermining proximally over the dorsum. **D:** Immediate postoperative result. **E:** Late postoperative result. (From Rousso, ref. 2, with permission.)

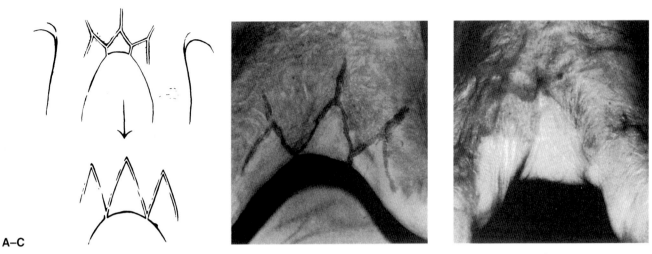

FIG. 5. A: Multiple V-Y-plasties used for incomplete release. **B:** Postoperative result after five–skin-flap technique. The three V-Y-plasties outlined. **C:** Postoperative result after three V-Y-plasties. (From Rousso, ref. 2, with permission.)

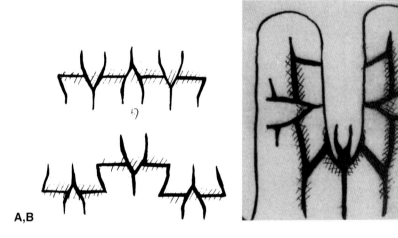

FIG. 6. Combinations of the five–skin-flap technique (cross-hatching marks the contracture). **A:** For linear contractures at different levels. **B:** For associated volar digitopalmar and interdigital web contracture. (From Rousso, ref. 2, with permission.)

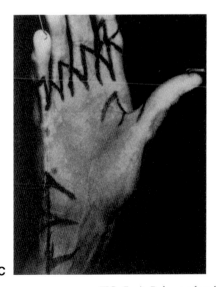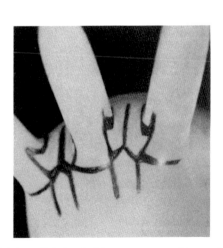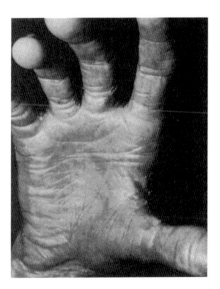

FIG. 7. A: Release of multiple interdigital web skin contractures with associated digitopalmar skin contractures. The interdigital contractures are alternately released in two stages. Note the five–skin-flap technique used for a contracture across the wrist. **B:** Glove model to help design the five–skin-flap release. **C:** Postoperative result after two stages completed. (From Rousso, ref. 2, with permission.)

If the injury results in a volar contracture of several adjacent webs, release of alternate webs in two stages is indicated (Fig. 7).

CLINICAL RESULTS

The result is predictable. The Z-plasties and V-Y-plasties adapt easily to the most frequent skin contractures. All flaps are smaller than when using a single Z-plasty, allowing scarred tissues to be elevated without resulting in necrosis at their tips.

Healthy flaps are interposed within the scarred area, helping prevent recurrence of contracture. Compression dressings or garments may be indicated postoperatively.

SUMMARY

The five-skin flap technique can be used to release many web space contractures. Further release can be obtained at a later stage with five V-Y-plasties. Various combinations and modifications can be used to treat particular cases.

References

1. Rousso M. Brûlures dorsales graves de la main: reconstruction de la commissure: technique à cinq lambeaux: I. La premiere commissure. *Ann Chir* 1975;29:475.
2. Rousso M. Brûlures dorsales graves de la main: II. Reconstruction des commissures 2, 3, et 4: modification à la technique à cinq lambeaux. *Ann Chir* 1975;29:1014.
3. Rousso M, Wexler MR. Secondary reconstruction of the burned hand. *Prog Surg* 1978;16:182.
4. Rousso M, Wexler MR. Management of the burned hand. In: Goldwyn RM, ed. *Long-term results in plastic and reconstructive surgery*, Vol. 2. Boston: Little, Brown, 1980;892–907.
5. Rousso M, Wexler MR. Burns of the upper limb. In: Tubiana R, ed., *The hand*, Vol. 2. Philadelphia: Saunders, 1981.
6. Mustardé JC. The treatment of ptosis and epicanthal folds. *Br J Plast* 1960; 12:252.

CHAPTER 316 ■ TRANSPOSITION FLAP FOR SOFT TISSUE ADDUCTION CONTRACTURE OF THE THUMB

M. SPINNER

EDITORIAL COMMENT

This and the subsequent chapter demonstrate excellent local flap techniques for first web-space reconstruction. However, the dorsal thumb flap allows for a much wider release of the first web space and uses an area that despite its relative insignificance from a functional standpoint, may be more apparent from a cosmetic standpoint. Both of these flaps are innervated ones, and consequently the first web-space widening is fully innervated. See also Chapter 317.

Loss of adduction of the thumb is a major handicap. Abdominal flaps of varying designs, local rotational flaps, Z-plasty, diamond split-thickness and full-thickness grafts—all have been suggested for correcting an adduction contracture of the thumb. A transposition flap from the index finger is an effective technique (1).

FLAP DESIGN AND DIMENSIONS

The adducted thumb is released by a planned incision that transposes skin from the radial aspect of the proximal phalanx of the index finger to the first web space (Fig. 1). The amount of contracture and release necessary is predetermined: the increased width desired determines the width of the base of the transposition flap taken from the radial side of the index finger.

The length of the flap is predetermined by the distance that is required for the apex of the flap to fit into the thenar eminence. A 1:1.5 ratio is ordinarily used but can be increased, if necessary, to a 1:3 ratio. The triangle of skin is outlined on the index finger.

OPERATIVE TECHNIQUE

The web is opened by continuing the volar radial aspect of the triangle into the adducted first web space and extending its midportion at right angles, into the volar aspect of the thenar eminence (Fig. 1C). The flap is elevated. It should be noted that this flap is well innervated by a branch of the superficial radial nerve (see Chap. 274). The underlying structures are easily visualized and the dorsal veins are preserved. The contracted fascia between the first and second metacarpals is released, as is the adductor muscle. (The fascia about the adductor is frequently scarred, and can be easily seen.)

The tailored flap is transposed into the defect created (Fig. 2). A split-thickness skin graft is used to cover the

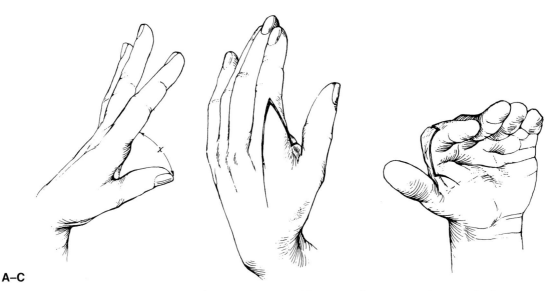

A–C

FIG. 1. **A:** Adduction contracture of the thumb (*X*). **B:** Oblique view, demonstrating the triangular flap based proximally on the dorsoradial aspect of the index finger. **C:** Volar aspect, demonstrating the thenar and index finger incision. (From Spinner, ref. 1, with permission.)

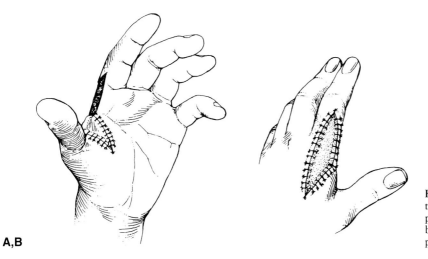

A,B

FIG. 2. **A,B:** Palmar and dorsal views. The adduction contracture has been released, and the transposition flap and split-thickness skin graft have been sutured in place. (From Spinner, ref. 1, with permission.)

defect on the radial side of the index finger and dorsal surface of the hand. The operative exposure gives free access to the shaft of the thumb, the index finger, and the metacarpophalangeal joints—as well as the adjacent contracted soft tissues.

CLINICAL RESULTS

Six hands have been treated with this procedure. In the cases treated, opponens transfer, arthrodesis of the thumb, metacarpophalangeal joint operations, and other local secondary operative procedures have been performed in conjunction with the release of the adducted thumb.

SUMMARY

A transposition flap for correction of soft-tissue adduction contracture of the thumb has two advantages. First, local tissue is used to correct the adduction contracture of the thumb. Second, the exposure is excellent for the simultaneous performance of other essential procedures, such as opponens plasty.

Reference

1. Spinner M. Fashioned transpositional flap for soft tissue adduction contracture of the thumb. *Plast Reconstr Surg* 1969;44:345.

CHAPTER 317 ■ DORSAL THUMB FLAP FOR THE THENAR WEB SPACE

B. STRAUCH AND M. FOX

The specialized nature of the first web space that allows for a wide range of thumb mobility is severely compromised when trauma or congenital deformity encroach on full web space expansion. Numerous procedures, including free skin grafts, distant flaps, and local flaps, have been described for correction of an adduction contracture of the first web space (1–5). Common to all of these procedures is a full release of the web space from dorsal to volar fulcrum at the base of the first and second metacarpals. Also common to these procedures is a residual area of less than normal sensation in the critical web space or key pinch contact area.

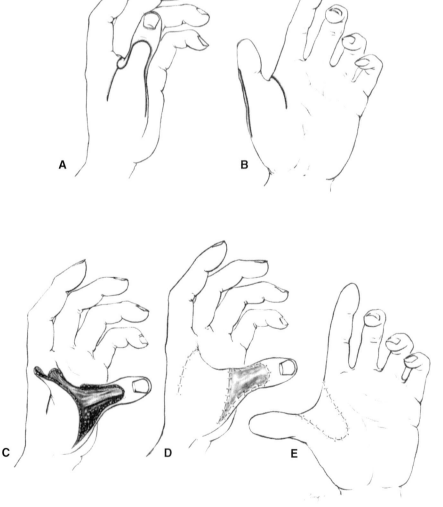

FIG. 1. A: The flap encompasses the entire dorsal skin of the thumb. The distal end extends 3 to 4 mm beyond the interphalangeal crease. The ulnar incision widens at the base to the middorsal area of the first web space. B: The volar incision extends from the free border of the web to the junction of the first and second metacarpals. C: Elevation of the flap affords full exposure of the underlying tissues. Abduction of the thumb leaves the flap properly oriented. D,E: Closure of the wounds and application of a split-thickness skin graft on the dorsum of the thumb. (Adapted from Strauch, ref. 4, with permission.)

920

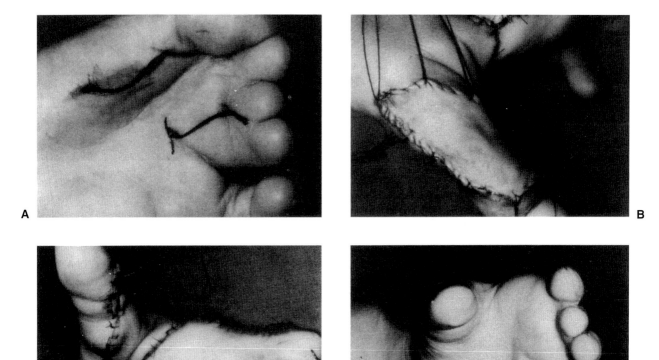

FIG. 2. A–D: A 6-year-old child with complete simple syndactyly of the first web space. Despite a completely encircling mantle of skin, the thumb had reasonably good mobility and was of normal length. The ulnar border of the flap was extended ulnarward, to compensate for the inability to extend the flap to the midaxial line on the ulnar side of the thumb. Full release with a dorsal thumb flap. Entire first web space and key pinch area covered with normally innervated full-thickness skin and soft tissue. (From Strauch, ref. 4, with permission.)

INDICATIONS

A local transposition flap, elevated over the dorsum of the thumb, allows for complete release of first web space contracture. This flap construction allows adequate visualization of underlying contracted tissues and a closure that provides full-thickness sensory skin coverage over the entire web space and key pinch contact area.

FLAP DESIGN AND DIMENSIONS

The flap is planned to encompass the entire dorsal skin of the thumb, from ulnar to radial midaxial lines (Fig. 1A). The distal extent of the flap is tapered and extends 3 to 4 mm beyond the interphalangeal (IP) joint. The radial midaxial line extends proximally to the basilar crease of the thumb.

OPERATIVE TECHNIQUE

An ulnar incision widens at the metacarpophalangeal joint to the middorsal area of the first web space and extends to the junction of the base of the first and second metacarpals. A volar incision is then extended from the free border of the web proximally to the junction of the first and second metacarpals (Fig. 1B). The flap is elevated at the level of the fascia, incorporating the superficial veins and the branches of the radial nerve into the flap. Full exposure of the adductor brevis, the insertion of the volar thenar intrinsics, as well as the entire ulnar side of the thumb, is attained. Fascial releases are accomplished after full integumentary release has been achieved.

Following complete soft-tissue release, the thumb is then fully abducted. The elevated flap, having been released from the thumb, now lies directly over the center of the first web space (Fig. 1C) and can be turned over into the palmar surface to close the skin defect (Fig. 1D). The radial volar side of the split web is rotated to close the defect on the thumb to a point dorsal to the midaxial line. A split-thickness skin graft is used to close the remaining defect on the dorsum of the thumb (Fig. 2).

SUMMARY

A flap designed from the dorsum of the thumb can be used not only to completely release an adduction contracture of the first web space but also to provide critical sensation.

References

1. Littler JW. The prevention and correction of adduction contracture of the thumb. *Clin Orthop* 1959;13:182.
2. Milford L. The hand, citing PW Brand. Evaluation of the hand and its function. *Orthop Clin North Am* 1973;4:1127. In: Edmonson AS, Crenshaw AH, eds. *Campbell's operative orthopedics*, 6th Ed. St. Louis: Mosby, 1980;274.
3. Spinner M. Fashioned transpositional flap for soft tissue adduction contracture of the thumb. *Plast Reconstr Surg* 1969;44:345.
4. Strauch B. Dorsal thumb flap for release of adduction contracture of the first web space. *Bull Hosp Joint Dis* 1975;36:34.
5. Sandzen SC Jr. Dorsal pedicle flap for resurfacing a moderate thumb-index web contracture release. *J Hand Surg* 1982;7:21.

CHAPTER 318 ■ DORSAL INDEX SKIN FLAP FOR THE THENAR WEB

E. J. HALL-FINDLAY AND B. STRAUCH

EDITORIAL COMMENT

The incorporation of the Z-plasty expands the Spinner flap potential of widening the first web space.

The use of the dorsal index skin as a flap for deepening a contracted web space was described by Brand for patients with leprosy (1–3). See Chapter 274 for a further discussion of this flap applied to the thumb.

FLAP DESIGN AND DIMENSION

This flap is designed for the thenar web space. The donor site can be closed primarily or with a skin graft, if more thumb abduction is required (Fig. 1).

If dorsal dissection alone is not sufficient to give a good web, a small Z-plasty may be added to give extra width to the web (Fig. 2). Brand cautions that an over-wide web produced weakness in pinch in leprosy patients since the web is necessary to stabilize the metacarpal when it is pushed by the index finger in the act of pinching (4). If a Z-plasty is necessary, its central limb must run along the free margins of the web for about 2 to 3 cm. Its dorsal limb will be the distal 2 to 3 cm of the dorsal incision already made and its ventral limb will run down the palmar side of the web from the other side of the central limb.

OPERATIVE TECHNIQUE

The dorsal skin and fascia must be incised to release the web space contracture. An incision is made along the full length of the index metacarpal starting from the index metaphalangeal (MP) joint and curving dorsally back toward the wrist. The skin over the web is elevated. While the thumb is held in abduction and opposition, the dorsal fascia is divided. In leprosy patients, Brand found it was not usually necessary, or indicated, to divide the paralyzed muscle. However, to get adequate abduction, the origins of the adductor pollicis and first dorsal interosseous muscles will often have to be divided.

A K-wire between the first and second metacarpals may be necessary to maintain some abduction during the postoperative period. This wire can be removed at the end of 6 weeks.

Once sufficient abduction is obtained, the skin defect is covered with either a split-thickness or a full-thickness skin graft.

CLINICAL RESULTS

The advantage of this particular method is that it places the skin grafted area over the dorsum of the hand where it causes less disability. Care must be taken during elevation of the flap to leave the paratenon over the extensor tendons (Fig. 3).

SUMMARY

A dorsal index skin flap can be used to deepen the first web space.

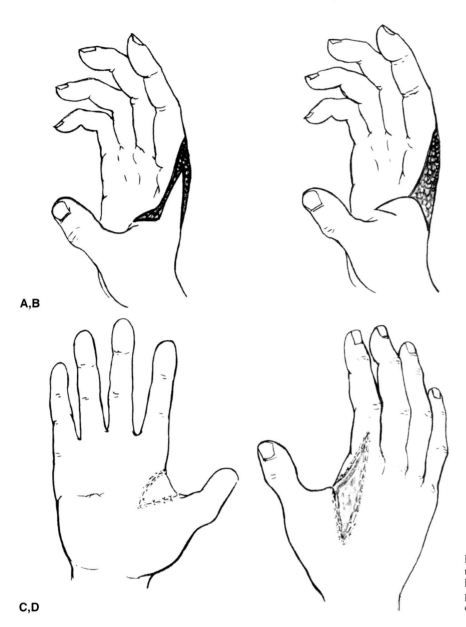

A,B

C,D

FIG. 1. A: The web has been released and the flap elevated. **B:** The apex of the flap (*x*) has been shifted into the palm. **C:** The flap in place seen from the palmar surface. **D:** The donor site is covered with a skin graft.

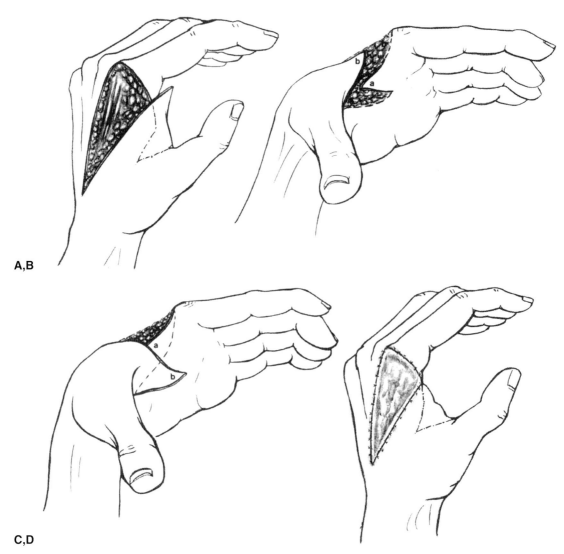

A,B

C,D

FIG. 2. **A:** Thumb web Z-plasty. A large posterior flap is created. **B:** The smaller palmar flap and the distal end of the posterior flap are shown. **C:** The flaps transposed. **D:** The donor site is covered with a skin graft.

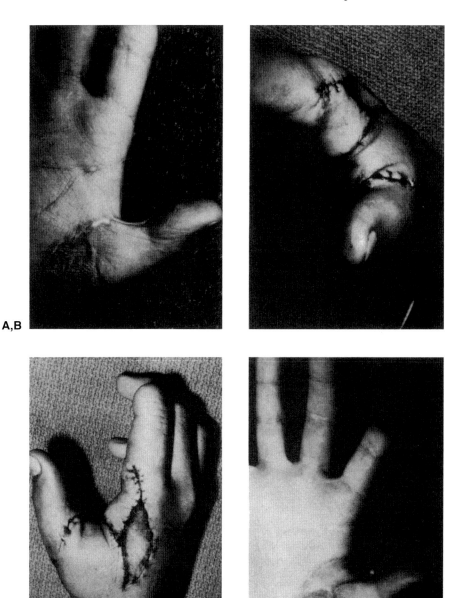

A,B

C,D

FIG. 3. A: This 12-year-old boy suffered total amputation of his thumb as a result of a motorcycle accident. The results of microvascular replantation were excellent (this is a case of Dr. Frank Forshew, Akron, OH), but the patient had a web space contracture of 38°. B,C: The dorsal flap has been transferred after release of the contracture. D: Final result. [These figures were provided by Drs. F. James Rybka of Carmichael, CA, and Frederick E. Pratt of Sacramento, CA (retired), for Chap. 274.]

References

1. Brand PW. Deformity in leprosy. In: Cochrane RG, ed. *Leprosy in theory and practice,* 2nd Ed. Bristol: John Wright, 1964;485.

2. Brand PW. The reconstruction of the hand in leprosy. *Ann R Coll Surg Eng* 1952;11:350.
3. Brand PW. Hand reconstruction in leprosy. In: Brand PW, ed. *British surgical practice: surgical progress.* London: Butterworths, 1954;124–125.
4. Brand PW. Personal communication with B. Strauch, 1988.

CHAPTER 319 ■ ARTERIALIZED PALMAR FLAP FOR FIRST WEB SPACE RECONSTRUCTION

L. O. VASCONEZ

Contracture of the thenar web space usually produces a disabling limitation of motion of the index finger and thumb, preventing grasping of larger objects. Causes of thenar web contracture include trauma, burns, hand infections, and systemic or local diseases, as well as paralysis in congenital malformations. Release of thenar web contractures to be effective usually requires a resurfacing with soft, pliable flap tissue.

INDICATIONS

An arterialized palmar flap to resurface the release of a thenar web contracture is best applicable to contractures secondary to burns of the dorsal skin, particularly when the index finger and thumb have suffered full-thickness burns and are covered with skin grafts. In such cases one cannot use the excellent "Brand flap" from the dorsum of the index finger (see Chap. 318) (1), and release by multiple Z-plasties is risky. A transposition flap from the palmar aspect of the hand that extends to the metacarpophalangeal joint of the index finger is most appropriate.

ANATOMY

A transposition palmar flap that is outlined adjacent to the defect on the thenar web space usually has its inferior margin extending along the metacarpophalangeal crease to the index finger. It is an arterialized flap that is supplied by cutaneous branches of the index digital artery as it crosses from the superficial arch toward the first web space. One or two branches, significant to supply the skin and subcutaneous tissue of the flap, emerge from the index digital artery in the thenar region.

FLAP DESIGN AND DIMENSIONS

The web contracture is first completely released and the index finger and thumb are held widely apart. A transposition flap is then outlined adjacent to the defect and extending along the radial aspect in the finger up to the metacarpophalangeal crease. The flap will lie over the course of the proper index

digital artery and its base will be proximally along the thenar region (Fig. 1).

OPERATIVE TECHNIQUE

The outlined flap is elevated superficial to the first lumbrical and adductor pollicis fascia and is raised sufficiently to allow a 60° to 90° angle of transposition to the recipient area of the thumb web space. Care is taken to avoid injury to the proper index digital nerve and artery. The flap is then sutured into the defect. The donor site, which is located along the palmar aspect of the hand extending to the radial aspect of the index finger, is covered with a split-thickness skin graft—preferably from the instep of the foot in black patients to avoid hyperpigmentation of the graft.

CLINICAL RESULTS

This arterialized flap is reliable and well vascularized from the vertically oriented branches of the digital artery. Recurrence of the contracture is unusual but a temporary splint may be needed for 2 to 3 months for web molding. The skin graft on the palmar aspect of the finger is well tolerated, although it is unsightly in black patients (Fig. 2).

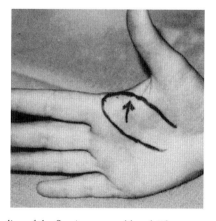

FIG. 1. Outline of the flap in a normal hand. The *arrow* points to the metacarpophalangeal crease.

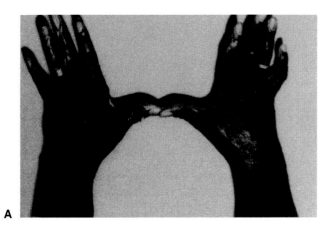

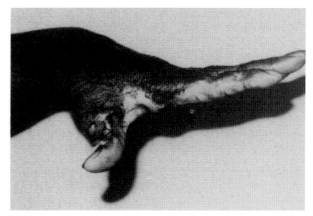

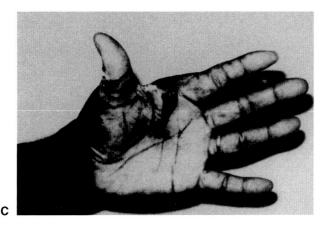

FIG. 2. **A:** Dorsal aspect of burned hands with moderate thenar web contracture on the left hand. The right hand thenar web contracture has been released with multiple Z-plasties. **B:** Released thenar web contracture with a palmar flap. Dorsal view. **C:** Palmar view. Note the hyperpigmented skin graft in the palm.

SUMMARY

The arterialized palmar flap is a local flap that provides enough good quality skin to release most of the moderate thenar web contractures.

Reference

1. Brand PW. Deformity in leprosy. In: Cochrane RG, ed. *Leprosy in theory and practice*, 2nd Ed. Bristol: John Wright, 1964;485.

CHAPTER 320 ■ FIRST WEB SPACE PSEUDO-KITE FLAP

P. LOREA, J. MEDINA, AND G. FOUCHER

EDITORIAL COMMENT

This is another good option for opening the first web space, particularly in patients with a congenital hand defect. The vascularized flap, although relatively small (if one is to close the defect primarily), does open up the web space for adequate functional rehabilitation.

Numerous flaps and plasties have been described to address functional limitations of the first web, which are present in several congenital or posttraumatic conditions. These flaps, although not perfectly adapted to congenital first-web deficiency, are dissected as islands from the web itself, the dorsal thumb or index finger, the dorsum of the hand, or the dorsal or palmar forearm. Because appearance is a major concern in congenital conditions, more so perhaps than in traumatic cases, a tetrahedral locoregional flap is described, which is designed to enlarge or to create a first web. The flap is dorso-radially harvested from the index finger and based on the axial vascularization of a kite flap. The donor site is closed primarily, avoiding the conspicuous scar of a skin graft on the dorsum of the hand.

INDICATIONS

In congenital cases, the pseudo-kite flap is an intermediate solution between local z-plasties and regional flaps from the dorsum of the hand (1), as well as distant flaps (e.g., posterior interosseous flap). We used this flap mainly in such congenital conditions as thumb hypoplasia (Blauth II and III), Apert syndactyly, amniotic band syndrome, and late-treated thumb in palm or symbrachydactyly (2), but we found it useful also in some posttraumatic conditions, such as in the sequelae of crush injuries (3). However, we do not use this flap after burn injury or in a Volkmann contracture, in which skin deficiency is sometimes too extensive, or when scars are present on the dorsum of the index finger.

We do not advocate the use of the pseudo-kite flap in every congenital condition with first-web deficiency. It is part of an armamentarium of flaps and plastic techniques, each of which is useful in selected conditions. The choice is dependent on many factors, as the design of the malformed first web is not the same in each patient (e.g., total absence, deficiency in length [distance between thumb and index metacarpophalangeal (MP) joints], or deficiency in depth [relative length of the thumb]). However, the flap has the successful ability to lengthen the first web without relative thumb lengthening (deepening of the web).

ANATOMY

The pseudo-kite flap is an axial-pattern flap perfused by the first dorsal interosseous artery, the axial vessel of the kite flap described previously (4). Numerous anatomic variations have been described, but these are not relevant in describing surgical technique (5). This artery consistently runs along the radial aspect of the second metacarpal, most of the time superficial to the aponeurosis of the first dorsal interosseous, sometimes deep to the aponeurosis, and sometimes both configurations are present together. Most of the cutaneous perforators are situated at the level of the neck of the second metacarpal, where the skin flap has its narrow skin bridge. During the proximal distal dissection, care must be taken underneath the skin paddle not to injure the first dorsal interosseous artery, which is tethered by a constant anastomotic circle around the neck of the second metacarpal.

FLAP DESIGN AND DIMENSIONS

The pseudo-kite flap is a rhomboid-shaped flap, corresponding to the tetrahedral aspect of the first web (Fig. 1). It is designed on the radial side of the dorsum of the first phalanx and MP joint of the index finger. The pivot point with a half-centimeter skin bridge is situated on the radial aspect of the neck of the second metacarpal bone, to include the first dorsal interosseous artery. The incision (AB) runs to the middle of the web (B). This incision continues straight on the palmar side (A'). The BC side of the rhombus is along the midlateral radial line of the index finger, with the length of BC usually equal to BA. The CD side is designed on the dorsal aspect of the proximal phalanx of the index finger, and DE on the dorsum of the hand, with point E situated along the second metacarpal some millimeters radial to point A, to preserve the narrow skin bridge. Dimensions vary according to the patient's age.

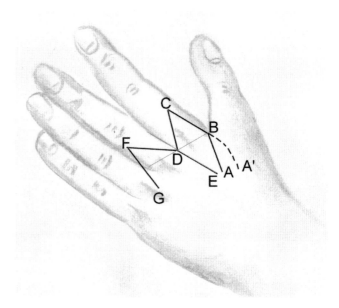

FIG. 1. Design of the flap.

Closure of the donor site is done by modification of a procedure described by Dufourmentel (6). BD and ED lines are prolonged ulnarly, and DF is drawn by bisecting this BD–ED angle. The length of DF is equal to the other sides of the rhombus. The last line (FG) is perpendicular to the extended BD and starts from point F. If more skin is necessary on the palmar aspect of the first web, a longer BA' line is possible; BC and DC lines may be extended by placing C more distally.

OPERATIVE TECHNIQUE

The incision begins with line AB extending palmarly to A'. Any fibrous band, fibrous tissue, or muscle tethering the first web is released by this exposure. The aponeurosis of the first dorsal interosseous and adductor muscles is incised, with care taken to preserve the nutrient artery. The first web opening may be maintained by a Kirschner wire. If necessary, this incision allows disinsertion of the first dorsal interosseous muscle from the first metacarpal. We avoid proximal transfer of the adductor muscle, favoring its disinsertion from the second and third metacarpals through a separate incision.

Lines BCDE are then incised to allow elevation of the flap. Care is taken to keep the dissection plane deep to the aponeurosis of the first dorsal interosseous muscle, to ensure inclusion of the first dorsal interosseous artery. It is not necessary to visualize the artery and is dangerous to skeletonize it. At the level of the metacarpal neck, one must be aware of the anastomotic branch, and if necessary, dissection must go deeper in the muscle to divide this branch and to avoid injuring the axial artery.

Elevation of a DFG flap is done in a more superficial plane, including only skin and subcutaneous tissue. The transfer of the flap allows closure of point C to point A' (Fig. 2). Closure of the donor site is done by transfer of the DFG triangle, F being sutured in the C position. Primary closure is possible when the index-finger MP joint is maintained in extension. If closure has to be done in flexion, a skin graft may be needed. If the rhombus was initially asymmetric, distal closure of the ABC angle is done in a V-Y fashion, until equalization of all sides of the rhombus is reestablished.

CLINICAL RESULTS

We reported previously on 16 flaps in 16 patients (2). Patient mean age at the time of surgery was 10 months (range, 6

degrees). Grasping ability was measured and compared with the normal side, with increasing-sized cylinders in eight patients. The web size was equal to that of the other side in five patients, 1 cm smaller in three patients, and 2 cm smaller in one. All patients (or families) were satisfied, and no patient needed reoperation.

Our experience with traumatic cases is not so extensive and includes six cases. Distal skin grafting of the donor site was required in three cases. No complications occurred, and patients were satisfied with the functional results and aesthetic improvement.

SUMMARY

The pseudo-kite flap is a rhomboid (diamond-shaped), axial-pattern, fasciocutaneous flap, useful in some cases of first-web insufficiency, mainly in congenital conditions. Most of the time, the donor site may be closed primarily, minimizing the scars on the "social" side of the hand.

References

1. Buck-Gramcko D. Syndactyly between the thumb and index finger. In: Buck-Gramcko D, ed. *Congenital malformations of the hand and forearm.* London: Churchill Livingstone, 1998;141.
2. Foucher G, Medina J, Navarro R, Khouri RK. Correction of first web space deficiency in congenital deformities of the hand with the pseudokite flap. *Plast Reconstr Surg* 2001;107:1458.
3. Foucher G, Cornil C, Braga Da Silva J. Le lambeau "pseudo-cerf volant" de l'index avec plastie LLL dans la reconstruction de la premiere commissure. *Ann Chir Plast Esthet* 1992;37:207.
4. Foucher G, Braun JB. A new island flap transfer from the dorsum of the index to the thumb. *Plast Reconstr Surg* 1979;63:344.
5. Sheriff MM. First dorsal metacarpal artery flap in hand reconstruction: I. Anatomical study. *J Hand Surg* 1994;19A:26.
6. Dufourmentel C. La fermeteur des pertes de substance cutaneé limitées "Le lambeau de rotation en L pour Losange." *Ann Chir Plast* 1962;7:61.

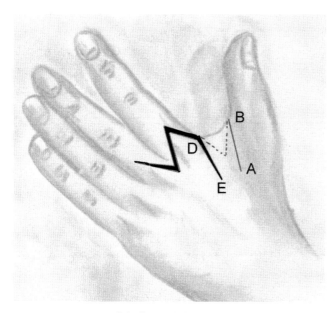

FIG. 2. Inset of the flap and closure of the donor site.

months to 6 years). A split-thickness skin graft was necessary in five cases. A dynamic flexion splint was necessary for the index finger in one case, and static night-splinting was used in 11 patients to maintain the first web opening. Complications included skin necrosis (one superficial), wound dehiscence, and skin-graft slough.

The mean lengthening of the web fold was 205%, compared with preoperative values. The first intermetacarpal angle was measured by radiograph, when available (seven patients), and increased from 11 degrees preoperatively (range, 6 to 17 degrees) to 75 degrees postoperatively (range, 54 to 89

CHAPTER 321 ■ MULTIPLE DORSAL ROTATION SKIN FLAPS FOR THE THENAR WEB

A. E. FLATT

The multiple dorsal flap technique was originally designed for the congenital mitten hand in which the thumbnail lies in the same plane as the fingers (1,2).

INDICATIONS

The usual indication for the use of these flaps is the need to supply sufficient skin for the thumb web space, to allow proper opposition of the thumb. The flaps can also be used to mobilize sufficient dorsal skin in a distal direction, to provide coverage for the metacarpal heads of patients who have suffered traumatic amputations at this level and who need strong protective coverage, either for the wearing of a prosthesis or during their ordinary work.

The commonest indication for these flaps is in the congenital mitten or five-fingered hand syndromes. In these patients there is not a true contracture of the web space, since the web

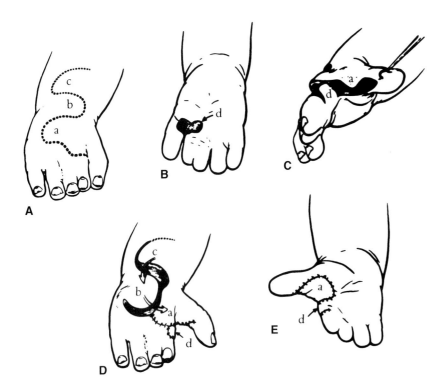

FIG. 1. A: Multiple dorsal rotation skin flap technique. The first flap (*a*) is based on the thumb and rotated into the opened web space. The second flap (*b*) is rotated into the defect left from (*a*). The third flap (*c*) is rotated into the defect left from (*b*). The defect from flap (*c*) is higher up on the forearm where there is more loose skin, so it can be closed in a curvilinear fashion. **B:** A small, square palmar flap (*d*) based on the index finger is used to cover the proximal radial portion of the index finger. (From Flatt and Wood, ref. 2, with permission.) **C:** Flap (*a*) rotated into the web space. Note that the palmar flap (*d*) is used to cover the index finger. **D:** Flap (*b*) is rotated to cover the defect by (*a*) and flap (*c*) is rotated into the defect by (*b*). Note flap (*a*) in position. **E:** Flaps (*a*) and (*b*) inset into position. A good release of the first web space can be achieved.

space has never really developed. The thumb is, in effect, trapped in an inadequate amount of skin, and its release by these flaps allows it to abduct, rotate, and assume the normal posture of the thumb immediately.

Other causes of contracture in the web space such as burn, skin avulsion due to scar contracture, or contracture due to neurologic disorder or to improper splinting, can also benefit from the use of these flaps. When a contracture is present, scarring must be dealt with at the same time.

OPERATIVE TECHNIQUE

The first, most distal, wide dorsal flap is based on the radial side of the dorsum of the thumb (Fig. 1 [a]), so that the venous drainage and radial nerve sensibility supply are intact. Next, a small square flap based on the index finger is raised from the palmar aspect of the skin between the thumb and the index finger (Fig. 1 [d]). This flap will provide coverage for the proximal and radial aspects of the index finger (Fig. 1).

The thumb web space can now be cleared of all tight fascia, the thumb can be widely abducted, and the dorsal flap can be laid in place. Both the dorsal flap and the index finger flap should be sutured in place before the second dorsal flap is raised. This second flap (Fig. 1 [b]) should be as wide as the others, but based on the ulnar side of the wrist. It is then rotated distally into the defect on the dorsum of the hand.

A third and final dorsal flap (Fig. 1 [c]) fills the defect created by the rotation of the second flap. This third flap is based radially on the most distal portion of the dorsal forearm. Undermining of the surrounding tissues and lining up of the skin edges will allow total closure of the area, resulting in a final single lazy-S scar running from the dorsal side of the index metacarpophalangeal joint to the lower portion of the forearm.

The use of these flaps can provide excellent web space coverage and freedom for a totally entrapped thumb (Figs. 2 and 3). The flap can also be used when there is, in effect, some adduction contraction and some definition of a true thumb. For instance, when the thumb is well developed distal to the interphalangeal joint, the dorsal flaps can be rotated as described

above; but on these occasions it may be possible to plan proper coverage without the use of the small, secondary index finger-based flap.

CLINICAL RESULTS

If a child is born with a total mitten hand, I believe that the thumb should be freed as soon as is reasonable and certainly by 6 months of age. Release of the thumb may not be delayed beyond 1 year, because by this age the child's cortex is sufficiently developed to make use of the thumb. A thumb must therefore be provided by this time.

Long-term results have been encouraging, and the flaps grow with the hand as the child increases in age. The scar is

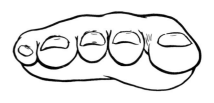

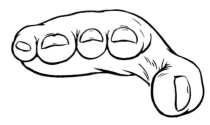

FIG. 2. (*Above*) In the child with a congenital mitten hand, the thumbnail lies in the same plane as the fingers. (*Below*) Opposition of the thumb is possible after providing adequate skin for the thumb web space. (From Flatt and Wood, ref. 2, with permission.)

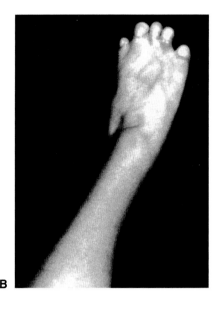
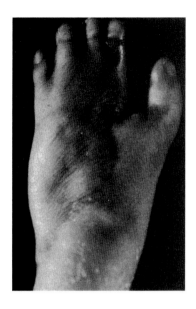

FIG. 3. A: Preoperative appearance of a congenital mitten hand. **B:** Postoperative result. (From Flatt and Wood, ref. 2, with permission.)

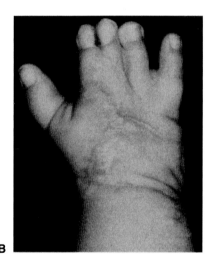
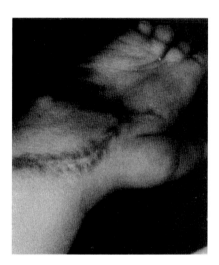

FIG. 4. Examples of multiple dorsal rotation skin flap results in two patients. Correction of the typical adducted and unrotated thumbs of the hypoplastic mitten hand has been provided by the flaps. Scarring is sometimes unattractive. (From Flatt and Wood, ref. 2, with permission.)

not always cosmetically pleasing and, on occasion, secondary excision and even Z-plasty have been needed to relieve particularly unpleasing, thickened scarring (Figs. 3 and 4).

panacea for the deepening of all thumb web clefts. Each adducted thumb contracture demands a careful evaluation of its specific problems and the selection of appropriate treatment from the many methods available.

SUMMARY

The multiple dorsal rotation skin flap technique as described here has worked well for selected cases. The principles have also been extended to other situations, such as providing coverage for loss of skin on the dorsum of the hand and metacarpophalangeal joints. This operation is not recommended as a

References

1. Brand PW. Deformity in leprosy. In: Cochrane RG, ed. *Leprosy in theory and practice*, 2nd Ed. Bristol: John Wright, 1964;485.
2. Flatt AE, Wood VE. Multiple dorsal rotation flaps from the hand for thumb web contractures. *Plast Reconstr Surg* 1970;45:258.

CHAPTER 322 ■ CROSS-ARM TRIANGULAR FLAPS FOR FIRST WEB SPACE RECONSTRUCTION

I. J. PELED, M. R. WEXLER, AND M. ROUSSO

Adduction contracture of the thumb is rather a frequent finding following trauma (lacerations, crush, burns), and may present as an early or late complication. Early splinting and physiotherapy are advisable, although not always feasible or effective.

The intrinsic muscles, adductor pollicis, and first dorsal interosseous, are contracted and are often included in the scarred fibrous tissue. The palmar fascia can also be involved in deep injuries or following infection.

INDICATIONS

When conservative treatment fails to correct the adduction contracture, a surgical procedure is needed to restore the proper relationship of the thumb to the fingers and palm. This is achieved by releasing the scarred skin and the fibrosed subcutaneous tissue, as well as by performing a myotomy of the intrinsic muscles to open the web space widely. During this procedure several important structures, such as the median nerve, flexor tendons of the index finger, and palmar arteries, may be exposed in the diamond-shaped defect that has been created.

Local flaps and Z-plasties may be used to close the defect in only a few cases. The local skin cover can have poor circulation, especially in burns. Skin grafts may succeed when the skin is the only structure that is contracted (1). In most cases the defect is large and deep, and distant flaps are the choice (2–6). One possibility is the use of two oppositely based, triangular, cross-arm flaps (7).

The inner aspect of the arm is an excellent donor area for hand resurfacing (8–12). The skin is thin, elastic, and scarce in adipose tissue and hair. The laxity and rich blood supply allow wide undermining and primary closure of the donor area in most cases.

ANATOMY

The rich blood supply of the inner arm is provided by two branches of the brachial artery: the superior and inferior ulnar collateral arteries (Fig. 1). The superior ulnar collateral artery crosses the deep fascia together with the ulnar nerve and supplies the brachialis anterior and triceps muscles and, by direct cutaneous branches, the skin of the upper inner arm. It anastomoses with the posterior recurrent branch of the ulnar artery.

The inferior ulnar collateral artery divides into two branches at the lower third of the arm. The anterior branch runs in front of the medial epicondyle and it anastomoses with the anterior recurrent branch of the ulnar artery. The direct cutaneous branches irrigate the lower inner arm (13).

FLAP DESIGN AND DIMENSIONS

The flaps are drawn in the inner aspect of the contralateral arm according to the size of the defect. One triangular flap is based superiorly and will cover the dorsal aspect of the web, and the other one is based inferiorly and will cover the ventral half of the defect. The base of each flap equals the width of the web defect (Fig. 2C).

OPERATIVE TECHNIQUE

The web is widely opened, incising and/or excising all the fibrous tissue and contracted muscle. The resulting defect has a diamond shape, with one of the axes lying along the web and the other crossing it perpendicularly from dorsal to palmar (Fig. 2B).

The flaps are raised in the plane of the loose areolar tissue space above the fascia. The two sides of the triangles are

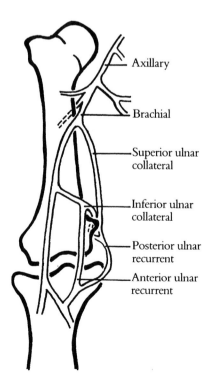

FIG. 1. Blood supply of the inner arm through the superior and inferior ulnar collateral branches of the brachial artery.

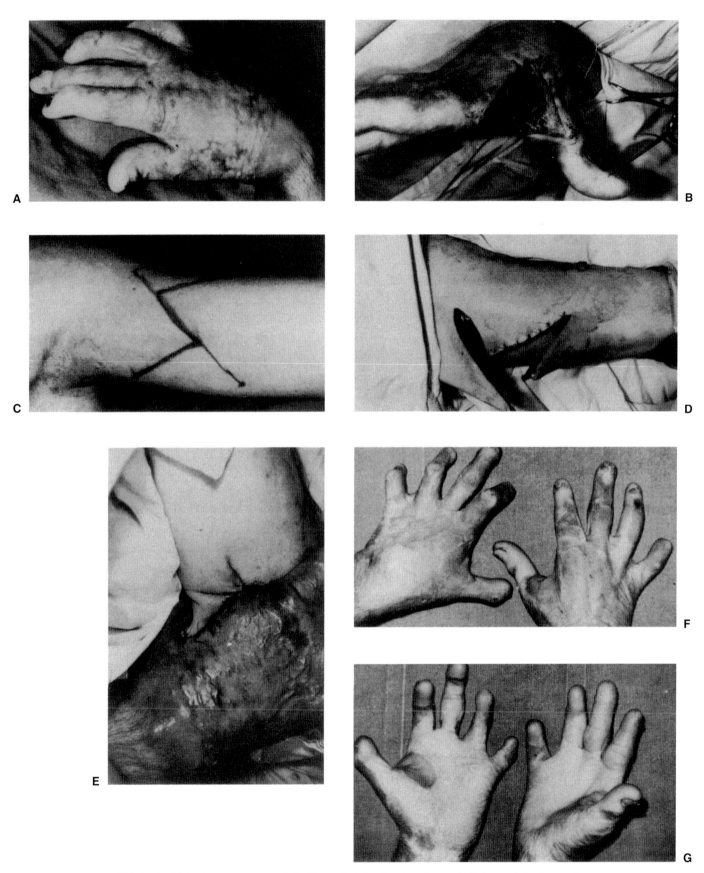

FIG. 2. A: Adduction contracture of the first web following deep burns. B: Release of the first web. C: Design of the contralateral triangular arm flaps. D: The opposed triangular flaps are raised and the donor area is closed primarily by undermining the lateral flaps. E: The two triangular flaps sutured to the created defect of the web. The hand grasps the contralateral arm. F: Dorsal view of the hands 1 year after bilateral release of the first webs. G: Volar view. (From Yeschua et al., ref. 7, with permission.)

sutured to the sides of the diamond while the hand grasps the arm (2,14).

The donor area is closed primarily by undermining the skin edges (Fig. 2D,E). Separation of the flaps is performed 10 to 14 days later, and the bases of the triangles are sutured to each other and form the arch of the web. When necessary, a Z-plasty is used to lengthen this scar. The position of the hand, grasping the opposite arm, is a good way of splinting and maintaining the abduction obtained by the release, without the need of internal Kirschner wire fixation (Fig. 2E).

CLINICAL RESULTS

The triangular cross-arm flaps are reliable, thin flaps that cover the whole defect. There is no need for a delay. The thumb is splinted in abduction by the grasping position on the arm. The only disadvantage is the lack of sensation of the flap.

The results have been excellent and no complications have been found. Except for the remaining scar at the donor area, there are no functional deficits (Fig. 2F,G).

With modern microvascular techniques, the same donor area can be used as a free flap (15–17), but conventional flaps are safe and may easily be carried out.

SUMMARY

Triangular cross-arm flaps can provide the skin and soft tissue needed to release severe first web space adduction contractures.

Sufficient release of the subcutaneous tissue and underlying fibrosed muscles can be performed.

References

1. Flynn JE. Adduction contracture of the thumb. *N Engl J Med* 1956;254:15.
2. Brown JB, McDowell F, eds. *Skin grafting*, 3d Ed. Philadelphia: Lippincott, 1958;108, 147.
3. Littler JW. The prevention and the correction of adduction contracture of the thumb. *Clin Orthop* 1959;13:182.
4. Flatt AE, Wood VE. Multiple dorsal rotation flaps from the hand for thumb web contractures. *Plast Reconstr Surg* 1970;45:258.
5. Grabb WC, Myers MB, eds. *Skin flaps.* Boston: Little, Brown, 1975;489.
6. Peacock EE. Burns of the hand. In: Converse JM, ed. *Reconstructive plastic surgery.* Philadelphia: Saunders, 1977;3376.
7. Yeschua R, Wexler MR, Neuman Z. Cross-arm triangular flaps for correction of adduction contracture of the first web space in the hand. *Plast Reconstr Surg* 1977;59:859.
8. Teich-Alasia S, Ambroggio G, Oberto E, Liguori G. Are traditional pedicle flaps really obsolete? *Chir Plast* 1980;5:77.
9. Delbet JP, Wallich E. La place du cross-arm flap dans la chirurgie de la main. *Ann Chir Plast* 1964;9:3.
10. Colson P, Janvier H. Le dégraissage primaire et total des lambeaux d'autoplastie à distance. *Ann Chir Plast* 1966;11:11.
11. Rouvière H. *Anatomie Humaine*, 4th Ed, Vol. III. Madrid: Bailly-Baillière, 1956;148.
12. Teich-Alasia S, Barberis ML. The value of the "cross-arm" flap in reconstructive surgery of the hand. *Chir Plast* 1972;1:134.
13. Sharpe C. Tissue cover for the thumb web: a review. *Arch Surg* 1972;104:21.
14. Gan KB. Inner arm flap for the reconstruction of nasal and facial defects. *Ann Plast Surg* 1981;6:277.
15. Dolmans S, Guimberteau JC, Baudet J. The upper arm flap. *J Microsurg* 1979;1:162.
16. Kaplan EN, Pearl RM. An arterial medial arm flap: vascular anatomy and clinical applications. *Ann Plast Surg* 1980;4:205.
17. Newsom HT. Medial arm free flap. *Plast Reconstr Surg* 1981;67:63.

CHAPTER 323 ■ MICRONEUROVASCULAR TRANSFER ON A FIRST WEB SPACE SKIN FLAP

B. STRAUCH AND E. J. HALL-FINDLAY

EDITORIAL COMMENT

This flap allows for a very high innervation density, so that two-point discrimination in the range of normal can be achieved.

The first web space skin flap from the foot may well be the ideal flap for providing sensory skin coverage to the hand (1–4). It can restore function to an anesthetic portion of a hand by supplying sensation with appropriate cortical representation. It is a thin flap with good texture and surprisingly large dimensions, and it results in minimal donor site morbidity.

INDICATIONS

Innervated flaps can be taken from other areas of the hand, depending on the nature of the injury, but the patient has difficulty interpreting signals. However, the first web space flap from the foot not only provides sensation, but sensation that has appropriate central representation. The texture of the flap is ideal, since toe plantar skin is so similar to the skin on the

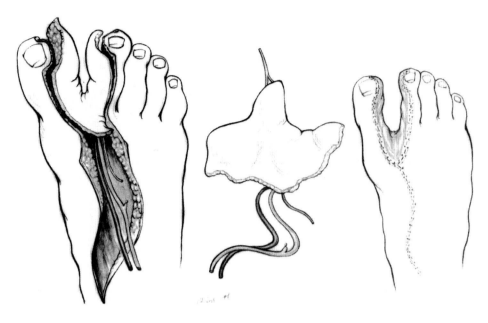

FIG. 1. Donor site preparation of the first web space skin flap. Note the deep peroneal nerve. The donor site is covered with a split-thickness skin graft.

volar surface of the fingers and hand. The flap also provides skin of good stability, essential for an adequate grip.

ANATOMY

The arterial supply to the first web space of the foot comes from both the dorsal and the plantar interconnecting arch systems (1,2,4). The first dorsal metatarsal artery, which leaves the dorsalis pedis artery as it passes between the first and second metatarsals to join the plantar arch, is used as the donor artery. The first dorsal metatarsal artery usually arises directly from the dorsalis pedis artery (in 88% of cases) (2). However, it may branch off at any level, while the dorsalis pedis artery passes toward the plantar system. Depending on its origin, the first dorsal metatarsal artery passes either superficial to or within the substance of the first dorsal interosseous muscle; the latter case makes dissection more difficult.

Venous drainage is by both venae comitantes accompanying the arteries, but mainly by superficial veins that drain into the saphenous system. Usually only one of these branches is used as the flap vein.

The first web space is innervated by both the deep peroneal nerve and the plantar nerves. The deep peroneal nerve lies adjacent to the first dorsal metatarsal artery. The plantar digital nerves are branches of the medial plantar nerve and therefore arise in the sole of the foot. They supply the medial surface and pulp of the second toe and the lateral surface and pulp of the big toe.

FLAP DESIGN AND DIMENSIONS

The dimensions of the flap can be unexpectedly large: 14 cm (medial to lateral) × 7.5 cm (plantar to dorsal) (4). The flap can also be extended in a dorsal direction to include all or part

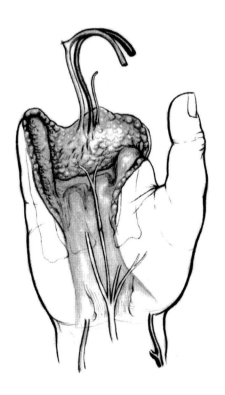

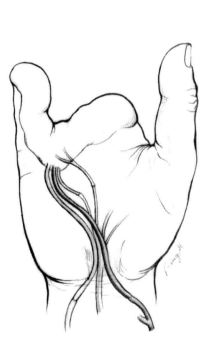

FIG. 2. The first web space flap used to provide sensory cover to the hand.

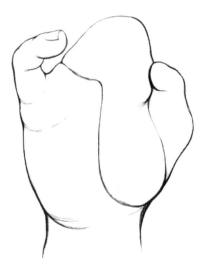 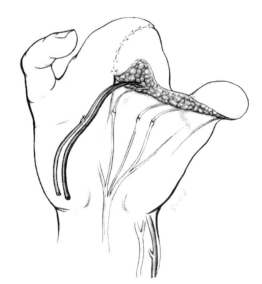

FIG. 3. The first web space flap can be used to provide sensation to the prehensile area in a hand that has been previously covered with an insensate flap. Note that the deep peroneal nerve and both digital nerves are being anastomosed to appropriate recipient nerves in the hand.

of the dorsalis pedis flap, depending on recipient site requirements. The skin with the greatest potential for good sensibility lies in the first web space itself (5 to 15 mm two-point discrimination in situ vs. 20 to 30 mm for the dorsalis pedis flap) (2,4) (Figs. 1 and 2).

The dorsalis pedis artery should be examined by palpation. The first dorsal metatarsal artery can be evaluated by both Doppler and lateral (preferably magnification type) arteriograms. Sensory testing, including two-point discrimination, should be assessed in situ. After making a pattern from the recipient site, one should outline the flap on the foot. The superficial veins are then mapped out, with the use of a tourniquet if necessary.

OPERATIVE TECHNIQUE

The flap dissection is begun dorsally, under tourniquet control and with the aid of loupe magnification. A curvilinear incision is made over the dorsalis pedis artery, carefully preserving all superficial veins. Once the dissection is in progress, the best donor vein can be selected, and the remaining veins ligated. (Some of these may be used for vein grafts later, if deemed necessary.)

The dorsalis pedis artery is identified and dissected distally until the origin of the first dorsal metatarsal artery is identified. All four branches (two plantar and two dorsal) of the first dorsal metatarsal artery should be carried with the flap. The deep peroneal nerve should also be found at this stage, lying adjacent to the first dorsal metatarsal artery. It is followed proximally until an adequate length can be obtained (Fig. 3) (1–4).

Once the arterial anatomy has been clearly defined, the deep branch of the dorsalis pedis artery that passes to the plantar arch can be ligated, as can the arcuate artery that passes laterally to supply the remaining dorsal metatarsal arteries.

The plantar digital nerves can be identified either through the incision made at the plantar border of the flap or while dissecting the skin flap away from the fascia of the toes as the dissection progresses in a dorsal to plantar fashion. At some point the dissection should be done from the plantar aspect, to dissect the nerves as far proximally as necessary, allowing tensionless recipient site anastomoses.

If the dorsalis pedis flap is to be included, the dissection should begin proximally, with careful preservation of the

dorsalis pedis artery within the flap (2,4). In this case the superficial peroneal nerve should be included with the flap.

CLINICAL RESULTS

Surprisingly, these flaps often develop better two-point discrimination on the hand than was ever present on the foot (2,4). This has not yet been adequately explained, but it could be the result of any of several hypotheses. First, the flap contracts after elevation, moving sensory receptors closer together. Also, the recipient site nerves are larger and may respond differently than nerves in the foot, or they may just have more axons available. The brain itself may play a role, as the cortical area representing the hand is larger than the area for the foot, and may therefore be able to discriminate impulses from the flap better than impulses from the foot.

The donor site is covered with split-thickness skin grafts, resulting in minimal morbidity. In some cases the graft becomes keratotic and forms irregularities that can be difficult to maintain from a hygienic viewpoint. If the dorsalis pedis flap is included, there may be some discomfort while wearing shoes. Weight bearing and walking are otherwise not adversely affected.

SUMMARY

Even when used for a small area, such as coverage for a thumb or pinching surface, this flap can turn a neglected hand into a functionally useful hand.

References

1. Gilbert A. Composite tissue transfers from the foot: anatomic basis and surgical technique. In: Daniller AT, Strauch B, eds. *Symposium on microsurgery.* St. Louis: Mosby, 1976.
2. May JW Jr, Chait LA, Cohen BE, O'Brien BM. Free neurovascular flap from the first web of the foot in hand reconstruction. *J Hand Surg* 1977; 2:387.
3. Morrison WA, O'Brien BM, MacLeod AM, Gilbert A. Neurovascular free flaps from the foot for innervation of the hand. *J Hand Surg* 1978;3:235.
4. Strauch B, Tsur H. Restoration of sensation to the hand by a free neurovascular flap from the first web space of the foot. *Plast Reconstr Surg* 1978; 62:361.

CHAPTER 324 ■ EXTENSOR CARPI ULNARIS AND FLEXOR DIGITORUM PROFUNDUS MUSCLE FLAP COVERAGE OF THE PROXIMAL ULNA

B. E. COHEN

With this procedure the flexor digitorum profundus muscle belly is freed and advanced and the extensor carpi ulnaris is transposed as a distally based muscle flap. The muscles remain in continuity distally and their neurovascular supply is not disrupted, thereby achieving single-stage coverage with no loss of hand function (1).

INDICATIONS

Coverage of the proximal ulna can be effected by two local forearm muscles without functional loss.

ANATOMY

The flexor digitorum profundus is a wide muscle in the deepest plane of the volar forearm muscles (Fig. 1). It arises from, and is the muscle most closely attached to, the anterior aspect of the ulna and the interosseous membrane. Its medial or ulnar portion is supplied by branches of the ulnar nerve and artery that enter its anterior (superficial) surface. There are no neurovascular structures between the muscle and the underlying ulna. The anterior interosseous nerve, a branch of the median nerve, supplies the lateral or radial portion of the muscle with branches that also enter anteriorly.

The extensor carpi ulnaris arises from the lateral epicondyle of the humerus and the posterior aspect of the ulna (Fig. 2). The main hilum, where branches of the posterior interosseous nerve and artery enter, is located on the deep aspect of the muscle, 8 cm distal to the olecranon. Although one or two small vessels may enter more proximally, the major pedicle can easily support the entire muscle belly.

OPERATIVE TECHNIQUE

The flexor digitorum profundus is freed from the ulna with sharp dissection and the use of a periosteal elevator over a length of 8 to 10 cm (Figs. 3B and 4B). This maneuver is safe, as there are no neurovascular structures between the muscle and the ulna. Once freed, the muscle may be easily advanced over the exposed portion of the ulna (Fig. 3C). The needed mobility may be obtained without dissecting over as far as the anterior interosseous vessels. The muscle is held in place with sutures to available soft tissue along the margin of the bone.

The extensor carpi ulnaris is approached distally where the intervals between the dorsal muscles are apparent. The radial border of the muscle is dissected free in a distal to proximal direction, up to the lateral epicondyle, from which it is now detached. The underside of the muscle is then freed from the ulna in a proximal to distal direction, until the main neurovascular pedicle is encountered, approximately 8 cm below the olecranon (Figs. 3B and 4B). The well-vascularized muscle belly can now be readily transposed and fixed to the adjacent soft tissue, thereby providing a second layer of coverage over the previously advanced flexor digitorum profundus (Figs. 3D and 4C).

Mobilization of the forearm skin on either side may be adequate to cover the transposed muscles (Fig. 4D). If not, skin grafts are applied to the muscles. A small suction drain may be used in the wound. To prevent pulling away of the muscle bellies, the extremity is splinted for 2 weeks in a neutral position, with the fingers in a functional position.

CLINICAL RESULTS

In using this technique, one should be aware that transposition of the extensor carpi ulnaris leaves the radiohumeral joint in a subcutaneous position (this has not been a problem), and that it does not appear to be capable of covering the olecranon. Choosing to use this, rather than an abdominal flap, shortens the hospitalization period and obviates the need for a second operation. Furthermore, there is no abdominal scarring and, if the skin can be closed over the muscles, one avoids a patch-like effect on the forearm surface.

SUMMARY

With this technique the proximal portions of the flexor digitorum profundus and extensor carpi ulnaris are moved without disturbing the vascular supply, the innervation, or the distal

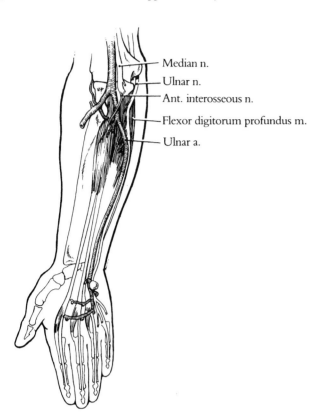

Median n.

Ulnar n.

Ant. interosseous n.

Flexor digitorum profundus m.

Ulnar a.

FIG. 1. Anatomy. The flexor digitorum profundus muscle is depicted in this anterior view of the right forearm. The ulnar portion of the muscle takes origin from the underlying ulna, while the neurovascular supply enters the muscle belly on its superficial surface. (From Cohen, ref. 1, with permission.)

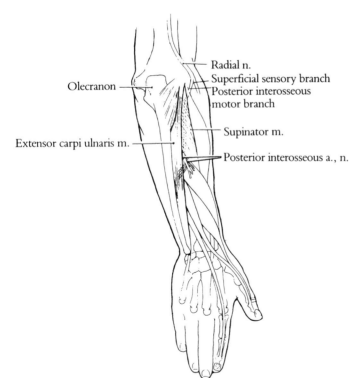

Radial n.

Superficial sensory branch

Posterior interosseous motor branch

Olecranon

Supinator m.

Extensor carpi ulnaris m.

Posterior interosseous a., n.

FIG. 2. Anatomy. The extensor carpi ulnaris muscle is shown on this dorsal view of the right forearm. The muscle arises from the lateral epicondyle of the humerus and the dorsal surface of the ulna. Its neurovascular supply enters its deep surface 8 cm distal to the olecranon. (From Cohen, ref. 1, with permission.)

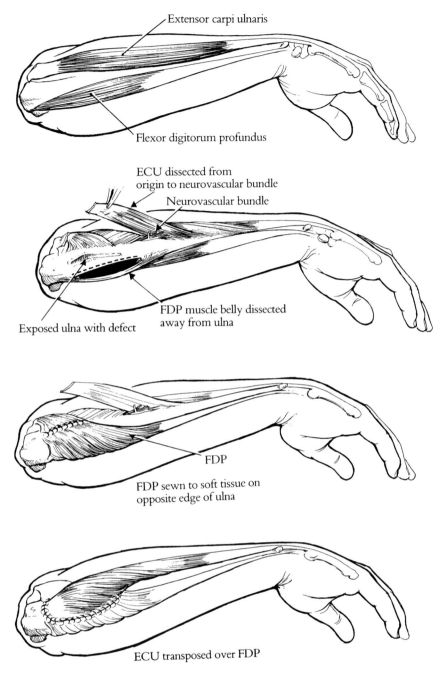

FIG. 3. A–D: Surgical technique. The operative steps for coverage of the proximal ulna by the extensor carpi ulnaris (*ECU*) and flexor digitorum profundus (*FDP*) are shown in this right forearm view from the ulnar aspect.

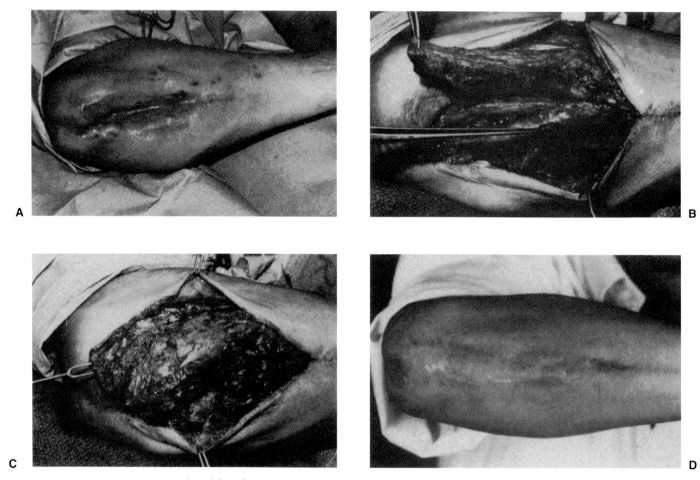

FIG. 4. **A:** A deep defect of the right ulna covered with thin epithelium and skin grafts. **B:** Thin coverage removed from ulna. The extensor carpi ulnaris and flexor digitorum profundus muscles have been elevated but not yet transposed (as in Fig. 3B). **C:** Muscles advanced and transposed over ulna (extensor carpi ulnaris superficial to flexor digitorum profundus) are sutured into place (as in Fig. 3D). Skin is mobilized for closure over muscle. **D:** Result at 1 year. (From Cohen, ref. 1, with permission.)

tendinous portions of these muscles. A portion of the origin is maintained, and the transposed portion is allowed to reattach in its new location. One-stage coverage of the proximal ulna is achieved, complete function is preserved, and an aesthetically pleasing result is obtained.

Reference

1. Cohen BE. Local muscle flap coverage of the proximal ulna without functional loss. *Plast Reconstr Surg* 1982;70:745.

CHAPTER 325 ■ ABDOMINOHYPOGASTRIC SKIN FLAP FOR HAND AND FOREARM COVERAGE

J. D. SCHLENKER AND E. ATASOY

The abdominohypogastric flap is an axial pattern flap with a dual axial blood supply (1). Anatomically, it lies parallel to and between the groin (iliofemoral) flap (2) and the transverse thoracoabdominal flap (3–5).

INDICATIONS

In our experience, the abdominohypogastric flap is indicated when flap coverage is needed for the forearm. The groin flap is frequently too short to reach these defects (6) and the transverse thoracoabdominal flap, located cephalad to the umbilicus, is too high for forearm coverage (3–5).

The abdominohypogastric flap is also indicated when the groin flap is not available. However, if the groin flap has already been used, the superficial inferior epigastric artery may have been divided during elevation of the groin flap, which would eliminate one of the arterial inputs to the abdominohypogastric flap and thereby increase the risk of ischemia. The deltopectoral flap is another alternative for hand and forearm coverage, but the deformity from grafting or scarring in the secondary defect is more apparent than that associated with either the groin or the abdominohypogastric flap (6).

ANATOMY

The dual cutaneous blood supply of the abdominohypogastric flap is derived from the superficial inferior epigastric artery, as is true of the hypogastric flap described by Shaw and Payne (6–8), and from the anterior perforators of the deep inferior epigastric artery (Fig. 1). These perforators are reported to be less numerous caudad to the umbilicus than those more cephalad that supply the thoracoabdominal flap (5).

The second supply to this flap, the superficial inferior epigastric artery, has been reported to be absent in 35% of dissections (8). However, when it is absent, a large branch of the superficial circumflex iliac artery often passes cephalad to the inguinal ligament to supply the region of the base of the abdominohypogastric flap (9,10).

FLAP DESIGN AND DIMENSIONS

The base of the abdominohypogastric flap lies between the umbilicus and the inguinal ligament. The upper border of the flap is drawn parallel to the 10th, 11th, or 12th ribs. The lower border is drawn with the aid of the Doppler probe to include branches of the superficial inferior epigastric artery (Fig. 2). The lower border is curved so that it lies 1 to 2 cm caudad to the laterally directed branches of the superficial inferior epigastric artery and does not extend medial to the main trunk of that artery. Laterally, the flap has been carried to the posterior axillary line. In our experience (four cases), the flap measures 10 to 15 cm in width and 20 to 24 cm in length.

OPERATIVE TECHNIQUE

The Doppler probe is essential to determine the course of the branches entering the base of the flap, in order to outline the lower border of the flap. Flow in the anterior perforators can be detected with the Doppler probe at the point at which the perforator penetrates the fascia. As the probe is moved away from this point of exit in any direction, the sound produced by the flow diminishes rapidly, indicating that the branches of the perforators are small. Usually three perforators have been identified between the pubis and the umbilicus.

In contrast to a thoracoabdominal flap that is elevated with the fascia over the serratus anterior muscle, the abdominohypogastric flap is raised superficial to the muscular fascia. The portion of the flap that covers the defect can be thinned so that a thickness of 0.5 cm or less of adipose tissue remains beneath the dermis.

CLINICAL RESULTS

We have employed this flap in four cases, all of which have been successful. In three patients the defect was on the wrist or forearm and in one it was on the dorsum of the hand. In two cases the flap was tubed (Fig. 3) and the skin edges of the donor defect were approximated without the need for a skin graft (1). In two patients the flap was employed after the groin flap had already been used on the same side.

SUMMARY

The abdominohypogastric skin flap can be reliably used for both hand and forearm coverage.

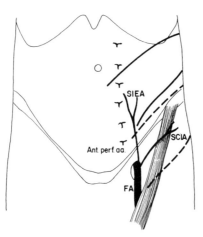

FIG. 1. The *dotted lines* outline the groin or iliofemoral flap supplied by the superficial circumflex iliac artery (*SCIA*). The abdominohypogastric flap is outlined by the *solid line*; it is supplied by anterior perforating branches of the deep inferior epigastric artery and by branches of the superficial inferior epigastric artery (*SIEA*). (From Schlenker et al., ref. 1, with permission.)

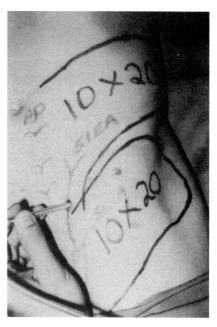

FIG. 2. The small Doppler probe is used to determine the course of the superficial inferior epigastric artery. The lower border of the abdominohypogastric flap is designed to include branches of this artery within the base of the flap. (From Schlenker et al., ref. 1, with permission.)

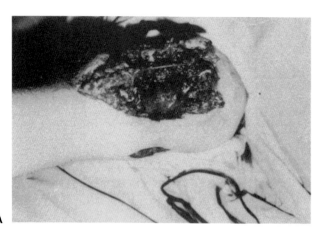

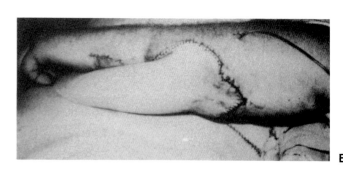

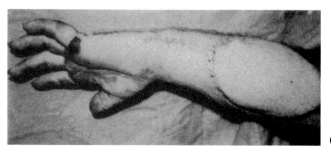

FIG. 3. A: Shotgun wound to the left forearm with division of the ulnar artery, ulnar nerve, and fracture of the ulna. The skin defect measured 10 by 15 cm. **B:** The defect in the forearm was primarily covered completely with a tubed abdominohypogastric flap. The flap was tubed and the donor and recipient sites were closed. The flap was divided and inset 3 weeks after the initial injury. **C:** One month after injury. There is complete healing of the skin over the forearm. (From Schlenker et al., ref. 1, with permission.)

References

1. Schlenker JD, Atasoy E, Lyon JW. The abdominohypogastric flap, an axial pattern flap for forearm coverage. *Hand* 1980;12:248.
2. McGregor IA, Jackson IT. The groin flap. *Br J Plast Surg* 1972;25:3.
3. Tai Y, Hasegawa H. A transverse abdominal flap for reconstruction after radical operations for recurrent breast cancer. *Plast Reconstr Surg* 1974;53:52.
4. Brown RG, Vasconez LO, Jurkiewicz MJ. Transverse abdominal flaps and the deep epigastric arcade. *Plast Reconstr Surg* 1977;55:416.
5. Davis WM, McCraw JB, Carraway JH. Use of a direct, transverse, thoracoabdominal flap to close difficult wounds of the thorax and upper extremity. *Plast Reconstr Surg* 1977;60:526.
6. McGregor IA. Flap reconstruction in hand surgery: the evolution of presently used methods. *J Hand Surg* 1979;4:1.
7. Schlenker JD, Averill RM. The iliofemoral (groin) flap for hand and forearm coverage: pitfalls, prevention and alternatives. *Orthop Rev* 1980;9:57.
8. Shaw DT, Payne RL. One stage tubed and abdominal flaps. *Surg Gynecol Obstet* 1946;83:205.
9. Taylor GI, Daniel RK. The anatomy of several free flap donor sites. *Plast Reconstr Surg* 1975;56:243.
10. Harii K, Ohmori K, Torii S, et al. Free groin skin flaps. *Br J Plast Surg* 1975;28:225.

CHAPTER 326 ■ TISSUE EXPANSION AND FLAPS OF THE UPPER EXTREMITY

G. G. HALLOCK

The development of large random flaps for the elimination of local arm defects (1–3), the augmentation of flaps prior to their transposition by gradual distension using inflatable silicone balloons (4,5), and the amelioration of donor site deformities (6,7), are all advantages not previously possible without the combination of tissue expansion with upper extremity flaps.

INDICATIONS

For all practical purposes, the scope of tissue expansion currently remains limited to skin augmentation (8–13). The following discussion is therefore limited to those named fasciocutaneous flaps that have a reasonably large territory and a constant, reliable anatomy that facilitate their dissection—the deltoid, lateral upper arm, and forearm flaps based on the radial or the ulnar artery or on their segmental perforators (Fig. 1). All are versatile microsurgical free tissue donor areas, while the lateral upper arm and forearm flaps may also be useful for coverage of ipsilateral upper extremity defects. Unless small dimensions are used, all ultimately require a skin graft of the donor area following transfer (14–17).

The immediate or delayed placement of expanders to allow later transformation of these defects into more acceptable linear scars has been particularly valuable for the distal radial forearm flap (7) where the residual nonaesthetic donor site is the most conspicuous (18,19). If required, pretransfer expansion may also create larger flaps.

OPERATIVE TECHNIQUE

For immediate expansion following flap transfer, the remaining medial or lateral skin and subcutaneous tissues are undermined above the muscle fascia to create a pocket that will accept the dimensions of the expansion envelope (Fig. 2A) (20,21). Usually a standard rectangular implant whose length exceeds that of the defect is satisfactory. Placement over bony prominences or joints is avoided so that mobility will not be impaired during expansion. The dermis at the defect edge is then carefully closed to the underlying tissues, as any gap will promote infection and subsequent extrusion of the implant. A remote valve prevents the risk of inadvertent implant puncture during fluid instillation. The expander can be placed directly under the flap, if pretransfer augmentation is elected.

Adequate wound healing is mandatory prior to commencing serial expansion and, not uncommonly, this must be delayed even up to 6 weeks. Then percutaneous saline is instilled on a weekly basis until skin capillary fill disappears or pain intolerance occurs. If rapid expansion or expansion of an anesthetic area is desired, objective monitoring of transcutaneous oxygen levels might be desirable for greater safety (22).

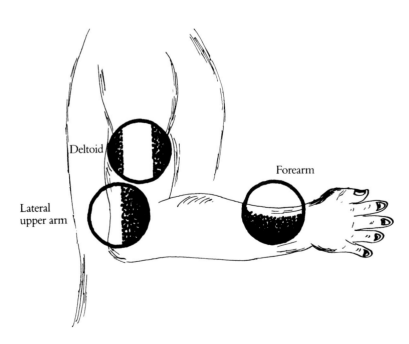

FIG. 1. Versatile fasciocutaneous donor sites of the upper extremity. *Shaded areas* are suitable for placement of expanders at the time of flap transfer.

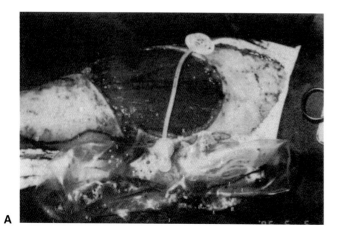
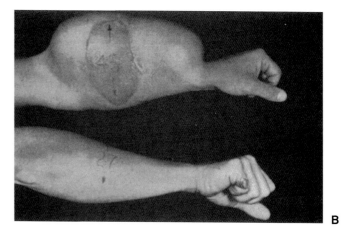
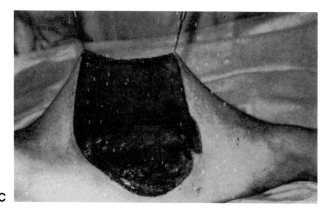
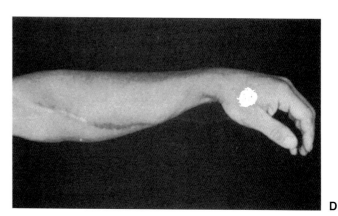

FIG. 2. **A:** Longitudinal curved expander placed in a dorsal pocket immediately after transfer of a radial forearm flap. **B:** Measurement of arm circumference allows determination of tissue gain required prior to implant removal. Note objectionable appearance of typical volar skin graft donor defect. **C:** Highly vascularized capsule on undersurface of the expanded dorsal flap, prior to its advancement to cover the skin graft defect depicted in **B**. Re-creation of the donor flap defect must await assurance that the augmented tissues will provide adequate coverage. **D:** Typical linear scar result following tissue expansion.

The difference in the circumference of the extremities from a given fixed point will determine the available tissue gain (Fig. 2B). When this exceeds coverage requirements, the expander may be removed. In many cases this requires expander overinflation well beyond the stated allowable volume, but at least twice this amount and probably more has been reported to be safe (23,24). Maximum inflation at the time of surgery will yield an additional 1 to 2 cm in length by way of acute load-cycling or skin stretching (25). A defect should not be created until confirmation that the expanded flap will provide adequate coverage (Fig. 2C), as it may be necessary to retain the expander for a second period of expansion.

CLINICAL RESULTS

Transforming an upper extremity deformity into a linear scar, or at least minimizing the size of a skin-grafted donor defect, have been usual sequelae of the appropriate use of tissue expansion (Fig. 2D). Complication rates are higher in extremity tissue expansion (11,12,26), and proper precautions and attention to wound healing must be adopted, if this concept is to be successful. A minimum of two surgical stages are required, regardless of whether pretransfer or post-transfer expansion is elected. Pretransfer expansion also carries additional risks to the flap: if the implant were to become infected,

the skin devascularized or thinned, or this pedicle compromised, the elective transfer might have to be aborted (13).

Caution must be observed with any attempt at extremity tissue expansion. Since the procedure requires a significant investment of both patient and surgeon time, the hazards as well as the advantages must be clearly outlined in advance.

SUMMARY

Although no universal flap yet exists that will meet every functional demand of the recipient area, while simultaneously minimizing the donor site defect, tissue expansion provides added advantages that allow use of many donor regions with the assurance that a linear scar will be the only residuum.

References

1. Morgan RF, Edgerton MT. Tissue expansion in reconstructive hand surgery: case report. *J Hand Surg* 1985;10A:754.
2. Mackinnon SE, Gruss JS. Soft tissue expanders in upper limb surgery. *J Hand Surg* 1985;10A:749.
3. Hallock GG. Tissue expansion techniques in burn reconstruction. *Ann Plast Surg* 1987;18:274.
4. Hallock GG. Tissue expansion. *Contemp Surg* 1986;29:34.
5. Leighton WD, Russell RC, Marcus DE, et al. Experimental pretransfer expansion of free flap donor sites: I. Flap viability and expansion characteristics. *Plast Reconstr Surg* 1988;82:69.

6. Hallock GG. Free flap donor site refinement using tissue expansion. *Ann Plast Surg* 1988;6:566.
7. Hallock GG. Refinement of the radial forearm flap donor site using skin expansion. *Plast Reconstr Surg* 1988;81:21.
8. Radovan C. Tissue expansion in soft-tissue reconstruction. *Plast Reconstr Surg* 1984;74:482.
9. Austad ED, Thomas SB, Pasyk K. Tissue expansion: dividend or loan? *Plast Reconstr Surg* 1986;78:63.
10. Sasaki GH, Pang CY. Pathophysiology of skin flaps raised on expanded pig skin. *Plast Reconstr Surg* 1984;74:59.
11. Manders EK, Schenden MJ, Furrey JA, et al. Soft tissue expansion: concepts and complications. *Plast Reconstr Surg* 1984;74:493.
12. Hallock GG. Extremity tissue expansion. *Orthop Rev* 1987;16:606.
13. Leighton WD, Russell RC, Feller AM, et al. Experimental pretransfer expansion of free-flap donor sites: II. Physiology, histology and clinical correlation. *Plast Reconstr Surg* 1988;82:76.
14. Russell RC, Guy RJ, Zook EG, Merrell JC. Extremity reconstruction using the free deltoid flap. *Plast Reconstr Surg* 1986;76:586.
15. Katsaros J, Schusterman M, Beppu M, et al. The lateral upper arm flap: anatomy and clinical application. *Ann Plast Surg* 1984;12:489.
16. Hallock GG. The radial forearm flap in burn reconstruction. *J Burn Care Rehabil* 1986;7:318.
17. Hallock GG. Soft tissue coverage of the upper extremity using the ipsilateral radial forearm flap. *Contemp Orthop* 1987;15:15.
18. Timmons MJ, Missotten FEM, Poole MD, Davies DM. Complications of radial forearm flap donor sites. *Br J Plast Surg* 1986;39:176.
19. Fenton OM, Roberts JO. Improving the donor site of the radial forearm flap. *Br J Plast Surg* 1985;38:504.
20. Hallock GG. Adjuvant use of the suction lipectomy cannula for blunt dissection. *Aesthet Plast Surg* 1985;9:107.
21. Hallock GG. Suction cannula assisted placement of traction sutures. *Ann Plast Surg* 1987;18:355.
22. Hallock GG, Rice DC. Objective monitoring for safe tissue expansion. *Plast Reconstr Surg* 1986;77:416.
23. Shively RE, Bermant MA, Bucholz RD. Separation of craniopagus twins utilizing tissue expanders. *Plast Reconstr Surg* 1985;76:765.
24. Hallock GG. Maximum overinflation of tissue expanders. *Plast Reconstr Surg* 1987;80:567.
25. Hirshowitz B, Kaufman T, Ullman J. Reconstruction of the tip of the nose and ala by load cycling of the nasal skin and harnessing of extra skin. *Plast Reconstr Surg* 1986;77:316.
26. Argenta LC, Marks MW, Pasyk KA. Advances in tissue expansion. *Clin Plast Surg* 1985;12:159.

CHAPTER 327 ■ MICRONEUROVASCULAR TRANSFER OF RECTUS FEMORIS MUSCLE AND MUSCULOCUTANEOUS FLAPS

R. R. SCHENCK

EDITORIAL COMMENT

The use of microvascular free transfer of muscles for restoration of both flexion and extension in the upper extremity has added a significant new dimension to the functional restoration of the upper extremity. At this time, the gracilis muscle appears to be the most useful for free transfer.

The rectus femoris muscle can be selected for a free muscle transfer to a patient's forearm, to replace traumatically destroyed digital flexors (1,2).

INDICATIONS

The rectus femoris musculocutaneous flap, whose length is ideal for forearm transplant, is particularly useful where strong motor power is necessary on the flexor aspect of the forearm. The technique offers the following advantages:

1. The single main arterial supply of the muscle simplifies arterial anastomosis at the recipient site. This is in contrast to the gracilis muscle that often has two arteries (3–6).

2. The femoral nerve branch is of adequate length for anastomosis.
3. The muscle is excellent in size and power for replacing lost forearm flexors. It can provide good grasp and strength. This is in spite of the anticipated 50% reduction in mass commonly observed after free muscle transfers.
4. There is adequate overlying skin for coverage of the muscle itself at the recipient site, yet primary closure at the donor site can be effected.
5. The muscle with its tendinous attachments is of appropriate length to reach from the new origin at the medial epicondyle to the new insertion site at the profundus tendons at the wrist.
6. There is no loss of effective quadriceps action in the donor leg. Complete and powerful knee extension is retained because of the remaining quadriceps muscle mass.

ANATOMY

The rectus femoris muscle originates from the anterior inferior iliac crest (Fig. 1). The neurovascular supply, consisting of the femoral nerve, artery, and vein, is found more medially.

The portion of the femoral nerve supplying the muscle can be most readily identified approximately 3 cm distal to the

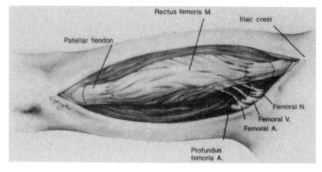

FIG. 1. The anatomy of the donor rectus femoris muscle is diagrammed to show its tendinous origin and insertion and its easily obtained arterial supply from one source, in contrast to the gracilis muscle, which may have multiple arteries supplying it. The overlying composite skin to be transferred is not shown in this diagram. (From Schenck, ref. 1, with permission.)

midpoint on Poupart's ligament, between the anterior inferior iliac crest and the lateral margin of the pubis. The femoral nerve can be identified under the sartorius muscle and traced there to its entry into the posteromedial margin of the rectus femoris muscle. There are usually two branches at the entry point.

The artery of the rectus femoris may arise from either the profunda femoris or the descending branch of the lateral circumflex femoral artery.

FLAP DESIGN AND DIMENSIONS

The flap can measure as much as 10 cm wide by 30 cm long. However, it is wise not to include the distal portion of skin near the knee.

OPERATIVE TECHNIQUE

The incision outline should be modified in a curvilinear manner near the superior portion of the muscle. The remainder of the incision encompasses the entire mass of the rectus femoris muscle, but care should be taken not to include skin that extends laterally or medially beyond the margins of the muscle belly itself (Fig. 2B).

The skin incisions are carried down vertically to the muscle fascia. After identifying the femoral nerve and the artery of the rectus femoris, the accompanying venae comitantes should be noted for later reference. The tendinous attachments of the rectus femoris are then divided proximally from the anterior inferior iliac crest and distally through the patellar tendon.

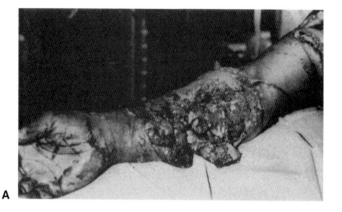

A

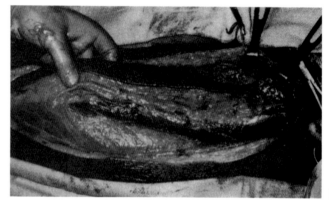

B

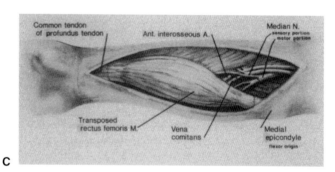

C

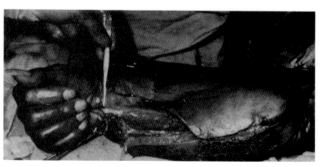

D

FIG. 2. A: The right arm of a 49-year-old man was severely injured in a milling machine, resulting in loss of all digital flexors by avulsion and the severing of the flexor carpi ulnaris, ulnar nerve and artery, median nerve, radial artery, and brachioradialis tendon. The two muscles, ulnar nerve, and radial artery were reapproximated and abdominal pedicle flap coverage was immediately provided. Eleven weeks later, bilateral sural nerve grafting was performed for both the median and the ulnar nerves. B: The left rectus femoris is being dissected, the origin being from the anterior inferior iliac crest on the right and the patellar tendon on the left. The elliptical composite skin flap is shown being taken carefully with the muscle, with its margins extending no farther than that of the muscle. C: The transferred rectus femoris muscle now lies in its new functional position, taking origin from the flexor origin at the medial epicondyle and inserting into the common mass of the flexor profundus tendons, just proximal to the partially divided transverse carpal ligament. D: The site of insertion of the transferred muscle can be seen, just prior to closure of all wound margins, using the composite skin. A small split-thickness skin graft (not visible) is necessary on the most ulnar aspect. (From Schenck, ref. 1, with permission.)

Finally, vascular clamps are applied to the artery and vein of the profunda femoris and the vessels and nerve are divided. A sufficient length of femoral nerve is critical. From 10 to 12 cm of the nerve's two branches can be obtained when the division is proximal to their common juncture. The donor site can be closed primarily.

Selection of the proper incision and exposure in the arm will depend on the existing scar and the previous flap margins. Owing to its location and size, the anterior interosseous artery is a convenient recipient vessel. However, a portion of a severed ulnar or radial artery, if patent, will serve the purpose just as well.

When the composite rectus femoris flap is transferred to the prepared arm, the proximal tendinous portion is sutured to the medial epicondylar fascia and the distal portion to the flexor profundus tendons near the wrist (Fig. 2C,D). The recipient arteries and nerves will vary according to the individual situation. Microneurovascular anastomoses should proceed with the vein being repaired first, then the artery. The motor nerve is repaired last.

When the distal rectus femoris muscle tendon is sutured to the flexor profundus tendons at the wrist, the transverse carpal ligament is divided in its proximal two-thirds. The wound is closed by suture of the cutaneous flap. If the composite skin does not fully cover the transferred muscle, a small split-thickness skin graft can be added. The dressing should be provided with a padded long arm posterior plaster splint for 90° of elbow flexion.

There is marked swelling of the transferred composite muscle-skin flap in the immediate postoperative period. There is apt to be slower than normal healing of the wound margins, and one should not be misled by the fact that the flap margins appear pink and bleed easily. Sutures should not be removed prematurely. Three to 6 months may be required before active motor end plate unit potentials can be noted on electromyography and/or correlated with clinical contractility (7,8).

CLINICAL RESULTS

In cases in which the author has personally performed the surgery, there have been no instances of residual donor defect.

In fact, full knee extension has been retained even against gravity or resistance. There has been no failure of the flap and no functional deficit. There was one instance of delayed healing at the wrist, when the skin in the suprapatellar area was included with the flap.

Among five cases reported by other surgeons who have used the rectus femoris muscle for a forearm composite graft, reinnervation was first detected by electromyography from 3 to 6 months following surgery. In these five cases, clinically detected reinnervation was also noted within the same 3-month time frame. These surgeons estimated excursion created by the transplanted muscle as ranging from 2 to 4 cm, and graded muscle activity at grade 3 or 4.

SUMMARY

The rectus femoris muscle or musculocutaneous flap can be used to replace the function of muscles such as the forearm flexors. Skin can be included with the flap or the muscle can be covered with a split-thickness skin graft.

References

1. Schenck R. Free muscle and composite skin transplantation by microneurovascular anastomoses. *Orthop Clin North Am* 1977;8:367.
2. Schenck R. Rectus femoris muscle and composite skin transplantation by microneurovascular anastomoses for avulsion of forearm muscles: a case report. *J Hand Surg* 1978;3:60.
3. Harii K, Ohmori K, Torii S. Free gracilis muscle transplantation with microneurovascular anastomoses for the treatment of facial paralysis. *Plast Reconstr Surg* 1976;57:133.
4. Harii K, Ohmori K, Sekiguchi J. The free musculocutaneous flap. *Plast Reconstr Surg* 1976;57:294.
5. Ikuta Y, Kubo T, Tsuge K. Free muscle transplantation by microsurgical technique to treat Volkmann's contracture. *Plast Reconstr Surg* 1976;58:407.
6. McCraw J, Dibbel D, Horton C, et al. Definition of new arterialized myocutaneous vascular territories. Paper presented at the 55th Annual Meeting of the American Association of Plastic Surgeons, Atlanta, Ga., 1976.
7. Tamai S, Komatsu S, Sakamoto H, et al. Free muscle transplants in dogs with microsurgical neurovascular anastomoses. *Plast Reconstr Surg* 1970;46:219.
8. Kubo T, Ikuta Y, Tsuge K. Free muscle transplantation in dogs by microneurovascular anastomoses. *Plant Reconstr Surg* 1976;57:495.

CHAPTER 328 ■ MICRONEUROVASCULAR TRANSFER OF THE LATISSIMUS DORSI MUSCLE AND MUSCULOCUTANEOUS FLAPS TO THE FOREARM

R. M. BARTON

The latissimus dorsi muscle offers the surgeon a formidable tool in reconstruction, as the muscle offers large bulk to cover significant defects, or it can be tailored to cover smaller ones. If needed, the overlying skin is dependable and may be oriented in any direction. The neurovascular pedicle has a predictable anatomic location, and the vessels have diameters that facilitate microvascular anastomosis.

INDICATIONS

Since the experimental groundwork for the successful transfer of functional muscle units was laid in 1970 (1), several criteria for free muscle transfer have evolved (2). Before restoration of the mechanical function of the hand and arm, the patient must have supple joints, a stable osseous skeleton, and an identifiable neurovascular supply. Moreover, free muscle transfer is indicated only when local tendon transfer cannot provide suitable functional restoration.

ANATOMY

The anatomy of the latissimus dorsi muscle has been well described (3). In nearly all patients, the thoracodorsal nerve, artery, and vein arise from or enter at a common hilum. The diameters of the artery and vein at their origin average 2.5 to 3.5 mm, respectively. The thoracodorsal artery then travels to the muscle, giving off one to three branches to the serratus anterior.

The length of pedicle that can be obtained is 9 cm. The nerve, artery, and vein enter the muscle on its inferior surface, approximately 2 cm medial to the lateral border and 10 cm inferior to the apex of the axilla. On entrance, the vessels and nerve bifurcate into transverse and longitudinal bundles. However, in 55% of patients there is no transverse branch, and the medial aspect of the muscle is supplied by many small branches from the posterior cord of the brachial plexus and lies proximal to the subscapular artery and vein before joining them in a common pedicle.

The intramuscular neural anatomy is similar to that of the artery and vein. Knowledge of the vascular and neural branching pattern makes it possible to take only part of the entire muscle or to split the muscle into two segments.

FLAP DESIGN AND DIMENSIONS

In transferring functional motor units, it is imperative to assess the amplitude of excursion required for motor function. For finger flexion the amplitude is at least 7 cm. Helpful technical points include marking the latissimus dorsi muscle in situ

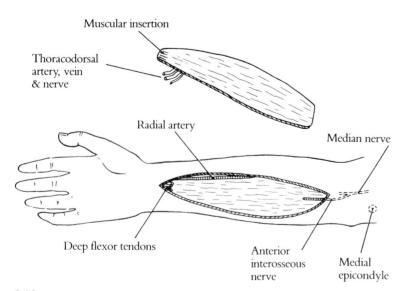

Muscular insertion

Thoracodorsal artery, vein & nerve

Radial artery

Median nerve

Deep flexor tendons

Anterior interosseous nerve

Medial epicondyle

FIG. 1. Transfer of a functional latissimus dorsi to the forearm.

with either indelible ink or suture material at standard intervals, to maintain this length when the muscle is transferred to the forearm. For restoration of finger flexion, the latissimus dorsi muscle is oriented with its insertion distally, to be attached to the flexor tendon(s), and its origin is oriented proximally, to be attached to the medial epicondyle (Fig. 1).

Preoperative planning must establish the integrity of the vascular and neural supply. Arteriography may be necessary. Intraoperative biopsy of the recipient nerve may be helpful to ensure its axonal content. Although the thoracodorsal nerve can be taken with an average length of 12 cm, it may be sectioned close to its muscular entrance to shorten the time for reinnervation.

When exploring the arm, it is helpful to design cutaneous flaps that will cover the musculotendinous junction after the insertion of the flap. The remainder of the latissimus dorsi muscle can either be transferred with its overlying skin paddle or grafted with a split-thickness skin graft.

CLINICAL RESULTS

The appearance of muscle function returns in approximately 6 to 12 months. The force of contraction of transferred

muscle has been measured at between 25% and 50% of its original functional strength. The rate of return of muscular function and its ultimate strength are closely related to the status of the recipient nerve. Although a pure motor nerve is preferable, a mixed nerve such as the anterior interosseous can be used.

SUMMARY

The latissimus dorsi muscle can be transferred to the upper extremity as an innervated flap, to restore function and to provide coverage.

References

1. Tamai S, Komatsu S, Sakamoto H, et al. Free muscle transplants in dogs with microsurgical neurovascular anastomoses. *Plast Reconstr Surg* 1970; 46:219.
2. Manktelow RT, McKee NH. Free muscle transplantation to provide active finger flexion. *J Hand Surg* 1978;3:416.
3. Tobin GR, Schusterman M, Peterson GH, et al. The intramuscular neurovascular anatomy of the latissimus dorsi muscle: the basis for splitting the flap. *Plast Reconstr Surg* 1981;67:637.

CHAPTER 329 ■ MICROVASCULAR FREE GRACILIS MUSCLE AND MUSCULOCUTANEOUS FLAP TO THE FOREARM

R. T. MANKTELOW AND R. M. ZUKER

There are many muscles that can be transferred from one location in the body to another through the use of microvascular techniques. The gracilis is the first muscle that was transferred in this manner (1,2). It remains one of the most useful muscles for microvascular transfer. The muscle is easy to remove, can be reliably transferred on its pedicle, produces no functional loss, and leaves an incisional scar on the upper medial portion of the thigh, where it is easily hidden. The potential for transferring a

muscle and having it function provides exciting reconstructive possibilities to the surgeon.

INDICATIONS

The muscle may be used for coverage of soft-tissue defects, for functional reconstruction in replacing missing skeletal musculature, and for facial reanimation in facial paralysis. When used for soft-tissue flap coverage, it may be transferred alone and a skin graft applied directly to the muscle, or it may be transferred with an overlying cutaneous island as a musculocutaneous flap (1–4). The gracilis muscle is well suited for small and medium-sized soft-tissue defects that cannot be adequately handled by simpler flap techniques. It will conform well to irregular contours, can be split longitudinally at both ends to allow placement into cavities and awkward spaces, and can be

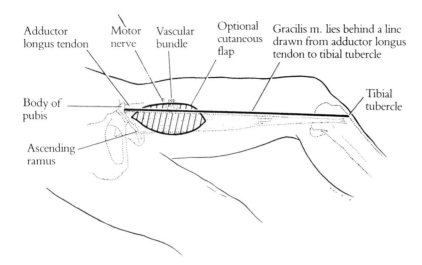

FIG. 1. The gracilis muscle lies in the medial thigh. The pedicle exits from the deep portion of the anterior surface in the proximal quarter of the muscle.

transferred in part or in whole. When one is transferring only a part of it, the transferred muscle will remain viable as long as the anterior margin of the muscle is transferred.

The muscle has been used for replacement of major muscular defects that result in significant functional loss (1,2,5,6). The commonest site of these defects is the forearm, usually in the flexor aspect. However, the muscle has also been used to replace the extensor musculature of the forearm, the anterior compartment of the upper arm, and the anterior compartment of the lower leg (see Chap. 497). This procedure is complicated and the time for functional recovery is prolonged. The procedure should not be used when simpler techniques of tendon transfer are available.

ANATOMY

The gracilis muscle is one of the superficial muscles on the medial aspect of the thigh. The proximal half of the muscle has a strap muscle configuration and the distal half a pennate configuration. It is broad above and tapers to a long, thin tendon below. Depending on the size of the individual, the muscle in an adult is 25 to 30 cm in length, with an additional 10 to 12 cm of tendon. The origin is the body of the pubis and its inferior ramus and the adjacent ramus of the ischium. The

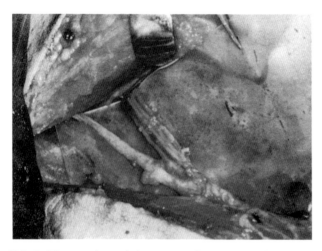

FIG. 2. The vascular pedicle consists of an artery and two venae comitantes. The nerve enters the muscle more obliquely proximal (on the left side) to the vascular pedicle.

muscle passes distally between the adductor longus and the adductor magnus, and ends in a tendon that passes medial to the condyle of the femur and inserts in the tibia just below the tibial tubercle.

The tendon lies between the sartorius and the semitendinosis. There is a single motor nerve, which is a branch of the obturator. This is composed of from two to six fascicles and enters the muscle obliquely (Figs. 1,2) just proximal to the dominant vascular pedicle. The nerve lies under the adductor longus. There are usually two or three vascular pedicles. The superior pedicle is dominant and, in almost all cases, the muscle will survive entirely on the superior pedicle alone. The artery in this pedicle is 1 to 2 mm in diameter, and there are two venae comitantes, one of which is usually larger than the artery.

OPERATIVE TECHNIQUE

Donor Site

Exposure of the gracilis is facilitated by abduction and external rotation of the hip with the knee flexed (Fig. 3). The gracilis muscle lies posterior to a line that is drawn from the adductor longus tendon to the tibial tubercle. When the knee is flexed, the muscle may be relaxed and sag posterior to this line.

An incision is carried through the skin immediately posterior to this line, and the dissection carried through the superficial thigh fascia to the muscle. The skin is elevated and the muscle is identified by separating the surrounding subcutaneous tissue from the muscle, and the anterior and posterior borders of the muscle are cleared.

The pedicle is identified by separating the adductor longus from the gracilis muscle. The pedicle will be found 8 to 12 cm from the muscle origin and will pass under the adductor longus muscle. The assistant can retract the adductor longus and display the pedicle. There are side branches from the venae comitantes and the artery to the adductor longus. If these are divided, it is possible to develop a 6 cm length of pedicle.

Dissection is then carried proximally and distally and the muscle is completely separated from its bed. Distally, there will usually be a second and often a third vascular pedicle entering the anterior border of the muscle at a distal point.

The incision is then carried as far distal as necessary to separate the muscle completely. If the tendon is required, a transverse incision is placed in the distal thigh, and the tendon is identified, retracted, and divided. The tendon should

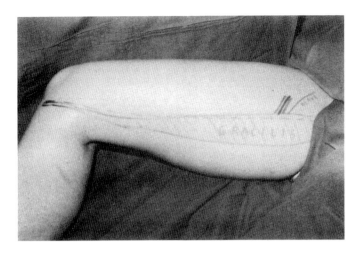

FIG. 3. The location of the gracilis is outlined in the medial thigh. The key structure to identify in the anterior border is the adductor longus tendon, which is easily palpated at its origin from the pubic tubercle.

be divided first and the origin second, in order that the pedicle will not be pulled out of the thigh.

If a cutaneous flap is desired with the muscle, care must be taken to place the flap directly over the muscle belly. There is usually one identifiable perforator that is approximately opposite the vascular pedicle. There are few, if any, perforators over the distal muscle belly. Our cadaver dissections have shown that there are significant interfascial vessels at this level that appear to provide the dominant blood supply to the skin of the middle and distal portion of the thigh.

Although the flap is reliable anteriorly and posteriorly in the proximal thigh, it is not reliable distal to 15 cm from the muscle origin, although it may occasionally survive in the middle third of the thigh. A musculocutaneous flap should not be used if the patient is obese, because of the difficulty in positioning the flap on the underlying gracilis muscle. The skin flap is not well attached to the muscle and should be tacked anteriorly and posteriorly to the gracilis muscle, in order that there is no shearing of the perforating vessels. The flap should be evaluated for the adequacy of circulation when the muscle and skin are separated and while the pedicle is still attached. The procedure involved in preparing the muscle for functional reconstruction is identical to that used when the muscle is prepared for coverage, except that the motor nerve is also taken with the muscle.

Recipient Site

The structures at the recipient site that must be prepared are the sites of origin and insertion for the muscle, a motor nerve, and a vascular pedicle. Care must be taken to raise suitable skin flaps that will adequately cover the muscle, to allow good muscle gliding. This is particularly important in the distal half of the muscle and at the point where the tendon is sutured to the recipient vessels. Preparation of the recipient site is frequently tedious, as the dissection usually involves an area of considerable scar tissue subsequent to muscle loss.

A pure motor nerve must be selected so that good reinnervation can be obtained. In the forearm, the anterior interosseous nerve is the first choice, although other branches of the median and ulnar nerves may be used. Good muscle function cannot be expected without a normal motor nerve and a good nerve repair.

The muscle is not transferred until the recipient site is completely prepared (Fig. 4). The usual ischemia is less than 2

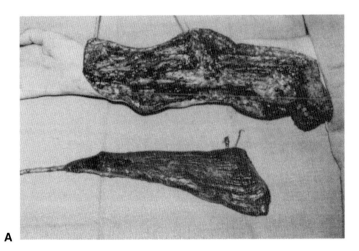

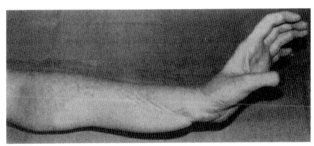

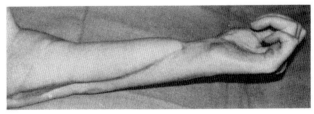

FIG. 4. A: The muscle should not be removed from the thigh until all structures in the forearm are prepared to receive it. B: The patient has the gracilis muscle transplanted to the forearm to replace the long flexors of all fingers. The muscle will stretch to allow full finger extension. C: Contraction of the muscle provides almost full finger flexion.

hours, although our experience in laboratory investigations suggests that an ischemia time of up to 3 hours is not harmful. When the muscle is separated from the thigh, it is positioned in the forearm and tacked into place. The muscle is then stretched out to its maximum expected size, and the relative positions of the muscle pedicle and the recipient vessels are identified. The vascular repairs are positioned in such a way that the nerve repair can be placed as close as possible to the muscle. The duration of muscle denervation will, to some extent, determine the degree of muscle atrophy, and this is directly proportional to the distance of the nerve repair from the neuromuscular junction. It is usually possible to do a nerve repair within 2 to 3 cm of the muscle. There is considerable connected tissue about the gracilis motor nerve, and this should be stripped back to allow a good fascicle-to-fascicle apposition with 11-0 nylon sutures.

The tension selected for the insertion of the muscle is important in the determination of eventual muscle function. If the muscle is being used to replace forearm flexors and there is some extensor and intrinsic function, the position of the fingers following a transfer will indicate the adequacy of the tension. When the gracilis tendon is sutured to the four profundus tendons, it will provide sufficient flexion so that the fingers are in slightly more flexion than in a position of function.

When adequate antagonistic muscles are not present, the technique of determining muscle tension is different. Prior to the removal of the gracilis from the leg, sutures reinforced with marking ink are placed at 5 cm intervals along the muscle belly when it is stretched to its maximum. This position is obtained by abducting the thigh and extending the knee.

Following the transfer of the muscle to the forearm, and with revascularization and nerve repair, it is firmly attached to the medial epicondyle with multiple mattress sutures. The tendon is then stretched distally toward the hand until the suture marks are once again 5 cm apart. This indicates the maximum length to which the muscle is normally stretched, and it should be placed within the forearm in such a way that when the wrist and fingers are extended the muscle will be stretched to approximately this location. Appropriate suture repair can be done between the flexor digitorum profundus tendons and the gracilis tendon with the fingers flexed, so that there will not be undue tension on the repair.

Care must be taken in suturing the muscle into its bed, so that the pedicle is not kinked. Good skin closure over the distal portion of the muscle and tendon-to-tendon juncture is important, to allow tendon gliding and to allow a tenolysis, if this should be necessary.

A window is placed in the dressing and in the underlying skin graft; this allows direct visualization of the muscle.

CLINICAL RESULTS

We have used the gracilis muscle as a free tissue transfer in 49 cases. In 24 cases the entire muscle was taken; in the others only a portion was taken for facial paralysis reconstruction. In all cases, all muscle was adequately perfused by the proximal pedicle. Occasionally the distal portion of the muscle will take a few minutes to develop a red color following revascularization, indicating that the blood supply may be very marginal distally.

The muscle has been used to motor extremities in 20 cases. It should be limited to those cases where there is a major functional deficit. The procedure is complex, and there are many areas where errors can be made that will result in inadequate function. These include, particularly, the vascular anastomosis, the selection of an adequate nerve and good nerve repair, and the positioning of the muscle under adequate tension. The return of muscle function appears to be improved with an exercise program that is given to the patient once reinnervation occurs. The results of muscle transplantation to the forearm have shown that the gracilis has a functional potential of providing up to 50% of normal grip strength and a full range of finger excursion (Fig. 4B,C)

SUMMARY

The gracilis is an excellent muscle to use for major functional deficits of either the flexor or the extensor aspect of the forearm. The procedure is complex and requires particular care in planning and execution.

References

1. Harii K, Ohmori K, Sekiguchi J. The free musculocutaneous flap. *Plast Reconstr Surg* 1976;57:294.
2. Manktelow RT, McKee NH. Free muscle transplantation to provide active finger flexion. *J Hand Surg* 1978;3:416.
3. Orticochea M. The musculocutaneous flap method. *Br J Plast Surg* 1972; 25:106.
4. McCraw JB, Massey FM, Shanklin KD, Horton CE. Vaginal reconstruction with gracilis myocutaneous flaps. *Plast Reconstr Surg* 1976;58:176.
5. Manktelow RT. Free muscle flaps. In: Green DP, ed. *Operative hand surgery*, 2nd Ed. New York: Churchill Livingstone, 1988;861–876.
6. Manktelow RT, Zuker RM, McKee NH. Functioning free muscle transplantation. *J Hand Surg* 1984;9A:32.

CHAPTER 330 ■ MICRONEUROVASCULAR FREE TRANSFER OF PECTORALIS MAJOR MUSCLE AND MUSCULOCUTANEOUS FLAPS

Y. IKUTA

The pectoralis major muscle, with or without skin, can be used as a microneurovascular transfer to replace muscles such as the powerful forearm flexors (1–4).

ANATOMY

The pectoralis major muscle has three origins—clavicular, sternal, and abdominal. In the first it arises from the medial half of the clavicle; in the second it arises from the anterior part of the sternum to the seventh rib; and in the last it arises from the anterior layer of the rectus abdominal muscle sheath and terminates at the lateral lip of the bicipital groove of the humerus (Fig. 1) (5).

It is a broad and flat fan-shaped muscle, innervated by the medial and lateral pectoral nerves extending from the medial and lateral cords that arise from the brachial plexus. The function of this muscle is to adduct the upper arm and to provide medial rotation. Deprivation of the muscle will result in some limiting of motor function, but to a degree that is very slight and will not interfere with daily life.

The main blood supply of the pectoralis major muscle is from the pectoral branch of the thoracoacromial artery that arises from the proximal portion of the axillary artery. The supply enters the undersurface of the muscle just lateral to the midclavicular line that corresponds to the upper border of the pectoralis minor muscle.

A branch of the thoracoacromial artery passes through the clavicular head of the pectoralis major muscle, becomes the cutaneous branch at the infraclavicular triangle, and ramifies outward to the acromial and deltoid areas of the shoulder (6).

The internal mammary artery that is a branch of the subclavian artery runs along the posterior aspect of the cartilages of the first to sixth ribs, distributes perforating branches through the intercostal spaces, and nourishes the pectoralis major muscle and its overlying skin. Among the skin flaps in which these arteries serve as a pedicle, the deltopectoral flap is well known and, of course, it can also be used as a musculocutaneous flap (6).

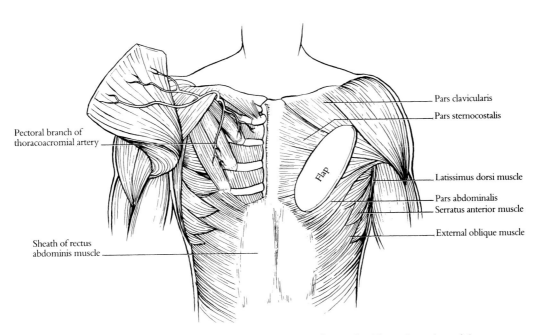

FIG. 1. The design of the pectoralis major musculocutaneous flap (*right*). The undersurface of the muscle with its thoracoacromial blood supply (*left*).

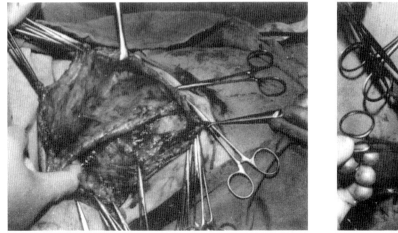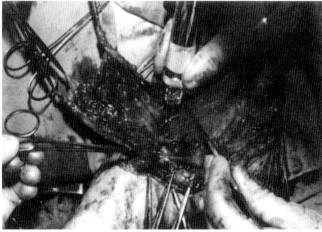

FIG. 2. **A:** The outer border or abdominal part of the right pectoralis major muscle is released (the head is to the left). **B:** By electrical stimulation applied to each of the branches, it is possible to confirm the area served by each. (From Ikuta et al., ref. 2, with permission.)

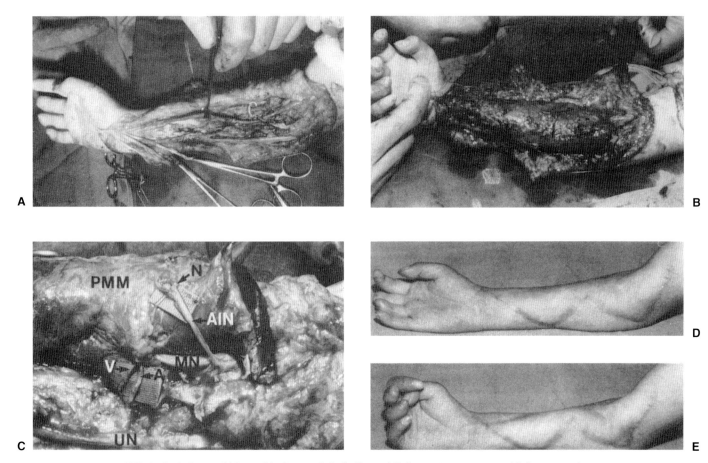

FIG. 3. **A:** A 6-year-old boy with characteristic findings of Volkmann's contracture. All flexor muscles were excised at a previous operation. **B:** The insertion of the pectoralis major muscle is sutured to the medial epicondyle of the humerus, and the muscular origin is sutured to the flexor tendons of the fingers and thumb. **C:** The vessel (A and V) and nerve (N) anastomoses are shown by turning over the muscle flap. *PMM*, pectoralis major muscle; *AIN*, anterior interosseous nerve; *MN*, median nerve; *UN*, ulnar nerve. **D,E:** Five months postoperatively finger sensation is almost normal and there is powerful active flexion of the thumb and the four fingers.

OPERATIVE TECHNIQUE

When the flap is to be used as an island or free musculocutaneous flap, it is raised from the acromion to the xiphoid, about 6 to 8 cm wide and about 30 cm long (5). In either case, the lateral border of the pectoralis major muscle is first identified and is then separated from the distal aspect of the sternum toward the proximal aspect; one must exercise care to isolate vessels to retain as the pedicle.

If the muscle is to be used as a musculocutaneous flap, it must be kept in mind that the location of the nipple will become slightly deviated, and difficulty may be encountered in preparing the flap because of the fatty tissue of the breast.

Fig. 2 shows the procedures for identifying the pectoralis major muscle. At first the origin of the right pectoralis major muscle is released and detached from the chest wall. The four nerve branches of the muscle are identified. By electrically stimulating each of the branches, it is possible to determine the area served by each. This method is useful when it is desirable to limit the amount of muscle transfer or to use it for more than two separate applications (7).

Fig. 3 shows the transplanted pectoralis major muscle in the forearm, as well as the postoperative results.

SUMMARY

The pectoralis major muscle flap can be transferred with or without skin to replace muscles such as the forearm flexors, where considerable exertion is required. There is minimal donor site morbidity.

References

1. Clark JMP. Reconstruction of biceps brachii by pectoralis muscle transplantation. *Br J Surg* 1946;34:180.
2. Ikuta Y, Kubo T, Tsuge K. Free muscle transplantation by microsurgical technique to treat severe Volkmann's contracture. *Plast Reconstr Surg* 1976;58:407.
3. Shanghai Sixth People's Hospital. Free muscle transplantation by microsurgical neurovascular anastomoses: report of a case. *Clin Med J* 1976;2:47.
4. Manktelow RT, McKee NH. Free muscle transplantation to provide active finger flexion. *J Hand Surg* 1978;3:416.
5. Ariyan S. The pectoralis major myocutaneous flap: a versatile flap for reconstruction in the head and neck. *Plast Reconstr Surg* 1979;63:73.
6. Mathes SJ, Nahai F. *Clinical atlas of muscle and musculocutaneous flaps.* St. Louis: Mosby, 1979;317–335.
7. Manktelow RT. Muscle transplantation. In: Serafin D, Buncke HJ, eds. *Microsurgical composite tissue transplantation.* St. Louis: Mosby, 1979; 369–391.

CHAPTER 331 ■ FREE FIBULAR TRANSFER

A. GILBERT

The free fibular transfer has revolutionized the reconstruction of long bone defects. Originally (1) the fibula was harvested by a posterior incision (2). I have found, however, that the lateral approach has several advantages (3).

INDICATIONS

Between 1975 and 1983, this approach was used 160 times with the following indications: for posttraumatic reconstruction in the upper and lower limb (6 and 43 times, respectively), for necrosis of the femoral head (63 times), for congenital pseudarthrosis (31 times), and for tumors (17 times). There were four cases of transfer with skin and two cases of transfer with the soleus muscle.

ANATOMY

The vascular anatomy of the fibula has been well described (4). The length of the fibula varies between 30 and 40 cm, with an average of 34 cm.

There are two types of vascularization to the fibula, provided primarily by the peroneal artery. One source is the nutrient artery, usually unique and branching 6 to 14 cm from the origin of the peroneal artery. The nutrient artery enters the bone in its middle third, usually at mid-diaphysis. It then divides into an ascending and a descending branch into the bone. Periosteal vascularization comes from a series of branches from the peroneal artery and the anterior tibial artery. These branches may be direct periosteal branches or musculoperiosteal arteries.

In my experience, the peroneal artery is seldom absent. In only one out of 160 clinical cases was it replaced by a direct branch from the posterior tibial artery to the bone.

OPERATIVE TECHNIQUE

The lateral approach has simplified free bone transfer and shortened operating time, so that harvesting takes between 30 and 50 minutes. The fibula may be harvested through a lateral approach in a patient who is supine, prone, or in a lateral position. The knee is slightly bent to relieve tension on the muscles (Fig. 1).

A line is drawn joining the head of the fibula and the lateral malleolus (Fig. 2A). At the middle of this line, a point will indicate the approximate location of the nutrient vessel. This point should be included in the graft.

Text continues on page 958.

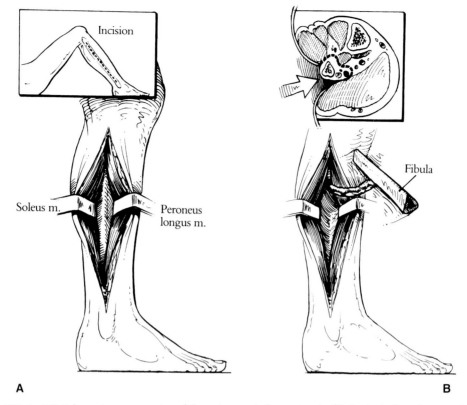

FIG. 1. A,B: Schematic representation of the main steps in harvesting the fibula via the lateral approach.

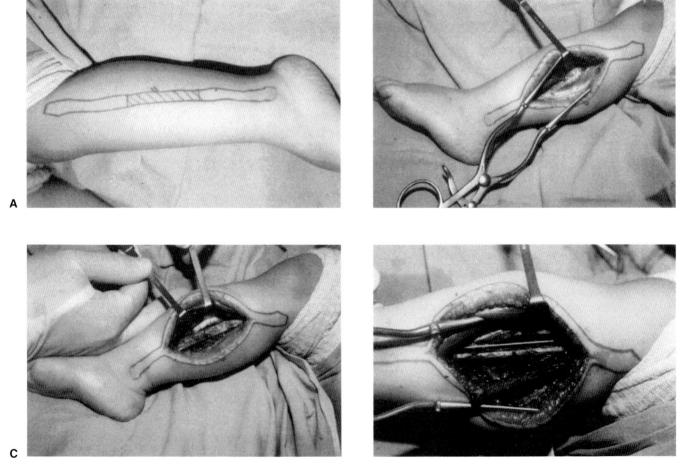

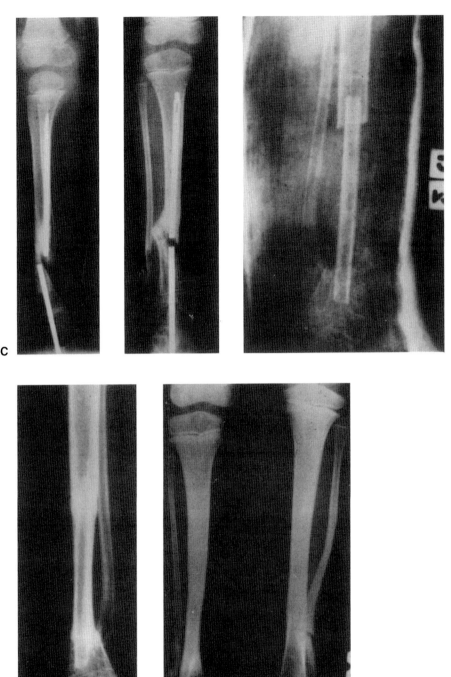

A–C

D,E

FIG. 3. **A,B:** A 5-year-old girl with congenital pseudarthrosis who had had several previous operations. **C:** Immediate postoperative result. **D:** Result at 3 months. **E:** Result at 1 year. Note the reconstruction of left (donor) fibula.

FIG. 2. The operative technique. **A:** The fibula is drawn on the skin and the middle third is preserved. **B:** After the peroneus longus is retracted anteriorly, the fibula is well exposed. **C:** After the muscles are detached from the bone, the aponeurosis is divided anteriorly. **D:** After the distal and proximal ends of the fibula are cut with the Gigli saw, the distal end of the peroneal vascular bundle is ligated. At this point, the proximal vessels can be identified and the peroneal artery transected just distal to the bifurcation.

The incision is slightly longer than the graft. After incision of the superficial aponeurosis, the dissection is directed straight toward the bone shaft, pushing the peroneal muscles and the musculocutaneous nerve forward and the soleus backward (Fig. 2C). The bone is reached quickly and the dissection then becomes extraperiosteal, but without keeping the musculotendinous cuff on the anterolateral two-thirds of the fibula.

Detachment continues forward up to the interosseous membrane, which is incised, and downward to the flexor hallucis longus. The graft is then measured and the bone sectioned at both ends, using a Gigli saw, although the peroneal artery has not yet been properly identified (Fig. 2D).

The graft can then be easily removed, taking the vascular bundle with it. This bundle is first located and tied at the distal portion of the graft, and the dissection continues toward the origin of the peroneal artery, keeping a minimal muscular cuff.

Using the dissection technique described and working under visual control, one can reach the peroneotibial bifurcation very quickly. The fibula is then isolated on its pedicle and the tourniquet is released, with testing for good bone vascularization. When the recipient site is ready, the pedicle (which has been kept in place) is sectioned just below the bifurcation.

The muscles are reinserted on the interosseous membrane with a few sutures, and the leg is closed on a suction drain. If the patient is in satisfactory condition, he can stand with his full weight on the grafted side after 3 to 4 days.

Variations in Technique

Recently, several modifications of the described bone transfer have been proposed. It has been shown that the transfer may include the soleus muscle, vascularized by its main pedicle, which depends on the peroneal artery (5).

It is also possible to take some skin with the fibula, either using the musculocutaneous branches of the peroneal artery (6), or as I have done in several cases, using only the direct cutaneous branches arising at the junction of the middle and distal thirds of the fibula.

CLINICAL RESULTS

Monitoring of the bone is difficult when it is not transferred with skin or muscle. Bone scans do not seem to be completely reliable, nor do arteriograms. In this series there has been no case of postoperative infection, but this does not mean that there were no failures. When there is no muscle with the bone, vascularization failure does not produce massive necrosis, but a nonvascularized bone graft is simply the result.

Very few complications were found at the donor site in adult patients. In six cases, there was a clinical absence of big toe extension. In children under 9 years of age, valgus deformity of the ankle occurs if the fibula is not reconstructed. I try always to reconstruct the donor bone using a corticoperiosteal tibial bone graft (Fig. 3). In 11 cases the graft resorbed or did not heal properly, and it was necessary to do a secondary procedure to obtain healing.

SUMMARY

Transfer of a vascularized fibula has become a well-established procedure for reconstruction of long bone defects. The use of a lateral approach to the donor site has greatly simplified the procedure.

References

1. Taylor G, Miller G, Ham F. The free vascularized bone graft: a clinical extension of microvascular techniques. *Plast Reconstr Surg* 1975;55:533.
2. Weiland A, Daniel R. Microvascular anastomoses for bone grafts in the treatment of massive defects in bone. *J Bone Joint Surg* 1979;61:98.
3. Gilbert AA. Free transfer of the fibular shaft. *Int J Microsurg* 1979;1:100.
4. Restrepo J, Katz D, Gilbert A. Arterial vascularization of the proximal epiphysis and the diaphysis of the fibula. *Int J Microsurg* 1980;2:48.
5. Baudet J, Panconi B, Caix P, et al. The composite fibula and soleus transfer. *Int J Microsurg* 1982;4:10.
6. Chung-Wei C, Wang Y. The study and clinical application of the osteocutaneous flap of fibula. *Microsurgery* 1983;4:11.

CHAPTER 332 ■ TRANSPOSITION SKIN FLAP TO THE ELBOW

M. B. CONSTANTIAN

Defects requiring flap coverage over the extensor surface of the elbow can be reconstructed with an anteriorly based transposition flap (1,2). Pressure ulcers often occur over the olecranon, commonly in patients who lie prone for long periods and prop themselves up on their elbows.

ANATOMY

Branches of the arteries that anastomose around the elbow joint supply this transposition flap: the middle and radial collateral and muscular branches of the deep brachial artery, the recurrent radial artery, the posterior ulnar recurrent artery, and the superior and inferior ulnar collateral (supratrochlear) arteries.

FLAP DESIGN AND DIMENSIONS

The flap should be designed large enough for the defect, remembering that its rotational arc does not easily exceed 4 to 6 cm and that the base cannot safely be backcut to ease closure. The usual undelayed flap dimensions are 8 to 12 cm in length and 6 to 9 cm in width. Flaps that are larger should be delayed.

OPERATIVE TECHNIQUE

If the olecranon bursa is involved (and it usually is), it must be completely excised. Joint involvement changes management and should be established preoperatively by probing and sinography. If a pyarthrosis exists, the joint may need to be curretted, resected, or arthrodesed. Flap closure over closed irrigation and suction catheters is an alternative management method for early pyarthrosis, and may succeed in experienced hands. Treatment of joint or bursa must be adequate. Failure to correct such abnormalities is the commonest cause of postoperative seroma, flap loss, infection, and ulcer recurrence.

The flap should be raised at the level of the deep fascia overlying the lateral head of the triceps and the proximal ends of the brachioradialis and extensor carpi radialis longus muscles. Drainage is advisable beneath the inset flap if bony modification has been necessary. A split-thickness skin graft is needed for the donor defect (Fig. 1).

CLINICAL RESULTS

As with many procedures, the success rate is high if each step is executed correctly. Aside from flap loss, the commonest complications are based on inadequate diagnosis or treatment of bursa or joint abnormalities that may lead to seroma, ulcer recurrence, or pyarthrosis. The surgeon may wish to use the brachioradialis muscle that lies beneath the flap as an additional or alternate source of vascularized tissue in the case of a pyarthrosis. Of course, a brachioradialis muscle flap is not advisable in quadriplegics, for whom this may be the only voluntary forearm muscle for transfer.

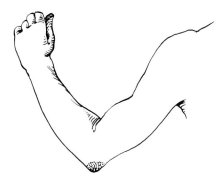

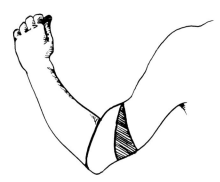

FIG. 1. Local transposition flap for closure of ulcer over olecranon. The secondary defect must be grafted with a split-thickness skin graft.

SUMMARY

A transposition skin flap should be considered as one of the alternatives for coverage of an elbow defect, especially over the olecranon.

References

1. Constantian MB, Jackson HS. Ulcers in less common sites. In: Constantian MB, ed. *Pressure ulcers: principles and techniques of management.* Boston: Little, Brown, 1980.
2. Hentz VR, Pearl RM, Kaplan EN. Use of medial upper arm skin as an arterialized flap. *Hand* 1980;12:241.

CHAPTER 333 ■ CEPHALIC VENOUS FLAP

R. L. THATTE AND M. R. THATTE

EDITORIAL COMMENT

This flap has limited clinical applications and, although the popularity of flow-through venous flaps has not entirely waned, it would not be the editors' first choice.

The cephalic venous island flap is a fasciocutaneous flap in the upper half of the radial side of the forearm (1). Based near the elbow, it has been shown to survive with only the cephalic vein as the feeding and draining vessel. All other structures, skin, subcutaneous tissue, and fascia are divided. The exact mechanism of the survival of venous flaps remains a matter for conjecture (2–4).

INDICATIONS

In the present state of its development the flap is useful to cover defects on the medial and posterior surfaces of the elbow like a standard fasciocutaneous flap. However, because it is based on a single vein as an island it is far easier to transpose.

FLAP DESIGN AND DIMENSIONS

The cephalic vein is marked on the lower two-thirds of the upper extremity after raising the tourniquet to occlude the venous flow. The tourniquet is then released. The arm is exsanguinated and the tourniquet is raised up to 250 mm Hg. A longitudinal flap is then marked along the forearm 5 cm on either side of the cephalic vein up to about the middle of the forearm, with its base at the elbow (Fig. 1).

OPERATIVE TECHNIQUE

The flap is cut along the longitudinal axis (i.e., *AB* and *DC*) as a fasciocutaneous flap, and the distal end (i.e., *BD*) is then cut after clamping and ligating the distal cephalic vein. The tourniquet is then released, obvious bleeders are cauterized and 100 units of heparin per kilogram of body weight are injected intravenously. After securing further hemostasis, the flap is then converted into an island (Fig. 2) by cutting across skin, subcutaneous tissue, and fascia (along *AC*; see Fig. 1) without severing the cephalic vein or its medial cubital tributary. (The medial cubital vein, however, may not be constant and is not a mandatory part of the flap design.) Neither of the veins are teased off of the flimsy soft envelope. The fasciocutaneous island hanging by the cephalic vein can now be transposed across the elbow medially or posteriorly as required.

CLINICAL RESULTS

As mentioned earlier, the flap is in its initial stages of development and is presented for its unique ability to survive on venous circulation alone without any apparent arterial input. We have used it in four cases for defects created by releasing contractures of the elbow on the medial side without any loss of flap. Because a flap was used, postoperative splinting was not needed.

SUMMARY

A fasciocutaneous island flap based only on cephalic venous circulation in the upper half of the forearm is presented in its early stages of development.

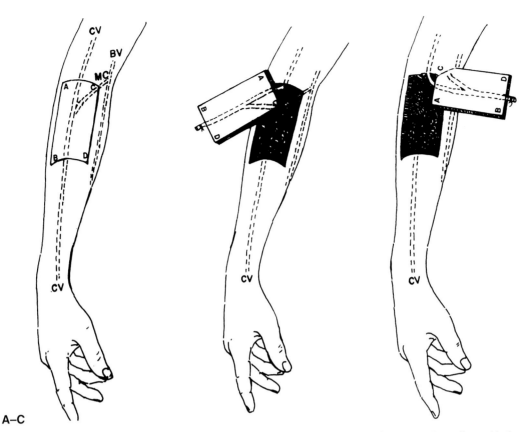

A–C

FIG. 1. **A:** Schematic drawing of flap design. CV, cephalic vein; BV, basilic vein; MC, median cubital vein. **B:** Flap raised retaining only its venous connections. **C:** Flap transposed through 90° with only proximal veins intact.

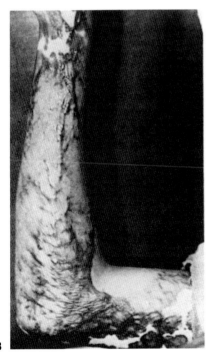
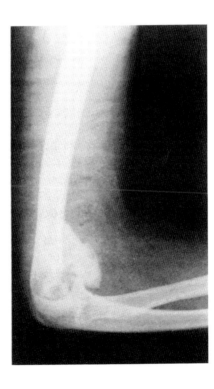

A,B

FIG. 2. **A:** Preoperative view showing the right elbow with a post-burn flexion deformity, in a 29-year-old man. **B:** The contracture was complicated by myositis ossificans. The elbow was fixed at 90°. *(Continued.)*

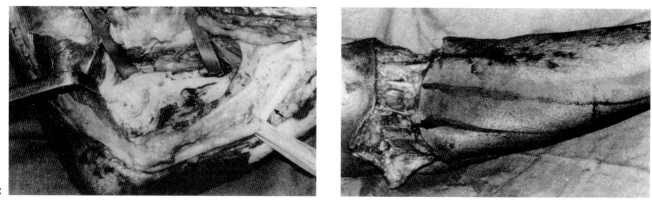

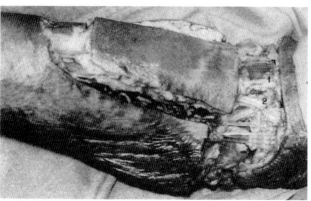
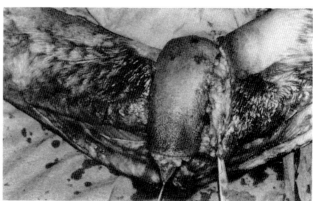

FIG. 2. *(Continued.)* **C:** The exposure by a long ulnar midneutral incision. The anterior block of bone was exposed by retracting all anterior structures and securing the ulnar nerve (*arrow*). A clear plane of dissection was available between the normal bone and the mature myositic bone mass, which was shelled out (5 × 5 cm). **D:** Once the scar tissue was excised, complete flexion of the elbow was possible, but extension was restricted by scar tissue straddling the medial side. The cephalic venous flap was then marked distal to the defect. **E:** The flap is attached to the body by (1) the cephalic vein, (2) the median cubital vein, and (3) the accessory cephalic vein. (Only the cephalic vein is necessary for survival of the flap.) **F:** The flap transposed into the defect.

References

1. Thatte RL, Thatte MR. Cephalic venous flap. *Br J Plast Surg* 1987;40:16.
2. Baek SM, Weinberg H, Song Y, et al. Experimental studies in the survival of venous island flaps without arterial inflow. *Plast Reconstr Surg* 1985;75:88.
3. Thatte RL, Thatte MR. A study of the saphenous venous island flap in the dog without arterial inflow using a non-biological conduit across a part of the length of the vein. *Br J Plast Surg* 1987;40:11.
4. Chavoin JP, Rogue D, Vachaud M, et al. Island flaps with an exclusively venous pedicle: a report of eleven cases and a preliminary haemodynamic study. *Br J Plast Surg* 1987;40:149.

CHAPTER 334 ■ SUPERIOR MEDIAL ARM FLAP

C. E. CARRIQUIRY

EDITORIAL COMMENT

The value of this chapter is the clear anatomy that the author outlines, so that the physical approach to the medial arm flap is possible. The flap is reliable as well.

The skin of the medial arm is thin, hairless, and barely pigmented, making it very suitable for coverage of the hand, face, neck, or flexor creases. Proper utilization of the direct septocutaneous branches of the brachial artery allow elevation of safe fasciocutaneous flaps. These can vary in size, design, orientation, pedicle position, and method of transfer, to meet a wide variety of clinical requirements.

INDICATIONS

Medial-arm septocutaneous flaps can be used for release of axillary and elbow-crease contractures, and can be deepithelialized for contour improvement of the anterior axillary wall and for subclavicular depression after mastectomy. As cross-arm flaps, they are useful for hand and digit coverage, particularly of the thumb, and for thenar-web reconstruction. They can also be utilized in the rare case of Tagliacotian nasal reconstruction.

ANATOMY

The brachial artery gives off three to four septocutaneous branches (1,2) that enter the medial arm septum at variable intervals. The uppermost branch origin is usually adjacent to the lower border of the pectoralis major tendon (Fig. 1), while the lowermost vessel emerges 2 to 4 cm above the medial epicondyle. On reaching the deep subcutaneous plane on top of the fascia, the septocutaneous vessels ramify into a few branches (see Fig. 1), which are interconnected by means of longitudinally oriented vessels, sometimes adjacent to the cutaneous nerves. This vascular arrangement allows safe elevation of longitudinal flaps that stretch along the whole length of the medial arm. They may be based on either the upper or lower septocutaneous perforator (Fig. 2).

Venous drainage is adequate through the venae comitantes of the septocutaneous arteries, although the basilic vein may also be included in some flaps.

The territories supplied by the superior ulnar collateral and the recurrent ulnar vessels overlap, to a considerable extent, with that of the brachial septocutaneous branches. Flaps based on the former (3,4) will not be described here.

FLAP DESIGN AND DIMENSIONS

Flaps can be either proximally or distally based and raised in either island or cross-arm fashion (2). Island flaps are usually for axillary or elbow release, and are based on the upper or lower septocutaneous vessels (see Fig. 2). The outline is centered on the groove between the biceps and triceps (Fig. 3B). The width is determined as needed; the flap can extend from midanterior to midposterior lines, and probably beyond. The base is positioned a few centimeters distal to the pectoralis tendon or proximal to the medial epicondyle (Fig. 3), where the septocutaneous vessels are predictably located. If an island design is not deemed necessary, a narrow skin pedicle can be preserved. The flaps can extend along the whole length of the middle aspect of the arm.

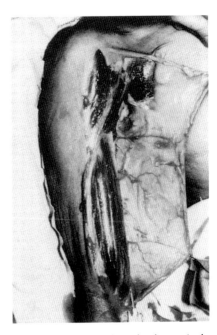

FIG. 1. The skin of a latex-injected arm has been raised at the subfascial plane from lateral to medial midlines and the fascia has been removed, so that three large septocutaneous perforators can be appreciated in detail. They emerge at the medial septum, just behind the brachialis muscle, and arborize in the deep subcutaneous fat. Longitudinal ramifications arise from the transverse trunks and course parallel to the axis of the arm. Note the position of the uppermost vessel, close to the pectoralis major insertion, and the most distal vessels at about 4 cm above the medial epicondyle. (From Carriquiry, ref. 2, with permission.)

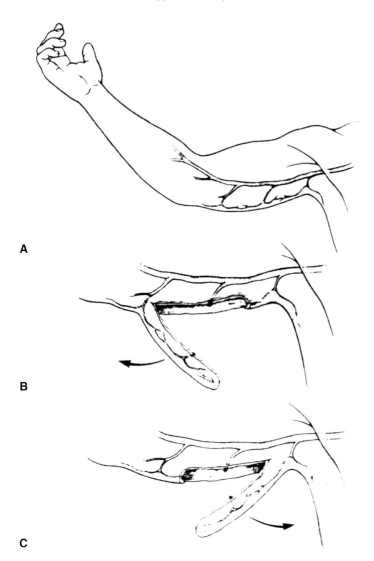

A

B

C

FIG. 2. A–C: Diagrammatic representation of the septocutaneous vessels of the medial arm as the basis for fasciocutaneous flaps. Flaps can be raised either distally (**B**) or proximally (**C**). One or more perforators must be severed to mobilize the flap; their territories are captured by the remaining pedicle. (From Carriquiry, ref. 2, with permission.)

Cross-arm flaps are similarly outlined, and their dimensions determined as required, allowing for a relatively long pedicle for better positioning and easier mobilization of the recipient hand (Fig. 4). In shorter flaps, oblique outlines radiating from the septum can be employed.

OPERATIVE TECHNIQUE

The incision is carried down to the subfascial areolar plane, and the septum is easily reached from both sides with blunt dissection. To obtain flap mobilization, the septum is severed from the tip toward the base. In longer flaps, one or two septocutaneous vessels included in the septum may have to be ligated (Fig. 2). Dissection proceeds carefully to preserve a segment of septum containing the nutrient vessels at the base (Fig. 3D). The skin incision can then be completed around the base of the flap, to achieve an island design, if necessary.

The donor site can be closed directly in flaps up to approximately 35 mm in width, if no skin flaccidity is present. For wider flaps, sheet skin grafts are needed, and they have a good take on the muscular surface of the donor defect.

It may be necessary to sever cutaneous nerves during flap mobilization, as well as superficial veins. As a rule, there is no need to preserve the basilic vein for improved drainage.

CLINICAL RESULTS

Care must be taken to preserve the fascial plexus by dissecting beneath the fascia. For flaps spanning the whole length of the medial arm, it is mandatory to preserve the feeding vessels at the flap base. On the whole, flap elevation is technically straightforward. Medial arm skin remains thin and pliable after transfer to recipient sites (Fig. 3E). Little or no redundance or flabbiness have been present in cases of digit or hand coverage.

Where direct closure of the donor site has been possible, scars have tended to widen. Sheet grafts applied to larger donor defects remain relatively inconspicuous. Numbness along the medial forearm is a frequent, if generally well-tolerated, sequela.

Distal necrosis and/or dehiscence as a consequence of pedicle torsion or excessive tension have occurred rarely in cross-arm flaps. The excellent vascularity of the flaps generally allows a choice of pedicle length and orientation best suited for each case (Fig. 4), so complications should remain rare. However, obese patients and children will tolerate the cross-arm position poorly, and should not be considered the best candidates for this procedure.

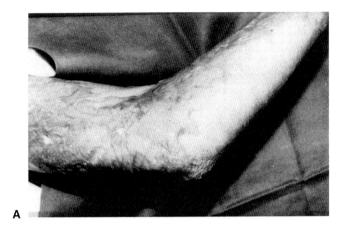

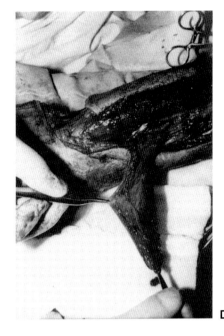

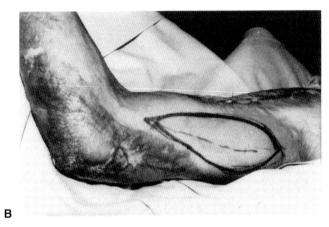

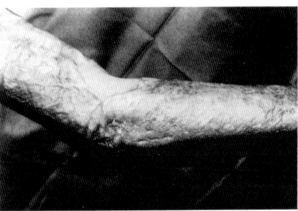

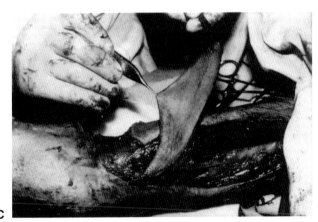

FIG. 3. **A:** Postburn contracture of the elbow crease; elbow extension is blocked. **B:** Outline of island fasciocutaneous flap on medial arm, which has been spared from burns. **C:** The flap elevated as an island. **D:** Undersurface of the flap is exposed. Note short segment of septum on which flap is based. **E:** One year postoperatively, extension and excellent contour have been achieved. (From Carriquiry, ref. 2, with permission.)

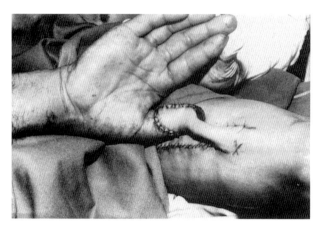

FIG. 4. Subtotal soft-tissue avulsion of volar surface of the thumb. A distally based cross-arm flap has been used for coverage. Note the long pedicle that prevents direct contact between the recipient hand and donor arm, and the direct closure of the donor site. (From Carriquiry, ref. 2, with permission.)

SUMMARY

The superior medial arm flap has proven highly reliable in terms of viability, either as an island or cross-arm flap. The flap is easy to raise, and a dependable vascularity allows variations in size, design, and method of flap transfer.

References

1. Salmon M. *Artères de la peau*. Paris: Masson, 1936.
2. Carriquiry CE. Versatile fasciocutaneous flaps based on the medial septocutaneous vessels of the arm. *Plast Reconstr Surg* 1990;86:103.
3. Kaplan EN, Pearl RM. An arterial medial arm flap: vascular anatomy and clinical applications. *Ann Plast Surg* 1980;4:205.
4. Maruyama Y, Onishi K, Iwahira Y. The ulnar recurrent fasciocutaneous island flap: reverse medial arm flap. *Plast Reconstr Surg* 1987;79:381.

CHAPTER 335 ■ FASCIOCUTANEOUS FLAPS FOR ELBOW COVERAGE

T. R. HEINZ AND L. O. VASCONEZ

EDITORIAL COMMENT

The fasciocutaneous flaps presented in this chapter and in Chap. 336 are excellent for traumatic defects with exposure of the elbow or elbow joint, as well as for resurfacing following excision of large olecranon type of ulcerations.

Local fasciocutaneous flaps form an important part of soft-tissue coverage for elbow defects, often following burns, but also as the result of trauma, tumor, or olecranon bursitis.

INDICATIONS

The options available among fasciocutaneous flaps for elbow coverage are numerous, given the rich collateral circulation of both the medial and lateral arm, which extends onto the forearm. The ideal flap, which may be derived from any of these territories, would be thin, pliable, and its donor site either entirely or partially closed primarily. Local flaps that satisfy these requirements may be derived from the medial or lateral arm.

ANATOMY

Lateral Arm Fasciocutaneous Flap

The standard lateral arm flap, which has been utilized as a free and pedicled flap, may be used in reverse fashion for elbow coverage based on the posterior radial collateral artery (PRCA) (1–4). Reversed lateral arm flaps for elbow coverage may be raised to at least 8 × 10 cm, based on injection studies with methylene blue. They are also based on the posterior radial collateral artery system taken, in this instance, as a reversed pedicle flap with a pivot point at the lateral epicondyle. This well-known flap pedicle is found in the lateral intramuscular septum and extends at least halfway up the arm proximally, giving off numerous perforators through the septum based on this vessel (Fig. 1). The radial nerve is found immediately adjacent to the pedicle, and care should be taken during dissection to avoid injury to this nerve.

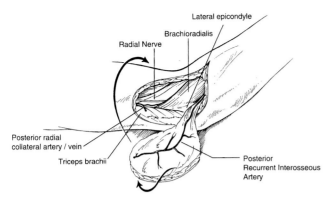

FIG. 1. Diagram of distally based lateral arm flap with pedicle lying over lateral epicondyle.

The venous return in this reversed island pedicle flap is presumably by multiple venae comitantes crossover (3).

Proximally Based Pedicle Lateral Forearm Flap

Careful anatomic studies of the forearm fascial extension of the well-known lateral arm flap have been carried out (5). This flap is found to divide into anterior and posterior divisions 4 cm proximal to the lateral epicondyle. The posterior division anastomoses with the interosseous recurrent artery and supplies the circulation about the elbow, including the joint and skin. The anterior division is of more interest, since it extends along the lateral forearm extensor surface in the axis of the brachioradialis muscle, for an average of 15 cm (Fig. 2). In cadaver studies, the artery extended from 13 to 18 cm.

Medial Arm Fasciocutaneous Flap

Flaps based on the medial circulation at the elbow have been studied and described (6). This is a fasciocutaneous reversed pedicle flap based on the ulnar recurrent artery, which, through a network of interconnecting fascial systems from perforators on the medial arm, can be harvested nearly up to the axilla. This provides very substantial flap coverage for anterior/cubital or posterior defects.

This fasciocutaneous flap is based on the network of the ulnar recurrent artery from the brachial artery, which travels distally through the larger posterior branch between the two heads of the flexor carpi ulnaris, to join the superior/inferior ulnar collateral arteries around the medial epicondyle (Fig. 3). It is found to travel posterior to the medial epicondyle and immediately posterior to the ulnar nerve, and must be separated from the nerve with meticulous dissection. Quite constant in at least 18 dissections is the network of five to six perforators that anastomose in a subfascial plane along the medial arm to the axilla. The ulnar recurrent artery itself branches from the ulnar artery just distal to the separation of the radial and ulnar arteries, as they leave the brachial artery and the antecubital area.

FLAP DESIGN AND DIMENSIONS

Lateral Arm Fasciocutaneous Flap

The midline of the flap should be placed on the longitudinal line between the deltoid insertion down to the lateral epicondyle of the humerus. A flap at least as large as 8×10 cm may be harvested, based on the PRCA. Primary closure is possible up to a flap width of 6 cm.

Lateral epicondyl

Pivot point - an extension of anterior division of post. radial collateral artery. This overlies and is coaxial with brachioradialis muscle.

Brachioradialis muscle

15 cm

FIG. 2. Layout and plan for proximally based lateral forearm flap based on extension of posterior radial collateral artery on axis of brachioradialis muscle.

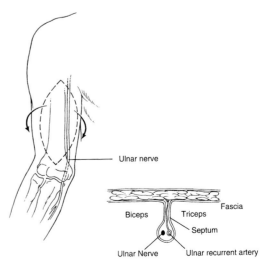

FIG. 3. Diagram of distally based medial arm flap, supported by septal perforators from ulnar recurrent artery. The ulnar nerve must be dissected carefully away.

Proximally Based Pedicle Lateral Forearm Flap

A thin, proximally based, pedicled fasciocutaneous flap may be harvested from the extensor forearm skin territories, typically with an elliptical design. It should be especially well suited to the antecubital area, such as for burn contracture release. The pivot point of this flap is again the lateral epicondyle and the territory immediately proximal to it. Flap design may be best done in a tongue-shaped fashion with primary closure of the donor site in most cases where an island is not required. In addition, anatomic and clinical studies have shown the potential for use of the lateral forearm flap in conjunction with the lateral arm flap, to provide a very substantial flap length, one that may or may not include the lateral antebrachial cutaneous nerve.

Medial Arm Fasciocutaneous Flap

The island skin margins should lie between the mid anterior and posterior lines of the arm itself. The flap size, on average, by methylene blue injections in cadaver studies, was 15 × 17 cm; clinically, however, flaps up to 29 × 8 cm have been raised without flap loss.

OPERATIVE TECHNIQUE

Lateral Arm Fasciocutaneous Flap

Flap design and markings are laid out on the involved arm, usually as an ellipse. Dissection is carried out posteriorly to the septum, followed by the anterior subfascial dissection, again to the septum. With the septum well delineated, the proximal pedicle vessels may be divided at the most proximal extent of the flap. Care should be taken to avoid injury to the radial nerve in this portion of the dissection. The deep fascia of the triceps posteriorly and biceps anteriorly, is included. Careful dissection allows elevation of the flap from the radial nerve and humerus, preserving the pedicle in the lateral intramuscular septum down to its pivot point at the lateral epicondyle. Careful planning should allow coverage of posterior anterior/cubital or even medial defects about the elbow. Sutures may be used to narrow or close the donor wound, and a skin graft may then be applied. Postoperative splinting of the limb at 130° to 150° at the elbow is recommended.

Medial Arm Fasciocutaneous Flap

The longitudinal portion of the predesigned flap should be incised through skin, subcutaneous fat, and fascia. The fascia may then be elevated from anterior and posterior to the septum between the brachialis and triceps muscles. The perforators that are distributed inferiorly and posteriorly in the subfascial plane may be identified and traced to the midline of the flap, and then to the pedicle itself, found in the interval between triceps and brachialis muscles adjacent to the ulnar nerve. The proximal pedicle may be divided at this time, and dissection of the pedicle itself from proximal to distal is carried out. Again, some care must be taken to avoid injury to the ulnar nerve that is immediately adjacent to the pedicle; this should be relatively easy. The pedicle may be dissected to just distal to the medial epicondyle, to allow easier rotation anteriorly or posteriorly, if coverage of the elbow is required.

The donor site may be primarily closed up to 6 cm or partially skin-grafted. Since the vessel lies deep between the muscles, even portions of the arm that have been burned and skin-grafted may be used around the pedicle itself or on the flap itself, given the very rich anastomotic network in the subfascial plane.

SUMMARY

The rich blood supply of the skin and fascia surrounding the elbow and antecubital fossa allows for the safe design of a variety of fasciocutaneous flaps, either proximally or distally based.

References

1. Culbertson J, Mutimer K. The reverse lateral arm flap for elbow coverage. *Ann Plast Surg* 1987;18:62.
2. Katsaros J, Schusterman M, Beppu M, et al. The lateral arm flap: anatomy and clinical applications. *Ann Plast Surg* 1984;12:489.
3. Lin S-D, Lai C-S, Chiu C-C. Venous drainage in the reverse forearm flap. *Plast Reconstr Surg* 1984;74:508.
4. Kincaid C, Banis J. The lateral arm flap. In: Gilbert A, Masquelet A, Hentz A, eds. *Pedicle flaps of the upper limb.* Boston: Little, Brown, 1992.
5. Lanzetta M, St. Laurent J-Y, Chollet A. The lateral arm flap: an anatomic and clinical study. Presented at the Annual Meeting, American Society for Reconstructive Microsurgery, Tucson, AZ, January, 1996.
6. Maruyama Y, Onishi K, Iwahira Y. The ulnar recurrent fasciocutaneous island flap: reverse medial arm flap. *Plast Reconstr Surg* 1987;79:381.
7. Cormack G, Lamberty B. The forearm angiotomes. *Br J Plast Surg* 1982;35:420.

CHAPTER 336 ■ RADIAL RECURRENT FASCIOCUTANEOUS FLAP FOR COVERAGE OF POSTERIOR ELBOW DEFECTS

F. C. AKPUAKA

The radial recurrent fasciocutaneous flap on the posterolateral aspect of the lower half of the upper arm is based on the radial recurrent artery, a constant branch of the radial artery. It is a useful flap for one-stage coverage of posterior elbow defects, and is superior to other alternatives (1).

INDICATIONS

The coverage of posterior elbow defects is usually difficult and time-consuming. Previously described local, distant, and free flaps (2–9), some of which are also one-stage procedures, have the disadvantages of difficulty of elevation, association with a significant degree of functional muscle loss, and, with the radial forearm or Chinese flap, complete division of the radial artery at the wrist that may be associated with a number of local complications (10–12). The radial recurrent fasciocutaneous flap has the advantages of decreasing donor site morbidity, preserving elbow flexion and a relative case of elevation and transfer.

ANATOMY

Very close to its origin, the radial artery gives off the radial recurrent artery, which supplies branches to the adjacent muscles such as the supinator, and to the elbow joint. It then runs upward between the brachialis and the brachioradialis muscles, to anastomose with the profunda brachii artery in the mid-upper arm, supplying these muscles (Fig. 1). The radial recurrent artery also supplies the fascia, subcutaneous tissue, and skin over the posterolateral aspect of the lower half of the upper arm.

FLAP DESIGN AND DIMENSIONS

The flap, which is a type B fasciocutaneous flap (13), is outlined over the course of the radial recurrent artery, which runs proximally across the lateral epicondyle toward the posterior border of the deltoid muscle. The base of the flap is at the elbow joint, and the proximal limit is at the mid-upper arm. The width of the flap depends on the size of the elbow defect, but the entire flap is taken on the posterolateral aspect of the upper arm (Figs. 2 and 3).

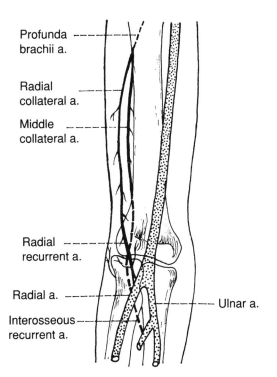

Profunda brachii a.

Radial collateral a.

Middle collateral a.

Radial recurrent a.

Radial a.

Interosseous recurrent a.

Ulnar a.

FIG. 1. Diagram demonstrating the anatomy of the radial recurrent fasciocutaneous flap and major arteries. (From Akpuaka, ref. 1, with permission.)

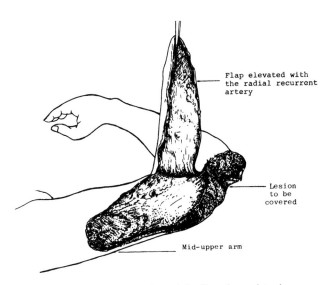

Flap elevated with the radial recurrent artery

Lesion to be covered

Mid-upper arm

FIG. 2. Schematic representation of the flap elevated in the upper arm. (From Akpuaka, ref. 1, with permission.)

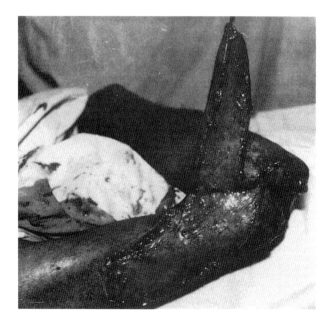

FIG. 3. Elevation of a 7 × 6 cm flap. (From Akpuaka, ref. 1, with permission.)

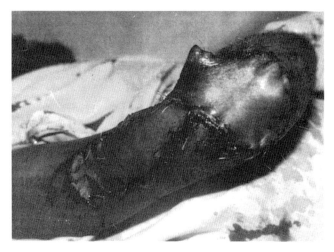

FIG. 4. Flap sutured into place. (From Akpuaka, ref. 1, with permission.)

OPERATIVE TECHNIQUE

The incision is begun on the lateral side and carried through the skin to beneath the deep fascia. The flap is freed by sweeping the finger up and down beneath the fascia, and then transposed over the defect, and sutured into position (Fig. 4). The wound is drained for about 48 hours, using corrugated or suction drains. With small-dimension tissue requirements, the donor defect can be closed primarily, but with a greater demand for replacement tissue, it is necessary to apply split-thickness skin grafts at the donor site.

CLINICAL RESULTS

A small series of cases, including post-olecranon fracture with wiring, left supracondylar compound fracture, and severe posttrauma defect, were treated with radial recurrent fasciocutaneous flaps, measuring from 4 × 4 cm to 7 × 6 cm. Donor sites were both sutured directly and covered by split-thickness skin grafts. Postoperative healing at the flap and donor sites, as well as elbow movement, were satisfactory. There were no complications.

SUMMARY

The radial recurrent fasciocutaneous flap is reliable, easy to elevate and transfer, and is associated with much less donor-site morbidity than other available procedures for posterior elbow reconstruction.

References

1. Akpuaka FC. The radial recurrent fasciocutaneous flap for coverage of posterior elbow defects. *Injury* 1991;22:332.
2. Abu Jamra FN. Repair of major defects of the upper extremity with a latissimus dorsi myocutaneous flap: a case report. *Br J Plast Surg* 1981;34:121.
3. Abu-Dalu K, Muggla M, Schiller M. A bipedicled chest wall flap to cover an open elbow joint in a burned infant. *Injury* 1982;12:292.
4. Fisher J. External oblique fasciocutaneous flap for elbow coverage. *Plast Reconstr Surg* 1985;75:51.
5. Sbitany U, Wary RC. Use of the rectus abdominis muscle flap to reconstruct an elbow defect. *Plast Reconstr Surg* 1986;79:988.
6. Grotting J, Walkinshaw M. The early use of free flaps in burns. *Ann Plast Surg* 1985;15:127.
7. Lendrum J. Alternatives to amputation. *Ann R Coll Surg Engl* 1980;62:95.
8. Lai MF, Krishna BV, Pelly AD. The brachioradialis myocutaneous flap. *Br J Plast Surg* 1981;34:431.
9. Nahai F, Mathes SJ. A selective approach to flap selection. In: Mathes SJ, Nahai F, eds. *Clinical application for muscle and myocutaneous flaps.* St. Louis: Mosby, 1982.
10. Yang C, Chen B, Gao Y, et al. Forearm free skin flap transposition. *N Med J China* 1981;61:139.
11. Fatah MF, Davis DM. The radial forearm island flap in upper limb reconstruction. *J Hand Surg* 1984;9B:324.
12. Timmons MJ, Missotten FEM, Poole MD, et al. Complications of radial forearm flap donor sites. *Br J Plast Surg* 1986;39:176.
13. Cormack GC, Lamberty BGH. A classification of fasciocutaneous flaps according to their patterns of vascularization. *Br J Plast Surg* 1984;37:80.

CHAPTER 337 ■ BRACHIORADIALIS MUSCLE AND MUSCULOCUTANEOUS FLAP FOR COVERAGE OF THE ELBOW

A. GILBERT AND J. RESTREPO

Coverage of the elbow can be difficult. Very few local flaps are safe and chest wall flaps can result in stiffness since the joint cannot be immediately mobilized. The brachioradialis muscle provides a small but effective local flap for coverage of the elbow (1–3).

INDICATIONS

This flap can cover completely the anterior aspect of the elbow, the lateral aspect and, depending on the length of the muscular belly, the olecranon and posterior aspect of the joint. It has been used in our experience for the treatment of flexion contractures of the elbow after burns and trauma. We have also used it as a free neurovascular muscle flap.

ANATOMY

Dissection and injection studies on 50 forearms have revealed the following.

The average length of the muscle, from its insertion on the humerus to its tendinous insertion on the radius is 30 cm (24 to 33 cm). This muscle is the most superficial muscle of the lateral border of the forearm. The average length of the tendon is 8 cm and the muscular part is approximately 22 cm.

The muscle is innervated by a branch of the radial nerve (C5–C6). There may be one or several branches. Their main entry point is usually 6 cm distal to the humeral insertion of the muscle. It is important to note that the nerve pedicle is different from the main vascular hilum.

The blood supply to the muscle consists of a main vascular pedicle and several accessory vessels. The main pedicle usually branches from the radial recurrent artery (Fig. 1) (78%) but may come from the brachial artery (12%), the radial artery (4%), or the ulnar recurrent artery (2%). This pedicle has an average length of 3.8 cm. The diameter of the direct branch is approximately 1.6 mm, but the radial recurrent artery has a diameter of 2 mm, which makes it a reason-able candidate for free microvascular transfer. The vascular hilum is situated from 6 to 16 cm (average 10 cm) distal to the humeral insertion.

FLAP DESIGN AND DIMENSIONS

The existence of direct musculocutaneous branches makes it possible to transfer the overlying skin with the muscle belly. Injection studies show that at least the proximal two-thirds of the skin overlying the muscle can be moved safely. The reasonable size of a proximally based flap would be 15 × 8 cm.

If the flap is taken as a musculocutaneous flap, the donor defect cannot be closed primarily. For this reason, the flap is usually used as a muscle flap and subsequently skin-grafted (Fig. 2).

OPERATIVE TECHNIQUE

An incision is made directly over the muscular prominence. The fascia is opened and the muscle is dissected free from its surroundings. A small distal incision is used to cut the tendon, taking care to preserve the cutaneous branch of the radial nerve. The dissection then progresses very quickly until it reaches the main pedicle. During this dissection, one or two secondary pedicles must be cut. A few branches of the radial recurrent artery will need to be transected to allow more mobility to the pedicle.

The muscle is then transferred and sutured over the defect. It is possible to "spread" the muscle, obtaining about one-third of extra width (Figs. 2 and 3).

SUMMARY

The brachioradialis muscle can be used with or without the overlying skin to cover anterior and lateral elbow defects.

971

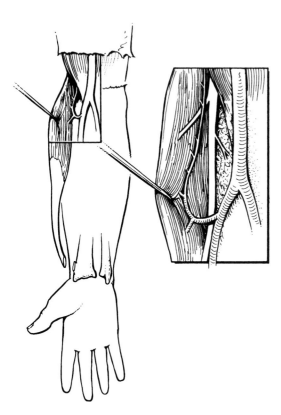

FIG. 1. The arterial supply to the muscle usually comes from the radial recurrent artery.

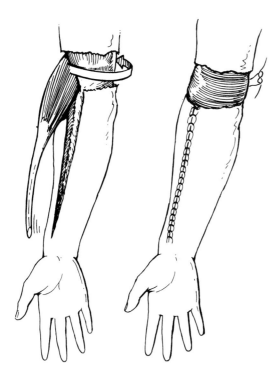

FIG. 2. The muscle is transferred and sutured into the defect.

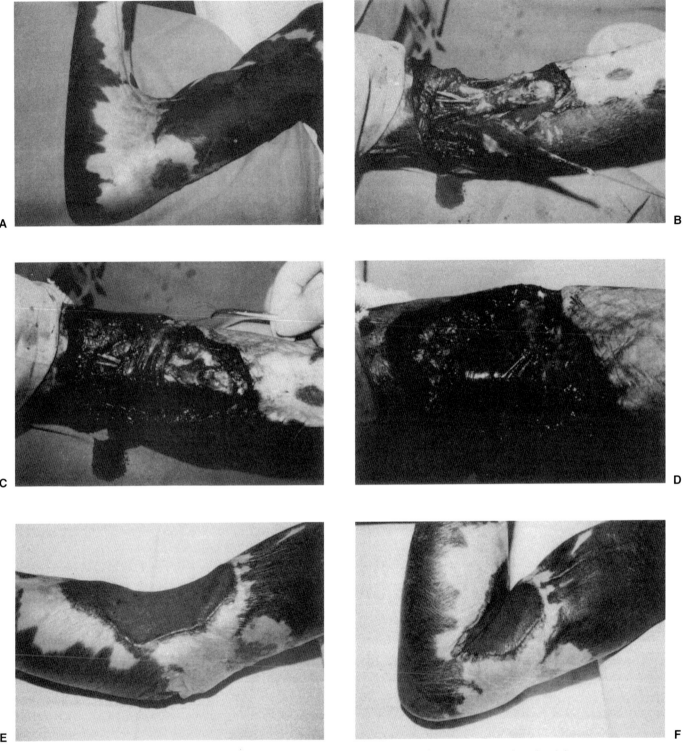

FIG. 3. A: Flexion contracture of the elbow in an 8-year-old child. B: The contracture is released and the biceps tendon is lengthened. C: The biceps tendon is covered by the brachioradialis muscle. D: The muscle can be spread to further cover the defect. E: Elbow extension at 6 months postoperatively. F: Elbow flexion at 6 months postoperatively.

References

1. Ger R. The coverage of vascular repairs by muscle transposition. *J Trauma* 1976;16:974.

2. Gilbert A, Restrepo J. Le long supinateur: anatomie et utilisation comme lambeau de rotation musculaire. *Ann Chir Plast* 1980;25:72.

3. Lai MF, Krishan BV, Pelly AD. The brachioradialis myocutaneous flap. *Br J Plast Surg* 1981;34:431.

CHAPTER 338 ■ EXTENSOR CARPI RADIALIS LONGUS MUSCLE FLAP FOR ANTERIOR ELBOW COVERAGE

R. V. JANEVICIUS

The extensor carpi radialis longus muscle, when elevated as an island flap, can cover large areas about the elbow joint, with minimum donor-site morbidity (1). It can be used alone or in conjunction with the brachioradialis muscle, to cover significant defects around the antecubital fossa.

INDICATIONS

Small defects about the elbow and antecubital fossa area can often be reconstructed with brachioradialis or flexor carpi ulnaris muscle flaps. When these muscles are not available, or when larger areas require coverage, the extensor carpi radialis longus (ECRL) muscle flap is indicated. Although it can be raised as a musculocutaneous unit (2), I prefer its use as a pure muscle flap, as its arc of rotation will be far greater, and donor-site morbidity will be minimal. The ECRL is a useful muscle for coverage about the elbow, including coverage of the radial and median nerves and the humerus, after trauma or tumor resection.

ANATOMY

The ECRL originates from the lower third of the lateral supracondylar ridge of the humerus, and inserts into the base of the index finger metacarpal. As it courses distally, it lies deep and ulnar to the brachioradialis and superficial to the extensor carpi radialis brevis (ECRB). Its muscle belly ends at the junction of the proximal and middle thirds of the forearm, its tendon then passing distally, superficial to the ECRB tendon. Its tendon then passes deep to the abductor pollicis longus and extensor pollicis brevis, then through the second dorsal compartment with the ECRB tendon, to insert into the dorsal base of the index metacarpal.

The ECRL is a Mathes type II muscle. Its proximal dominant vascular supply arises from the radial recurrent artery 80% of the time, directly from the radial artery 10% of the time, and directly from the ulnar artery 10% of the time (3).

The proximal vascular pedicle arises within 4 cm of the antecubital crease. Minor pedicles occur distal to this point.

Motor innervation of the ECRL arises from the radial nerve and enters the muscle proximally close to the proximal vascular pedicle.

Wrist extension occurs by synergistic contraction of the ECRL, ECRB, and extensor carpi ulnaris (ECU) muscles. When the ECRB and ECU are present, the ECRL is an expendable muscle, as evidenced by its utility in tendon transfers for median- and ulnar-nerve palsies (4,5). Moreover, its successful use in tendon transfers has demonstrated the predictability of its proximal vascular anatomy.

FLAP DESIGN AND DIMENSIONS

Because of its single dominant proximal vascular pedicle, the ECRL muscle arc of rotation is approximately 4 cm distal to the antecubital crease. Disinserting the muscle from the index metacarpal will allow radial and ulnar transposition, but limited antecubital and elbow coverage. Disoriginating the muscle from the humerus and fashioning a pure island flap, will allow for a more extensive arc of rotation and more proximal coverage.

OPERATIVE TECHNIQUE

The defect about the antecubital fossa and/or olecranon is defined and measured (Fig. 1). The ECRL is harvested via a longitudinal incision, extending distally from the soft-tissue defect, and overlying the midportion of the ECRL. The brachioradialis muscle is retracted radially to facilitate exposure. The ECRL is disinserted from the index metacarpal and elevated off the ECRB (Fig. 3). Dorsal traction as one dissects proximally will reveal the minor vascular pedicles.

The proximal dominant vascular pedicle should be identified approximately 4 cm distal to the antecubital crease. The radial nerve will be encountered in this area and must be carefully preserved (Fig. 2). Minor distal pedicles, distal to 4 cm beyond the antecubital crease, may be safely ligated.

The origin of the muscle is detached from the humerus to create a pure island flap. Neural branches from the radial nerve may be divided to denervate the muscle and diminish bulk within the antecubital fossa. The muscle is transposed and covered with a split-thickness skin graft (Fig. 4). The donor site is closed primarily.

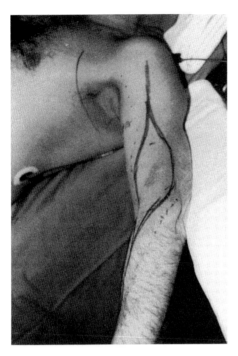

FIG. 1. A 5-cm margin with an underlying muscle-group resection is outlined. (From Janevicius and Greager, ref. 1, with permission.)

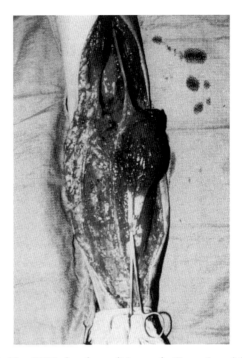

FIG. 3. The ECRL has been disinserted. (From Janevicius and Greager, ref. 1, with permission.)

CLINICAL RESULTS

A biopsy-proven malignant fibrous histiocytoma of the distal arm was resected with 5-cm margins, and an underlying muscle-group resection included removal of the brachialis and brachioradialis muscles (Fig. 1). This resulted in a defect exposing the radial nerve for a distance of 15 cm, as well as the distal humerus (Fig. 2). The ECRL was elevated and fashioned as a pure island flap (Fig. 3), then rotated 180° to fill the defect and to cover the exposed radial nerve and humerus (Fig. 4).

Thirty months postoperatively, the patient has normal elbow flexion and extension (Figs. 5 and 6), normal radial nerve and hand function, and a stable skin graft. He has continued to work full time in his previous job as a jackhammer operator.

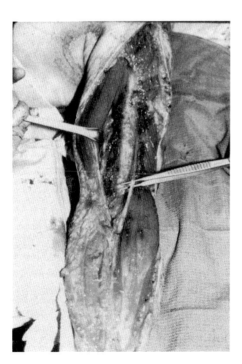

FIG. 2. The resection exposes a 15-cm segment of the radial nerve, as well as the distal humerus. (From Janevicius and Greager, ref. 1, with permission.)

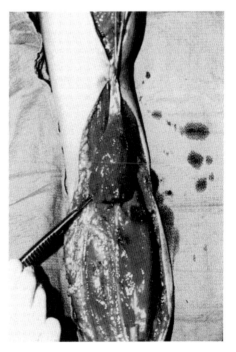

FIG. 4. The ECRL island flap has been rotated 180°. (From Janevicius and Greager, ref. 1, with permission.)

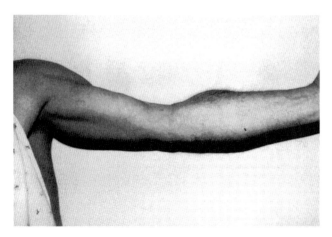

FIG. 5. Full extension is demonstrated postoperatively. (From Janevicius, Greager, ref. 1, with permission.)

SUMMARY

The extensor carpi radialis longus muscle is well suited for reconstruction about the antecubital fossa. Substantial defects can be covered, resulting in minimal donor-site morbidity.

References

1. Janevicius RV, Greager JA. The extensor carpi radialis longus muscle flap for anterior elbow coverage. *J Hand Surg* 1992;17A:102.

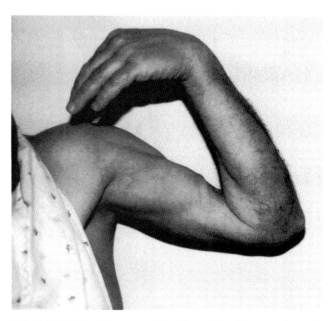

FIG. 6. Full flexion is present. (From Janevicius, Greager, ref. 1, with permission.)

2. Ohtsuka H, Imagawa S. Reconstruction of a posterior defect of the elbow joint using an extensor carpi radialis longus myocutaneous flap: case report. *Br J Plast Surg* 1985;38:238.
3. Parry SW, Ward JW, Mathes SJ. Vascular anatomy of the upper extremity muscles. *Plast Reconstr Surg* 1988;81:358.
4. Burkhalter WE. Median nerve palsy. In: Green DP, ed. *Operative hand surgery*, 2nd ed. New York: Churchill Livingstone, 1988;1499–1534.
5. Omer GE. Ulnar nerve palsy. In: Green DP, ed. *Operative hand surgery*, 2nd ed. New York: Churchill Livingstone, 1988;1534–1554.

CHAPTER 339 ■ MICROVASCULAR FREE TRANSFER OF A COMPOUND DEEP CIRCUMFLEX GROIN AND ILIAC CREST FLAP TO THE UPPER EXTREMITY

G. I. TAYLOR AND R. J. CORLETT

The composite deep circumflex iliac flap provides a large bloc of bone, and in some situations advantage may be taken of its curvature (1–3). In the upper limb, it would seem most appropriately suited for stabilization of the various joints, viz., the shoulder, elbow, or wrist, particularly if there is associated extensive soft-tissue loss.

Our experience with the use of the deep circumflex iliac osteocutaneous flap in the upper extremity is limited. It does provide a large amount of bone. However, the curvature of the crest and the associated soft-tissue bulk make it a less attractive solution for those problems that involve a long segmental defect of the radius, ulna, or humerus. In these situations we have found that the fibula is the flap of choice (3). Our experience with the flap is restricted to two cases that required skin and bone replacement at the wrist and at the elbow joint (Figs. 1 and 2).

See Chap. 204.

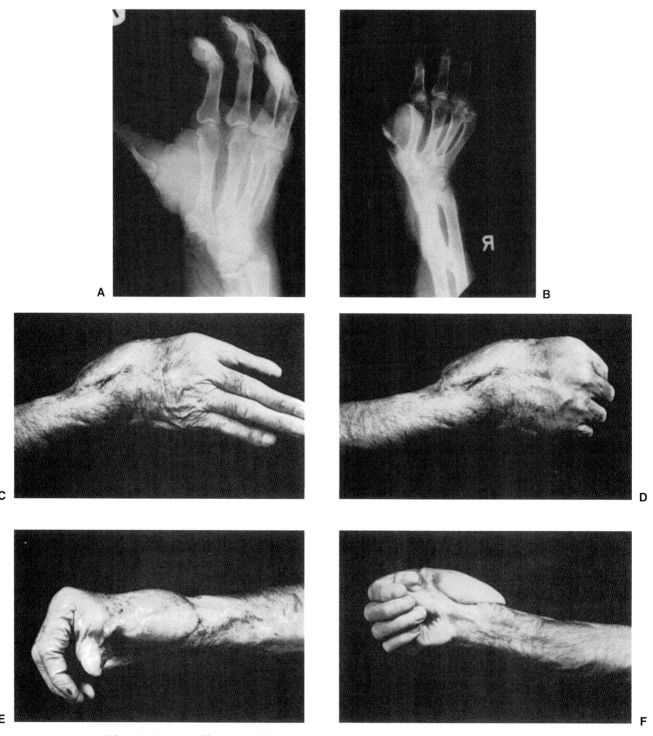

FIG. 1. A: A 62-year-old patient with the dorsal and radial part of his hand ablated. The defect included the first metacarpal, the proximal phalanx of the thumb, the scaphoid, the trapezium, and the radial styloid process. There was an associated oblique fracture of the lower end of the radius. The dorsal skin, the radial wrist extensors, the extensor tendons of the thumb, and the ligamentous structures of the wrist were lost. A composite iliac crest muscle and skin flap was raised, based on the deep circumflex iliac artery. The skin flap measured 8 × 4 cm and the bone 14 × 3 cm. The wrist was arthrodesed, using the vascularized bone graft to bridge the skeletal defect between the dorsal surface of the radius, the remaining carpal bones, the second metacarpal, and the tip of the terminal phalanx of the thumb. An osteotomy of the bone graft was performed at the level of the first metacarpophalangeal joint, to obtain the correct position of the thumb. Postoperatively, the patient developed a wound infection and subsequently a small portion of the distal bone graft was lost. Following debridement of this area of bone and grafting with a split-thickness skin graft, the graft healed without further complication. B: Radiograph of the result at 12 months. C, D, E, F: The graft has provided a stable wrist, the hand is in good alignment, and there is an excellent range of movement of the fingers at the metacarpophalangeal and proximal interphalangeal joints. The thumb, although foreshortened, has remained stable and has required no further surgical intervention.

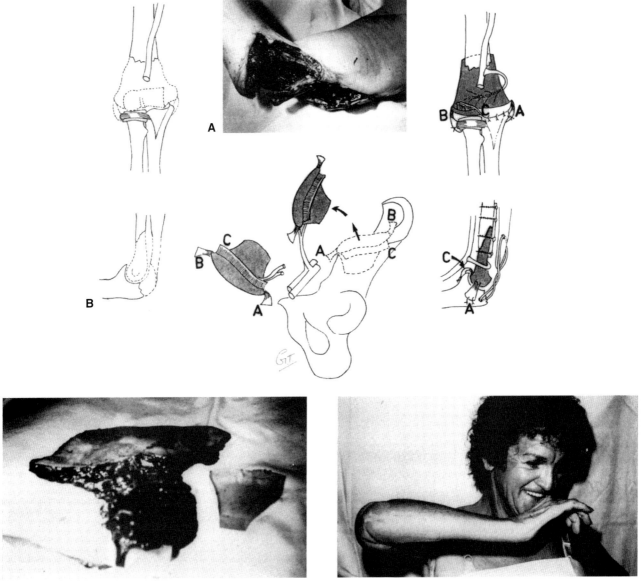

FIG. 2. **A:** A 53-year-old woman suffered a shotgun injury to the region of her right elbow. There was loss of the distal 5 cm of her humerus, the proximal 2 cm of the olecranon, the attached triceps muscle and tendon, and an 8 cm gap in the ulnar nerve, together with loss of the overlying skin (see Fig. 2F). **B:** A segment of iliac crest was chosen, using the anterior portion of the contralateral hip to simulate the lost segment of the distal humerus (*dotted lines*). The curvature of the crest was designed to fit the curvature of the articular surfaces of the head of the radius and the olecranon. Various soft-tissue attachments to the iliac crest were used to reconstruct the elbow joint capsule and ligaments. A segment of attached inguinal ligament provided the ulnar collateral ligament (A) and a flap of thick periosteum was elevated to reconstruct the radial collateral ligament (B). A fringe of fascia lata (C) reconstructed the anterior joint capsule. The loose areolar layer on the surface of the external oblique muscle at its attachment to the crest offered a convenient gliding layer for joint articulation. The blade of the ilium was sculptured to resemble the lower end of the humerus. (*Continued*)

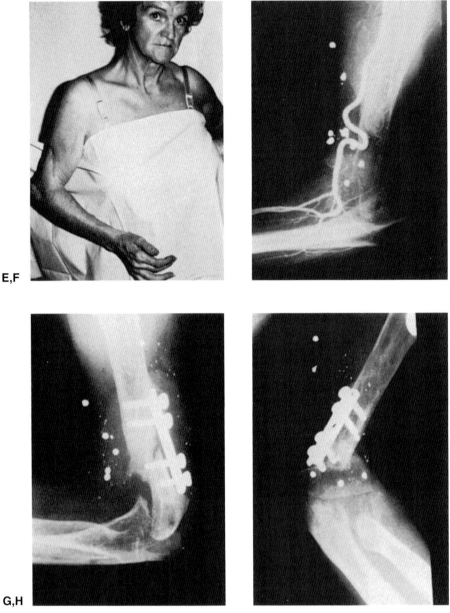

E,F

G,H

FIG. 2. *Continued.* **C:** The flap was detached (shown here with a model of the deficient distal humerus), secured to the distal humerus, and revascularized to the brachial artery and its vena comitans. The triceps mechanism was reconstructed with tendon grafts to the remaining olecranon. The ulnar nerve was repaired with three sural nerve cable grafts, and the skin defect closed with a flap. The elbow was immobilized at 90° **D, E:** The postoperative course was uneventful. At 6 weeks gentle mobilization of the elbow commenced. At 8 weeks there was a range of elbow movement of 25° to 30°, and the preoperative range of supination and pronation had been regained. The elbow is painless and stable. **F:** Preoperative angiogram. **G, H:** Postoperative radiographs at 8 weeks.

References

1. Taylor GI, Townsend P, Corlett RJ. Superiority of the deep circumflex iliac vessels as the supply for free groin flaps. *Plast Reconstr Surg* 1979;64:745.

2. Taylor GI, Townsend P, Corlett RJ. Superiority of the deep circumflex iliac vessels as the supply for free groin flaps: experimental work. *Plast Reconstr Surg* 1979;64:595.

3. Taylor GI. The current status of free vascularized bone grafts. *Clin Plast Surg* 1983;10:185.

CHAPTER 340 ■ THORACO-EPIGASTRIC SKIN/FASCIA FLAP TO THE ARM

V. L. LEWIS, JR.

Flaps based on the midline of the body have played an important role in reconstructive plastic surgery. Webster (1) in 1937 designed a flap based on the superior epigastric artery. Braun et al. (2) and Cannon and Trott (3) oriented epigastric flaps transversely for application to the upper extremity. Tai and Hasegawa (4) recognized the contribution of the superior epigastric perforators to the transverse flap, and successfully designed longer flaps for chest wall coverage.

With the success and versatility of the thoracoepigastric flap, it is interesting that a recently proposed schema for upper extremity reconstruction makes no mention of it (5). However in upper extremity trauma, the demonstration that microsurgical reconstruction could be done early (6,7) and the development of criteria for wound closure (8) have undoubtedly decreased the frequency of use of pedicled thoracoepigastric flaps.

INDICATIONS

The thoracoepigastric flap has been successfully used to cover losses from burns (9,10), penetrating trauma (11,12), extravasation, and pressure injuries. The flap has been applied to the arm, elbow, forearm, wrist, and hand by adjusting the level at which it is designed. The flap can be applied to the anterior, medial, and posterior arm, and dorsal and volar forearm, wrist, and hand.

The flap may be applied immediately to traumatic defects for coverage of blood vessels, nerves, or tendons, if the wound is completely debrided and bacterial counts low. In repair of dirty wounds and burns, it is most successfully applied secondarily. Secondary defatting can be safely performed.

ANATOMY

Early reports on medially based thoracoepigastric flaps focused on length-to-width ratios, emphasizing short lengths and wide bases (2,13). The work of Milton (14) initiated the idea that it was more important that a flap be designed to contain expectable vessels than that it be designed to certain rigid ratios. The observation of Brown et al. (11) that, in an upper abdominoplasty, no bleeding is encountered from the rectus sheath to the latissimus border suggested that the epifascial blood supply of the abdomen radiated from perforators in the rectus abdominus muscle.

The work of Taylor et al. (15) and Boyd et al. (16) definitively clarified the anatomic basis of the transverse thoracoepigastric flap (Fig. 1A). Boyd et al. reported, "The deep epigastric arcade forms the abdominal portion of a ventral vascular railroad, linking the subclavian and external iliac arteries." The deep inferior epigastric artery supplies blood to the majority of major perforating vessels leaving the rectus abdominus muscle and running laterally to the area of the latissimus dorsi muscle. These vessels are in the plane above the fascia, making flap elevation in the subfascial plane mandatory.

The superior epigastric artery, though smaller than the inferior epigastric, contributes to the upper abdominal and thoracic flap (16). Derived primarily from the internal thoracic (internal mammary) artery (17), it also receives contributions from (1) terminal branches of the intercostals (18), (2) the superficial inferior epigastric (11), and (3) meets the inferior epigastric in a complex of spiral vessels within the rectus muscle (19). Damage to the internal thoracic artery by trauma, operation or radiation, significantly reduces reliability of the flap.

FLAP DESIGN AND DIMENSIONS

The flap includes skin, subcutaneous tissue, and muscular fascia of the lateral thoracic and upper abdominal areas. The base is the lateral border of the rectus sheath, and the undelayed lateral border is the posterior axillary line, or anterior edge of the latissimus dorsi muscle. Both delayed and undelayed extensions beyond this line are described (10,12,20). With delay, the flap has been extended to within 5 cm of the dorsal midline (20,21).

The upper limit of the flap base is the areola in men or the inframammary fold in women. However, upward (10) and downward (22) movement of the base, in accordance with the principle of known perforator inclusion, is possible. The flap width is in accordance with defect size, but widths of 10 to 15 cm are usual (23), and a width of 30 cm reported (12) (Fig. 1B). The length of the flap from the lateral rectus border to the posterior axillary line averages 20 to 25 cm in the adult, varying with gender and size of the torso. It is not necessary to raise the full length of the flap if a shorter flap will cover the defect. Davis et al. (20) found that a 16-cm donor defect could be closed in a chubby individual, and a 10-cm defect in a thin person.

The rotation point of the thoracoepigastric flap has been described as the lateral margin of the rectus abdominis fascia, near the underportion of the flap base (20). The rotation point is not the lower portion of the base, because upward flap mobility is gained when the abdominal wound is closed by reversed abdominoplasty advancement. A key to closure is cited (20) as being release of the dense fascia overlying the iliac crest.

When applied to the upper extremity, the flap usually isn't rotated. If it is rotated, without a delayed random extension, the flap will reach the upper axilla and the anterior chest wall. With a delayed addition, it will reach the apex of the axilla and clavicle (21,23).

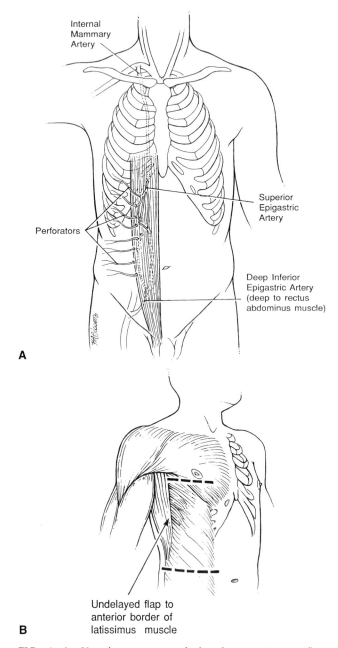

A

B

Undelayed flap to
anterior border of
latissimus muscle

FIG. 1. **A:** Vascular anatomy of the thoracoepigastric flap.
B: Dimensions and limits of undelayed flap.

OPERATIVE TECHNIQUE

The flap is elevated in a lateral to medial direction, with division of approximately ten muscular intercostal perforating vessels, mostly over the serratus anterior muscle. Depending on the design and width of the flap, elevation exposes the serratus anterior, external oblique and pectoralis major muscles. Elevation of the flap from the posterior axillary line medially is in the subfascial plane. The random delayed portion over the latissimus is raised superficial to the fascia. The lateral border of the rectus abdominis sheath is determined by palpation before the flap is elevated, and is marked on the skin. No elevation is carried out medial to this line (Fig. 1). The perforating vessels that support the flap may or may not be visible when this point is reached. These vessels must never be divided. Doppler identification may, if necessary, be used to protect the perforating vessels. The viability of the flap is assessed with fluorescein if there is any concern.

The flap is placed over the defect on the upper extremity, either the anterior or posterior surface, and sutured in two layers. If the donor defect cannot be closed, it and the inner surface of the flap base may be covered with meshed skin graft or membrane dressing.

Active wrist and hand motion are maintained with physiotherapy. If necessary, wrist dorsiflexion is maintained with a volar splint. The upper extremity may be supported with a sling or shoulder immobilizer.

The pedicle is divided in stages, beginning at 14 to 21 days postoperatively. The guidelines for this are primarily historic and empirical (3). Division is begun at the later time if the flap lacks a border on the arm consisting of normal, well-vascularized soft tissue (13). Division of the pedicle is accomplished in two or three stages by measured quarters or thirds, with the division completed in 7 to 10 days. The axial vessels are identified and ligated as part of the division. When there is doubt about the adequacy of the blood supply to the flap from the arm, the flap base may be clamped with a noncrushing clamp and fluorescein given.

The divided flap margin is not inset into the arm, but allowed to contract and form a contour, making surgical inset usually unnecessary and preventing marginal necrosis. At flap division, the graft is removed from the flap base and bed, and remaining flap returned to its bed.

CLINICAL RESULTS

With proper design, and undamaged blood supply, the thoracoepigastric flap has proved highly reliable in upper extremity reconstruction (Fig. 2A and B). Combining the results of reports that listed number of cases (9,11,12,20), of 25 flaps transferred, 23 succeeded. Experience with the flap in chest wall and breast reconstruction is also good. Flap reliability decreases with damage to the longitudinal blood supply, and undelayed extension beyond the posterior axillary line. Abdominal scars that have not damaged the perforating vessels (i.e., midline laparotomy scars) have not influenced flap survival.

Wide flap donor defects covered with skin grafts, though unsightly, are acceptable in limb salvage (Fig. 2C). Immobilization of the shoulder while the flap heals has not resulted in stiffness that could not be resolved by physical therapy. However, arthritis or preexisting stiffness might relatively contraindicate this flap choice.

SUMMARY

The thoracoepigastric flap, which has been expanded due to recent understanding of the blood supply, can provide coverage for large areas of the arm and forearm.

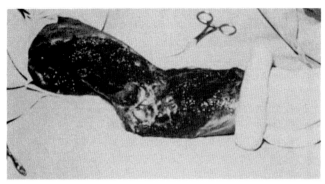

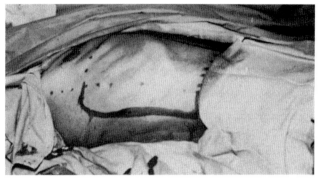

A   **B**   **C**

FIG. 2. **A:** Electrical burn defect. **B:** Extended thoracoepigastric flap coverage of defect. **C:** Long-term follow-up of coverage. (From Lewis and Cook, ref. 10, with permission.)

References

1. Webster JP. Thoracoepigastric tubed pedicles. *Surg Clin North Am* 1937;17:145.
2. Braun JB, Cannon B, Graham WC, et al. Direct flap repair of defects of the arm and hand. *Ann Surg* 1947;122:706.
3. Cannon B, Trott AW. Expeditious use of direct flaps in extremity repairs. *Plast Reconstr Surg* 1949;4:415.
4. Tai Y, Hasegawa H. Transverse abdominal flap for reconstruction after radical operations for recurrent breast cancer. *Plast Reconstr Surg* 1974;53:52.
5. Hallock GG. A schema for local flap selection in the upper extremity: a hypothesis. *Ann Plast Surg* 1990;25:479.
6. Godina M. Early microsurgical reconstruction of complex trauma of the extremities. *Plast Reconstr Surg* 1986;78:285.
7. Lister G, Scheker L. Emergency free flaps to the upper extremity. *J Hand Surg* 1988;13A:22.
8. Breidenbach WC. Emergency free tissue transfer for reconstruction of acute upper extremity wounds. *Clin Plast Surg* 1989;16:505.
9. Hallock GG, Dingeldein GP. The thoracoepigastric flap as an alternative for coverage of the burned elbow. *J Burn Care Res* 1982;3:393.
10. Lewis VL, Cook JQ. The nondelayed thoracoepigastric flap: coverage of an extensive electric burn defect of the upper extremity. *Plast Reconstr Surg* 1980;65:492.
11. Brown RG, Vasconez LO, Jurkiewicz MJ. Transverse abdominal flaps and the deep epigastric arcade. *Plast Reconstr Surg* 1975;55:416.
12. Kalisman M, Wexler MR, Yeshua R, et al. Comparison between the early use of skin flap and skin graft for the correction of large tissue loss at the elbow. *Ann Plast Surg* 1978;1:474.
13. Kelleher JC, Sullivan JG, Barbak GJ, et al. Use of a tailored abdominal pedicle flap for surgical reconstruction of the hand. *J Bone Joint Surg* 1970;51A:1552.
14. Milton SM. Pedicled skin-flaps: the fallacy of the length:width ratio. *Br J Surg* 1970;57:502.
15. Taylor GI, Corlett RJ, Boyd JB. The versatile deep inferior epigastric (inferior rectus abdominis) flap. *Br J Plast Surg* 1984;37:330.
16. Boyd JB, Taylor GI, Corlett R. The vascular territories of the superior epigastric and deep inferior epigastric systems. *Plast Reconstr Surg* 1984;73:1.

17. Moore KL. *Clinically oriented anatomy.* Baltimore: Williams and Wilkins, 1984;75.
18. Kerrigan CL, Daniel RR. The intercostal flap: an anatomical and hemodynamic approach. *Ann Plast Surg* 1979;2:411.
19. Scheflan M, Dinner MI. The transverse abdominal island flap: Part I. Indications, contraindications, results and complications. *Ann Plast Surg* 1983;10:24.
20. Davis WM, McCraw JB, Carraway JH. Use of a direct, transverse, thoracoabdominal flap to close difficult wounds of the thorax and upper extremity. *Plast Reconstr Surg* 1977;60:526.
21. Cronin TD, Upton J, McDonough JM. Reconstruction of the breast after mastectomy. *Plast Reconstr Surg* 1977;59:1.
22. Seitchik SM, Granick MS, Soloman MP, et al. Post-traumatic upper extremity wound coverage utilizing the extended deep inferior epigastric flap. *Ann Plast Surg* 1992;28:465.
23. Bostwick J, Vasconez LO, Jurkiewicz M. Breast reconstruction after a radical mastectomy. *Plast Reconstr Surg* 1978;61:682.

CHAPTER 341 ■ MEDIAL ARM FLAP

E. N. KAPLAN, R. PEARL, AND V. R. HENTZ

EDITORIAL COMMENT

The attractiveness of the thin, pliable skin and of a most acceptable donor site on the inner aspect of the arm would make this flap a favorite one. Unfortunately, the blood supply is quite variable, particularly as it relates to the ulnar collateral artery. In a great number of cases, that artery is not present and the flap would be random and thus less reliable.

The physical quality, location, and blood supply of medial arm skin make it useful for reconstructive procedures in various clinical situations. The thinness, pliability, and hairlessness of the skin commend it as an excellent choice for resurfacing of the face, neck, and hands (1–4).

INDICATIONS

The medial arm flap has been used for rotation into the axilla for release of burn and radiation scar contractures, for augmentation of soft-tissue defect of the chest, and for treatment of upper arm lymphedema. As a distant flap, it provides excellent coverage for the contralateral upper extremity, especially the thumb, as well as for much of the head and neck region. As a free flap, this tissue may be transferred to any recipient site requiring less than 20 × 12 to 15 cm of thin, pliable, hairless tissue (Fig. 1).

ANATOMY

Vascular

In addition to the direct cutaneous blood supply, there is an overlapping with the musculocutaneous perforators from the biceps and triceps (1,3). Although one could use the musculocutaneous flow as the basis for flap design, the supplying muscles would need to be included, and this would obviate the thin and pliable quality of the flap and could produce unacceptable functional deficits. The use of the fascia, however, as the primary vascular source may obviate the need for inclusion of direct cutaneous arteries (1,4–6) (Fig. 2).

Arterial

The *brachial artery* is the continuation of the axillary artery beyond the teres major. The artery courses in the intermuscular septum between the biceps and the triceps (Fig. 3).

The *profunda artery* is a musculocutaneous artery that is usually the first branch off the brachial. It arises 2 to 3 cm beyond the teres major and passes posteriorly between the humerus and the triceps to accompany the radial nerve. The branches from the profunda brachii supply the triceps, then perforate into the skin. Small (0.1 to 0.3 mm) cutaneous branches perforate the muscular fascia at 2- to 3-cm intervals, to supply the skin of the posterior two-thirds of the arm.

The *superior ulnar collateral artery* is an axial cutaneous vessel that arises 4 to 6 cm beyond the pectoralis major and courses distally through the subcutaneous tissue to enter the medial arm skin 6 to 12 cm beyond the pectoralis (Fig. 4). The arterial diameter is from 0.8 to 1.5 mm. In 60% of dissections this artery originates from the profunda artery, and in 20% it originates directly from the brachial artery. In the other 20% there is a double system with a direct cutaneous vessel exiting from both the brachial artery and the profunda artery. In this latter situation the vessel size is inadequate for free flap transfer but can be used for local or distant pedicle flaps.

The *biceps musculocutaneous artery* arises 6 to 8 cm distal to the pectoral muscle. After penetrating the biceps muscle, two or three major perforating vessels vascularize the anterior arm skin. The size of these vessels is variable.

The *inferior ulnar collateral artery* is an axial cutaneous artery that arises 5 to 10 cm from the elbow and may form collaterals either around the elbow or with the superior ulnar collateral artery. In 6 out of 16 dissections, a 0.4 to 0.6 mm direct cutaneous artery supplied the skin of the distal third of the arm.

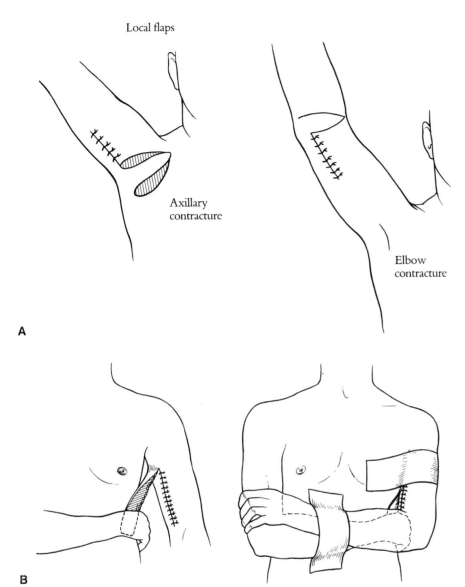

FIG. 1. A: Medial arm skin can be used for replacement of local axillary or elbow skin. Tissue deficiency caused by burn contracture, injury, radiation, and infection has been corrected. B: The thin, pliable inner arm skin is ideal for resurfacing the contralateral hand and fingers.

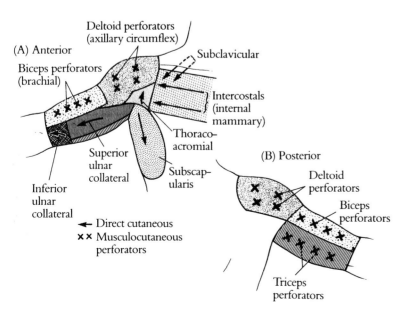

FIG. 2. The vascular territories of the medial arm are depicted. The primary supply is from the direct cutaneous vessels. The remainder of the arm is supplied by musculocutaneous perforators.

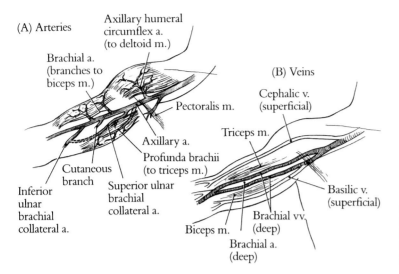

FIG. 3. This was the most common pattern of vascular anatomy. The superior ulnar brachial collateral artery was a branch of the brachial artery. It can also branch off the profunda artery (or both). (From Hentz et al., ref. 1, with permission.)

Venous

Venous drainage tends to follow the superior ulnar collateral or other branches into the paired brachial veins on each side of the brachial artery. However, there is separate venous drainage through the cephalic and/or basilic veins.

FLAP DESIGN AND DIMENSIONS

The proximally based medial arm flap can be designed to extend from the midanterior to midposterior line. A flap of this extent will require a skin graft for the donor site, but narrow flaps can be primarily closed (Fig. 5). The flap will consistently survive to three-quarters the length of the upper arm (20 to 30 cm), but can extend to the elbow if a delay procedure is first performed.

Preoperative flap planning includes both identification of the superior ulnar collateral artery, using the Doppler flowmeter, and marking of the large subcutaneous veins (Fig. 4B). The flap is centered along the axis of the superior ulnar brachial cutaneous collateral artery, as determined by Doppler, and includes at least one large superficial vein.

OPERATIVE TECHNIQUE

Flap Elevation

The skin boundaries are incised down through and including the areolar plane overlying the muscular fascia. The deep plane of elevation includes the areolar fascia to protect the superior brachial collateral artery. Dissection on the muscular fascia can be rapid until the point of penetration of the vessel into the skin, beginning distally at the flap tip, as determined by the Doppler study (about 6 to 10 cm from the anterior axillary fold). *Care is taken to avoid the intermuscular septum that contains the ulnar and median nerves and the brachial artery.* Protection is facilitated by marking the brachial artery course between biceps and triceps. Proximal to the point where the superior ulnar collateral artery penetrates the skin, the dissection requires more care, so as not to transect this direct cutaneous artery as it exits the intermuscular septum. The dissection is terminated as soon as enough elevation has been completed to allow transfer to the recipient site. Although this flap can be elevated as an island flap, only minimal increase in arc of rotation is achieved, while markedly increasing the difficulty of the dissection and the risk to the vascular pedicle.

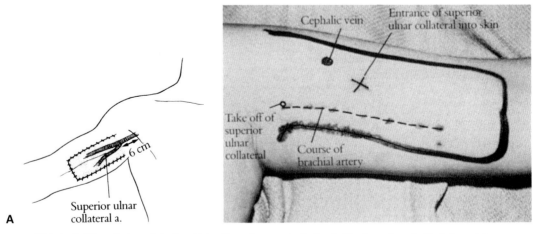

FIG. 4. **A:** The relation of the brachial collateral artery is depicted. The branch typically is found 4 to 6 cm beyond the axillary fold. **B:** A Doppler (presurgical) evaluation can often identify the artery and its course. These relationships were confirmed intraoperatively. (From Hentz et al., ref. 1, with permission.)

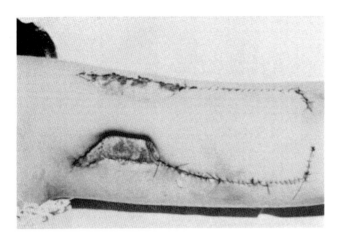

FIG. 5. The preferred method for distant flap design and elevation includes tubing of the base and grafting of the bed for large flaps. In this patient a delay procedure was performed.

Flap Delay

Flap delay increases survival potential for the distal quarter of the proximally based arm flap (7). This distal area is independent territory and is supplied by the inferior ulnar collateral system and by musculocutaneous perforators that must be transected. Theoretically, the distal quarter can be carried as a random dermal flap at the end of the arterial flap, without a delay procedure. However, we do not have sufficient case numbers to estimate the risk for distal flap loss. Therefore, we have adopted a conservative attitude.

Flap Transfer and Inset

When the flap is to be used at a distant site, such as the hand or face, the distal end is configured and inset to fit the defect, and the proximal flap is tubed. Local flaps to the axilla or elbow are directly transposed and inset. The donor site is either grafted or closed directly, depending on flap width and other local conditions.

Flap Takedown

When the flap is used as a pedicled distant flap, we recommend an assessment of the adequacy of flap vascularization from the recipient site, prior to takedown. After application of a tourniquet, the flap is evaluated both clinically and with fluorescein. One week prior to flap transection, the superior ulnar brachial collateral artery can be identified and ligated at the pedicle base.

Free Flap

If the flap is being used as a free flap, the superior ulnar brachial collateral artery must be identified where it exits the brachial artery, 4 to 6 cm distal to the pectoralis insertion. The medial brachial cutaneous nerve can also be included, to create a neurovascular flap that runs with this tissue. If the nerve can be sutured to an available sensory nerve at the recipient site, it allows protective sensation (Fig. 6).

This flap serves as an alternative to the use of the dorsum or the first web space of the foot in patients requiring a neurosensory flap. Its advantages are the ability to close the donor site primarily, the lack of functional sequelae associated with skin grafts of the foot, and the inconspicuous location of the donor site. The main disadvantages are the inconsistent location and variable size of the superior ulnar collateral artery. Moreover, in those areas that require sensation, the medial brachial cutaneous nerve may not be as efficacious as the common plantar nerve (8).

The design of the flap is the same as in the pedicle technique, with inclusion of one of the subcutaneous veins for providing venous drainage if the venae comitantes are not chosen for anastomosis. The anterior incision is deepened to the biceps muscle and the fascia of this muscle is included in the flap. The lateral aspect of the brachial artery is identified and the profunda brachii artery noted approximately 4 cm distal to the pectoralis major insertion. If a second large vessel is seen, 1 to 2 cm more distally, this is the superior ulnar collateral artery, and it can be followed distally as it supplies the medial arm skin. Unfortunately, its course is usually under the ulnar nerve. Care must be taken to identify and preserve the ulnar nerve.

In those situations in which the superior ulnar collateral artery is a branch of the profunda artery, there will usually not be a direct artery from the brachial artery. Instead, a large branch will exit from the profunda artery toward the medial skin, which can be identified by following the profunda brachii artery distally. In those rare situations where there is both a direct cutaneous artery from the brachial artery, as well as a superior ulnar collateral artery from either the profunda or the brachial artery, a free flap is less feasible because of vessel size. Preoperative angiograms can obviate this uncertainty and allow better definition of the supplying vascular system. Whether the extremely large basilic veins or smaller venae comitantes are chosen, venous drainage is determined by the size of the recipient vessels.

CLINICAL RESULTS

In over 30 applications of this flap, there has been no loss of flap length due to vascular compromise. When we have limited the length of the flap to three-quarters the length of the upper arm (Fig. 7), only one partial slough occurred, and this was at the time of pedicle division. In this case, neither superior ulnar collateral artery identification, assessment of flap vascularization, or ligation was performed, prior to detaching the flap from its direct arterial supply.

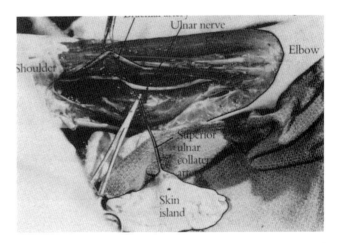

FIG. 6. The anatomic relations of the superior brachial collateral artery are shown. This dissection is essential for free flap transfer. Note the vessel in the intermuscular septum and its course under the ulnar nerve.

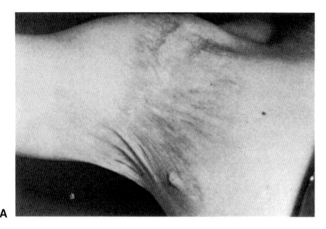
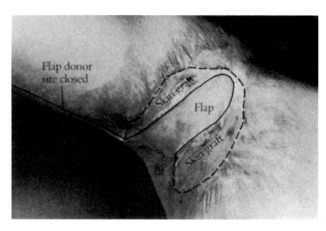

FIG. 7. A: A 12-year-old girl with axillary burn contracture. A proximally based arterial arm flap measuring 3 by 12 cm (less than three-fourths of the arm length) was elevated and transposed into the axilla in one stage. **B:** A skin graft is used on one or both sides of the flap, depending on the flap and defect size.

By incorporating the superior ulnar brachial collateral artery, the flap may be transferred as a proximally based undelayed flap extending three-quarters the length of the arm with complete reliability. If the artery is not identified or is inadvertently injured, the rich fascial network can sustain the flap. In addition, the skin can be transferred as a free flap from the same vascular system. The major limitation of this tissue as a pedicled flap is the need for shoulder immobilization. For distant transfer, the major drawback of this flap as a free flap is the inconsistent and occasionally small size of the donor vessel.

Medial arm skin has proved to be thin, pliable, and hairless, and the flap dependable. However, in comparison with surrounding recipient site skin, medial arm skin has sometimes been inappropriate in color.

SUMMARY

The medial arm flap can provide thin, pliable coverage from the axilla to the hand. It can be used as a direct, distant, or free flap, depending on the recipient site. By including the medial brachial cutaneous nerve, the free flap can also provide protective sensation.

References

1. Hentz VR, Pearl RM, Kaplan EN. Use of the medial upper arm skin as an arterialized flap. *Hand* 1980;12:241.
2. Kaplan E, Buncke H, Murray D. Distant transfer of cutaneous flaps in humans. *Plast Reconstr Surg* 1973;52:301.
3. Song R, Song Y, Yu Y, et al. The upper arm free flap. *Clin Plast Surg* 1982;9:27.
4. Budo J, Finucan T, Clarke J. The inner arm fasciocutaneous flap. *Plast Reconstr Surg* 1984;73:629.
5. Daniel RK, Taylor GI. Distant transfer of an island flap by microvascular anastomoses. *Plast Reconstr Surg* 1973;52:111.
6. Taylor GI, Daniel RK. The anatomy of several free flap donor sites. *Plast Reconstr Surg* 1975;56:243.
7. May H. *Plastic and reconstructive surgery,* 3rd Ed. Philadelphia: FA Davis, 1971.
8. Daniel R, Terzis J, Schwarz G. Neurovascular free flaps. *Plast Reconstr Surg* 1975;56:13.

CHAPTER 342. Lateral Trunk Flaps *E. G. Zook and R. C. Russell*

www.encyclopediaofflaps.com

CHAPTER 343 ■ LATISSIMUS DORSI FUNCTIONAL TRANSFER TO THE ARM

W. Y. HOFFMAN AND L. O. VASCONEZ

With its vascular supply and innervation left intact, the latissimus dorsi can be transferred to the arm for restoration of either flexion or extension at the elbow (1–9). A skin island may be included in the design of the flap for coverage of the additional bulk from the muscle transfer or for closure of soft-tissue defects.

INDICATIONS

It is important to assess the strength of the latissimus preoperatively: the muscle may have been weakened by the same process that affected the arm, such as brachial plexus injury or poliomyelitis. Preoperative conditioning has been used to strengthen the latissimus. In some neurologic disorders, it is well to consider the function of the latissimus in stabilizing the hip for gait. Other operations on the upper extremity, such as joint fusion or tendon transfer, should be incorporated in the overall reconstructive plan.

OPERATIVE TECHNIQUE

Incisions are required over the latissimus posteriorly, in the axilla over the elbow anteriorly, over the olecranon for extension and flexion, and over the coracoid process if the insertion of the muscle is transferred. The lateral portion of the muscle may be used in order to diminish bulk or to preserve normal latissimus function.

The serratus anterior branches and sometimes the circumflex scapular vessels must be ligated to allow sufficient mobilization of the muscle that is converted into an island. The muscle is then passed under the pectoralis tendon to reach the arm.

For flexion, the divided origin of the muscle is sutured to the distal biceps tendon; for extension, to the triceps tendon. Including a rim of the thoracodorsal fascia with the muscle and fixation to the radial tubercle or the olecranon process will make this juncture more secure.

The insertion of the latissimus on the humerus has been transferred to the proximal biceps or triceps tendon for a more direct line of pull. By extending the muscle with strips of fascia lata, finger flexion can also be restored.

Muscle tension is critical in this procedure, as in any functional muscle transfer. Measuring the distance between two or more sutures placed in the muscle before its division may provide a guide to reestablishing physiologic muscle length. Overcorrection is preferred, bringing the arm to 90° to 100° for flexor repairs and to full extension for extensor repairs.

CLINICAL RESULTS

The results of this operation have been satisfactory. If the latissimus has normal function preoperatively, a fair degree of strength is achieved, with one patient reportedly lifting 15 pounds. If the muscle is weakened before surgery, there is still substantial functional gain from being able to position the hand upward for working and eating.

SUMMARY

The latissimus dorsi muscle, with or without skin, can be transferred with its neurovascular supply left intact, to restore flexion or extension to the elbow.

References

1. Schottstaedt ER, Larsen LJ, Bost FC. Complete muscle transposition. *J Bone Joint Surg* 1955;37A:897.
2. Hovnanian AP. Latissimus dorsi transplantation for loss of flexion or extension at the elbow. *Ann Surg* 1956;143:493.
3. Axer A, Segal D, Elkon A. Partial transposition of the latissimus dorsi: a new operative technique to restore elbow and finger flexion. *J Bone Joint Surg* 1973;55A:1259.
4. Zancolli E, Mitre, H. Latissimus dorsi transfer to restore elbow flexion. *J Bone Joint Surg* 1973;55A:1265.
5. Landra AP. The latissimus dorsi musculocutaneous flap used to resurface a defect on the upper arm and restore extension to the elbow. *Br J Plast Surg* 1979;32:275.
6. Bostwick J III, Nahai F, Wallace JG, Vasconez LO. Sixty latissimus dorsi flaps. *Plant Reconstr Surg* 1979;63:31.
7. Tobin GR, Man D, Meadows K, et al. Split latissimus dorsi motor transfer (Abstract). *J Bone Joint Surg* 1981;5:104.
8. Steven PJ, Neale HW, Gregory RD, Kreikin JG. Latissimus dorsi musculocutaneous flap for elbow flexion. *J Hand Surg* 1982;7:25.
9. Brones MF, Wheeler ES, Lesavoy MA. Restoration of elbow flexion and arm contour with the latissimus dorsi myocutaneous flap. *Plast Reconstr Surg* 1982;69:329.

CHAPTER 344 ■ TISSUE EXPANSION IN CONJUNCTION WITH FLAPS OF THE UPPER EXTREMITY

G. G. HALLOCK

EDITORIAL COMMENT

This is an attractive concept in an effort to enlarge the surface area of an available flap. However, the recoil phenomenon of expanded flaps should not be forgotten.

Pre- or posttransfer tissue expansion, as an adjunct to upper-extremity flaps, can augment the potential available surface area for wound coverage, and can minimize donor-site morbidity by permitting only a solitary linear scar.

INDICATIONS

Major advantages not previously possible without a combination of tissue expansion and the increased anatomic knowledge of reliable upper-extremity flaps (Fig. 1), include pretransfer augmentation of reliable flap territories, and the amelioration of donor-site morbidity (1–11). These developments were possible only after the commercial introduction of medical-grade inflatable silicone balloons, now used commonly for chronic and gradual tissue distension.

The current scope of tissue expansion in the upper extremity remains limited to skin augmentation (12–15). Of the numerous reliable fasciocutaneous flaps that have been identified in the upper limb and are available for local flap transfer, many are limited in size (Fig. 1). Unless restricted to relatively small dimensions or taken strictly as fascial flaps, all the known donor areas have previously required a skin graft to maintain skin integrity following flap harvesting.

The immediate or delayed placement of tissue expanders adjacent to existing defects, now allows the secondary transformation of the defect into a more acceptable linear scar. This has been particularly valuable for the more distal radial forearm flap, in which a conspicuous unaesthetic or unstable skin graft over the flexor tendons has heretofore been considered a major detriment (Fig. 2B). Under elective conditions, pretransfer expansion not only increases the potential flap surface area, but also allows primary closure of the donor site at the time of flap transfer, thereby avoiding any need for a skin graft (Fig. 3).

OPERATIVE TECHNIQUE

Immediate tissue expansion can begin at the time of flap transfer, or expander placement can follow total wound healing, although this is more inconvenient (Fig. 2). Any remaining skin and subcutaneous tissue adjacent to the donor site are undermined above the muscle fascia and preferably under the deep fascia to preserve all collaterals to the residual fascial plexus in the area. The pocket created should be made through as narrow an opening as possible. This can be done either by blind dissection with a blunt instrument (e.g., a cervial dilator or liposuction cannula) (16), or more carefully and sharply under direct endoscopic guidance (17). The dimensions of the cavity should approximate those of the chosen expander envelope to ensure no edge infolding. Normally, a standard rectangular implant should prove satisfactory, when its length exceeds that of the defect. Sometimes, a custom-designed implant may be more appropriate, to minimize the total required number of expanders (Fig. 2A).

Implantation over bony prominences or joints is avoided, so that mobility will not be impaired during the period of expansion. The access incision to underlying tissues must be carefully closed, preferably in several layers, to minimize the risk of dehiscence leading to implant infection or exposure, and invariably resulting in extrusion. A remote valve, rather than an intrinsic one, prevents the risk of inadvertent implant puncture during later fluid instillation. Although the port can be left totally external (18), internal placement at least theoretically lessens the risk of contamination or damage over a long course of expansion, even if retrieval can be more difficult.

Totally elective flap transfers allow for consideration of pretransfer expansion. Great care must be observed in placement of the expander, to protect against damage to the perforators responsible for flap viability. Color duplex imaging, a repeatable, rapid, noninvasive diagnostic modality, can identify the presence of cutaneous perforators, their caliber, and flow. This allows for the construction of a preoperative map, ensuring the retention of essential perforators during undermining of the territory, just prior to insertion of the expansion envelope (Fig. 3). Direct dissection of the pocket, with endoscopic visualization to avoid the perforators, would be the most minimally invasive approach.

Adequate wound healing prior to the beginning of serial expansion is necessary; a delay of even up to 6 weeks is possible. Normal saline is then instilled on a convenient schedule, frequently once or twice a week, via percutaneous injection into the remote port, until skin capillary refill disappears or pain intolerance occurs. Accelerated expansion (19) or expansion of an anaesthetic region may be more safely controlled with monitoring by laser Doppler flowmetry (20).

Accrued tissue gain in the extremities is readily approximated as a difference in their circumferences from a given, fixed point (Figs. 2B and 3B). Once desired coverage requirements are exceeded, the expander can be removed. In clinical

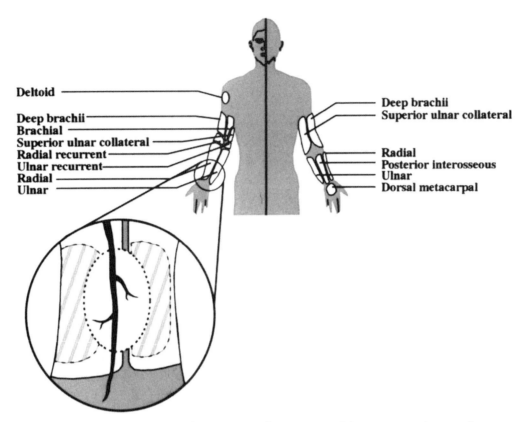

FIG. 1. Diagram of the described fasciocutaneous flap territories of the upper extremity, according to their source vessels. All are versatile for local transfer; many are possible candidates for consideration as free flaps. *Shaded regions in inset* demonstrate suitable areas for expander placement adjacent to the vascular pedicle of a radial forearm flap, which cannot be undermined to ensure flap viability, whether pre- or posttransfer expansion is selected. (Modified from Hallock, ref. 29, with permission.)

practice, this may demand overinflation well beyond the vendor's maximum allowable volume. However, safety has been validated beyond twice these amounts in in vitro experiments (21), and confirmed in humans (22). Maximal inflation again at the time of final envelope removal will yield an additional 1 to 2 cm in all dimensions, by acute load cycling or skin stretching (23,24).

No defect should be reconstructed until advancement of the expanded flap confirms that adequate coverage is possible. Occasionally, it may be necessary to retain the expander for a second course of expansion, if achievement of the initial goal proves to be incomplete (25).

CLINICAL RESULTS

Although an actual gain in epidermal surface area can be measured during chronic expansion, concurrent subcutaneous fat atrophy occurs with flap thinning; this can sometimes be used to advantage, if bulk is not essential at the recipient site (13,26).

Complication rates can be relatively high in extremity tissue expansion, and more precautions and meticulous tissue handling are essential, if success is to be achieved.

Pretransfer expansion has additional risks, specific to the flap itself, including skin necrosis from flap thinning, implant extrusion, or infection. In addition, obligatory capsule formation around the implant and adjacent edema, can compromise identification of the vascular pedicle, risking devascularization, and can even lead to aborting an elective transfer (8). A minimum of two surgical stages is always required, whether it is pretransfer or posttransfer expansion that is selected.

Since the technique requires a significant time investment by both patient and surgeon, all potential hazards must be clearly and fairly outlined in advance. Simpler methods of acute tissue expansion, such as presuturing (27), wide undermining (28), or use of skin-stretching devices may be more suitable (24).

SUMMARY

The augmentation of reliable flap territories, and the amelioration of donor-site deformity, are major advantages of tissue expansion, used as an adjunct to random, local skin flaps for upper-limb defects.

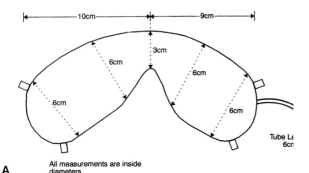

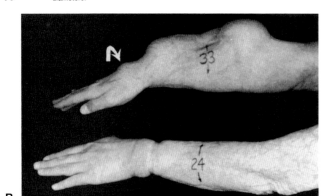

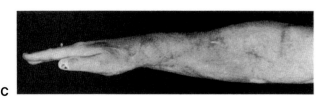

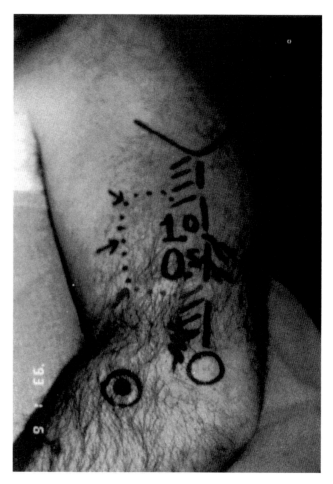

FIG. 2. A: Diagrammatic blueprint of custom-designed envelope with remote valve, intended to circumscribe the apex of a triangular-shaped, skin-grafted radial forearm free flap donor site, which otherwise would have required two rectangular expanders. **B:** Comparison of forearm circumferences allows estimation of tissue gain prior to implant removal. Note protrusion of remote valve positioned on the dorsal right hand for convenient access for injections (*arrow*). The inflated right forearm expander surrounds a contour depression after flap harvest. This defect was annoying to the patient, even though most of the remaining extremity had previously also been skin-grafted for burns. **C:** Flattening and reduction of some of the skin-grafted area of the forearm, providing the desired improvement in appearance 8 months following the commencement of posttransfer delayed expansion. (From Hallock, ref. 10, with permission.)

FIG. 3. Mapping the location and caliber of all perforators through the lateral intermuscular septum of the arm, as identified by color duplex imaging. The area within the dots was considered safe for undermining, for placement of an expander, to allow pretransfer expansion of a lateral arm free flap, with no risk of damage to the nutritive perforators within the cross-hatched zone.

References

1. Morgan RF, Edgerton MT. Tissue expansion in reconstructive hand surgery. *J Hand Surg* 1985;10A:754.
2. Mackinnon SE, Gruss JS. Soft tissue expanders in upper limb surgery. *J Hand Surg* 1985;10A:749.
3. Hallock GG. Extremity tissue expansion. *Orthop Rev* 1987;16:606.
4. Ogawa Y, Kasai K, Doi H, Takeuchi E. The preoperative use of extra-tissue expander for syndactyly. *Ann Plast Surg* 1989;23:552.
5. Hallock GG. Color duplex imaging for identifying perforators prior to pretransfer expansion of fasciocutaneous free flaps. *Ann Plast Surg* 1994;32:595.
6. Masser MR. The pre-expanded radial free flap. *Plast Reconstr Surg* 1990;86:295.
7. Shenaq SM. Pretransfer expansion of a sensate lateral arm free flap. *Ann Plast Surg* 1987;19:558.
8. Leighton WD, Russell RC, Feller AM, et al. Experimental pretransfer expansion of free-flap donor sites. II. Physiology, histology, and clinical correlation. *Plast Reconstr Surg* 1988;82:76.
9. Hallock GG. Free flap donor site refinement using tissue expansion. *Ann Plast Surg* 1988;6:566.
10. Hallock GG. Refinement of the radial forearm flap donor site using skin expansion. *Plast Reconstr Surg* 1988;81:121.
11. Hallock GG. Complications of fasciocutaneous flaps including donor site treatment. In: Hallock GG, ed. *Fasciocutaneous flaps*. Boston: Blackwell Scientific, 1992;157–171.
12. Radovan C. Tissue expansion in soft-tissue reconstruction. *Plast Reconstr Surg* 1984;74:482.
13. Austad ED, Thomas SB, Pasyk K. Tissue expansion: dividend or loan? *Plast Reconstr Surg* 1986;78:63.
14. Manders EK, Schenden MJ, Furrey JA, et al. Soft-tissue expansion: concepts and complications. *Plast Reconstr Surg* 1984;74:4933.
15. Cohen BE, Ruiz-Razura A. Acute intraoperative arterial lengthening for closure of large vascular gaps. *Plast Reconstr Surg* 1992;90:463.
16. Hallock GG. Adjuvant use of the suction lipectomy cannula for blunt dissection. *Aesth Plast Surg* 1985;9:107.
17. Eaves FF, Price CI, Bostwick J, et al. Subcutaneous endoscopic plastic surgery using a retractor-mounted endoscopic system. *Perspect Plast Surg* 1993;7:1.
18. Dickson WA, Sharpe DT, Jackson IT. Experience with an external valve in small volume tissue expanders. *Br J Plast Surg* 1988;41:373.
19. Pietila JP, Nordstrom REA, Virkkunen PJ, et al. Accelerated tissue expansion with the "overfilling" technique. *Plast Reconstr Surg* 1988;81:204.
20. Hallock GG, Rice DC. Increased sensitivity in objective monitoring of tissue expansion. *Plast Reconstr Surg* 1993;91:2217.
21. Hallock GG. Maximum overinflation of tissue expanders. *Plast Reconstr Surg* 1987;80:567.
22. Hallock GG. Safety of clinical overinflation of tissue expanders. *Plast Reconstr Surg* 1997.
23. Hirshowitz B, Kaufman T, Ullman J. Reconstruction of the tip of the nose and ala by load cycling of the nasal skin and harnessing of extra skin. *Plast Reconstr Surg* 1986;77:316.
24. Mackay DR, Saggers GC, Kotwal N, Manders EK. Stretching skin: undermining is more important than intraoperative expansion. *Plast Reconstr Surg* 1990;86:722.

25. Sellers DS, Miller SH, Demuth RJ, Klabacha ME. Repeated skin expansion to resurface a massive thigh wound. *Plast Reconstr Surg* 1986;77:654.
26. Pasyk KA, Argenta L, Hassett C. Quantitative analysis of the thickness of human skin and subcutaneous tissue following controlled expansion with a silicone implant. *Plast Reconstr Surg* 1988;81:516.
27. Liang MD, Briggs P, Heckler FR, Futrell JW. Presuturing—a new technique for closing large skin defects: clinical and experimental studies. *Plast Reconstr Surg* 1988;81:694.
28. Hirshowitz B, Lindenbaum E, Har-Shai Y. A skin-stretching device for the harnessing of the viscoelastic properties of skin. *Plast Reconstr Surg* 1993;92:260.
29. Hallock GG. Territories of fasciocutaneous flaps by source and subtype. In: Hallock GG, ed. *Fasciocutaneous flaps*. Boston: Blackwell Scientific, 1992;181–193.

Page numbers followed by *f* indicate illustrations; *t* following a page number indicates tabular material.

Donor site (*contd.*)
　of intestinal transfer, 654–655
　of microvascular free transfer of omentum, 32
　of pectoralis major muscle flap, 373–375
　of radial forearm free flap, 581–583
Dorsal branch of digital nerve innervated cross-
　　finger flap for finger reconstruction, 739
　anatomy of, 739
　clinical results for, 741
　first-stage operative technique for, 739
　indications for, 739
　second-stage operative technique for, 739–740
　summary about, 739
Dorsal burn, 912
Dorsal cross-finger flap for finger reconstruction,
　　733
　anatomy of, 733
　clinical results for, 734–735
　design and dimensions of, 733
　indications for, 733
　loss of
　　dorsal finger tissue and, 733
　　volar finger tissues and, 733
　major fingertip amputations and, 733
　operative technique for, 734
　summary about, 735
Dorsal finger tissue, loss of, 733
Dorsal index skin flap for thenar web, 922
　clinical results for, 922, 925*f*
　design and dimensions of, 922, 923–924*f*
　operative technique for, 922
　summary about, 922
Dorsal interosseous (DIO) fascia, 875
Dorsal rectangular skin flap for web space
　　reconstruction, 910
　clinical results for, 911
　design and dimensions of, 910–911
　indications for, 910
　operative technique for, 911
　summary about, 911
Dorsal scapular island flap, 358–360
　anatomy of, 358–359, 359*f*
　clinical results of, 359–360
　design and dimensions of, 359
　indications for, 358
　operative technique for, 359, 360*f*
　summary about, 360
Dorsal thumb flap for thenar web space, 920
　design and dimensions of, 920*f*, 921
　indications for, 921
　operative technique for, 920*f*, 921
　summary about, 921
Dorsal to volar transposition skin flap of finger
　　for thumbtip reconstruction, 783
　anatomy of, 783–784
　clinical results for, 784
　design and dimensions of, 784
　indications for, 783
　operative technique for, 784
　summary about, 784
Dorsalis pedis (skin) flap
　with extensor tendons; microvascular free
　　transfer of, for hand reconstruction, 888
　anatomy of, 890
　clinical results for, 888, 890
　indications for, 888, 890
　operative technique for, 890
　summary about, 890
　for eye socket reconstruction, 97
　anatomy of, 97
　clinical results for, 97, 98*f*
　design and dimensions of, 97, 98*f*
　donor site for, 97
　indications for, 97
　operative technique for, 97
　recipient site for, 97
　summary about, 97
　for foot and ankle reconstruction, 1483
　anatomy of, 1484–1485
　design and dimensions of, 1485
　indications for, 1484
　operative technique for, 1485, 1486*f*, 1487
　summary about, 1488
　to heel, for foot and ankle reconstruction, 1527
　anatomy of, 1527
　design and dimensions of, 1527–1528

　indications for, 1527
　operative technique for, 1528–1529
　summary about, 1529
　for hypopharyngeal reconstruction, 665
　anatomy of, 666
　clinical results for, 667
　design and dimensions of, 666
　donor site of, 667
　indications for, 665–666
　operative technique for, 666–667
　recipient site of, 667
　summary about, 667
　for intraoral lining, 571
　anatomy of, 571
　clinical results for, 571–572
　design and dimensions of, 571
　indications for, 571
　operative technique for, 571
　summary about, 572
　microvascular and microneurovascular free
　　transfer of, for hand reconstruction, 891
　anatomy of, 891
　design and dimensions of, 891
　indications for, 891
　operative technique for, 891, 892*f*
　summary about, 891–892
Dorsalis pedis myofascial flap for foot and ankle
　　reconstruction, 1488
　anatomy of, 1488
　clinical results for, 1489–1490
　design and dimensions of, 1488, 1489*f*
　indications for, 1488
　operative technique for, 1488–1489
　summary about, 1490
Dorsolateral island skin flap to fingertip and
　　thumb tip, 786
　anatomy of, 786
　clinical results for, 786, 788
　design and dimensions of, 786, 787*f*
　indications for, 786
　operative technique for, 786, 787*f*
　summary about, 788
Dorsolateral neurovascular skin flap of finger for
　　finger reconstruction, 726
　anatomy of, 726
　clinical results for, 727–728
　design and dimensions of, 726–727
　donor site for, 727
　indications for, 726
　operative technique for, 727
　recipient site for, 727
　summary about, 728
Double breasting of raw surfaces, 1232
Double-bump deformity, 493
Double-opposing-tab flap, 1089
Double triangular subcutaneous pedicle skin flap,
　　266–267
Double-Z rhomboid plasty for facial wound
　　reconstruction, 283
　anatomy of, 283
　clinical results for, 285
　design and dimensions of, 283–285
　indications for, 283
　operative technique for, 285
　summary about, 286
Dufourmentel flap, 1283
Dupuytren's contracture, 713, 715*f*, 733
Dura mater, 12*f*
Dynamic abductor digiti minimi
　　musculocutaneous flap for thumb, 813
　anatomy of, 814
　clinical results for, 815
　design and dimensions of, 814
　indications for, 813, 814*f*
　operative technique for, 814–815
　summary about, 815
Dysplasia, 1299

E
Ear
　chondrocutaneous conchal flap to, 239
　external, subcutaneous pedicle flap and, 244
　　anatomy of, 244
　　clinical results for, 247
　　design and dimensions of, 246
　　indications for, 244, 245

　　operative technique for, 246
　　summary about, 247
　helix-scapha defects of, 231, 232*f*
　retroauricular dermal pedicle skin flap to, 247
　　anatomy of, 247
　　clinical results for, 247
　　design and dimensions of, 247
　　operative technique for, 247
　　summary about, 247
　temporoparietal fascial flap to, 259
　　anatomy of, 259
　　clinical results for, 261
　　design and dimensions of, 259
　　indications for, 259
　　operative technique for, 259–261
　　summary about, 262
Ear helix free flap, nasal alar reconstruction
　　with, 192
　anatomy of, 192
　clinical results for, 193, 194*f*
　design and dimensions of, 193
　operative technique for, 192–193
　summary about, 193
Ear reconstruction, 225
　partial, retroauricular bipedicle skin flap for, 237
　　anatomy of, 237
　　design and dimensions of, 237
　　indications for, 237
　　operative technique for, 237
　　summary about, 237
　partial, retrograde auricular flap for, 241
　　anatomy of, 241
　　clinical results for, 243
　　design and dimensions of, 241
　　operative technique for, 242–243
　　summary about, 243
Earlobe
　cleft, repair of, 255
　torn, skin flap to, 253
　　anatomy of, 253
　　clinical results for, 254
　　design and dimensions of, 253
　　indications for, 253
　　operative technique for, 253
　　summary about, 254
Earlobe contracture, roll-under flap for release of,
　　257
　anatomy of, 257
　clinical results for, 258
　design and dimensions of, 257
　indications for, 257
　operative technique for, 258
　summary about, 258
Earlobe reconstruction, lateral neck skin flap for,
　　ONLINE
Eave skin flap for helical reconstruction, 225
　clinical results for, 226
　design and dimensions of, 225
　indications for, 225
　operative technique for, 225–226
　summary about, 226
Eisler's fat pad, 52
Elastoplast bandage, 904, 1514
　for holding omentum and implant, 1024*f*
Elbow, anterior coverage of, 974–976
Elbow reconstruction
　brachioradialis muscle and musculocutaneous
　　flap for, 971
　anatomy of, 971, 972*f*
　design and dimensions of, 971, 972*f*
　indications for, 971
　operative technique for, 971, 972–973*f*
　summary about, 971
　cephalic venous flap for, 960
　clinical results for, 960
　design and dimensions of, 960, 961*f*
　indications for, 960
　operative technique for, 960, 961–962*f*
　summary about, 960
　fasciocutaneous flaps for coverage of elbow for,
　　966
　anatomy of, 966–967
　design and dimensions of, 967–968
　indications for, 966
　operative technique for, 968
　summary about, 968